Perceptual Learning

Perceptual Learning

edited by Manfred Fahle and Tomaso Poggio

A Bradford Book
The MIT Press
Cambridge, Massachusetts
London, England

This book was set in Bembo on '3B2' by Asco Typesetters, Hong Kong, and was printed and bound in the United States of America.

Library of Congress Cataloging-in-Publication Data

Perceptual learning / edited by Manfred Fahle and Tomaso Poggio.
   p. ; cm.
 "A Bradford book."
 Includes bibliographical references and index.
 ISBN 0-262-06221-6 (hc : alk. paper)
 1. Perceptual learning. 2. Visual cortex. 3. Auditory cortex.
4. Neuroplasticity. I. Fahle, Manfred. II. Poggio, Tomaso.
[DNLM: 1. Perception—physiology. 2. Learning—physiology.
3. Visual Perception—physiology. WL 705 P42875 2001]
QP408 .P47 2001
612.8′2—dc21   2001044333

To my mother, Helma Fahle, who was always there to help in many ways, small and large

Contents

IV Modeling *335*

Introduction

A Definition

The present book deals with "perceptual learning," adding another volume to the already enormous pile of paper devoted to the topic of learning. Is this necessary? I think it is, since perceptual learning is a new and exciting aspect of learning and one that has seen tremendous progress during the last decade—without any textbook available to bring together the by now large body of knowledge assembled during these years. But what is perceptual learning, after all? In what respect does it differ from other forms of learning? A good starting point is a definition following Gibson 1963: "Any relatively permanent and consistent change in the perception of a stimulus array following practice or experience with this array will be considered perceptual learning." In the framework of this book, we will concentrate on those types of learning that are relatively independent from conscious experience and do not lead to "knowing that" (Ryle 1949) and declarative forms of memory, which can be true or false. Perceptual learning leads to implicit memory, to "knowing how," to a "memory without a record" and is often very specific for rather low-level attributes of the stimulus learned. Contrary to declarative forms of learning, and similar to motion learning, perceptual learning seems to directly modify the neuronal pathways active during processing of the task, and not to require an intermediate consolidation storage, such as the hippocampus. Contrary to associative learning, perceptual learning does not bind together two pro-

cesses that were separated but improves discrimination between stimuli that could not be discriminated before the learning; observers may learn to perceive something new that they could not perceive before. Recently, it became clear that some forms of perceptual learning are highly specific, e.g., for the exact stimulus orientation. This finding suggests that perceptual learning takes place on a rather "early" stage of cortical information processing. The importance of modifications on relatively "early" levels, such as the primary visual cortex, constitutes a profound break with the views generally held until recently regarding (non)plasticity of primary sensory cortices and the basis of learning in perceptual tasks.

Older Views on Plasticity in the Nervous System

Let us consider as an example the primary visual cortex. Suppression of one eye's input in squinting patients will cause this eye to become amblyopic, and it will attain low visual acuity. Improvement is possible only if treatment starts, in humans, during the teen years. This concept of a critical phase in early childhood during which the (primary) visual cortex is still plastic agrees well with the results obtained primarily by Wiesel and Hubel (1965) (cf. chapter 15) on the development of the visual cortex in cat and monkey. By patching one eye in young kittens, most neurons in the primary visual cortex could be made to connect primarily or even exclusively with the open eye, while only a small percentage was activated through the patched eye. Removing the patch from one eye early in life (in cats, during the first few months of life) and transferring it to the partner eye reversed this cortical modification. It appeared that the primary visual cortex was indeed plastic during the early parts of childhood, but not thereafter, both in humans and other vertebrates. Consequently, Marr's (1982) view of the adult primary visual cortex as a rather hardwired preprocessing module extracting certain elementary features from visual scenes reflected a common belief of this time. And it made sense that the first stage would be "hardwired" in adult life, since changing preprocessing of visual information based on learning of one task would inevitably change preprocessing of many other tasks in every strictly feedforward system. Hence, the experimental results on the specificity of some forms of perceptual learning obtained during recent years, from the specificity of perceptual learning for the eye trained, the orientation of the stimulus and the visual field position used (cf. chapters 9 to 12), as well as the electrophysiological results on plastic changes of the adult visual (chapter 3), auditory (chapter 8), and somatosensory system (chapter 2) mean a radical change of our views on the primary visual cortex compared to one or two decades ago, while plasticity of the somatosensory system had been known for a much longer time. We have to accept that the primary sensory cortices are much more plastic than hitherto believed—and this new insight has implications not only for our views on the functioning of the healthy brain but also for the rehabilitation of patients after cortical damage. At the same time, we learn that the primary sensory cortices are not only quite plastic but that their neurons can change their functional properties in a task-dependent way and integrate information over considerable areas of the visual field, far beyond their classical receptive fields (e.g., Allman et al. 1985; Gilbert 1998).

Perceptual Learning and Related Terms

Perceptual learning differs from other forms of learning in that it can be highly specific, that is, transferring little to very similar tasks, and hence at least partly involves structural and/or functional changes in *primary* sensory cortices. This type of "early" and "specific" perceptual learning is of paramount importance also for computer vision—the majority of all attempts in computer vision rely on exactly this improvement in discrimination between similar stimuli through (prolonged) training and feedback. It certainly relates to long-term memory, since improvement obtained through perceptual learning lasts for months, and it clearly is not of the declarative type of learning, since it does not consist of consciously memorized facts or events. Quite to the contrary, most observers will be unable to formulate what exactly do they differently *after* compared to *before* the learning process. So perceptual learning is a form of implicit learning, similar in several respects to procedural (motor) learning of skills and habits but which are thought to be based on changes in the striatum, not the cortex (e.g., Milner, Squire, and Kandel 1998). Perceptual learning also differs from associative learning because it relies neither on mechanisms of classical nor on operant conditioning, which involve the amygdala and cerebellum, respectively. Nonassociative learning usually involves reflex pathways while perceptual learning does not lead to simple reflex responses. The type of implicit learning most closely related to perceptual learning is priming, as we will see below when considering the relation between perceptual learning and other forms of change in the nervous system such as plasticity, adaptation, habituation, aftereffects, sensitization, priming, development, maturation, and even memory and improvement through insight.

Plasticity is defined here as modifiability of the brain leading to more appropriate function. The term most often describes the neuronal substrate of changing behavior, such as changes in synaptic weights or formation of new synapses. Plasticity, for example, serves to adjust the functional and anatomical organization of the central nervous system as a result of sensory experience or other factors. The term also describes functional and anatomical changes by which the central nervous system alleviates limitations caused by lesions. The term *adaptation* is most often used in relation to changes of information processing on relatively peripheral levels in the central nervous system, as a result of extended presentation of a stimulus, or after a change in environmental conditions. A classic example is light adaptation. There, the working range of the visual system is shifted to the most appropriate level to deal with the changes in ambient light intensity. Hence, adaptation usually means an adjustment within a predefined working range, with no long-term changes of the nervous system. (In psychology, "adaptation" tends to be used also for long-lasting changes.) *Habituation* (called *satiation* in the context of rewards) seems to be a special case of adaptation, namely a shift of working range towards *lower* sensitivity, as in the case of decreased reflex response after repeated stimulation while *sensitization* indicates a temporal increase in sensitivity, for example, after a painful stimulus. *Aftereffects* can be considered, in many cases, as the result of adaptation, most often habituation, in cases where perception is the result of antagonistic neuronal channels. Duration of aftereffects is usually short. *Priming* describes the effect of a (sometimes subliminal) stimulus on subsequent perception of (other) stimuli and/or behavioral responses. The effect of priming is usually short, vanishing after a few tens of seconds, while some effects usually called priming, such as the ones obtained by means of the Gollin Figures (Gollin 1960), and when perceiving the Dalmatian dog or depth in random-dot stereograms (Julesz 1971), can last for months and should rather be considered as perceptual learning.

Development and *maturation* are also coupled with changes of (cortical) information processing and of behavior. These terms, unlike learning, ascribe the main thrust of the changes in a behavior to genetics, not the environment. Hence, changes in observable behavior are seen as the consequences of the growing and maturation of the organism along a largely predefined path rather than as a consequence of information gathered through interaction with the outside world (in practice, of course, genetics and environmental influences strongly interact in determining behavior).

Improvement through *insight*, as the name indicates, is a term that should be reserved for more effective information processing based on cognitive processes and incorporating an abrupt change, such as one-shot learning does (cf. also chapters 13, 14). Such processes play a role also in perceptual learning but come close to declarative forms of learning. *Memory* usually is a consequence of learning. It implies the coding, storage, and retrieval of information. While perceptual learning certainly is based on some form of information storage, this information is stored implicitly by changing the way the stimuli are analyzed.

Stimulus Specificity of Perceptual Learning Causes a "Paradigm Change"

Visual recognition of objects improves through training, and "practice makes perfect" (Volkmann 1863; Best 1900). For beginners in the study of histology, all specimens look quite similar (for example, liver, lung, or kidney). Sooner or later, however, the advanced student wonders how one could possibly miss the difference. This type of visual classification is a relatively complex visual task, but it has also been known for decades that performance in much simpler perceptual tasks improves through practice, as for example vernier discrimination (McKee and Westheimer 1978), stereoscopic depth perception (Ramachandran and Braddick 1973), and discrimination between line orientations (Vogels and Orban 1985). Generally, however, these improvements in discriminative power were not attributed to changes on the peripheral or early levels of information processing, but were, implicitly or even explicitly, considered to be based (exclusively?) on cognitive, that is, high-level changes of visual information processing.

During the last decade, however, a number of electrophysiological and psychophysical experiments have shed some doubts on this purely cognitive interpretation, suggesting that even the adult primary sensory cortices show much more plasticity than was hitherto believed. The first evidence of this was the specificity of improvement through learning for stimulus orientation. Fiorentini and Berardi (1980; chapter 9, this volume) were the first to describe such orientation specificity, finding that practice improved discrimination between complex gratings, but that the improvement did not transfer to stimuli rotated by 90 degrees. Poggio, Edelman, and Fahle (1991; chapters 11, 15, 18) described a similar orientation specificity for a vernier discrimination task where observers had to indicate whether the right segment of a horizontal vernier was above or below the left segment, or whether the lower segment of a vertically oriented vernier stimulus was offset to the right or to the left relative to the upper segment. Both groups of observers improved performance highly significantly during training but their performance returned to base level when the stimulus was rotated by 90 degrees. Hence, the improvement obtained through training was specific for stimulus orientation (cf., however, Ball and Sekuler 1987).

A similar specificity of improvement even for the retinal position and the eye used during training was observed in a texture discrimination task where observers had to discriminate a figure from its surround based on the orientation of the stimulus elements (Karni and Sagi 1991; chapter 10). Moreover, improvement did not transfer between a three-dot vernier and a three-dot bisection task, although the stimuli of both tasks differ by approximately one photoreceptor diameter only, thus excluding all explanations based on better accommodation or fixation (Fahle and Morgan 1996). Hence, the changes of the nervous system underlying this form of perceptual learning should occur on a quite early level of cortical information processing where the neurons are already selective for different stimulus orientations (unlike in the retina), but still partly monocularly activated unlike in all cortical areas beyond the primary visual cortex. In particular, the eye specificity of the improvement as well as its high positional and orientation specificity (less than 5-degree bandwidth, cf. chapter 11) point to the primary visual cortex as the most probable site for at least a large part of the changes underlying this form of perceptual learning. Perceptual learning, however, is not restricted to these rather simple visual stimuli, but extends to more complex line figures (chapter 15), simple objects (chapter 16) and faces (chapter 17). Training observers with repeated presentations of iso-oriented (parallel) lines increases detection sensitivity for these stimuli, probably by strengthening lateral interactions that exist in the primary visual cortex between the corresponding neurons (von der Heydt and Peterhans 1989; Dresp and Bonnet 1991; Polat and Sagi 1994; Dresp 1999; chapter 10).

Recent neuroanatomical (see chapter 1) and electrophysiological evidence (chapters 2–7) supports this conclusion. The first indications for plasticity in the wiring of the adult primary sensory cortex stem from the somatosensory cortex, where Merzenich and collaborators found an amazing amount of change in the distribution of receptive fields after lesions (Merzenich et al. 1988; see also chapters 2 and 7). And in the somatosensory system, perceptual improvement was associated with a highly selective cortical reorganization in the primary somatosensory cortex, S1, with high stimulus selectivity (Recanzone et al. 1992; and chapter 2). Single-cell recordings in adult monkeys demonstrated that receptive fields in the primary visual cortex can change position after retinal lesions (Gilbert and Wiesel 1992; Eysel and Schweigart 1999; chapter 3). Apart from their location, receptive fields also can radically change their receptive field sizes within minutes after retinal lesions. The increase in size is about an order of magnitude for cortical receptive fields close to the lesion's border (Gilbert and Wiesel 1992). Accordingly, the distribution of mass potentials evoked by visual stimulation in humans changes as a result of training, especially pronounced for short latencies over the primary visual cortex (Fahle and Skrandies 1994). Even more complex single cell properties change as a function of training, and shifts of receptive field position, which amount to about 2 mm of cortical distance for short-term learning, can increase to about 8 mm for long-term learning (Pons et al. 1991). Animals trained to discriminate pitches around a defined standard frequency improve specifically for this frequency band, and the corresponding representation in primary auditory cortex increases (Recanzone, Schreiner, and Merzenich 1993). Training to discriminate the main motion direction in dynamic random dot patterns improves both performance of the animal and the response characteristics of single cells in area MT (Zohary et al. 1994), and neurons in inferotemporal cortex change their receptive field properties according to complex stimuli

they were trained with (Kobatake, Wang and Tanaka 1998; Tanaka, chapter 4, this volume; Logothetis, Pauls, and Poggio 1995; Sheinberg and Logothetis, chapter 6, this volume). The effects of structural lesions of the retina can be mimicked by presenting an artificial scotoma, that is, by preventing visual input to part of the retina. The consequences are similar to if less pronounced than those of structural lesions (Volchan and Gilbert 1994). Presenting one stimulus within a cortical receptive field and another one simultaneously close by produces expansion of the receptive field towards the outside stimulus (Eysel, Eyding, and Schweigart 1998; see chapters 4 and 6). Similar, but far more pronounced changes occur after coactivation in the somatosensory cortex (Diamond, Armstrong-James, and Ebner 1993; Wang, Merzenich, Sameshima, and Jenkins 1995; Godde, Stauffenberg, Spengler, and Dinse 2000), indicating that the extent of adult plasticity may differ between the two systems. As a consequence of these experimental results, we now know for sure that even the adult primary sensory cortices have a fair amount of plasticity to perform changes of information processing as a result of training. These results have far-reaching implications for the concept of memory, too. "Memory" in perceptual learning is not a property of one or a few assemblies of cortical neurons in specialized parts of the brain, but all cortical areas seem to be able to change and adapt their function both on a fast and a slow time scale.

Multiple Levels of Learning and Top-Down Influences

The earlier insight is still true that changing the very front end of information processing as a result of learning one perceptual task would necessarily change processing of many other stimuli presented to the same sensors. The speed and amount of learning depends strongly on attentional control (Ahissar and Hochstein 1993; chapter 14), as well as on "insight" (Rubin, Nakayama, and Shapley 1997; chapter 13)—that is, on top-down influences within the brain. Receptive fields of cortical neurons even in the primary visual cortex change in a task-dependent way, influenced by the actual perceptual task presented to the animal (Gilbert 1998; Gilbert et al., 2001; Crist, Li, and Gilbert, 2001)—another indication for the importance of top-down influences. Hence, present models of perceptual learning increasingly emphasize that learning occurs at a number of different levels of information processing and that top-down influences from "higher" levels play a crucial role in adjusting, in a task-dependent way, the processing of the "lower" levels. Indeed, recent experiments have provided direct evidence for strong top-down influences caused by error feedback and attentional processes on perceptual learning (Ahissar and Hochstein 1993; Weiss, Edelman and Fahle 1993; Herzog and Fahle 1997; see also chapters 18 and 20). Different observers may use (slightly) different strategies to solve the same task, possibly involving different levels of cortical stimulus representation, and may improve at different speeds. These differences may cause one of the unsolved problems in perceptual learning: Why is it that some observers improve vigorously while others not at all?

It seems that the high specificity of perceptual learning in vision is partly lost if relatively easy tasks are learned, while specificity of improvement is highest for very difficult tasks. A possible explanation is that "easy" tasks are learned on a relatively "higher" level of information processing, where the information extracted from the visual scene is better used than was possible before training and hence show interocular transfer of improvement. Difficult tasks, on the other hand, may require additional changes on lower levels of processing that are specific for the

eye trained for exact visual field position and for stimulus orientation (Ahissar and Hochstein 1997; chapter 14).

To conclude, perceptual learning differs from other forms of learning in that it can be very task- and stimulus-specific and probably involves functional and anatomical changes even in primary sensory cortices. Although perceptual learning, at first glance, seems to rely mostly on relatively complex cognitive processes, the specificity of improvement for quite low-level attributes such as visual field position, stimulus orientation, and the eye used for training a visual task indicates a strong and crucial involvement of primary (visual) cortex, where neurons are still partly monocularly activated. However, monocular neurons in V1 usually lack orientation specificity (Hubel and Wiesel 1977), hence specificity cannot be explained in a strictly feedforward system. Dependence on attention, error feedback, and "insight," on the other hand, demonstrates that strong top-down influences play a major role in perceptual learning and that perceptual learning, of course, also involves more cognitive levels of the brain. Hence, the study of perceptual learning processes not only shows us the amazing amount of plasticity even in adult sensory information processing at a relatively peripheral level but also leads to a view of cortical information processing not as a feedforward system of sequential neuronal layers but as a complex and plastic feedback system with strong and important top-down influences on "lower" or "early" parts of information processing.

Recent Advances in Research on Perceptual Learning

Perceptual learning is a quite active area of research, and the extensive list of references at the end of this book is testimony to this activity. Some of this activity is outside the scope of the individual chapters of this book. On the following pages, I will briefly referee important contributions to perceptual learning, most of which are not cited elsewhere in the book. The fast progress in research on perceptual learning is documented by quite a number of reviews highlighting different aspects of this research (Gibson 1963; Wohlwill 1966; Hall 1991; Sagi and Tanne 1994; Gilbert 1994; Walsh and Both 1997; Goldstone 1998; Wiggs and Martin 1998; Hurlbert 2000). Perceptual learning has a number of *different aspects*, ranging from sensorimotor (e.g., tactile) to purely sensory learning in all sensory submodalities such as olfaction, taste, hearing, and vision.

The interplay between sensory input and motor output was tested, for example, in maze discriminations in animals (Trobalon, Sansa, Chamizo, and Mackintosh 1991; Trobalon, Chamizo, and Mackintosh 1992; cf. also Prados, Chamize and Mackintosh 1999), indicating the importance of visual context on some forms of motor learning. Spatial learning, as tested with a prism adaptation task, revealed the existence of different levels of learning. More complex spatial remapping can be learned on a cognitive level but not on a perceptual level (Bedford 1993; cf. also Howard 1971). The cerebellum may play a role in this type of learning (cf. Daum et al. 1993; Vaina, Belliveau, Des Roziers, and Zeffiro 1998). Several studies proved the intricate relation between visual perception and motor learning in which demonstrations of a motion allowed human observers to adequately reproduce this motion (Vogt 1995; cf. also Meegan, Aslin and Jacobs 2000; cf. Kodman 1981 for visual-motor learning in retarded persons).

Distinct perceptual learning occurs in the *somatosensory system*, for example with vibrotactile stimulation (Epstein, Hughes, Schneider, and Bach-y-Rita 1989; Hughes, Epstein, Schneider, and Dudock 1990), but also with other tasks such as tactile reversal and oddity learning (Krekling, Tellevik, and Nordvik 1989; Benedetti 1991; cf. also Layton 1972). This tactile learning is highly task specific while generalizing between different body locations (Sathian and Zangaladze 1997; cf. also Nagarajan, Blake, Wright, Byl, and Merzenich 1998; Sathian and Zangaladze 1998; Harris and Diamond 2000; cf., however, Godde, Stauffenberg, Spengler, and Dinse 2000). These psychophysical studies are in agreement with the plasticity of the somatosensory system found in both sum potential recordings (Pascual-Leone and Torres 1993; Spengler, Roberts, Poeppel, Byl, Wang, Rowley, and Merzenich 1997) and recordings from single neurons and small clusters of neurons (Recanzone, Merzenich, Jenkins, Grajski, and Dinse 1992; Wang, Merzenich, Sameshima, and Jenkins 1995; Diamond, Amstrong-James, and Ebner 1993; Godde, Spengler, and Dinse 1996).

Perceptual learning of taste and olfaction leads to bias-free improvement in wine discrimination (Owen and Machamer 1979; Bende and Nordin 1997; for a review, see Granger and Lynch 1991). Generalization of a conditioned aversion reaction to lemon-saline to presentation of lemon-sucrose was substantially reduced by prior exposure to the individual compound solutions (Mackintosh, Kaye, and Bennett 1991; cf. also Bennett and Mackintosh 1999; Bennett, Levitt, and Anton 1972; Bennett and Anton 1992; Anton, Player, and Bennett 1981 for the effects of stimulus preexposure on perceptual learning in rats).

Auditory learning concerns either more basal or else complex functions, such as understanding of language. On a basal level, training to discriminate between different frequencies increases precision of performance especially for the trained frequency band in humans (Demany 1985; Irvine, Martin, Klimkeit, and Smith 2000) as well as the cortical representation of this frequency band in the monkey auditory cortex (Recanzone, Schreiner, and Merzenich 1993). Performance in several auditory tasks improves through learning (Grunke and Pisoni 1982; Tomblin and Quinn 1983), with complex tasks requiring longer learning times (Watson 1980; cf. also Leek and Watson 1988). Comparisons between monaural and binaural loudness estimates indicate the basis of learning during calibration of a loudness estimate (Marks, Galanter, and Baird 1995). Language comprehension improves through training (reviewed by Kuhl 1994), and training with sentences improves performance more than training with isolated words (Greenspan, Nusbaum, and Pisoni 1988; Nygaard and Pisoni 1998; cf. also Harpur, Estabrooks, Allen, and Asaph 1978, for perceptual learning in language acquisition). Improvement may last for a long time (Bradlow, Akahane-Yamada, Pisoni, and Tohkura 1999), a finding important for perceptual learning with cochlear implants (Watson 1991; Pisoni 2000; see Clark, chapter 8, this volume).

Not only in the somatosensory but also in the visual system, *receptive field properties* change as a result of perceptual learning (Eysel, Eyding, and Schweigart 1998; Gilbert 1994; Zohary, Celebrini, Britten, and Newsome 1994; Logothetis, Pauls and Poggio 1995; Gilbert, Das, Ito, Kapadia, and Westheimer 1996; Tovee, Rolls, and Ramachandran 1996; Gilbert, Ito, Kapadia, and Westheimer 2000; Eysel, chapter 3, this volume). Consistent with this plasticity on the single-cell level, sum-potentials over the human occipital pole change after training of motion- and stereo-discrimination tasks (Fahle and Skrandies 1994; Skrandies and Fahle 1994; Skrandies 1995; Skrandies, Lang, and Jedynak 1996; Skrandies and Jedynak 1999; Skrandies, Jedynak, and Fahle 2001), as well as during associative learning (Miltner, Braun, Arnold, Witte, and Taub 1999) and sensorimotor learning (mirror-star learning task:

Gliner, Mihevic, and Horvath 1983). Training an orientation-discrimination task led to a decrease of activity in striate and extrastriate visual cortex during task execution, as measured with positron emission tomography (Schiltz, Bodart, Dubois, Dejardin, Michel, Roucoux, Crommelinck, and Orban 1999), while it increased activity in prefrontal cortex during an associative sensory learning task (McIntosh, Rajah, and Lobaugh 1999). Bilateral electroconvulsive therapy had a greater impact on perceptual learning than right unilateral ECT (Daniel, Crovitz, and Weiner 1984).

Animal models of perceptual learning on the behavioral level found that mixing exposure of stimuli to be discriminated accelerated perceptual learning compared to separate exposure (Honey and Bateson 1996; cf. also Honey, Bateson, and Horn 1994). Different animal studies demonstrated effects of animal population density on perceptual learning (Levitt and Bennet 1975), investigated the relationship between imprinting and perceptual learning in chicks (Kovach, Fabricius, and Fält 1966), led to insights into the perceptual learning of monkeys (Humphreys and Keeble 1976; Gaffan 1996), and showed that early visual deprivation impairs visual discrimination learning (Zernicki 1999).

The *mechanisms* underlying perceptual learning have been extensively investigated and discussed. One central question is specificity versus generalization: while perceptual learning is quite specific, certain aspects nevertheless generalize. For example, a second, similar task may start at the same low performance level as the initial task, but performance may improve *faster* than in the initial task (Liu and Weinshall 2000). This finding is interpreted using a model based on limited computational capacity. Abrupt learning can be interpreted as either being based on different mechanisms than gradual learning (Ahissar and Hochstein 1997, chapter 14, this volume) or else on the same mechanisms (Nakayama and Shapley; Rubin, Nakayama, and Shapley 1997; Rubin et al., chapter 13, this volume), but it seems clear that different levels of cortical processing are involved (cf. also Watanabe et al., 2001). Other experiments indicate that the target signal changes during perceptual learning while the level of internal noise stays constant (Gold, Bennett, and Sekuler 1999; cf., Dosher and Lu 1998; Dosher and Lu 1999). Incomplete pictures are far better recognized after perceptual learning that probably takes place on a rather cognitive level (Gollin 1965), and one study reports on the relationship between autobiographical (explicit) and perceptual (implicit) learning (Jacoby and Dallas 1981).

Attention exerts a significant influence on many types of perceptual learning (e.g., Adcock and Mangan 1970; Ahissar and Hochstein 1993; Ito, Westheimer, and Gilbert 1998). It has been discussed whether long-term changes in perception should be explained by association or perceptual learning (Bedford 1995, 1997) and whether inhibitory processes may be involved in perceptual learning (Killcross, Kiernan, Dwyer, and Westbrook 1998). The dimensionality of internal object representations is reduced in peripheral vision but can be increased by perceptual learning (Jüttner and Rentschler 1996). Some forms of perceptual learning may require REM sleep (Karni, Tanne, Rubenstein, Askenasy, and Sagi 1994; cf. also Karni and Sagi 1993). A large literature exists on so-called prism adaptation effects that compensate for the changes induced by wearing prism spectacles (cf. Epstein 1975; Melamed and Arnett 1984). This type of perceptual learning seems to rely mostly on changes in the motor system and is therefore not dealt with in this book.

Based on these and other aspects of the mechanisms possibly underlying perceptual learning, and, of course, based on the experimental results, several

more *formal models* of perceptual learning have been proposed (see chapters 15, 18, and 20, this volume). Some of these are focussed on receptive field organization (e.g., Kalarickal and Marshall 1999), while most are concerned with more complex features (Peres and Hochstein 1994; Rentschler, Jüttner, and Caelli 1994; Stone 1996; Jüttner, Caelli, and Rentschler 1997; Stone and Harper 1999; Saksida 1999).

Improvement through training occurs for several *low-level tasks* such as motion perception (Liu and Vaina 1998; Liu 1999; Zanker 1999), orientation discrimination (Rivest, Boutet, and Intriligator 1996; King, Shanks, and Hart 1996; Fahle 1997; cf. Baldassi and Burr 2000 for the relation between visual search and orientation identification versus target location), discrimination of spatial frequencies (Fiorentini and Berardi 1980, 1997) and textures (Karni and Sagi 1991), as well as in seeing form from motion (Vidyasagar and Stuart 1993) and spatiotemporal interpolation (DeLuca and Fahle 1999). Visual hyperacuity denotes the fact that discrimination thresholds in several visual tasks such as stereoscopic depth perception, vernier acuity, and orientation discrimination are far below the diameter of foveal photoreceptors and thus are sensitive probes for perceptual learning. Several studies found improvement through training with these tasks to be highly specific for most stimulus parameters such as visual field position, size, orientation, and even the eye used during training (Freeman 1966; Schoups, Vogels and Orban 1995; Crist, Kapadia, Westheimer, and Gilbert 1997; Matthews, Liu, Geesaman, and Qian 1999; cf., however, Beard, Levi, and Reich 1994). Stereoscopic depth perception also dramatically improves through training (Ramachandran and Braddick 1973; McKee and Westheimer 1978; O'Toole and Kersten 1992; Sowden 1995; Sowden, Davies, Rose, and Kaye 1996; van Ee 2001). Interobserver variance is sometimes high in these tasks (Fahle and Henke-Fahle 1996). Details on the specificity versus generalization in these types of tasks can be found in chapters 11, 12, 18, and 20. It should be noted that depending on training regime, specificity of learning may be strongly decreased (Liu and Vaina 1998).

The effects of *masking* may change after training (Dorais and Sagi 1997; cf. also Saarinen and Levi 1995), as does the perception of illusory contours (Gellatly 1982; Rubin, Nakayama, and Shapley 1997), and learning of a visual search task involving motion information can be adversely affected by transcranial magnetic stimulation (TMS) (Stewart, Batelli, Walsh, and Cowey 1999). This technique also demonstrated cortical plasticity in perceptual learning (Walsh, Ashbridge, and Cowey 1998).

Not surprisingly, improvement through training occurs for *higher-level tasks*, too. Some examples are the improvement of length estimation in the horizontal-vertical illusion which is faster under feedback conditions than without feedback (Brosvic, Rowe-Boyer, and Dihoff 1991), perceptual-motor skills in dentistry (Birch 1976), and rehabilitation of handicapped children (Scott 1974). Perception of more complex forms and objects such as textures, complex graphical signs, objects, and faces improves through practice (McLaren 1997; Espinet, Almaraz, and Torres 1999; Fine and Jacobs 2000; Furmanski and Engel 2000; cf. Dolan, Fink, Rolls, Booth, Holmes, Frackowiak, and Friston 1997 for a functional neuroimaging correlate: enhanced activity in inferior temporal cortex). Visual classification, such as the sexing of young chickens (Biederman and Shiffrar 1987), also improves as a result of training (Hock, Webb, and Cavedo 1987; Wills and McLaren 1998).

Visual search, that is, the decision whether or not a defined target is present in a display, is another favorite task to test perceptual learning. For this task,

improvement transfers completely between eyes (Schoups and Orban 1996) but is specific to orientation, size, and position (Ahissar and Hochstein 1995; cf. also Epstein 1967; Ahissar, Laiwald, Kozminsky, and Hochstein 1998). These results indicate that perceptual learning for visual search may be less specific than learning of visual discriminations and may take place on another level of cortical processing (Sireteanu and Rettenbach 1995, 2000; cf., however, Ellison and Walsh 1998; Lobley and Walsh 1998). Parallel visual search achieved through perceptual learning may be fast but nevertheless effortful (Leonards, Rettenbach, and Sireteanu 1998). Task-specific attention seems to play an important role in these learning processes (Ahissar and Hochstein 2000; cf. also Stadler 1989 for the role of awareness in learning during visual search).

Perceptual learning is a potential hope for *patients* suffering from different disorders of visual perception, ranging from amblyopia (Levi and Polat 1996) over prosopagnosia (cf. Greve and Bauer 1990 for implicit face learning; cf., however, Sergent and Villemure 1989) to brain damage with visual field defects (Kasten and Wuest 1998; Kasten, Wuest, and Sabel 1998; cf. Markowitsch and Härtling 1996 for the effects of visual priming), and Alzheimer's disease (Postle, Corkin, and Growdon 1996), and Grafman, Weingartner, Newhouse, Thompson, Lalonde, Litvan, Molchan, and Sunderland (1990) report positive "implicit" perceptual learning. The same is true for the somatosensory domain (see chapter 2).

One study finds better discrimination between novel stimuli in autistic patients than in normals but lack of perceptual learning for these stimuli in the autistic patients (Plaisted, O'Riordan, and Baron-Cohen 1998). Several studies agree that even amnesic patients can be primed in visual perception that lasts for up to 12 months (and hence should be considered as perceptual learning) (Crovitz, Harvey, and

Clanahan 1981; Gabrieli, Milberg, Keane and Corkin 1990; Tulving, Hayman, and Macdonald 1991; Kapur, Abbott, Footitt, and Millar 1996; Chun and Phelps 1999; cf. Yamashita 1993 for perceptual-motor learning in amnesic patients and Squire and Zola 1997 for an overview of amnesia and memory).

Age dependence of perceptual learning was addressed by a few studies (Fahle and Daum 1997: fine-grain spatial memory; Gilbert 1996: visual search; Rockstroh, Dietrich, and Pokorny 1995: reaction time for visual stimuli). Generally, performance deteriorates slightly with increasing age. A number of additional studies addressed perceptual leaning specifically in infants and children, both normal (Jensen 1966; Kerpelman 1967; Odom, McIntyre, and Neale 1971; Turnure 1972) and abnormal (Brodlie and Burke 1971; Zelniker and Oppenheimer 1976; De Filippo Lutzer 1986), with generally positive results.

Aims and Scope of This Book

The aim of the present book is twofold: first, to review the advances made during the last decade in the field of perceptual learning, presented by some of the most prominent and competent researchers in the field; second, to combine this information to allow a clearer understanding of where we stand, which questions have been answered, and which ones still await a solution. So while the book can only illustrate the present state of knowledge on perceptual learning, it also demonstrates the ways in which information can be gathered, what the basic questions are—independent of the present state of knowledge, and where we presently stand in the attempt to answer these fundamental questions. In a fast-changing field such as perceptual learning, no single person oversees all the newest results and developments.

Therefore, the present book has many authors, each presenting a part of the field. This, moreover, allows the reader to spot some more or less subtle differences between the interpretations of different experts in the same field. It is no secret that there is a bit of controversy among researchers on perceptual learning regarding such issues as the exact model for the mechanisms underlying perceptual learning, and the reader may become aware of a couple of smaller controversies regarding the best strategy to further examine the phenomena and mechanisms of perceptual learning. On the other hand, I was surprised when reading all the chapters by how much agreement has been reached among different groups on all the main issues (and most of the small ones).

The topics dealt with in the book cover the field of perceptual learning in a rather broad and extensive way, starting from the anatomical and physiological changes that correspond on a neuronal level to the changes of behavior observable on the systems level. Starting on a neuroanatomical level, we look at the development of interneuronal connections during ontogenesis and at the changes induced by lesions or external influences (chapter 1). Chapter 2 then presents an overview of the changes induced by lesions and especially perceptual learning in the somatosensory system. The electrophysiological correlate of (perceptual) learning as evidenced by the plasticity of visual receptive fields after lesions and training, as well as the probable underlying mechanisms, are described in chapter 3, followed, in 4 through 6, by the description of development of complex receptive field properties through training in temporal (chapter 4) and parietal as well as occipital visual cortices (chapters 5 and 6). An account on cortical reorganization and perceptual learning and their perceptual correlates as evidenced by non-invasive methods in humans (chapter 7) finishes this first part of the book.

The second part of the book deals mostly with learning on a systems level as investigated mainly by psychophysical methods. Chapters 8 to 12 concentrate on more low-level aspects of perceptual learning, such as auditory learning (chapter 8), the adaptation and improvement through learning in discriminating simple visual stimuli such as gratings (chapter 9), the long-lasting and fast modifications of low-level visual networks (chapter 10), and the invariance versus specificity of perceptual learning (chapters 11 and 12). The chapters in part III deal with higher-level perceptual learning and address the relations between cognitive aspects of learning and perceptual learning (chapter 13) and summarize the evidence for a bidirectional relationship between perceptual learning and cognition (chapter 14), followed by accounts on higher learning of early visual tasks (chapter 15) and learning to recognize objects in general (chapter 16), or specifically to recognize faces (chapter 17).

The three chapters of part IV finally put it all altogether, by modeling perceptual learning in general (chapter 18), providing an independent component analysis for perception (chapter 19), and by listing some problems encountered in modeling perceptual learning that command the development of "feedback" models of learning (chapter 20).

The glossary defines some of the central terms of the book, and a single reference list for the entire book will help the reader get a rapid overview. For the hurried reader, the take-home message of the book is given here, in order to save him or her from reading the entire book:

Perceptual learning is a new field in the general domain of "learning." More specifically, it is a form of implicit learning and denotes a lasting modification of behavior following sensory stimulation caused by previous experience with a perceptual task. In many instances, perceptual learning is very specific for quite elementary stimulus attributes such as position in the visual field, orientation, and for the eye used during learning (if one eye is covered). This specificity indicates a neuronal substrate for some forms of perceptual learning partly on the level of the primary visual cortex. Present models assume a plasticity of this primary visual cortex even in adults, triggered by appropriate stimuli under strong top-down influences from more "cognitive" levels of the cortex. These findings promise to develop better therapies for patients suffering from cortical lesions after stroke (infarction) or trauma, based on the insights gained by studying the mechanisms of perceptual learning.

Manfred Fahle

Anatomy and Physiology

I

Experience-Dependent Plasticity of Intracortical Connections

Siegrid Löwel and Wolf Singer

Abstract

One of the basic features of visual scene analysis is to assemble the components of objects into a unified percept and to segregate them from background. In addition, we store information about previous experience partly through perceptual learning and test our interpretations of the visual world against incoming sensory input. In recent years, evidence has accumulated indicating that long-range neuronal connections within visual cortex mediate the influences of context and experience, possibly also those of expectation. Focusing on the "hardware" of these important computations, namely on the layout and plasticity of long-range connections in young and adult cortex, this chapter addresses the following questions. What is the extent and laminar specificity of these long-range connections? What does their layout look like? Which types of neurons are involved? What is the functional role of the connections? How do they develop? How does experience modify their layout? Is plasticity also possible in adult brains? What are the underlying mechanisms?

Acknowledgments

It is with pleasure that we thank Charles Gilbert, Kevan Martin, Bill Bosking, and Rainer Goebel for providing us with original versions of their published figures; Renate Ruhl and Steffi Bachmann for help with the figures; John M. Crook and Sven Meyburg for critical reading of the manuscript; and the Max-Planck-Society and the Wissenschaftsgemeinschaft Gottfried Wilhelm Leibniz for their support.

1.1 Introduction

One of the basic functions of the cerebral cortex is the representation and analysis of relations among components of sensory and motor patterns. To correctly interpret visual scenes, for example, the cortex must, on the one hand, assemble components of an object into a unified percept and, on the other, segregate these components from the background. Neurons in the primary visual cortex fire action potentials in response not only to the appearance of a particular stimulus within their classical receptive field but also to more global characteristics of a visual scene, such as the contours and surfaces within which a stimulus is embedded. Contrary to long-standing belief, recent physiological and anatomical evidence suggests that spatial integration occurs in part already at the level of the primary visual cortex. The anatomical substrate for integrative capabilities at this level and for their possible experience-dependent modifications are long-range tangential connections formed by excitatory cortical neurons. Because these horizontal connections span a cortical region much larger than that corresponding to the classical receptive field of an individual neuron, the connections are thought to be important for context-dependent modifications of neuronal responsivity and thus to be essential for the integration of information from widely distant points in the visual field. And because the architecture of long-range connections has been shown to be modifiable by visual experience during early development, it follows that the criteria for perceptual integration or grouping are at least partly acquired through experience and learning. In addition, in the adult, the effectiveness of intracortical interactions continues to be modifiable on timescales ranging from seconds to months, and long-range horizontal connections have been implicated in these processes, too.

We will first focus on the layout of long-range intracortical connections, then discuss experience-dependent modifications observed during early postnatal development, and finally summarize available evidence for the role of these connections in adult plasticity. Because most of the relevant published data are from the mammalian visual system, we will concentrate on long-range connections in the primary visual cortex, also termed *area 17* by the anatomist Korbinian Brodmann (1909), who divided the human cortex into consecutively numbered cyto-architectonic areas.

1.2   Layout of Intracortical Connections

A fundamental characteristic of the cerebral cortex is the similarity of its gross morphological organization across different areas. In all mammals, the neocortex consists of six layers extending over about 2 mm from layer I, which lies next to the pial surface of the brain, down to the lower margin of layer VI, which directly faces the underlying white matter, a more or less cell-free region containing axons both entering and leaving the cortex. The cortex itself is referred to as "gray matter" and is composed of neuronal cell bodies, dendrites, axon terminals, and glial cells (for a general introduction to neuroscience see, for example, Purves et al. 1997).

1.2.1   Extent and Laminar Specificity of Long-Range Connections

The classical view of cortical connectivity, derived mainly from the impregnation of single neurons with silver salts (the so-called Golgi technique used in the classical studies of Santiago Ramón y Cajal and Camillo Golgi), is that axons tend to run perpendicularly to the cortical surface, from layer to layer, with relatively little spread parallel to the cortical surface (e.g., Lund 1973). Findings of this kind supported the famous columnar concept of the visual cortex, which was based on the classical electrophysiological experiments of Hubel and Wiesel (1962), and which particularly emphasizes vertical connections (see also Gilbert 1983). However, more than twenty-five years ago, it was demonstrated that long-range connections are also a prominent feature of visual cortical connectivity: after cortical lesions in macaque monkeys, degenerating terminals were observed up to a distance of 3.5 mm from the lesion sites (Fisken, Garey, and Powell 1975; see also Szentágothai 1973; Creutzfeldt et al. 1977). Experiments using more modern tracer techniques (i.e., extra- and intracellular injections of the enzyme horseradish peroxidase, HRP; injections of biocytin or fluorescent latex microspheres) have clearly established that extensive horizontal connections do span distances of several millimeters (up to 8 mm) within individual cortical layers (Rockland and Lund 1982; Gilbert and Wiesel 1983; Martin and Whitteridge 1984; Kisvárday and Eysel 1992; Luhmann, Martínez-Millán, and Singer 1990; for a review, see Gilbert 1992). Called "long-range horizontal," "tangential," or "intralaminar," these connections are especially prominent in cortical layers II/III and V; their synapses exhibit the morphology of excitatory synapses and contact dendrites of spiny and nonspiny cells in the same proportion that these cell types occur in the cortex (80% and 20%, respectively; Kisvárday et al. 1986; McGuire et al. 1991).

1.2.2 Types of Neurons Involved in Long-Range Connections

Axon collaterals of spiny stellate and pyramidal neurons, the two types of cortical excitatory cells (Gilbert 1983), form the anatomical basis for long-range intracortical connections. Pyramidal cells constitute the main cell type in the visual cortex and their somata are distributed in all cortical layers, except layer I. They are characterized by a triangular cell body and a large apical dendrite directed radially toward the pial surface. Typically, all their dendrites (apical as well as basal ones) are covered with a high density of spines, dendritic protrusions that receive at least one excitatory synapse (Peters and Kaiserman-Abramof 1969). Spiny stellate cells lack a dominant apical dendrite but—as the name indicates—have spiny dendrites. In contrast to pyramidal neurons, however, spiny stellate cells are present exclusively in layer IV of primary sensory areas (Lund 1973; Valverde 1986). Therefore they are the major target neurons of thalamocortical afferents (in case of visual cortex, afferents from the lateral geniculate nucleus, a thalamic nucleus that receives information from the retinas) that terminate in the cortical input layer IV (Gilbert 1983).

About 20% of the total number of cortical neurons are immunopositive for gamma-aminobutyric acid (GABA), the major inhibitory neurotransmitter in the cerebral cortex. These neurons are categorized into at least eight different classes according to morphological criteria. Among these, only large basket and dendrite-targeting cells provide lateral inhibitory connections extending up to 1.5 mm; all other cell types have predominantly local axon collaterals.

Thus the inhibitory network is at least two to three times smaller in extent than the excitatory network

(Kisvárday et al. 1997; Crook, Kisvárday, and Eysel 1998). Because we are interested in long-range connections that are involved in integrating visual information across columnar boundaries from distant points in the visual field, we will concentrate on excitatory long-range connections.

1.2.3 Patchy Nature of Long-Range Connections

Intracellular injections of HRP reveal that the axon collaterals of individual neurons are not distributed homogeneously across the cortex but—as viewed from the cortical surface—form numerous discrete terminal clusters. These collateral clusters measure about 300 μm–600 μm in diameter. Extracellular injections of a variety of other tracers result in a similar picture of patchy intracortical connections (figure 1.1). These patchy connections are reciprocal: small intracortical injections of both anterograde and retrograde neuronal tracers label clusters of (retrogradely labeled) neurons and (anterogradely labeled) axon terminals that are spaced at regular intervals (about 1 mm) in the visual cortices of cats, ferrets, tree shrews, and primates (Rockland and Lund 1982, 1983; Rockland 1985; Gilbert and Wiesel 1983; Boyd and Matsubara 1991; Kisvárday and Eysel 1992; Burkhalter, Bernardo, and Charles 1993; Livingstone and Hubel 1984). Thus long-range tangential axon collaterals interconnect regularly spaced clusters of cells.

1.2.4 Modular Selectivity

Because neurons that respond to similar visual stimuli, for example, to lines of a particular orientation presented at a particular location in the visual field (within their receptive field), are not distributed randomly across the cortex but are arranged in columns extending from layer I to layer VI (the so-called orientation columns; Hubel and Wiesel 1962;

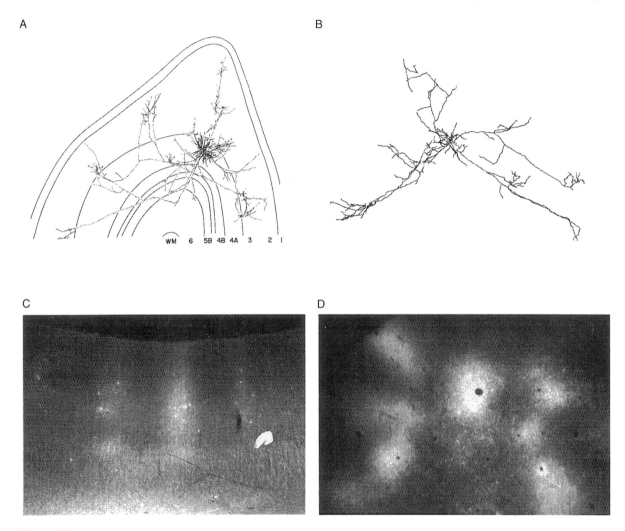

Figure 1.1
Patchiness of long-range intracortical connections in the cerebral cortex. (*A*) Camera lucida reconstruction of a spiny stellate cell of cortical layer 4 displaying an extensive and patchy axonal distribution. The cell body of this neuron is located in layer 4A, whereas most of the collateral branches are restricted to cortical layers 2 and 3. Frontal section through the primary visual cortex of a cat. (Modified from Martin and Whitteridge 1984.) (*B*) Reconstruction of the axon arbors of a pyramidal cell of layer 2 projected onto a plane parallel to the cortical surface. The cell body is located in the center of the reconstruction. Again the clustered nature of the collateral branches is clearly visible. (Modified from Gilbert and Wiesel 1983, 1120, figure 2b.) In panels A and B, neurons were intracellularly injected with the enzyme horseradish peroxidase. (*C, D*) Patchy intracortical connections visualized after extracellular injections of the fluorescent carbocyanine dye DiI. Fluorescent photographs of a section cut perpendicularly to the cortical lamination (panel C) and a section cut parallel to the cortical surface (panel D) of cat visual cortex. The dye DiI labels both axon terminals (visible as the more homogeneous white labeling) and neuronal cell bodies (the small brightly fluorescent dots seen in panel C). Scale bar: 500 μm (panels C, D).

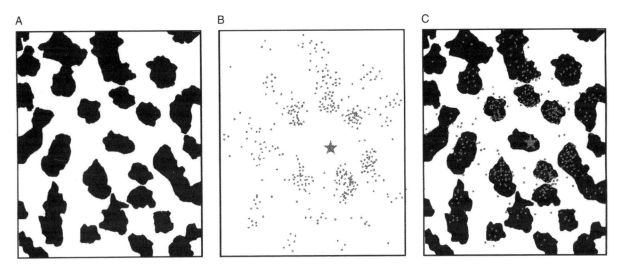

Figure 1.2
Columnar specificity of long-range tangential connections. Schematic drawing of the topographic relationship between intrinsic connections and orientation columns in the primary visual cortex of cats. (*A*) Pattern of orientation columns (black regions represent cortical regions stimulated with horizontal moving contours). (*B*) Patchy distribution of retrogradely labeled neurons (gray dots) in the same region of cortex (labeled from the injection site, marked with a star). (*C*) Superposition of panels A and B. Note that the injection site of the fluorescent neuronal tracer was located in a black column (i.e., a horizontal orientation column) and that labeled neurons are predominantly but not exclusively distributed within columns of the same functional preference (other dark columns).

Blasdel and Salama 1986), the question arises, do interconnected cells share similar functional properties? Within the last ten to fifteen years, evidence has accumulated that this is indeed the case with respect to preference for stimulus orientation or color (Ts'o, Gilbert, and Wiesel 1986; Ts'o and Gilbert 1988; Gilbert and Wiesel 1989; Gray et al. 1989; Hata et al. 1991; Malach et al. 1993; Malach, Tootell, and Malonek 1994; Kisvárday et al. 1997; Bosking et al. 1997). The relationship between horizontal connections and cortical functional architecture was determined through cross-correlation analysis and by combining the labeling of both intracortical connections and cortical columns, among other techniques. Anatomically, it was shown that the clustering

of long-range connections shows a clear relationship to the system of orientation columns: injections of fluorescent latex microspheres into, for example, a horizontal orientation column revealed retrogradely labeled neurons that were concentrated in the same and other horizontal orientation columns (figure 1.2). In agreement with these data, the statistical technique of cross-correlation analysis, used to analyze the timing of action potentials in pairs of neurons and to measure the effective connection strength between two cells, showed that neurons with correlated action potentials had similar orientation preference. These findings do not mean that horizontal fibers exclusively connect neurons with identical response properties—cells with differing

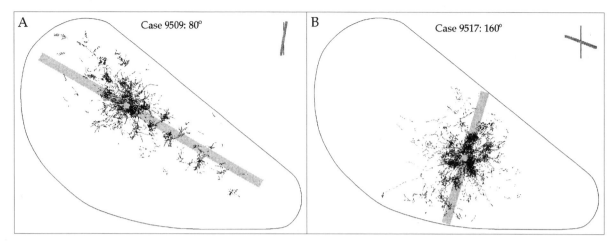

Figure 1.3
Axial selectivity of long-range intracortical connections. (*A*, *B*) Distribution of labeled synaptic boutons resulting from focal extracellular injections of biocytin into functionally characterized sites of tree shrew visual cortex (area V1). The preferred orientation at the injection site is shown in the inset of each panel. The outline of the dorsal portion of V1 is indicated by a thin black line. Along the central portion of the border between areas V1 and V2, this line corresponds to a vertical line in the map of visual space. The axis in cortex corresponding to the preferred orientation is indicated by the gray rectangle underlying each distribution. Each black dot indicates an individual labeled bouton. There is a dense and fairly uniform distribution of boutons found near each injection site. At longer distances the distributions are patchy, contacting other sites that have similar orientation preference as the injection site. Note in addition that in both panels A and B the distributions are elongated along an axis that corresponds to the preferred orientation of the injection site. (Modified from Bosking et al. 1997, figures 8A and 8C.)

properties are also contacted, although to a smaller extent—but rather that, on average, like tends to connect to like.

1.2.5   Axial Selectivity

Interestingly, the long-range horizontal fibers do not distribute isotropically across the visual cortex. In addition to the modular specificity, they exhibit axial specificity, that is, there is a systematic relationship between a neuron's orientation preference and the distribution of its axon arbors across the cortical map of visual space: horizontal connections extend for longer distances and give rise to a larger number of terminal boutons along an axis of the visual field map

that corresponds to the neuron's preferred orientation (Fitzpatrick 1996; Bosking et al. 1997; see also Schmidt, Goebel, et al. 1997; figure 1.3). Thus long-range horizontal connections preferentially link neurons with cooriented, coaxially aligned receptive fields.

1.2.6   Possible Functions of Long-Range Horizontal Connections

These anatomical data suggest a close relation between the topology of tangential intracortical connections and the perceptual grouping criterion of colinearity. Dating back to the time of the Gestalt psychologists at the beginning of the last century, it

A   B

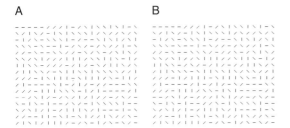

Figure 1.4
Example of perceptual grouping on the basis of colinearity.
(*A*) Colinear line segments that define the edges of a
rhombus are grouped together and stand out from the
randomly distributed line segments of the background. (*B*)
Line segments are arranged as in panel A except for those
defining the outline of the rhombus, which are now parallel to each other and hence orthogonal to the corresponding segments in panel A. (Modified from Schmidt,
Goebel, et al. 1997.)

has been known that perceptually salient contours
consist of line segments that are adjacent, colinear,
and of similar orientation (Wertheimer 1938; Grossberg and Mingolla 1985; Ullman 1990; Field, Hayes,
and Mess 1993). Given the observed specificity in
the functional architecture, the connections are ideally suited to support perceptual grouping according
to the Gestalt criterion of colinearity by modulating
the saliency of distributed cortical responses in a
context-dependent way (Schmidt, Goebel, et al.
1997). Figure 1.4 illustrates that our visual system has
the tendency to group contour segments that share
the same orientation, especially if these are colinear
(Field, Hayes, and Hess 1993; Polat and Sagi 1993,
1994; Kapadia et al. 1995). Human observers are
much better at detecting a contour composed of
small oriented line segments that are aligned colinearly along the contour path than when the segments that are aligned orthogonally to the contour,
which implies that somewhere in the processing
hierarchy, neuronal responses to colinearly aligned

contours must be distinguished from responses to the
other, physically identical contours. The only cues
for this distinction are the relations between the location and orientation of the surrounding contours.
Selection of responses must therefore occur in a
context-dependent way at a level of processing where
neurons have orientation-selective receptive fields.
Because neither the perceived location nor the general appearance of individual contour elements is
influenced by context, (1) the grouping operation
must occur at a level where neurons have receptive
fields whose size is equal to or smaller than that of
the pattern elements, and (2) response selection must
not alter the feature selectivity of the neurons. These
two requirements make it likely that colinear
grouping occurs at an early stage of cortical processing. Taken together, available evidence is thus supporting the hypothesis that the criteria for perceptual
grouping operations are determined by the architecture of the tangential connections.

In addition, several other functions have been
attributed to these connections (see, for example,
Mitchison and Crick 1982), but which of them prevail under which conditions is still a matter of debate. Long-range connections have been proposed
to (1) contribute to the generation of large composite
receptive fields (Singer and Tretter 1976; Gilbert and
Wiesel 1985; Bolz and Gilbert 1990; Schwarz and
Bolz 1991); (2) mediate inhibitory and subthreshold
excitatory effects from beyond the classical receptive
field (Blakemore and Tobin 1972; Nelson and Frost
1978; Morrone, Burr, and Maffei 1982; Allman,
Miezin, and McGuinness 1985); (3) contribute to
orientation and direction selectivity (Eysel, Wörgötter, and Pape 1987; Eysel, Crook, and Machemer
1990); (4) be responsible for adaptive changes in
cortical maps after deafferentation (Kaas et al. 1990;
Heinen and Skavenski 1991; Gilbert and Wiesel
1992; Darian-Smith and Gilbert 1994); and (5) syn-

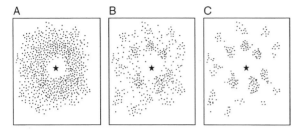

Figure 1.5
Schematic drawing of the development of clustered long-range connections in cat visual cortex. (*A, B, C*) Distribution of retrogradely labeled neurons (black dots) after tracer injections at postnatal day (PND) 1, 15, and 50, respectively. Injection site is indicated by a star. Note that the emergence of patchy intracortical connections (panel C) from an initially random distribution of interconnected cells (panel A) proceeds via a phase of "crude" clusters (panel B) characterized by a large number of neurons located in the spaces between the "adult" clusters.

chronize the responses of spatially distributed neurons as a function of stimulus coherence (Gray et al. 1989; König et al. 1993; Singer et al. 1997).

1.3 Development of Long-Range Intracortical Connections

In kitten visual cortex, tangential fibers develop mainly after birth and attain their adult specificity within the first six to eight weeks (Luhmann, Martínez-Millán, and Singer 1986; Price 1986; Callaway and Katz 1990; Galuske and Singer 1996). When kittens and humans are born, clustered horizontal connections are absent (Burkhalter, Bernardo, and Charles 1993; Callaway and Katz 1990; Luhmann, Singer, and Martínez-Millán 1990). Injections of retrograde tracers (such as fluorescent latex microspheres; see Katz, Burkhalter, and Dreyer 1984) into the superficial layers of the cat visual cortex within the first postnatal week reveal a homogeneous dis-

tribution of retrogradely labeled neurons extending over a limited tangential domain (figure 1.5). Similarly, injections of DiI (a lipophilic dye that stains cell bodies, dendrites, and axonal arborizations; see Honig and Hume 1989) in the neonatal human cortex up to an age of four months, result in a cluster-free labeling. In cats, during the second postnatal week, between postnatal day (PND) 8 and PND 10, the earliest perceptible and still crude clusters of retrogradely labeled cells appear, distributed over a somewhat greater tangential area than they were just a few days earlier (Price 1986; Callaway and Katz 1990; Luhmann, Singer, and Martínez-Millán 1990; Lübke and Albus 1992). The emergence of "crude" clusters means that many retrogradely labeled neurons are present in the spaces between clusters. In the next few weeks, the number of labeled cells between the clusters gradually declines until the adult pattern consisting of distinct clusters of labeled neurons with few cells between the clusters emerges. At the end of the fourth postnatal week, axon length has reached its maximal extent (Galuske and Singer 1996).

What is the mechanism of cluster refinement? Use of an ingenious double-injection paradigm (injections of fluorescent microspheres at a single cortical site at two different times during postnatal development), demonstrated that neurons located between clusters, which were labeled by early tracer injections (at PND 15), were still clearly visible after clusters had refined (at PND 29), but no longer made connections with the original injection site (neurons were not double-labeled with both the early and late tracer; see Callaway and Katz 1990). This observation indicated that cells between the clusters selectively lose a certain set of their horizontal long-range collaterals. Available data thus suggest that selective retraction of a subset of connections produces cluster refinement (see also Ruthazer and Stryker 1996). Reconstructions of individual pyramidal cells from cat visual cortex demonstrate that early in development, cells extend long, relatively unbranched axon collaterals. At this time, axonal arbors lack distinct collateral branches. Between three and six weeks postnatally, when clearly segregated clusters of retrogradely labeled neurons are emerging, the long-range axon collaterals become grouped and distal collateral branches are elaborated, as seen in the adult (Katz and Callaway 1992).

Taken together, the emergence of patchy intracortical connections from an initially random distribution of interconnected cells early in life can be divided into at least two distinct phases: (1) crude cluster emergence, followed by (2) arbor refinement, consisting of both selective retraction of "inappropriate" connections and the elaboration of "appropriate" axonal branches (see also Durack and Katz 1996; Ruthazer and Stryker 1996).

1.3.1 Patchy Connections and Orientation Columns during Development

Because of the close relationship between clustered long-range connections and orientation columns, neurons located between the crude clusters in early postnatal development must receive inputs from different orientation columns. This is likely to account for the observation that orientation tuning is much broader in young cats than in adults: adult values for tuning emerge at the same time clusters achieve their adult level of refinement (about one month postnatally; Imbert and Buisseret 1975; Albus and Wolf 1984; Braastad and Heggelund 1985). Similarly, in ferrets, the second phase of cluster refinement coincides with the emergence of mature orientation tuning and maps (Ruthazer and Stryker 1996; Durack and Katz 1996). In summary, in the early phase of crude cluster emergence, neurons make connections with a larger-than-normal range of orientation columns. Thereafter, when adultlike clusters appear, axon collaterals projecting to "incorrect"

orientation columns are thought to be selectively eliminated and collaterals to "correct" orientation columns, to be added (Katz and Callaway 1992).

1.4 Plasticity of Long-Range Connections during Development

The emergence of well-segregated clusters of interconnected cells in a developmental period when visual experience is known to profoundly influence cortical development (the "sensitive period"; see, for example, Wiesel, 1982) indicated that the specificity of the long-range connections might also depend on visual experience. In particular, the anatomical observation that clusters refine by the elimination of one set of connections (the "inappropriate" ones) and the stabilization of another set of connections (the "appropriate" ones) raised the possibility that selective stabilization is influenced by neuronal activity and is not genetically determined.

1.4.1 Development of Patches

Experiments with visually deprived animals confirmed this hypothesis. In cats that were dark-reared or binocularly deprived (lid-sutured), the selectivity of long-range intracortical connections was severely reduced, and the "normal" and selective adult pattern of connectivity did not appear (Katz and Callaway 1992; Luhmann, Martínez-Millán, and Singer 1986; Luhmann, Singer, and Martínez-Millán 1990). Nevertheless, crude clusters were present, so that the initial phase of cluster refinement does not seem to require patterned visual activity. This does not necessarily indicate that neuronal activity plays no role in cluster development. Indeed, chronic infusion of tetrodotoxin (TTX, a sodium channel blocker that prevents neurons from firing action potentials) into the visual cortex of ferrets resulted in a spatially random distribution of retrogradely labeled cells, whereas removal of the eyes did not prevent the initial development of crude clusters (Ruthazer and Stryker 1996). Thus blockade of cortical but not of retinal activity prevented the initial development of clustered horizontal connections. These observations indicate that spontaneous activity patterns in the primary visual cortex, the lateral geniculate nucleus (its main afferent nucleus), or other afferent sources are sufficient to organize the emergence of crude clusters.

The refinement of clusters, however, is clearly dependent on visually driven patterned activity. Both dark-rearing and prolonged binocular deprivation prevent the normal progression from "crude" to "refined" clusters. Experiments using retrograde tracers injected into area 17 revealed patterns of retrogradely labeled neurons in binocularly deprived cats at PND 38 that very much resembled patterns obtained in normally raised animals at PND 14 (Katz and Callaway 1992), although intracellular injections showed that individual "deprived" axon arbors resembled normal arbors of similar age, displaying both clustered and elaborate distal branches. Thus neurons are likely to restructure their axonal arbors but to connect to a larger than normal range of orientation columns.

Taken together, the development of patchy long-range intracortical connections is characterized by an early period of crude cluster formation that is activity- but not experience-dependent and a later period that is experience dependent and causes cluster refinement.

What are the mechanisms underlying this experience-dependent stabilization of intracortical connections? According to Hebb's postulate (1949) for associative learning and its modern extension by Stent (1973) and Changeux and Danchin (1976), synaptic contacts between synchronously active pre- and postsynaptic neurons are selectively strength-ened, whereas synaptic contacts between asynchronously active pre- and postsynaptic neurons will be weakened. Correlation-based mechanisms inspired by Hebb's original ideas about the modification of synapses have been implicated in a variety of systems, including the development of ocular dominance columns in the visual cortex (Hubel and Wiesel 1965) and in the development of the retinotectal projection in goldfish and frogs (Constantine-Paton, Cline, and Debski 1990).

Direct evidence for the hypothesis that long-range horizontal connections are also stabilized selectively between cells exhibiting correlated activity was obtained in strabismic cats. In these animals, the optical axes of the two eyes are not aligned, and the images on the two retinas cannot be brought into register. As a result, the responses mediated by anatomically corresponding retinal loci in the two eyes are not correlated. During a critical period of postnatal development, the connections between the afferents from the two eyes and their common cortical target cells are malleable and become destabilized if their activity is not sufficiently correlated (Singer 1990; Wiesel 1982; Swindale 1981; Miller, Keller, and Stryker 1989). As a consequence, strabismus, also called "squint," accentuates the segregation of the geniculocortical afferents from the two eyes in layer IV (Shatz, Lindström, and Wiesel 1977; Löwel 1994), and most of the cells in the visual cortex become responsive exclusively to stimulation of either the left or the right eye (Hubel and Wiesel 1965). Although each of these monocularly driven cell populations is capable of subserving normal pattern vision, strabismics are unable to combine information coming from the two eyes into a single percept; to avoid double vision, they use only one eye at a time and suppress the signals from the other eye (Duke-Elder and Wybar 1973; von Noorden 1990). Thus, the coherence of responses to visual patterns is likely to be the same in strabismics as in normal animals for cells driven from the same eye, but much lower for cells driven from different eyes. Anatomical experiments in the primary visual cortex of divergently squinting cats (cats with a divergent squint angle use alternating fixation to avoid double vision) revealed that cell clusters were driven almost exclusively from either the right or the left eye and that tangential intracortical fibers preferentially connected cell groups activated by the same eye (Löwel and Singer 1992). After injections of retrograde tracers into the primary visual cortex, retrogradely labeled neurons were distributed in well-segregated clusters up to 5 mm from the injection site. The locations of cell groups preferentially activated by either the right or the left eye (the so-called ocular dominance columns; Hubel and Wiesel 1962) were visualized using the radioactive tracer [^{14}C]2-deoxy-glucose (2-DG; Sokoloff et al. 1977): after monocular visual stimulation, regions of increased neuronal activity take up more of the radioactively labeled glucose analog than less active regions. Because they accumulate the radioligand, they can be visualized autoradiographically: regions of increased neuronal activity and thus of increased radioactivity show up as darker on X-ray films exposed to brain sections. Comparing the patterns of retrogradely labeled neurons to those of ocular dominance columns labeled with 2-DG revealed that cell clusters were located preferentially within the same ocular dominance territories as the injection site (figure 1.6). Analyses of normally sighted control animals provided no evidence for an eye-specific selectivity of tangential connections. This agreed with other evidence that in normally sighted cats, tangential connections are related to orientation but not to ocular dominance columns (Gilbert and Wiesel 1989; Schmidt, Kim, et al. 1997). These results suggested that the development of long-range intracortical connections depended on experience-dependent selection mechanisms similar to those in the development of thalamocortical connections (see, for example, Wiesel 1982): neurons "wire together if they fire together."

In summary, these anatomical results are all compatible with the idea of a selective stabilization of tangential fibers between coactive groups of neurons. They support the hypothesis that the strength of intrinsic connections in the primary visual cortex reflects the frequency of previous correlated activation. The experimental evidence appears convincing for the "ocular dominance selectivity" of the tangential fibers: these fibers tend to connect cell groups activated by the same eye in strabismic but not in normally sighted cats. The role of visual experience in fine-tuning the "orientation selectivity" and the "axial selectivity" of the tangential fibers is less clear. Experiments in strabismic cats indicate that strabismus does not interfere with the tendency of long-range horizontal fibers to link predominantly neurons of similar orientation preference (Schmidt, Kim, et al. 1997).

Recently, modular and axial selectivity of tangential fibers was reported in the visual cortex of very young tree shrews as early as one to three weeks after eye opening (Crowley et al. 1996). It thus seems that either a small amount of visual experience is already sufficient or that visual experience is not needed at all for establishing the modular and axial specificity of horizontal connections as seen in adult animals, although further experiments are needed to clarify this issue.

1.5 Development and Plasticity of Callosal Connections

In the visual system, the left visual hemifield is represented in the right visual cortex and the right visual hemifield is represented in the left visual cortex. Nevertheless, everyday experience tells us that we do

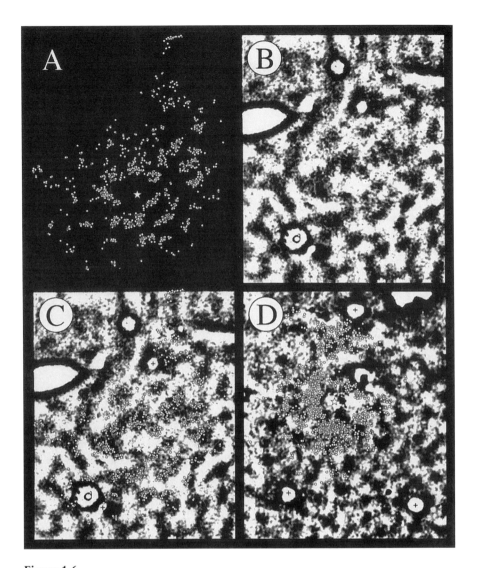

Figure 1.6

Experience-dependent selection of long-range intracortical connections. Topographic relations between ocular dominance columns and intrinsic connections in the primary visual cortex of strabismic (panels A–C) and normally raised cats (panel D). (*A*) Distribution of retrogradely labeled cells after an injection with fluorescent latex microspheres. White dots indicate the position of individual cells; a star, that of injection site. (*B*) 2-deoxyglucose pattern showing the topography of ocular dominance territories in the region containing the retrogradely labeled cells in panel A. The black regions represent the domains of the right eye. (*C*) Superposition of panels A and B. Most of the retrogradely labeled cells are located within zones of high 2-DG uptake (black regions). The injection site was located in a right eye domain as verified by the location of retrogradely labeled cells in the lateral geniculate nucleus. (*D*) Superposition of ocular dominance domains (black regions) and retrogradely labeled neurons (white dots) in normally raised cats. Note the absence of a systematic topographic relationship between the two patterns. (Modified from Löwel and Singer 1992.)

not see a break at the connection between left and right visual hemifield, the vertical meridian. How is this achieved? The two hemispheres of the brain are connected by large axon bundles, one of which is the corpus callosum. It is by far the largest fiber tract in the brain and consists almost exclusively of axons linking cortical neurons. The main function of the callosal fibers is to ensure that the two hemifields are combined into a single percept of the outside world without a noticeable break at the vertical meridian.

Callosal fibers share a number of features with long-range intracortical connections. They originate from and terminate on similar classes of cells, are reciprocal, and exhibit topological specificity (for a review, see Innocenti 1986). In the adult, callosally projecting neurons are restricted to a strip (a few millimeters wide) at the cortical representation of the vertical meridian (the border between areas 17 and 18). Neurons located close to the representation of the vertical meridian have receptive fields that cross the midline of the visual field, and the responses to stimuli in the ipsilateral hemifield are conveyed by callosal input. The ipsilateral and contralateral halves of the crossing receptive fields have the same orientation and direction preference (Berlucchi and Rizzolatti 1968; Lepore and Guillemot 1982; Blakemore et al. 1983), suggesting that the orientation preference of the callosal afferents is matched with that of their respective target cells. Callosally projecting neurons in sensory, motor, and association areas of many species exhibit a columnar distribution (Innocenti 1986), and the axon arbors of callosal neurons are patchy (Houzel, Milleret, and Innocenti 1994).

In young kittens, callosally projecting neurons are not confined to the representation of the vertical meridian but distribute across the entire area 17 (Innocenti, Fiore, and Caminiti 1977; Innocenti and Caminiti 1980). Thus callosal axons in cats are ini-

tially imprecise and exuberant and attain their adult specificity by elimination of ectopic axon terminals (Innocenti and Caminiti 1980). As with horizontal fibers, visual callosal connections can be modified by manipulating early visual experience: early strabismus, monocular deprivation, and short periods of binocular deprivation interfere with the developmental process that eventually confines the callosal projection zone to the vertical meridian, so that callosally projecting neurons come to occupy a broader strip along the border between areas 17 and 18 (Innocenti and Frost 1979; Berman and Payne 1983; Elberger, Smith, and White 1983; Lund, Mitchell, and Henry 1978; Cynader, Lepore, and Guillemot 1981). Thus both tangential intrinsic fibers and callosal connections exhibit a high degree of selectivity in the adult, and both projections are susceptible to experience-dependent modifications. Studying callosal fibers in the primary visual cortex of strabismic cats, it was shown that the selection mechanisms for stabilizing callosal connections are similar to those responsible for specifying the tangential intracortical connections: comparing the pattern of retrogradely labeled neurons to that of domains sharing the same ocular dominance and orientation preference labeled by the radioactive 2-DG technique revealed that 60% of the transcallosally labeled neurons were located in the monocular orientation domains labeled with 2-DG (Schmidt, Kim, et al. 1997). Callosal fibers thus interconnect neurons exhibiting the same ocular dominance and orientation preference, with similar selectivity as the intrinsic fibers, so that both fiber systems seem to be equally susceptible to the effects of strabismus. The development of the interhemispheric pathway and that of long-range intracortical connections are therefore likely to be governed by similar experience-dependent organizing principles; neurons exhibiting decorrelated activation patterns lose their corticocortical connections (Schmidt, Kim, et al. 1997). This observation agrees with previous suggestions that interhemispheric and intrahemispheric connections serve similar functions and should therefore be organized similarly (Hubel and Wiesel 1967; Innocenti 1986).

1.6   Plasticity of Long-Range Intracortical Connections in the Adult

Until recently, it was widely assumed that the "wiring" of the mature cortex is stable. Plasticity in the adult cerebral cortex was thus largely ignored as a scientific topic, in contrast to the "rewiring" of neuronal circuitry in developing systems or phenomena such as long-term potentiation (LTP) and long-term depression (LTD) in the cortex, hippocampus and cerebellum (see Eysel, chapter 3.6.1, and Sterr et al., chapter 7.1, this volume). This has changed dramatically since the pioneering experiments of Michael Merzenich, Jon Kaas, and their colleagues, who demonstrated that receptive fields in the adult somatosensory system can change both their size and arrangement within sensory maps in response to peripheral lesions (for a review, see Buonomano and Merzenich 1998a; Dinse and Merzenich, chapter 2, and Sterr et al., chapter 7, this volume). In the somatosensory system, the body surface is mapped topographically onto the primary somatic sensory cortex, much as in the visual system, where the visual field is represented in the primary visual cortex. In a series of experiments Merzenich and colleagues examined the cortical representations of the hand in owl monkeys before and after amputation of a digit (Merzenich et al. 1984). Two to eight months after this peripheral manipulation, the body map in the somatosensory cortex was changed substantially such that neurons within the cortical area originally occupied by the missing finger (cortex that

before the lesion responded only to the skin surfaces on the digit to be amputated) now responded to stimulation of the adjacent, intact fingers (Merzenich et al. 1983a,b, 1984). Thus the cortical representation of the intact fingers changed and expanded in size at the expense of the amputated digit's representation. Although this expansion was significant, representational changes remained relatively local and applied only to the representation of intact, immediately adjacent digits.

Further experiments demonstrated that representational plasticity in the somatosensory cortex did not necessarily require amputation. When adult owl monkeys were trained to use a particular digit for a behavioral task that was repeated several thousand times, the cortical representation of that digit expanded at the cost of the other, less often used digits (Jenkins et al. 1990). Thus practice alone was sufficient to enlarge the region of cortex containing neurons that were activated during the repetitive behavioral task.

In the following years, a large body of evidence accumulated indicating that in adult cortex of all sensory modalities and in the motor system, neuronal response properties and the functional architecture can display experience-dependent changes in the fine-grain representation of the sensory surface (for a review, see Dinse and Merzenich, chapter 2, and Eysel, chapter 3, this volume). In the visual system, map reorganization was demonstrated with retinal lesions in the primary visual cortex of both cats and monkeys. Because most visual cortical neurons have binocular receptive fields, it was necessary to lesion both retinas to effectively deprive the visual cortex of all its normal input. Immediately after the lesion, the cortical region receiving input from the lesioned part of the retina was silenced, although it recovered over the next few months. Within days or weeks, cells in the initially silent cortical region (the cortical "scotoma") began to fire action potentials when retinal loci outside the lesion were stimulated. Thus receptive fields of cells in the cortical scotoma shifted from representing the lesioned part of the retina to retinal zones surrounding the lesion. As in the somatosensory system, the representation of the lesioned area decreased, whereas the representation of the areas around the lesion increased (Kaas et al. 1990; Chino et al. 1992; Gilbert and Wiesel 1992; Heinen and Skavenski 1991, see also Schmid et al. 1996; for reviews, see Kaas 1991; Buonomano and Merzenich 1998a; Gilbert 1998). In a related experiment, monkeys were fitted with prisms that reversed the visual field. After a few months, neurons in the primary visual cortex developed novel receptive fields in the ipsilateral hemifield that normally only activates neurons in the contralateral cortex (Sugita 1996). These results indicated that (1) visual cortical neurons can acquire new inputs not only from neighboring retinal areas but also from distant areas; and that (2) changes in the visual input—not necessarily lesions—are sufficient to induce changes in the visual field map.

1.6.1   Underlying Mechanism and Substrate

One of the major questions raised by these investigations was where in the nervous system the cortically recorded changes actually take place. Although it is now clear that virtually every level of the nervous system is able to exhibit plasticity under certain circumstances, visual system experiments indicated that in many cases the primary site of change is located in the cortex itself. In principle, both retina and the lateral geniculate nucleus could be sites of plasticity. If this were the case, one would expect that the silent zones in these structures would shrink in parallel with the observed cortical changes (see chapter 11.7 this volume). This was not the case,

however: areas of the lateral geniculate nucleus corresponding to the cortical scotoma remained silent two months after lesioning (Gilbert and Wiesel 1992). In addition, conditioning experiments in the cortex produced clear evidence that plastic changes can occur in adult cerebral cortex (Greuel, Luhmann, and Singer 1988; Frégnac et al. 1992; Cruikshank and Weinberger 1996b). Because cortical reorganization was observed to extend over more than 10 mm laterally (Pons et al. 1991), the long-range horizontal connections were considered the most likely candidates to mediate these changes. In the visual system, the spread of thalamocortical afferents is roughly 2 mm and thus much smaller than the extent of the observed plastic changes in the cortex. In a series of experiments aimed at elucidating the respective roles of cortical versus subcortical sites for cortical reorganization, electrophysiological recordings were performed at various stages along the visual pathway. Even after cortical reorganization was completed, a large and silent region approximating the size of the normal representation of the lesioned retinal area remained in the lateral geniculate nucleus, indicating that most of the reorganization must be intrinsic to the cortex (Gilbert and Wiesel 1992; Darian-Smith and Gilbert 1995). Anatomical analysis in these animals demonstrated that the thalamocortical afferents did not sprout into the cortical scotoma, so that their physical extension (1.5–2.0 mm laterally in cortex) was insufficient to account for the observed cortical reorganization. In contrast, long-range horizontal connections displayed sprouting. Using extracellular injections of the anterograde tracer biocytin into cortex just outside the boundary of the original cortical scotoma, Darian-Smith and Gilbert (1994, 1995) compared the density of lateral projections into reorganized visual cortex to that of lateral projections into normal (nondeprived) visual cortex and found that axon collaterals from cortical neurons surrounding the visual cortical scotoma predominantly branched into the deprived as opposed to the normal cortical area: axon fibers were always denser within reorganized than within normal cortex, with fiber densities 57–88% greater in reorganized than in normal cortex. Because morphological changes consisted in an enrichment of fiber clusters (both axon collaterals and synaptic boutons were added) rather than an extension of fibers beyond the normal level (Darian-Smith and Gilbert 1994), reorganization was most probably mediated by modifications in the preexisting framework of long-range intracortical connections. Similarly, in the motor cortex, functional reorganization was mediated and constrained by the anatomical framework of preexisting, horizontal projections (Huntley 1997). On the other hand, a recent study (Florence, Taub, and Kaas 1998) indicated that sprouting in the somatosensory system may also occur beyond the framework of preexisting connections: analysis of the distributions of thalamic and cortical connections in macaque monkeys with long-standing accidental trauma to a forelimb revealed that thalamocortical projections were relatively normal, whereas connections in the somatosensory cortex (areas 3b and 1) were markedly more widespread in lesioned than in normal animals.

The receptive field shift of neurons in the original cortical scotoma indicates that the role of horizontal long-range connections changes from modulating a neuron's response (subthreshold) to driving it (suprathreshold). Normally, visual cortical neurons respond best to stimulation of a small portion of the visual field (their "classical" receptive field), but nevertheless receive synaptic connections from outside their classical receptive field. When the principal afferent input to a visual or somatosensory cortical neuron is removed (as in the case of retinal lesion or digit amputation experiments), subthreshold inputs are thought to become unmasked, to be strengthened with time, and eventually to become the neuron's major excitatory drive. Taken together, the consensus from many studies is that activity-dependent representational plasticity arises from a combination of unmasking of widespread, normally subthreshold connectivity and the formation of new functional connections through axonal sprouting. Strengthening the effectiveness of existing connections may involve, on a timescale of minutes to hours, use-dependent facilitation of the effectiveness of preexisting synaptic connections, whereby the modifications may be initiated by phenomena such as LTP and LTD (Singer 1995; see also Eysel, chapter 3, this volume). Over longer time periods (weeks to months), cortical reorganization involves the formation of new synapses and the sprouting of additional axon collaterals and thus the establishment of entirely new connections.

Unexpected just a few years ago, adult plasticity thus displays properties previously thought to be restricted to so-called critical periods early in development. Contrary to long-standing belief, cortical representations in adult animals are thus highly dynamic entities, continuously modified by experience and adjusted to current environmental demands: whenever a particular peripheral input is used proportionally more than other inputs, more cortical area seems to be allocated to the representation of that input. A prime example of these plastic changes is a recent fMRI study (Karni et al. 1995) in the human primary motor cortex showing a more extensive representation of a practiced versus unpracticed sequence of finger movements after several weeks of daily training sessions. Persisting for several months, these changes suggest that a long-term experience-dependent reorganization of the adult motor cortex may underlie the acquisition and retention of a new motor skill.

Adaptation of Inputs in the Somatosensory System

2

Hubert R. Dinse and Michael M. Merzenich

Abstract

This chapter summarizes evidence that cortical maps and cortical response properties are in a permanent state of use-dependent fluctuations, where "use" includes training- and learning-induced changes. In their simplest form, use-dependent changes are input driven. Although attention and other high-level processes may contribute and enhance use-dependent neural changes by specific pathways conveying top-down information, reorganization can occur in the absence of high-level processes. The current experimental data imply that altered performance is based on altered forms of neural representations, and that all forms of perceptual learning can therefore be assumed to operate within the framework of cortical adaptivity.

2.1   Introductory Remarks

2.1.1   Two Forms of Plasticity

Postontogenetic plasticity describes the capacity of adult brains to adapt to internal or environmental changes. It is useful to distinguish between two different forms of adult plasticity:

1. Lesion-induced plasticity, which subsumes cortical reorganization after injury or lesion, induced either centrally or at the periphery, refers to compensation for and repair of functions acquired before the injury or lesion.

2. Training- and learning-induced plasticity, often called "use-dependent plasticity," refers to plastic changes that parallel the acquisition of perceptual and motor skills.

Because, for example, amputation changes the pattern of use entirely, a more accurate distinction would be between "lesion-induced" and "non-lesion-induced" plasticity. To what extent the two forms are based on different or perhaps even on similar mechanisms is a matter of ongoing debate.

In contrast to developmental plasticity, adaptations of adult brains do not rely on maturation or growth. For learning-induced alterations, there is agreement on the crucial role played by so-called functional plasticity based on rapid and reversible modifications of synaptic efficacy, although large-scale amputations have been shown to involve sprouting and outgrowth of afferent connections into neighboring regions at cortical and subcortical levels (Florence, Taub, and Kaas 1998; Jain et al. 2000).

2.1.2   Sites of Changes

Perceptual learning is often highly specific to stimulus parameters such as the location or orientation of a stimulus, with little generalization of what is learned to other locations or to other stimulus configurations (see chapters 9, 11, 12, 14). Selectivity and locality of this type implies that the underlying neural changes are most probably occurring within early cortical representations that contain well-ordered topographic maps to allow for this selectivity (see chapter 1). In addition, a transfer of the newly acquired abilities is often considered an important marker of the processing level at which changes are most likely occur: limited generalization is taken as evidence for high locality of effects in early representations. In contrast, transfer of learned abilities is taken as evidence for the involvement of higher processing levels often observed in task and strategy learning (see chapters 13, 14). There is increasing evidence that changes in early cortical areas might be more directly linked to perceptual learning than previously thought (Karni and Sagi 1991; Recanzone, Jenkins, et al. 1992; Schoups, Vogels, and Orban 1995; Crist et al. 1997; Fahle 1997, chapter 10).

In fact, most of what we know today about adaptation of the somatosensory system comes from the investigation of the somatosensory areas characterized by extended and ordered neural representations of the body surface (box 2.1). In contrast, less is known about both the role of higher areas and the interaction between sensory association areas for perceptual learning. In any case, the conjecture that perceptual learning affects early areas provides an important conceptual link to somatosensory adaptational processes (see chapters 9–14).

2.1.3   Driving Forces That Lead to Adaptational Changes

What factors might induce changes in neural representations? Let us assume a dynamically maintained steady state of representations emerging from learning during development and adulthood that reflects the adaptation history to a "mean environment," defined as the accumulated and idiosyncratic experience of an individual. Adaptational processes are assumed to operate on these representations, and long-lasting changes are likely to occur when sensory input patterns are altered such that they deviate from the mean environment. The average steady state can be altered in three principal ways:

1. By changing the input statistics. Specifically effective in driving adaptational changes are simultaneity, repetition, and, more generally, spatiotemporal proximity (see chapters 14, 20). Because these changes in input do not involve attention or processing for meaning, they induce a class of noncognitive adaptations based largely on bottom-up processing.

2. By drawing attention to certain aspects of a stimulus, thereby selecting it in comparison to others. The relevance of a stimulus can also change, depending on context, history, and behavioral task, thereby modifying how physically defined attributes are processed. There is general agreement that modification of early sensory processing by attention and stimulus relevance reflects top-down influences arising from cognitive processes (see chapters 13, 14, 20).

3. By using reward or punishment to reinforce learning. Such influences usually accelerate adaptational processes and are assumed to be mediated by specific brain regions modifying early sensory processing (see chapter 20).

2.1.4   The Hebbian Metaphor

A central paradigm in the description and analysis of cortical plasticity is built around the Hebbian concept (1949): episodes of high temporal correlation between pre- and postsynaptic activity are prerequisite for inducing changes in synaptic efficacy. Historically, the idea that cooperative processes are crucially involved in generating long-lasting changes in excitability can be traced back to the nineteenth century (James 1890).

Indeed, since Hebb, the aspect of simultaneity has become a metaphor in neural plasticity, although the exact role of Hebbian mechanisms in use-dependent plasticity remains controversial (Carew et al. 1984; Fox and Daw 1993; Granger et al. 1994; Montague and Sejnowski 1994; Joublin et al. 1996; Buonomano and Merzenich 1996; Edeline 1996; Cruikshank and Weinberger 1996a,b; Ahissar et al. 1998). It has been suggested that the definition of Hebbian mechanisms

Box 2.1

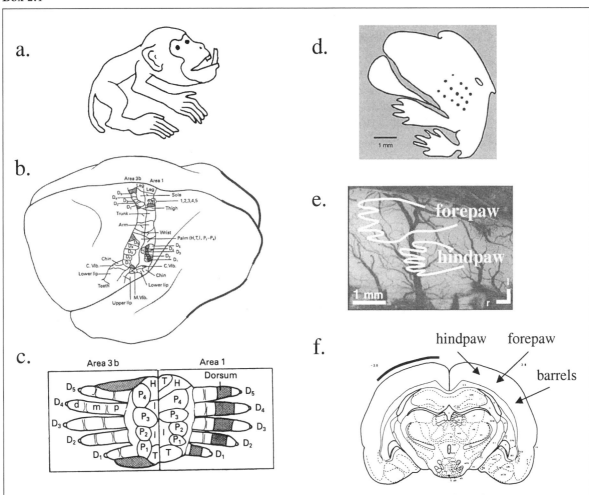

Higher mammals contain complete and ordered topographic maps of the skin of the body surface giving rise to a "homunculus." Adjacent locations on the skin are represented at adjacent locations in the cortex. Exceptions such as face-hand border arise from the problem of mapping a three-dimensional object onto a two-dimensional surface. (*a, d*) Examples of "homunculi" for monkey and rat. Monkeys are characterized by "multiple" representations. (*b*) Mirror-like arranged body surface representations of areas 3b and 1 in an owl monkey. (*c*) Detailed map of the hand representation often used for assessment of adaptational changes. In rats, most of our knowledge about the body representation is from primary somatosensory cortex that is mapped along the dorsolateral aspect of the cortex. (*f*) Locations of hind paw, forepaw, and barrel system. (*e*) Video image of the dorsal surface of the brain, as indicated by the thick dark line in panel *f*, with the locations of the hind and forepaws marked in white. (Panels *a–c* reprinted with permission from Kandel et al. © [1992] McGraw-Hill Companies; *f* reprinted with permission from Pellegrino et al. [1986]).

must be extended beyond simultaneity in the sense of strict coincidence to cover all facets arising from learning processes. Such a definition must include a large number of pre- and postsynaptic patterns as well as a broad time window of what neural systems regard as "simultaneous."

2.1.5   Use-Dependent Plasticity as a Basis of Perceptual and Motor Skills

One of the striking features of use-dependent plasticity is the correlation of cortical changes with performance. The acquisition of skills has often been used as an index for the buildup of implicit memories. There are a number of crucial properties that distinguish implicit from explicit memory. Implicit memories are acquired automatically and unconsciously. Many repetitions over a long time without higher-level cognitive processes are sufficient to improve perceptual and motor skills. That the repetitions are noncognitive and many represents an important aspect of use-dependent neural plasticity. It has therefore been speculated that use-dependent plasticity might be strongly related to, if not a substrate for, implicit memory function.

2.1.6   Input Statistics versus Attention

As outlined above, attention plays an important role in learning and adaptational processes (Ahissar and Hochstein 1993; Recanzone, Merzenich, et al. 1992; Goldstone 1998; Buchner et al. 1999). It has been suggested that specific high-level attentional mechanisms modify early sensory processing levels (Ahissar and Hochstein 1993), although recent experiments (Ito, Westheimer, and Gilbert 1998) indicate that attentional mechanisms themselves can be changed by practice (see also chapter 14). Similarly, researchers (Sireoteanu and Rettenbach 1995) have shown that

training can transform a serial search to a parallel search task (see chapters 13, 14, 20).

On the other hand, there is little doubt about the significant contributing role of input statistics. Many studies have demonstrated that neural changes and parallel improvement of performance can be evoked by a specific sensory input pattern without involving attentional mechanisms, provided the statistics are sufficiently altered (see also section 2.4.2).

2.1.7   Top-Down Modulation of Plasticity

There are many brain centers that play a role in modulating cortical responsiveness. The major source of cholinergic inputs long implicated in learning and memory comes from several groups of neurons within the basal forebrain, which receives inputs from limbic and paralimbic structures. For example, in animal experiments, pairing of sensory stimulation with electrical stimulation of the nucleus basalis has been shown to result in rapid and selective reorganization (Rasmusson and Dykes 1988; Edeline et al. 1994; Bakin and Weinberger 1996; Bjordahl, Dimyan, and Weinberger 1998; Kilgard and Merzenich 1998). On the other hand, lesion of the cholinergic system has been shown to prevent plastic reorganization (Baskerville, Schweitzer, and Herron 1997; Sachdev et al. 1998). Consequently, cholinergic inputs have been assumed to represent one example of a top-down system providing modulatory information of higher-order, presumably cognitive processes (cf. chapters 13, 14 and 20).

2.1.8   Synopsis

The present chapter summarizes recent work on somatosensory adaptations with special emphasis on behavioral and perceptual consequences of use-dependent plasticity as defined above. (For reviews covering all facets of cortical plasticity, see Merzenich et al. 1988; Kaas 1991; Garraghty and Kaas 1992; Sameshima and Merzenich 1993; Donoghue 1995; Weinberger 1995; Cruishank and Weinberger 1996a; Edeline 1996; Merzenich, Wright, et al. 1996; Dinse et al. 1997; Kaas and Florence 1997; Sanes and Donoghue 1997; Buonomano and Merzenich 1998a; Nicolelis, Katz, and Krupa 1998.)

We first survey studies of training and use in a variety of animal models, then discuss recent studies of somatosensory adaptations in humans by researchers using noninvasive imaging technologies. These imaging studies provide compelling evidence for the relevance of adaptational changes to everyday life. Next, we consider approaches that, by varying input probability, explore how "driving factors" induce adaptational changes. We review the increasing evidence for "maladaptive" aspects of neuroplasticity and touch on the role of "subcortical" plasticity. Finally, we critically examine what is changed during adaptations, as this relates to the coding and decoding of sensory information during adaptations needed to alter perceptual and motor performance.

2.2 Role of Training, Differential Use, and Behavior

It is common wisdom that perceptual skills improve with training (see Gibson 1953). Recent studies in "perceptual learning" have focused on problems and questions associated with skill acquisition. One of the most stimulating questions in cortical plasticity is how cortical changes are linked to changes in performance, a question requiring simultaneous assessment of both neurophysiological and behavioral changes.

For example, Recanzone, Jenkins, and coworkers (1992) showed that tactile frequency discrimination training in adult owl monkeys over several months leads to a significant reduction of frequency discrimination threshold. When the cortical areas representing the skin of the trained fingers were mapped, large-scale cortical reorganization became apparent, which included changes in receptive fields and in the topography of cortical representational maps (Recanzone, Merzenich, et al. 1992). After training, sinusoidal stimulation of the trained skin elicited larger-amplitude responses, peak responses earlier in the stimulus cycle, and temporally sharper responses, than did stimulation applied to control skin sites. Analysis of cycle histograms for area 3b neuron responses revealed that the decreased variance of each stimulus cycle could account for behaviorally measured frequency discrimination improvements (Recanzone, Merzenich, and Schreiner 1992). These studies demonstrated for the first time a direct relation between cortical plasticity and improvement of performance (see also figure 2.1), establishing a tight link between neurophysiological experiments and psychophysical tasks and making it possible to correlate precisely defined aspects of use with plastic changes.

A related approach was taken by Xerri et al. (1999), in which monkeys were trained to pick up food pellets from wells of different sizes. Although all monkeys exhibited a gradual improvement in digital dexterity, each monkey developed an individual retrieval strategy. In area 3b, the cortical magnification of the differentially engaged glabrous fingertip surfaces was nearly twofold larger than it was for control digits. Receptive fields of neurons representing the engaged digital surfaces were less than half as large as those representing the corresponding surfaces of control digits. These results confirmed that behaviorally important skin surfaces are represented in a much finer representational grain than normal.

Use-dependent plasticity has been investigated in a more natural context as well, where the link between behavior and cortical reorganization is often

a

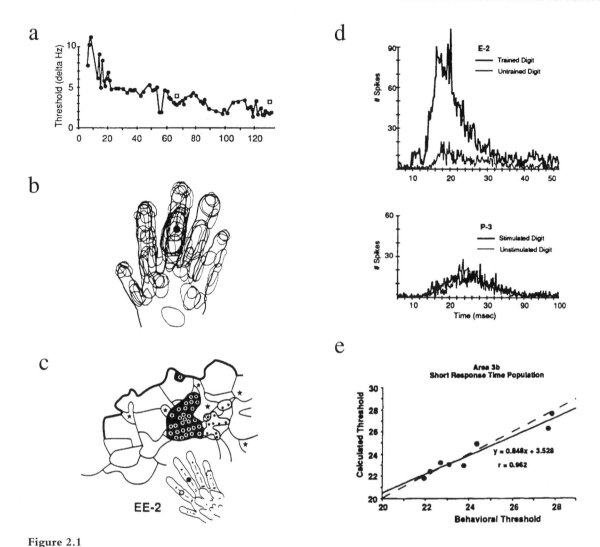

b

c

EE-2

d

e

Figure 2.1
Adult owl monkeys were trained to detect differences in the frequency of a tactile flutter vibration stimulus above a 20 Hz standard. All stimuli were delivered to a constant skin site on a small segment of one finger. (*a*) Changes of psychophysical performance in terms of threshold over successive sessions indicate progressive improvement with training that was highly selective for the trained skin site. (*b*) Representative receptive fields defined in area 3b on the trained hand of the same monkey shown in panel a. Filled circle denotes the area of skin trained in the behavioral task. The size of receptive fields increased in the zone of representation of the trained digit as compared to adjacent digits or the control hand. (*c*) Cortical representational map highlighting all penetrations that included some or all of the trained skin (dark stipple), the homologous skin on the adjacent digit (light stipple) or both skin surfaces (hatched). The inset shows the stimulated skin site (black dot) and its equivalent on the adjacent finger (stippled dot). This analysis revealed that the representation of the stimulated skin was larger than the control skin site. (*d*) To study the temporal response characteristics, neurons were stimulated using

less quantifiable, although still intuitively obvious. In their study of lactating rats, Xerri, Stern, and Merzenich (1994) showed the implications of episodic differential use following normal nursing behavior: the area SI representation of the ventral trunk skin was significantly larger in lactating rats than in matched postpartum nonlactating or virgin controls. The greatest representational change was a twofold increase of the cortical representation of the nipple-bearing skin between the forelimbs and hind limbs.

Housing rodents in an enriched environment has been shown to inhibit spontaneous apoptosis, prevent seizures, and produce general neuroprotective effects (Young et al. 1999). Furthermore, in the hippocampus of even senescent mice, an enriched environment induced neurogenesis (Kempermann, Kuhn, and Gage 1997). The areal extent of the forepaw cutaneous representation was significantly larger in rats housed in enriched environments promoting differential tactile experience (EE rats) for 71–113 days from weaning than in control rats housed under standard conditions (Coq and Xerri 1998). In addition, the receptive fields tended to progress in more orderly fashion across the digit glabrous skin of EE rats than they did in control rats, corroborating the view that cortical cutaneous maps are maintained in a permanent state of use-dependent fluctuation.

In adult rats, a tendon of a hind limb was cut, leading to slight changes in walking behavior. Analysis of receptive fields (RFs) and cortical representational maps of the hind paw revealed an increase of RF size and a shrinkage of the cortical map within a few days. Both behavioral effects and cortical changes were reversible within weeks (Jürgens and Dinse 1997a; Zepka, Jürgens, and Dinse 1996), demonstrating that even modest modification in behavior can lead to rapid and large-scale cortical changes. These findings extend the results of Fox and coworkers (1994), who studied adult rats under space flight conditions after complete prevention from use or hind limb suspension. Both approaches resulted in modified posture and gait, which returned to normal after about two weeks. Behavioral adaptations were paralleled by a reduction in the number of GABA-immunoreactive cells (D'Amelio et al. 1996).

For the human motor system, similar fast adaptational regulations have been reported. Using transcranial magnetic stimulation (TMS) mapping, Licpert, Tegenthoff, and Malin (1995) have shown that, in patients who had unilateral immobilization of the ankle joint without peripheral nerve lesions, the area of motor cortex representing the tibial anterior muscle was significantly smaller for the immobilized than for the unaffected leg. The reduction in area was correlated with the duration of immobilization, an effect rapidly reversed by voluntary muscle contractions.

The framework of modified use as a determinant of cortical organization has been tested in an in-

sinusoidal tactile stimuli in the range of 20 to 26 Hz corresponding to the frequency range tested behaviorally. Upper population cycle histogram (E-2) was constructed from summing neural responses of trained and stimulated digits (heavy line) recorded at all area 3b locations, superimposed with histograms for stimulation of adjacent untrained digits (thin line), in the monkey shown in panels a–c; bin width was 0.1 msec. Note entrained and faster response characteristics for the trained digit, an effect missing for the passively trained monkey shown in lower population cycle histogram (P-3). (e) Regression analysis for the calculated threshold based on the overlap of the second cycle in the cycle histograms as a function of behaviorally threshold, indicating that the training-induced temporal processing characteristics can explain behavioral performance to a considerable degree. (Modified from Recanzone, Jenkins, et al. 1992; Recanzone, Merzenich, et al. 1992; Recanzone, Merzenich, and Schreiner 1992. Reprinted with permission from the American Physiological Society.)

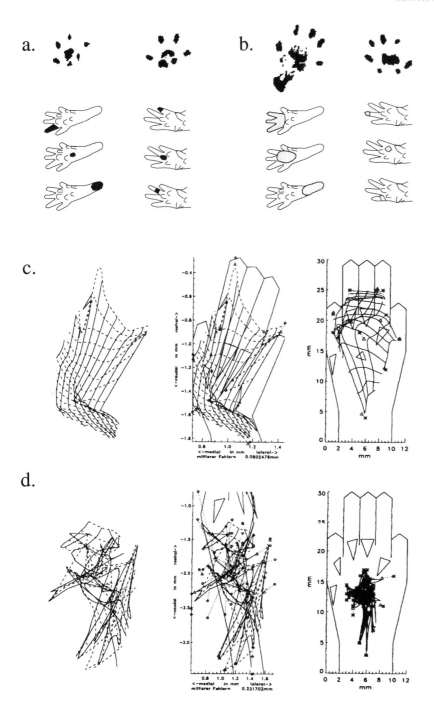

vestigation of age-related modifications of cortical representational maps in old rats, known to show a number of age-related changes. The characteristic impairment of the sensorimotor state is most strikingly expressed in a walking impairment of the hind limbs (Schuurman et al. 1987; Ingram 1988; Stoll et al. 1990). Using electrophysiological recordings, researchers (Jürgens and Dinse 1995; Spengler, Godde, and Dinse 1995) demonstrated that behavioral changes in old rats were paralleled by massive reorganization of the somatosensory cortex (figure 2.2). Age-related changes were characterized by an enlargement of receptive fields of the hind paw representation, an increase of RF overlap and a deterioration of the topography of the cortical maps. It has been suggested (Dinse et al. 1995) that certain aspects of these age-related behavioral changes reflect plastic changes resulting from prolonged disuse of the hind limbs rather than from age-related cortical degeneration. Sensorimotor behavior of the forelimbs remains largely unaffected even in animals of high age.

Accordingly, in the case of neural degeneration, one would expect comparable changes to occur in both the forepaw and the hind paw representation. Indeed, analysis of RFs in the cortical forepaw representation of animals of high age revealed no alterations (Jürgens and Dinse 1997b). The results imply that age-related changes can be regionally very specific, thereby arguing against an unspecific origin for such changes, and that age-related neural changes and specific age-related behavioral alterations are linked.

Interestingly, enriched environment has been shown to prevent age-related decrease in synaptic density in the aged brain (Saito et al. 1994); indeed, when old rats were kept in an enriched environment for several months, no comparable age-related alterations of sensory (Churs et al. 1996) and motor hind paw representations (Reinke and Dinse 1999) were found. These results indicate that the beneficial outcome of an enriched environment, namely, reinforced mobility and agility, occurs even in animals of high age.

Figure 2.2
Specific effects of age on receptive fields of the hind paw recorded in somatosensory cortex of aged rats. (*a, b*) Representative examples of behavioral changes of walking pattern derived from footprint analysis for young, control animal, left hind paw and right forepaw and for old animal, left hind paw and right forepaw, respectively. Note selectivity of walking impairment restricted to hind leg. Examples of receptive fields (RFs) recorded in the hind paw representation (panels a and b, lower left) and in the forepaw representation (panels a and b, lower right) in young and old animal, respectively. Age-related changes are limited to the behaviorally impaired extremity. To visualize the effects of aging on the topography of the underlying cortical maps, we reconstructed somatosensory maps using a computer-based interpolation algorithm based on a linear least square approximation of sampling coordinates of penetration sites and corresponding receptive field centers. (*c, d*) Reconstructions of a cortical hind paw representation are shown for control and for old rat, respectively. Examples of cortical topographies represented as a regular lattice within somatosensory cortex (*left*). Extrapolated cortical representation of a schematic and standardized drawing of the hind paw (*middle*). Dashed lines indicate horizontal, and solid lines the vertical, components of the lattice. One square of the lattice represents 1 mm^2 skin area. Diamonds indicate penetration sites; squares give the interpolated RF centers. Dotted lines give the deviation between them. Backprojection of the regular lattice of the cortical map onto the hind paw (*right*). Squares give the interpolated, and stars the measured, RF centers. One square of the lattice represents the skin portions that is represented by 0.01 mm^2 cortical area. According to these reconstructions, maps of the hind paw representation recorded in old animals, characterized by a selective impairment of the hindlegs show a dramatic distortion of their representational maps and a loss of topographic order. (Modified from Spengler, Godde, and Dinse 1995; Jürgens and Dinse 1997b. Panels *c* and *d* reprinted with permission from Spengler et al. © [1995] Lippincott Williams & Wilkins.)

Taken together, these studies suggest that small alteration in behavior due to special demands imposed in everyday life alters early cortical representations rapidly and reversibly. The summarized studies imply that wearing a cast for some weeks due to a broken limb should be sufficient to alter associated maps of somatosensory and motor cortex (for discussion of perceptual consequences, see section 2.3).

From a more general point of view, the findings on age-related changes in the somatosensory system extend the concept of use-dependent plasticity to high age. There is growing evidence from human studies that sensorimotor processing is more closely related to cognition than previously thought (Grady and Craik 2000). Aging gives rise to an increasingly strong association between sensory and cognitive functioning (Baltes and Lindenberger 1997).

2.3   Relevance of Adaptational Changes from Noninvasive Imaging Studies in Humans

The recent development of noninvasive imaging techniques has made it possible to study the impact of modified use and practice in humans. (For an overview of the modern imaging techniques currently employed in human studies, see, chapter 7, this volume.) Imaging studies have provided overwhelming evidence that extensive use and practice result in substantial changes of associated cortical representations in blind Braille readers (Pascual-Leone and Torres 1993; Sterr et al. 1998a,b), in players of string instruments (Elbert et al. 1995), in other musicians (Pantev et al. 1998), and in subjects given long-term perceptual training in tactile discrimination (Spengler et al. 1997). Of particular interest are findings on cross-modal plasticity in blind subjects (Sadato et al. 1996; Cohen et al. 1997, 1999; Röder, Rösler, and Neville 1999; Röder et al. 1999).

Furthermore, cortical reorganization of the finger representation extending several millimeters was observed in adults studied before and after surgical separation of webbed fingers (syndactyly; Mogilner et al. 1993), a finding reminiscent of what had been reported some years ago for artificial induction of syndactyly in monkeys (Clark et al. 1988).

Taken together, human studies confirm the close relation between intensified use and enlargement of associated cortical representational maps thus supporting the relevance of the concept of cortical plasticity for everyday life.

What are the functional implications of these changes? Although, as discussed above (see section 2.1.5), the observed effects are assumed to be the substrate mediating the altered performance, there is controversy about the specificity of the neural changes that accompany perceptual changes. According to one view, the adaptational changes are highly specific, allowing for improvement of the trained motor or perceptual skill only: neural changes arising during training are assumed to have little effect on information processing beyond that skill. According to an alternative view, neural changes result in a widespread modification of sensory processing overall; changes in perceptual and cognitive skills generalize widely beyond the trained task. In other words, there is controversy over whether a specific improvement is paralleled by other perceptual changes, independent of the trained performance. There is evidence, for example, that many aspects of auditory processing in blind subjects are superior to those in normally sighted subjects (see Hollins 1989; see also Röder, Rösler, and Neville 1999, 2000). Pascual-Leone and Torres (1993) reported increased sensory representation of the reading finger in blind Braille readers, but no change in their spatial two-point discrimination abilities, whereas Axelrod (1959) found evidence of improved discrimination performance in such readers. More studies are needed to resolve this controversy and to clarify how far perceptual changes extend across different forms of specific adaptations and skills (see also section 2.8).

Although extremely beneficial in revealing signatures of cortical plasticity, human studies of the type discussed cannot determine the "driving factors" behind cortical reorganization. The exact nature of inputs in a physical stimulus pattern is difficult, if not impossible, to assess. What is needed, therefore, are complementary studies that investigate cortical reorganization induced by a systematic variation of input pattern.

2.4   Role of Input Statistics

Although many lines of evidence have shown that the somatosensory system adapts to input pattern of different probabilities, whether—without cognitive processes—variation of input statistics alone suffices to reorganize cortical maps is a matter of long-standing debate. Accordingly, studies that directly address the role of input probabilities for adaptational processes are needed to provide insight into principles and constraints governing adaptational processes.

2.4.1   *Intracortical Microstimulation*

A technique to evoke selective motor responses by applying current through microelectrodes inserted into defined regions of motor representations, intracortical microstimulation (ICMS) has more recently been employed to study short-term and reversible plastic changes in motor, somatosensory, auditory, and visual cortex as well as thalamic relay nuclei of the somatosensory system (Nudo, Jenkins, and Merzenich 1990; Dinse, Recanzone, and Merzenich 1990, 1993; Recanzone, Merzenich, and Dinse 1992;

Spengler and Dinse 1994; Sil'kis and Rapoport 1995; Gu and Fortier 1996; Kimura, Melis, and Asanuma 1996; Maldonado and Gerstein 1996a,b; Joublin et al. 1996; Xing and Gerstein 1996; Dinse et al. 1997). ICMS allows researchers to investigate the properties of functional plasticity locally—independently of the peripheral and subcortical pathways and independently of the constraints provided by particularities of a sensory pathway and its preprocessing. In a typical ICMS experiment, repetitive electrical pulse trains of very low currents (usually less than 10 µA) are delivered via a microelectrode. Based on theoretical calculations, ICMS of that intensity was assumed to activate a cortical volume of only 50 microns in diameter (Stoney, Thompson, and Asanuma 1968) supporting the locality of the changes. Synchronized discharges are generated, which are assumed to play a crucial role in mediating plastic changes. The short timescale and reversibility of ICMS effects supported the hypothesis that modulations of synaptic efficiency in neuronal networks occur very rapidly without necessarily involving anatomical changes.

In the rat motor cortex, border shifts in movement representations exceeding 500 microns were observed after a few hours of ICMS (Nudo, Jenkins, and Merzenich 1990). Application of ICMS in the hind paw representation of the adult rat somatosensory cortex caused an overall but selective expansion of receptive field size (Recanzone, Merzenich, and Dinse 1992; Dinse, Recanzone, and Merzenich 1993; Spengler and Dinse 1994). Receptive fields close to that of the stimulation site were enlarged, and comprised large skin territories always including the RF at the ICMS site, revealing a distance-dependent, directed enlargement toward the ICMS receptive field. Early ICMS-related reorganization could already be detected after 15 minutes of ICMS, and much greater effects emerged after 2 to 3 hours. Changes were reversible within 6 to 8 hours after termination of ICMS (Dinse, Recanzone, and Merzenich 1993; Spengler and Dinse 1994).

Neural groups and assemblies are thought to be subject to modification during reorganizational processes. Using ICMS, researchers can directly address the question of dynamic changes of neural assembly membership (cf. 2.7). ICMS resulted in a significant enhancement of correlated, synchronized neural activity that paralleled changes of cortical RFs and cortical maps (Dinse, Recanzone, and Merzenich 1990, 1993). Similar results have been obtained for plastic changes in auditory cortex (Maldonado and Gerstein, 1996a,b). Where cortical neurons exhibited highly synchronous oscillatory firing patterns that were enhanced by ICMS, depending on the anatomical distance between the two neurons: ICMS changed the strength and the local number of such correlations. Overall, the results obtained with intracortical microstimulation demonstrated the capacity for cortical plasticity in the absence of peripheral stimulation.

2.4.2 Coactivation Studies

To study the effects of input statistics systematically, a number of protocols have been introduced in which the neural activity needed to drive plastic changes was generated by simultaneous, associative pairing (Diamond, Armstrong-Jones, and Ebner 1993; Wang et al. 1995; Godde, Spengler, and Dinse 1996; Godde et al. 2000). In a pioneering study by Frégnac et al. (1988), functional persistent changes in response properties of single neurons of cat visual cortex were induced by a differential pairing procedure, during which iontophoresis was used to artificially increase the visual response for a given stimulus and decrease the response for a second stimulus. In contrast, the protocols described below used a pairing of adequate (tactile) stimuli.

In Diamond, Armstrong-Jones, and Ebner 1993, sensory experience was altered by a few days of "whisker pairing": whiskers D2 and either D1 or D3 were left intact, whereas all other whiskers were trimmed. Reorganizational changes were assessed in terms of response amplitude evoked by single neurons recorded in the corresponding barrel field representations of somatosensory cortex. During the period of whisker pairing, the RFs of cells in barrel D2 changed in distinct ways: the response to the center RF, whisker D2, increased. The response to the paired surround RF whisker nearly doubled, and the response to all trimmed, unpaired surround RF whiskers decreased. After whisker pairing, the response to the paired neighbor of D2 was more than twice as large as the response to the trimmed neighbor of D2. These findings indicate that a brief change in the pattern of sensory activity induced by pairing of tactile stimuli can alter the configuration of cortical RFs of adult animals.

To test the hypothesis that consistently noncoincident inputs may be actively segregated from one another in their distributed cortical representations, monkeys were trained to respond to specific stimulus sequence events (Wang et al. 1995). Animals received temporally coincident inputs across fingertips and fingerbases, but distal versus proximal digit segments were noncoincidentally stimulated. Electrophysiological mapping experiments in area 3b showed that synchronously applied stimuli resulted in integration of inputs in the cortical maps, whereas stimuli applied asynchronously were segregated. In contrast to those in normal control animals, cortical maps in trained animals were characterized by two bandlike zones in which all neurons had multiple digit RFs representing the stimulated skin surfaces. These two zones were separated by a region containing normal single-digit RFs. This segregation was further augmented by a band of units responding

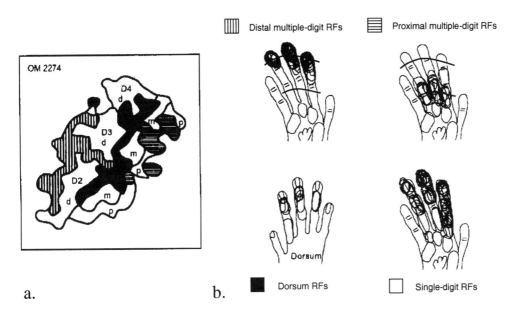

Figure 2.3
Typical reorganized cortical map of a hand in area 3b and receptive fields derived in an owl monkey engaged in a behavioral training to discriminate tactile stimulus sequences delivered to the hand by two narrow bars. One bar stimulated a narrow line of skin across the distal segments of the digits 2, 3, and 4; the second bar excited a narrow line of skin crossing the proximal segments of the same three digits (thin lines in panel b). The training resulted in temporally coincident inputs across fingertips and finger bases, whereas the distal versus proximal digit segments were noncoincidentally stimulated. (*a*) The reorganized map shows that in contrast to normal maps, a significant portion of the map exhibited multiple receptive fields that were specific to either the proximal (horizontal striping) or distal (vertical striping) portions of the digit. Interestingly, both regions representing the trained skin surfaces became segregated by a band of single-digit receptive fields (white) and a band of receptive fields located on the dorsum of the hand (black). (*b*) The corresponding receptive fields are sorted according to the four classes observed: distal multiple-digit, proximal multiple-digit, dorsum, and single-digit receptive fields. (Modified from Wang et al. 1995; Buonomano and Merzenich 1998a. Reprinted with permission from the *Annual Review of Neuroscience*, vol. 21 © 1998 by Annual Reviews www.AnnualReviews.org. Physiological Society. Reprinted by permission from *Nature* © 1995 Macmillan Magazines Ltd.)

to dorsal skin inputs, both features are normally not present in area 3b finger representations (figure 2.3). Interestingly, maps derived in the ventroposterior portion of the thalamus (VPL) were not equivalently reorganized suggesting that this particular type of representational plasticity appears to be cortical in origin.

In Godde, Spengler, and Dinse 1996, non- or only partially overlapping receptive fields on the hind paw of adult rats were used for coactivation in order to study effects of simultaneous stimulation. The authors reported reversible reorganization, namely, selective enlargement of the cortical territory and of the receptive fields representing the stimulated skin fields, as well as emergence of a large representation that included a joint representation of both sites (figure 2.4). A control protocol of identical stimulus patterns applied to only a single skin site evoked no changes,

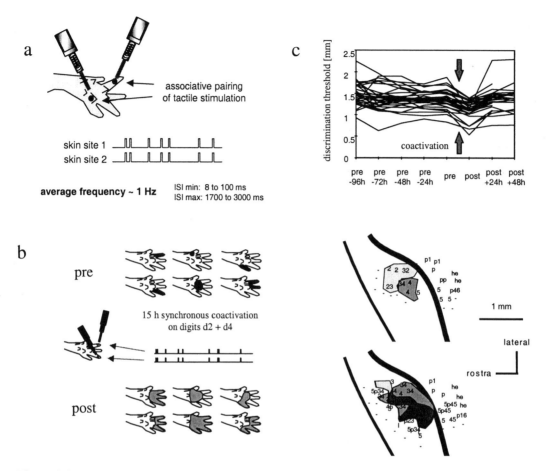

Figure 2.4

Scheme of the tactile coactivation protocol as utilized by Godde et al. (1996, 2000). (*a*) Two locations on the skin were simultaneously stimulated for several hours with computer-controlled tactile stimulators. Example of the time course of stimulation is shown. Average frequency is about 1 Hz. (*b*) Changes of receptive fields (RFs) as compared to control condition (*top left*) after coactivation (*bottom left*) performed on d2 and d4 are characterized by a dramatic enlargement of RF size. Note that, after coactivation, digit RFs cover always all of the skin surface of the coactivated digits d2 and d4. Cortical maps derived before (*top right*) and after (*bottom right*) coactivation on d2 and d4. Black lines indicate blood vessels, penetration sites are marked. Numbers indicate digits 1 to 5, p, pads; he, heels. Bars indicate locations where cells could not be driven by low threshold cutaneous inputs. Cortical territories representing d2 or d4 are denoted by different grays. Dark gray indicates zone of overlap between both representations, that is, a common representation of d2 and d4. After coactivation, cortical territory representing the coactivated skin sites increased significantly; new skin representations containing the stimulated skin fields emerged up to 400 microns beyond the control boundaries, whereas recording sites that were more rostral maintained their unresponsiveness. Note also the emergence of a large common representation of both skin sites not present under control conditions. (*c*) Tactile two-point discrimination thresholds of the index finger of the right hand as measured in a two-alternative forced-choice discrimination experiment in thirty-five right-handed human subjects. Thresh-

indicating that coactivation was essential for induction. The selective and local changes within the cortical map imply that early sensory cortical processing was affected: only those areas undergoing a specific alteration in input reorganized.

To demonstrate the perceptual relevance of neural changes induced by the coactivation protocol, Godde et al. (2000) investigated spatial discrimination performance in human subjects given similar passive costimulation of the tip of the index finger. Using discrimination thresholds to mark reorganizational effects due to variation of input statistics on human perception, they found that two hours of coactivation sufficed to drive a significant improvement of the spatial discrimination performance. These results demonstrated the potential role of pure input statistics in inducing cortical plasticity without involving cognitive factors such as attention or reinforcement (figure 2.4; see also section 2.8). A combined assessment of discrimination thresholds and recording of somatosensory evoked potentials in human subjects revealed that the individual gain of discrimination performance was correlated with the amount of cortical reorganization in primary somatosensory cortex as referred from the shifts of the location of the N20 dipole (Pleger et al. 2001).

The coactivation protocol allows complete control of timing and amount of stimulation. Using asynchronous rather than synchronous stimulation resulted in reorganizations characterized by a large separation of both stimulated skin sites (Zepka, Godde, and Dinse 2000).

Similarly, Liepert, Terborg, and Weiller (1999) reported that about an hour of synchronous movements of the thumb and foot resulted in a reduction of the distance of the center of gravity of their respective output maps in area MI as measured by TMS, whereas asynchronous movements evoked no significant changes, indicating that similar principles of coactivation hold for both the sensory and motor system.

Recanzone, Merzenich, et al. (1992) recorded only modest increases in topographic complexity in cortical hand representations for passively stimulated hands and no effects on RF size or overlap. On the other hand, the coactivation studies discussed above showed a clear effect on both cortical and perceptual levels, even though attention was not involved. In the human discrimination experiments, subjects were instructed not to attend the stimulation; indeed, during the several hours of coactivation all subjects continued their normal business work. Conceivably, the engagement in normal day work had not been possible without the simultaneous attentive engagement in other perceptual and motor tasks. One explanation is that during the coactivation protocol, which was, on average, applied at a rate of 1 Hz for several hours, selected skin regions were stimulated 10,000 times or more, a much higher frequency of stimulation than that given the monkeys during the passive discrimination training. Conceivably, the intensity of the stimulation protocol might be the crucial factor responsible for its effectiveness. As stated in section 2.1.6, adaptational changes and parallel improvement of performance can be evoked by changes in input statistics provided the statistics are sufficiently altered.

Coactivation studies of this type are instrumental in providing insight into the role of timing parameters

olds were measured five days before and immediately after coactivation (arrows) and on two subsequent days. In all subjects, thresholds were reduced immediately after coactivation but returned to control values one day after coactivation, revealing a time course of reversibility similar to that described for the electrophysiological reorganizational changes in rats. Control experiments performed on the index finger of the opposite hand, which received no coactivation, showed no changes. (Modified from Godde, Spengler, and Dinse 1996. Reprinted with permission. © [1996] Lippincott Williams & Wilkins.)

that control reorganization in animals and humans: they allow researchers to experimentally assess the time window that defines simultaneity; to relate neural changes as measured in animals with psychophysical performance as assessed in humans; and thereby to explore the perceptual relevance of simple paradigms that successfully induce adaptational changes at the neuron level.

2.5 Therapeutic Consequences of Somatosensory Adaptations

The final outcome of reorganizational process need not be beneficial. There is increasing evidence that abnormal perceptual experiences such as the phantom limb sensation arise from reorganizational changes induced by the amputation of the limb. A strong relationship has been reported, but not for nonpainful phantom phenomena experienced after arm amputation, implying that these changes are maladaptive rather than adaptive (Flor et al. 1995). By contrast, neuromagnetic source imaging revealed minimal reorganization of primary somatosensory cortex in congenital amputees and in traumatic amputees not suffering from phantom limb pain (Flor et al. 1998). These data indicate that phantom limb pain is related to, and may be a consequence of, plastic changes in primary somatosensory cortex. Interestingly, recent studies reported a decrease of phantom limb pain associated with prosthesis-induced use of the stump (Weiss et al. 1999) and with less related reorganization in the motor cortex (Lotze et al. 1999). The precise topographic mapping of the phantom limb onto the face area was explained in terms of the topography of the border of the face-hand maps (Ramachandran, Stewart, and Rogers-Ramachandran 1992; Halligan et al. 1993; Aglioti et al. 1997).

The power of the early evoked magnetic field elicited by painful stimulation was elevated in pa-

tients with chronic pain relative to that elicited by painful back stimulation in healthy controls. Furthermore, this enlargement showed a linear increase with chronicity of pain (Flor et al. 1997), suggesting that the cortical reorganization that accompanies chronic pain may serve an important function in its persistence.

Repetitive strain injuries including occupationally induced focal dystonia have a high prevalence in workers who perform heavy schedules of rapid alternating movements or repetitive, sustained, coordinated movements. It has been hypothesized that use-dependent plastic changes such as those reviewed above may cause repetitive strain injuries characterized by sensory dysfunction and impairment of motor control (Byl, Merzenich, and Jenkins 1996; Byl et al. 1997). This view is supported by studies showing that monkeys trained in repetitive hand closing and opening developed typical movement control disorders indicated by a 50% drop in motor performance. Electrophysiological mapping within the primary somatosensory cortex revealed a dedifferentiation of cortical representations of the skin of the trained hand, manifested by receptive fields 10 to 20 times larger than normal, as well as by a breakdown of the receptive field topography (Byl, Merzenich, and Jenkins 1996). Thus repetitive, highly stereotypic movements can actively degrade cortical representations of sensory information guiding fine motor hand movements. Using MEG, Elbert et al. (1998) found a smaller distance between the representations of the digits in somatosensory cortex for the affected hand in musicians suffering from focal hand dystonia than for the hands of nonmusician control subjects, indicating that central reorganization develops as a consequence of repetitive strain injuries in humans as well (see also chapter 7).

The maladaptive consequences of cortical plasticity have become increasingly acknowledged as a major factor in various forms of dysfunctions. For example, a negative outcome of neuroplasticity may play a major role in some forms of age-related changes. Jürgens and Dinse (1997b) found that walking impairments that develop in rats of high age as a secondary response to muscle atrophy and to other factors promoting limited agility were the result of maladaptive cortical reorganizations.

2.6 Subcortical Plasticity

Studies of subcortical and brain stem structures have clearly shown that reorganizational changes occur along the entire sensory pathway (Wilson and Snow 1987; Garraghty and Kaas 1991; Nicolelis et al. 1993; Pettit and Schwark 1993; Florence and Kaas 1995; Faggin, Nguyen, and Nicolelis 1997; Jones and Pons 1998; Nicolelis, Lin, and Chapin 1997; Hubscher and Johnson 1999; Xu and Wall 1997, 1999; Woods et al. 2000). On the other hand, cortical changes have been reported in the absence of parallel subcortical changes. Accordingly, there are still many open questions about the role of subcortical substrates. For example, Wang and coworkers (1995) did not find topographic changes in the thalamic relay nucleus comparable to those in area 3b after co-activation, as described in section 2.4.2. Similarly, Tinazzi et al. (1997) could not find parallel subcortical changes after transient deafferentation in humans. Dinse et al. (1997) found that applying microstimulation in the thalamus had little effect on RF size when compared to applying such microstimulation directly in cortex.

Of course, the central question behind these studies is exactly what role cortices play in the overall processes of reorganization (Darian-Smith and Gilbert 1995; Fox 1994; Florence, Taub, and Kaas 1998; Kaas and Ebner 1998; Kaas 1999; Kaas, Florence, and Jain 1999). Much of the plasticity encountered at a subcortical level may depend on feedback connections from the cortex (Ergenzinger et al. 1998; Krupa, Ghazanfar, and Nicolelis 1999). Furthermore, the usually extensive cortical reorganizations may in part depend on activation of the widespread horizontally connected network that is lacking in thalamic nuclei.

2.7 Beyond Receptive Fields

Earlier work on cortical reorganization concentrated largely on the analysis of receptive fields and on the areal extent of representational maps. Both variables still figure widely in current research, and abundant data have allowed researchers to make valuable comparisons between different species and modalities (box 2.2). In addition, new imaging techniques, such as fMRI, have allowed them to study adaptational changes in humans more precisely, to describe changes in neural representations in terms of the activation size of cortical maps, and thereby to link human and animal studies. Temporal aspects of coding have become increasingly prominent; consequently, synchronicity and correlated activity have been intensively studied (see 2.4.1, figure 2.5). There is now substantial evidence that cooperativity among many neurons is subject to modification during plastic reorganization, implying that changes in temporal coding are important or even crucial to use-dependent plasticity. This evidence supports the hypothesis that neural assembly membership is organized along primarily dynamic lines (for theoretical work, see Edelman and Finkel 1984; Braitenberg 1986; von der Malsburg 1987; Aertsen et al. 1989; Abeles 1991; Shenoy et al. 1993; for experimental work, see Dinse, Recanzone, and Merzenich 1990, 1993; Ahissar et al. 1992, 1998; Nicolelis et al. 1993; Nicolelis, Lin, and Chapin 1997; Maldonado

Box 2.2

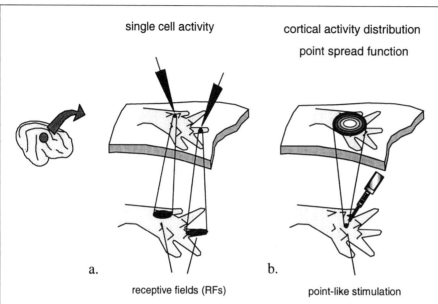

Two different ways to assess cortical maps, activity distributions, and receptive fields. (*a*) Action potentials from single neurons or from small clusters of neurons are measured by inserting microelectrodes into the middle layers of the cortex. The receptive field on the skin surface is defined as that region where stimulation evokes action potentials. This procedure maps activity recorded in the cortex into the stimulus space that allows an easy and systematic way of parametric analysis. When moving the electrode to an adjacent location in the cortex, a systematic shift in the corresponding receptive field location will be encountered. A complete topographic map can be obtained when a large number of electrode penetrations are combined such that the penetration coordinates are related to the corresponding receptive field coordinates. (*b*) Cortical activity distributions are measured. In contrast to panel *a*, a fixed stimulus, ideally a small, "pointlike" stimulus, is applied, and the entire activity in the cortex evoked by that stimulus is measured. This type of activity distribution if often referred to as "point spread function" (PSF). Technologies used for this kind of analysis are optical and functional magnetic resonance imaging. It should be noted, however, that the PSF can be obtained using microelectrodes, in which case the activity of single or multiple neurons evoked by the "pointlike" stimulus is recorded and its spatial distribution is derived from a systematic mapping of that response at different locations.

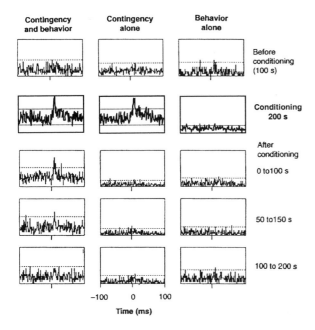

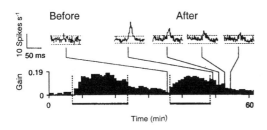

Figure 2.5

Pairs of neurons were recorded in a monkey performing an auditory discrimination task. The dependence of functional plasticity on the contingency between activities of two neurons and on behavior was tested by a combination of cellular conditioning and behavioural paradigms. The activity of one neuron in each pair (CS neuron) was regarded as the conditioned stimulus (CS); the activity of the other neuron (CR neuron), as the conditioned response (CR). An auditory stimulus capable of eliciting or suppressing activity in the CR neuron was used as unconditioned stimulus (US), which was used both for pairing the activities of the two neurons and for guiding the monkeys performance in an auditory discrimination task.

and Gerstein 1996a,b; Faggin, Nguyen, and Nicolelis 1997; Ghazanfar, Stambaugh, and Nicolelis 2000; Laubach, Wessberg, and Nicolelis 2000).

Nevertheless, temporal processing, that is, the computation of sequential events, is still poorly understood. The severe temporal constraints imposed by timing and sequencing modulate neuron responses and reveal response properties not apparent under steady state conditions using solitary stimulation: moreover, the analysis of timing and order effects allows researchers to directly link cortical with behavioral studies. Indeed, there is clear experimental evidence that repetitively applied stimuli evoke cortical responses that differ from those evoked by a single stimulus isolated in time (Gardner and Costanzo 1980; Lee and Whitsel 1992; Dinse 1994;

There were three conditions: conditioning with behavior (contingency and behavior), conditioning without behavior (contingency alone), and pseudoconditioning (behavior alone) that occurred when the monkey performed the task but the contingency between neurons was not affected. *Top*, cross-correlograms (top) show effect of modification of functional connections between neuron pairs. Uppermost row shows control condition, with no significant correlations between the shown neuron pair; second row shows conditioning condition, with correlated activity both for contingency and behavior and for contingency alone. Interestingly, persistent changes in functional connectivity require the establishment of contingency together with behavior. *Bottom*, example of functional plasticity as a function of time, with periods of conditioning indicated by the filled horizontal bars. Cross-correlograms before and after the second conditioning are presented above to indicate changes in functional plasticity. Gain of connection was defined as peak area in correlograms. As shown, the gain was enhanced during the first conditioning period (left) and remained strong after conditioning was stopped (right). The potentiation was extinguished during the next minutes of spontaneous activity; the second conditioning was then applied, yielding similar results. (Modified from Ahissar et al. 1992.) Reprinted with permission. © [1992] American Association for the Advancement of Science.)

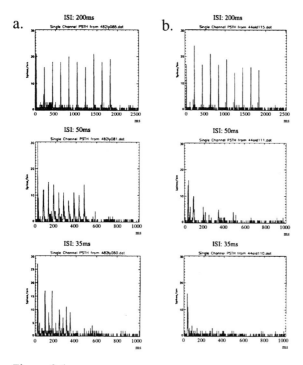

Figure 2.6
The effect of aging on temporal sequence representation was investigated using trains of 10 tactile stimuli of variable interstimulus intervals (ISIs). (*a, b*) Examples of post-stimulus-time histograms (PSTHs) recorded in young and in old rat, respectively. ISIs used were 200 msec, 50 msec, and 35 msec. Bin size was 1 msec; neural activity in spikes per bin is plotted on the ordinate, time on the abscissa. Each PSTH gives the response accumulated over 32 trials; pause between each single trial was 5 sec. For a slow repetition rate of tactile stimuli, neurons recorded in young and old rats follow truthfully each stimulus, which evoked about the same peak activity. Whereas neurons recorded in the young rat can still represent the sequence of stimuli delivered at an ISI of 50 msec, those recorded in the old rat manifest a significant deterioration in their ability to follow this sequence. This failure to represent fast sequences becomes even more dramatic at an ISI of 35 msec. In addition to massive changes of topography developing during aging (see figure 2.2), there is also a significant deterioration of temporal processing abilities, which are also corre-

Merzenich et al. 1993; Tommerdahl et al. 1996, 1998; Polley, Chen-Bee, and Frostig 1999a).

Thus far, few researchers have related changes in temporal processing to parallel changes in perception. Recanzone, Merzenich, and Schreiner (1992) demonstrated that behavioral training of a frequency discrimination task affected entrainment of repetitive stimuli (see figure 2.1). Jürgens and Dinse (1995; see figure 2.6), using trains of repetitive tactile stimuli of variable interstimulus intervals (ISIs), observed dramatic impairment of repetition coding and input sequence representations in the hind paw representation of old rats as compared to young controls. They found comparable changes of the neural input sequence representation in rats with artificially induced walking alterations (Jürgens and Dinse 1997a). Other researchers (Buonomano 1999; Buonomano and Merzenich 1998b), in their in vitro studies, demonstrated a different susceptibility between first and later excitatory postsynaptic potentials (EPSPs) to time-varying stimuli for neocortical slices, indicating that the balance of different time-dependent processes can modulate the state of networks in a complex manner.

It has been suggested that a dysfunction in normal phonological processing, which is critical to the development of oral and written language, may derive from difficulties in perceiving and producing basic sensorimotor information in rapid succession. Indeed, children with language-based learning impairments of this type, when given adaptive training in temporal processing, showed marked improvement in their ability to recognize brief and fast sequences of non-

lated to the behavioral status of the hind limb: the temporal deficits can be ameliorated by housing the animals in an enriched environment. (Modified from Jürgens and Dinse 1995; Churs et al. 1996.)

speech and speech stimuli, suggesting that the re-organizational changes are specifically sensitive for temporal parameters of the input. (Tallal, Miller, and Fitch 1993; Merzenich, Jenkins, et al. 1996; Tallal et al. 1996).

Thus adaptational processes alter both spatial and temporal aspects of sensory processing, which has implications for all forms of perceptual learning, and specifically for tasks involving spatiotemporal proximity such as interval or saltation learning (Geldard and Sherrick 1972; Cholewiak 1976; Kilgard and Merzenich 1995).

2.8 Coding of Adaptational Changes

Changes in receptive fields, cortical maps, correlated activity, and temporal sequence processing (see figure 2.7) clearly suggest that use and training alters cortical processing. Yet, in most cases, the causal link between neural changes and changes in performance remains to be clarified. Recanzone, Merzenich, and co-workers (1992) pointed out that there was no correlation between increased RF size and performance. In contrast, the enhancement of temporally coherent responses correlated strongly with the discriminative performances (Recanzone, Merzenich, and Schreiner 1992).

Indeed, many studies have reported an increase in receptive field size in response to a broad spectrum of different forms of induction of adaptational changes. This frequently observed phenomenon makes it difficult to attribute a specific coding aspect to RF size. It could be that strengthening of synapses during a Hebbian learning process inevitably leads to RF enlargement with little bearing on behavior. From a methodological point of view, assessment of RF size is usually done by hand-plotting techniques that provide scant information about the internal organization of receptive fields and their spatial

substructures. Accordingly, subtle but highly task-specific and more complex changes in RF organization that are easy to miss experimentally may contribute to an improvement of perceptual performance. On the other hand, several potential mechanisms can result in RF enlargement: downregulation of inhibitory surrounds; strengthening of excitatory, previously subthreshold RF regions; enhanced, synchronized discharge resulting in lowering of thresholds; or a mixture of all these putative mechanisms. In any event, monitoring RF size without monitoring the mechanisms underlying changes in RFs will yield only limited insight into the meaning of the changes.

For the tactile coactivation protocol described above, Godde and coworkers (Godde, Spengler, and Dinse 1996; Godde et al. 2000) observed an RF increase in rats and a lowering of the discrimination threshold in human subjects. Assuming that the coactivation protocol results in comparable changes in both man and rat, the enhancement of the discrimination performance appears at first sight to contradict the reported receptive field enlargement. A discrepancy between perceptual thresholds and single-neuron properties is not a new finding, however. For example, Westheimer (1979) found that hyperacuity could not be explained in terms of the receptive field sizes of single cells. Coactivation-induced plasticity included enlargement of receptive fields, accompanied by increased receptive field overlap and enlargement of the representational maps, which, in turn, reflected an increase in the total number of neurons activated by the stimulation and thus of processing resources. Temporal aspects of neuron responses were also changed in terms of response duration and paired pulse behavior. It appears reasonable that all these changes, in concert, enable cortical networks to perform a faster and more elaborate decoding and processing of information.

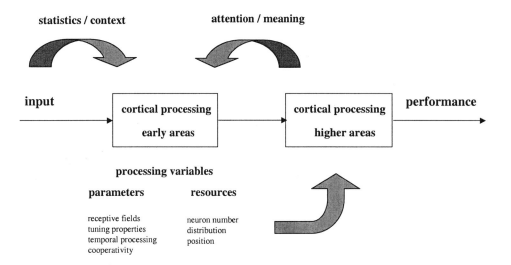

Figure 2.7
Scheme of adaptational processes and interaction with information processing. The main driving forces of adaptations are input statistics and context, on the one hand, and attention and meaning, on the other; by acting bottom-up and top-down, respectively, these modify information processing. Among the parameters subject to modification by adaptational processes are the typical descriptors of cortical processing such as receptive fields, tuning properties, and various aspects of temporal processing and cooperativity among many neurons. In addition to training- or use-specific alteration of such parameters, processing resources can be adjusted according to the requirements of the behavioral status.

In the psychophysical experiments performed by Godde and coworkers (2000), spatial discrimination, but not localization abilities were tested. Evidence for a trade-off between localization and discrimination can be inferred from Sterr et al. 1998a, which reported that stimuli were more often mislocalized on the reading fingers of three-finger Braille readers than on control fingers (see chapter 7). This finding suggests that spatial discrimination performance might benefit from enlarged receptive fields at the expense of localization performance. Thus further understanding of what is coded requires not only detailed analysis of neural changes, but also a broad battery of psychophysical and behavioral tests to find out what really is changed, what is improved, and what may become impaired.

From a theoretical point of view, the "coarse coding" principle (Hinton, McClelland, and Rumel-

hart 1986; Baldi and Heiligenberg 1988; Eurich and Schwegler 1997; Eurich et al. 1997) has been used to explain high-resolution performance by a population of neurons with broad tuning characteristics: given sufficient overlap between tuning curves, each desired resolution can be achieved. If we assume that it is not the property of a single cell that determines behavior, the coarse coding principle can be considered a variant of the more general population coding approach. Neural population analysis implies that large ensembles of neurons contribute to the cortical representation of sensory or motor parameters. Early formulations of this idea postulated that complex stimuli are represented by the simultaneous activation of elementary feature detectors (see Erickson 1974). In primary motor cortex, ensembles of neurons broadly tuned to the direction of movement have been shown to accurately represent the current value of that parameter (Georgopoulos, Schwartz, and Kettner 1986). When Nicolelis and coworkers (1998) used simultaneous multisite neural ensemble recordings to investigate the representation of tactile information in areas 3b, SII, and 2 of the primate somatosensory cortex, they found that small ensembles consisting of 30–40 broadly tuned somatosensory neurons were able to identify correctly the location of a single tactile stimulus in a single trial. Similarly, for visual cortex, Jancke et al. (1999) showed that a population of neurons represented the actual position of a stimulus with deviations several times smaller than average receptive field size. Recently, it has become evident that a critical step in learning how distributed cell assemblies process behaviorally relevant information is identifying functional neuronal interactions within high-dimensional data sets (see Nicolelis 1999). By chronically recording neuronal ensembles in the rat motor cortex throughout the period required for rats to learn a reaction time task, Lauberg, Wessberg, and Nicolelis (2000) demonstrated an increase in the experimenter's ability to predict a correct or incorrect single trial based on measures such as firing rate, temporal patterns of firing, and correlated firing.

Thus there appears to be at least one simple rule of thumb: extensive use leads to an enlargement of representational areas, whereas limited or no use leads to a reduction in such areas, indicating a form of proportionality between representational area and use (see figure 2.8). As discussed above, representational size correlates with the number of neurons activated by a given task or stimulation, which suggests that enhanced performance is at least partially achieved by recruitment of processing resources.

Recent animal studies have challenged this view, however. Combining electrophysiological mapping and optical imaging of rat somatosensory cortex, Polley, Chen-Bee, and Frostig 1999b observed a large-scale expansion of a single whisker's functional

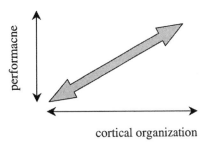

Figure 2.8
According to the summarized experimental evidence, there appears to be a proportionality between changes in behavioral performance and cortical organization, although the exact mapping of cortical changes into performance remains unclear.

representation after innocuous removal of all neighboring whiskers, but a large-scale contraction of the representation after the same procedure when the animal was given a brief opportunity to use its whiskers for active exploration of a different environment. Thus allowing the animal to use its deprived receptor organ in active exploration can determine the direction of plasticity in the adult cortex. Further studies are needed to explore whether a similar potential for a use-dependent direction of reorganizational changes holds true in normal (nondeprived) animals. From a more general point of view, this study suggests that the outcome of adaptations in the somatosensory system might depend on far more subtle constraints imposed by the individual task than previously thought.

Of course, part of the problem is the simple fact that even under normal conditions—without involving adaptive processes—sensory processing and the coding of performance are only poorly understood. That is why it is not clear what receptive field size means. Is it "good" when a tuning curve gets sharper? "Good" for what? The exploration of adaptivity should help us, not only to unravel the mechanisms of learning, but also to better understand sensory coding and processing.

2.9 Conclusions

It is now well acknowledged that use-dependent plasticity can have a significant "negative" impact. Many forms of maladaptive consequences of cortical reorganization have been described. There are more and more examples of highly successful therapeutical intervention based on these findings about use-dependent plasticity. Yet many open questions remain. Among them are the origin and contributing role of subcortical plasticity, the link and interaction between cortical and higher cortical adaptations, and, most important, the coding and decoding of adaptational processes. Comparison of adaptations taking place in auditory and visual systems may shed light on how far somatosensory adaptations generalize in the typical learning processes of the adult brain.

Plasticity of Receptive Fields in Early Stages of the Adult Visual System

Ulf T. Eysel

3

Abstract

Receptive fields (RFs), the windows through which the visual nerve cells "see" the outside world, are produced when sensory information from the retina is processed in excitatory and inhibitory networks. Originally regarded as spatially defined (retinal) areas that go through a critical period of postnatal refinement and that later remain essentially static and based on anatomical connectivity, RFs have in recent years been shown to exhibit considerable plasticity in the mature central nervous system. Such plasticity can be elicited by repetitive use or by disuse of the retina, and can also arise as a result of damage to the visual cortex. This chapter explores how these different conditions may be connected with each other and with the basic principles of perceptual learning, whether we can experimentally influence this plasticity, and whether related training procedures can help patients improve recovery from visual deficits.

3.1   Introduction

The plasticity of receptive fields (RFs) in the early stages of the visual system is closely related to perceptual learning, especially to the basic mechanisms of perceptual learning that can be induced experimentally even in anesthetized animals. Plasticity in the adult visual cortex enables the system to reorganize and compensate for lost functions after damage to the visual system. This chapter seeks to explain how the normal ability of the visual system to reorganize and the pathophysiological aspects of recovery from lesions are related. After summarizing how RFs in the cat primary visual cortex can be changed

by repetitive associative stimulation, we will outline the effects of disuse due to retinal lesions or retinal stabilized images (artificial scotomas). Cells in the primary visual cortex respond to changes in retinal input with acute and chronic RF plasticity that is suited to fill in a retinal scotoma by means of central mechanisms. The same happens chronically and to a lesser extent in the subcortical dorsal lateral geniculate nucleus. Next, we will show the early effects of visual cortex lesions and how the visual field loss caused by the lesions can be partially compensated by chronic RF size plasticity. We will touch on the use-dependent RF plasticity that can be elicited at the border of acute cortical lesions, which closely resembles the plasticity previously described for the normal adult visual cortex, and we will address the underlying cellular mechanisms such as up- and downregulation of excitatory and inhibitory transmitter systems, possible effects of growth factors, morphological reactions, and synaptic learning (long-term potentiation, or LTP). We will argue that recent findings on the link between perceptual learning and the improvement of lost functions can be used to improve recovery from sensory defects by appropriate training.

3.2   Effect of Repetitive Visual Stimulation on Receptive Fields in Adult Striate Cortex

Fast associative cellular plasticity of visual cortical cells has been shown in vitro with electrical stimulation as well as in vivo by pairing of natural stimuli with artificial depolarization. Adult sensory cortices (visual, somatosensory, and auditory) are capable of considerable plasticity (Kaas 1991; Eysel 1992; Weinberger 1995; Cruikshank and Weinberger 1996b; Gilbert 1998; see also chapter 1). Cellular correlates of long-term use-dependent changes in attentive learning have been shown in the auditory and somatosensory cortices of awake, behaving animals using natural sensory stimuli given over days to weeks (Recanzone et al. 1992, 1993; Bakin and Weinberger 1990; see also chapter 2). To induce changes in cellular responses in vivo on a faster timescale, natural sensory stimuli have been paired with electrical or pharmacological stimulation of cells in the visual, auditory, and somatosensory cortices of anesthetized animals (Frégnac et al. 1988, 1992; Cahusac 1995; Cruikshank and Weinberger 1996a; Frégnac and Shulz 1999). These experiments have provided in vivo evidence that the modifiability of mature visual cortical connections follows the Hebbian learning rule, which requires both pre- and postsynaptic activity within a defined time window (Hebb 1949). However, none of the above approaches answered the question as to whether LTP-like activity-dependent changes—as seen in adult visual cortical cells in vitro (Artola and Singer 1987; Kimura et al. 1989; Hirsch and Gilbert 1993; Kirkwood and Bear 1994)—can be obtained with purely natural sensory stimulation in vivo.

We approached this issue by recording from single cells in the visual cortex of the anesthetized adult cat and showed that long-lasting changes in receptive field size and substructure can indeed be obtained within minutes (Eysel, Eyding, and Schweigart 1998). To elicit "associative" synaptic changes, visual costimulation was applied to the central parts of an excitatory RF and its immediate unresponsive surround. Our aim was to stimulate visual cortical cells so that they would specifically "learn" to respond to an originally subthreshold region outside their exci-

tatory RF or to change their subfield composition within the RF of simple cells. By carefully mapping the RF with averaged post-stimulus-time histograms (PSTHs) in response to optimally oriented on-off stimuli, we were able to determine the exact size of the RF and to identify an adjacent completely unresponsive region on one side of the RF as test region by repetitive stimulation and statistical evaluation; another region, located just outside the RF or in the minimal discharge field at the opposite border of the RF, was selected as control region so as to detect even minimal unspecific changes (figure 3.1A). The experimental conditioning stimulation, which we called "visual costimulation," consisted of repetitive 1/sec "on-off" stimuli covering parts of the excitatory RF (including its highly responsive center) and the unresponsive test region just outside the RF (figure 3.1B). In about one-third of all cells, a specific widening of the RF into the unresponsive region was observed when the previously unresponsive region was tested 15 to 180 min after 15 min of costimulation (figure 3.1C). In general, this effect was observed after 10 to 75 min of costimulation and persisted from 20 min to more than 3 hours. In none of these cases did we see a change of the response in the nonstimulated control region. In addition to the associative plasticity seen at the border of receptive fields, potentiation of responses inside the classical RF was often observed. For example, after costimulation, which elicited a strong "off" response, an initially small "off" response in the central region of an excitatory RF increased and changed the center response from a predominantly "on" to an "on-off" response after 60 min of repetitive stimulation. We observed no differences for any of these effects between areas 17 and 18 or between simple and complex cells. In addition, the findings were independent of RF size and eccentricity within 10° around the area centralis.

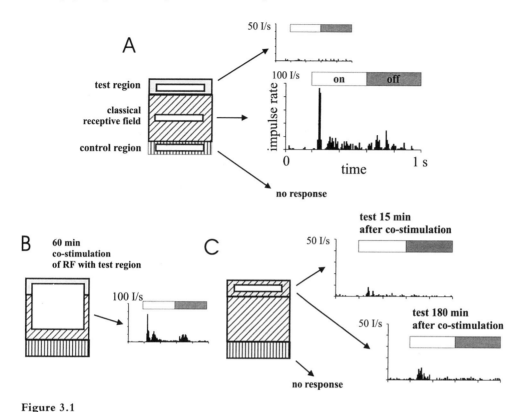

Figure 3.1

Receptive field expansion as consequence of associative costimulation of the classical receptive field with an unresponsive adjacent region. (*A*) Schematic drawing of the classical receptive field (RF; oblique hatching), the unresponsive test region (gray) on one side and the unresponsive control region (vertical hatching) on the other. The white bars represent the light stimuli used for stimulation. The post-stimulus-time histograms (PSTHs) to the right show the missing response in the test region and the strong "on" and weaker "off" response in the center of the classical RF prior to the experiment. Like the test region, the control region shows no response. (*B*) The associative visual costimulation is applied for 15 minutes (900 "on-off" stimuli). The stimulus covers a large part of the classical RF and the test region. The "on-off" response during costimulation resembles the response from the RF center. (*C*) The expansion of the RF toward the costimulated test region is proven by the clear "on" responses in the PSTHs obtained from that region 15 minutes and 3 hours after costimulation.

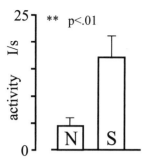

Figure 3.2
Peak activity during associative costimulation in impulses per second (I/sec) is shown for the S group ($n = 22$), which afterward had a specific widening of the receptive field and for the N group ($n = 22$), which showed no effect. The S group displays significantly higher activity ($p \leq 0.01$).

The widening of the RF was specifically dependent on costimulation: there was no change in excitability at the nonstimulated opposite side of the excitatory RF, and controls with 60 min stimulation of the RF alone did not show any increase in RF size. The widening of RFs was activity dependent. When responses were very small during costimulation or when inhibition prevailed during costimulation, no widening of RFs could be obtained. The peak response rates during costimulation as a direct measure of activity during visual costimulation in cells that showed a specific widening of the RF (S group, $n = 22$, 17.08 ± 3.85 impulses/sec) and in cells that showed no changes in RF size (N group, $n = 22$, 4.34 ± 1.21 impulses/sec; figure 3.2) were quite different. Statistical tests using both response rates during costimulation and facilitation indices (Eysel, Eyding, and Schweigart 1998) revealed a significant dependence ($p < 0.01$) of specific RF plasticity on stimulus-locked postsynaptic activity during associative costimulation. The response type ("on" or "off") developing in the coactivated test

region was as a rule the same as that found at the nearby border of the RF. In mapping studies of visual cortical RF, blockade of GABAergic inhibition with bicuculline revealed a more extended distribution of subthreshold synapses than suprathreshold "on" and "off" inputs both within and close to the borders of the classical RF (Pernberg, Jirmann, and Eysel 1998). This indicates that coincident activation of subthreshold synapses with suprathreshold inputs could lead to increasing synaptic weight in the sense of associative LTP at the subthreshold synapses and a long-term increase of RF size.

The presumed underlying increase in synaptic efficacy seems to follow the Hebbian learning rule. A certain activity during costimulation proved to be a necessary condition; it can provide postsynaptic depolarization coincident with the arrival of normally subthreshold excitation from the region outside the RF. The large variation in activity observed during successful coactivation may be due to local features of signal processing such as shunting by dendritic conductances or by active dendritic processes; that is, the activity seen with extracellular recording during costimulation need not reflect the local currents at the dendritic sites where strengthening of synaptic efficacy takes place. The observed receptive field changes can last for hours and we therefore consider these changes as evidence for synaptic plasticity in vivo similar to long-term potentiation described for layer II/III cells in the cat and rat visual cortex in vitro (Artola and Singer 1987; Kimura et al. 1989; Hirsch and Gilbert 1993; Kirkwood and Bear 1994). Where excitation during costimulation is weak or absent and specific excitatory enlargement of RF size does not occur, intracortical inhibition may play a special role: inhibitory synapses at layer III neurons may reduce visual cortical LTP by shunting excitatory postsynaptic currents (Artola and Singer 1987); a central role may also be played by inhibitory intracortical circuits in gating of visual cortical plasticity at the network level (Kirkwood and Bear 1994). Long-term potentiation was successfully induced in cat visual cortex slices by stimulation of long-ranging horizontal fibers when the elicited responses were predominantly excitatory, but not when the composite responses contained significant inhibitory potentials (Hirsch and Gilbert 1993).

In our first attempt (Eysel, Eyding, and Schweigart 1998) to show RF plasticity in anesthetized cat visual cortex in vivo by applying repetitive natural visual stimulation, we exclusively investigated cells in layers II/III shown to be capable of LTP in in vitro experiments (Artola and Singer 1987; Kimura et al. 1989; Hirsch and Gilbert 1993; Kirkwood and Bear 1994) and used simple, unspecific large field conditioning stimuli and optimally oriented test stimuli to look for significant results with a minimal number of experimental variables. To determine the specificity of the effect and whether it can be observed in cortical layers other than II/III, further experiments will be needed, using different orientations and variable temporal coherence of conditioning stimuli in different parts of the RF and recording from other cortical layers.

Pathways that might be involved in the effects observed here in layer II/III cells include collaterals of geniculocortical afferents (Gilbert and Wiesel 1979; Freund, Martin, and Whitteridge 1985) acting via interneurons of the same cortical column; long-range excitatory axons of cells in layers II/III/IV (Gilbert and Wiesel 1979; Hirsch and Gilbert 1993; Kisvárday and Eysel 1992; see also chapter 1); and interactions between areas 17 and 18 and higher visual areas.

In psychophysical experiments with adult humans, training has been shown to significantly improve performance in visual perceptual tasks (Fiorentini and Berardi 1980; Fahle, Edelman, and Poggio 1995; see also chapters 9–12). Our finding that repetitive visual stimuli rapidly induced long-lasting RF modifications could provide the basis for modeling the cellular mechanisms that underlie this fast visual learning, which is most probably rooted in early visual processing.

Although visual RFs are characterized by suprathreshold inputs, subthreshold synapses within the RF and close to the borders may also be activated. Associative coactivation of sub- and suprathreshold synapses—presumably converging on common somatic or dendritic sites—appears to lead to specific synaptic strengthening and to locally changed RF substructure and enlarged RFs. Thus mature visual cortical cells can "learn" to respond to previously subthreshold inputs during synchronous coactivation in an anesthetized state in vivo, a correlate of perceptual learning at the level of the single cell or cortical network.

3.3 Effect of Deafferentation on Cortical Receptive Fields and Retinotopy

Fast changes in visual receptive field properties also follow acute disuse associated with retinal lesions (Chino et al. 1992; Gilbert and Wiesel 1992) and are elicited when selective surround stimulation is applied to artificial retinal scotomas (Pettet and Gilbert 1992; Das and Gilbert 1995b; DeAngelis et al. 1995).

Retinal lesions lead to an interruption of visual signal flow from the destroyed region. Cells in the thalamus (lateral geniculate nucleus) and the primary visual cortex are locally deprived of their normal input. Because of the predominantly binocular innervation of visual cortical cells, only homonymous, binocular lesions can cause deafferentation of the cortical cells. Circumscribed retinal lesions introduce a characteristic imbalance in the target regions: cells with normal afferent input are situated in the immediate neighborhood of visually silenced cells.

This situation leads to changes in cortical cell RF size and topography when the active cells gain influence on their inactive neighbors through the long-range intracortical horizontal fiber system (Darian-Smith and Gilbert 1995; Das and Gilbert 1995a). This possible basis for the perceptual filling in of "artificial" and "real" retinal scotomas will be addressed in greater detail below. Such reorganization after a retinal lesion occurs at the cortical level with redundant information from the border of the retinal lesions, that is, the response to a stimulus at the border of the lesion is represented in its correct cortical location as well as laterally displaced in the originally deafferented region (reorganization with redundant information; figure 3.3); it has been described in the cat and monkey visual system (Kaas et al. 1990; Heinen and Skavenski 1991).

3.3.1 Effect of Artificial Scotomas and Acute Retinal Lesions on Receptive Fields

Psychophysical observations yielded an immediate filling-in phenomenon for retinal scotomas (Gerrits and Timmermann 1969) and a delayed filling-in phenomenon for stabilized retinal images (Yarbus 1957; Millodot 1965; Gerrits, de Haan, and Vendrick 1966) that can be regarded as "artificial retinal scotomas" (Gerrits and Vendrick 1970). A stabilized image follows all eye movements, hence the contours of its borders are not enhanced by the continuous motion. Such an image vanishes with time, it is filled in from the surround with redundant information similar to the (instantaneous) filling in of the blind spot or a retinal scotoma.

In recent years, artificial scotomas were introduced into experimental neurophysiology (Pettet and Gilbert 1992). Short-term RF size changes were found in the cells within an artificial scotoma. When single-cell receptive fields were recorded from the

center of an artificial retinal scotoma (a masked region of the retina surrounded by moving pattern stimuli), significant increases of RF size were measured (Pettet and Gilbert 1992; Das and Gilbert 1995b). This is equivalent to a filling in of the masked region with information from the surround. Although DeAngelis et al. (1995) questioned the RF size increases reported in these studies, arguing that there was primarily a general increase in responsiveness and that normalization of the activity resulted in unchanged receptive field dimensions, further experiments showed a genuine RF expansion, with cells responding to parts of the visual field, where previously they could not be excited (Gilbert et al. 1996).

Similar effects were seen when unilateral or bilateral retinal lesions were applied. Within minutes after homonymous binocular retinal lesions, the RFs in primary visual cortex of monkeys and cats expanded at the border of the cortical representation of the lesions (Gilbert and Wiesel 1992). RFs reached, on average, five times their original area (growing from 0.07 to 0.37 degree^2); these early changes were also accompanied by shifts in retinotopy and map reorganization when retinal lesions were smaller than 5° of visual angle (Chino 1995, 1997).

3.3.2 Lesion-Induced Changes in Excitability in the Surround of the Scotoma

The retinotopic projections of homonymous retinal lesions (panel A of figure 3.3) cause a cortical region devoid of retinal input from the homonymous visual field area from both eyes (deafferented visual cortex; panel B), which is associated with a blind region in the visual field (scotoma; panel C). To measure the changes of cortical excitability introduced by the retinal lesions, we recorded spontaneous activity and visually evoked activity inside and outside the deaf-

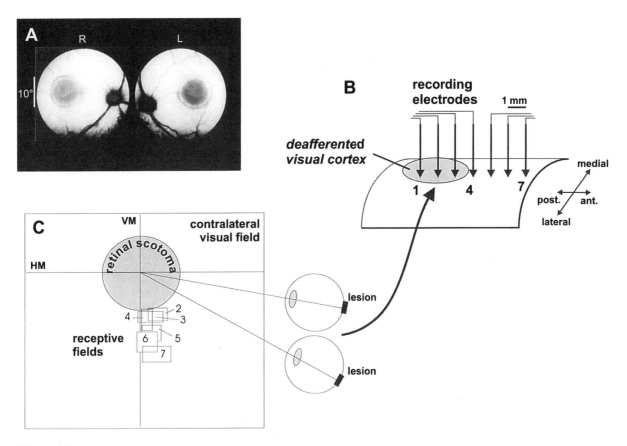

Figure 3.3
Methods and basic topographical reorganization a month after bilateral central retinal lesions. (*A*) Fundus photographs of homonymous 10° diameter retinal lesions in the right (R) and left (L) eye. (*B*) Schematic drawing of the lesioned eyes and one hemisphere of the visual cortex. The bilateral, homonymous lesions in the eyes (black rectangles) lead to a region of deafferentation in the visual cortex (gray area). The electrode array covers the deafferented region and a part of cortex anterior to it. The individual electrodes are spaced by 1 mm and are numbered from 1 to 7 from posterior to anterior. Fields are mapped with an array of recording electrodes (1–7). (*C*) The receptive fields (RFs) of cells recorded in the visual cortex are drawn in the contralateral visual field. The four anterior electrodes (4–7) are located outside the deafferented region and have receptive fields migrating upward along the vertical meridian (VM) up to the border of the retinal scotoma. The three posterior electrodes (1–3) are located within the deafferented cortex. RFs 2 and 3, obtained at these cortical locations, are displaced in the visual field and are found at the border of the scotoma.

ferented visual cortex (Arckens et al. 2000) with a
linear array of electrodes two weeks after photocoagulation of both central retinas (10° diameter) of
cats (figure 3.3). In three cats, an array of seven
electrodes set 1 mm apart was placed so that the
most posterior electrode recorded in deafferented
cortex, whereas the most anterior electrode recorded
in normal cortex. Both the spontaneous activity and
the visual evoked activity were minimal within the
deafferented cortex and maximal just outside, approaching normal values at larger distances from
the deafferented region. Because the distance of
recording tracks might have missed subtle distance-
dependent changes, in another experiment, with a
fourth cat, the electrodes in the multiunit array were
spaced 0.3 mm apart along a mediolateral line, with
all electrodes having the same anterior-posterior position. The electrodes were moved down the medial
bank of area 17 (figure 3.4A) and closely spaced cells
were recorded along each track, first in the deafferented cortex, then in the border region, and finally
in the adjacent normal cortex. Again a clear peak of
increased activity was seen just adjacent to the deafferented cortex in both spontaneous and visually
evoked activity, and both were significantly lower in
the deafferented cortex than in the more distant
normal cortex (figure 3.4B).

3.3.3 Chronic Changes in Receptive Field Size and Cortical Topography Induced by Retinal Lesions

Retinal lesions cause chronic reorganization in the
afferent visual pathway of the cat. After a monocular
photocoagulator lesion, the excitability of primarily
deafferented cells in the thalamic relay nucleus (dorsal lateral geniculate nucleus, or dLGN) changes in a
characteristic way: the cells showing a loss of visual
drive and a significant decrease in spontaneous
activity in the dLGN regain visual input from the
retina directly adjacent to the lesion after about three

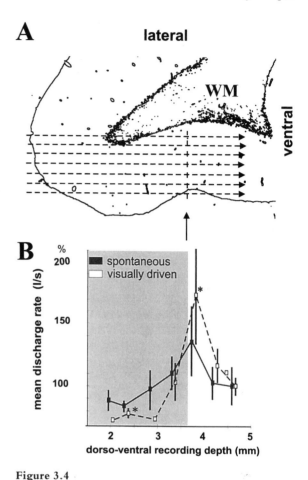

Figure 3.4
Recordings along the medial bank of the primary visual
cortex of the cat reveal changes of excitability at the border of the deafferented cortex. (*A*) Schematic drawing of a
coronal section of area 17 with the tracks of seven electrodes indicated by dotted lines with arrowheads. The arrow
and the dashed line indicate the border of the deafferented
cortex. The cortical surface is to the left. WM = white
matter. (*B*) Mean discharge rate (mean ± s.e.) at different
depths in relation to the border of the deafferented region
(gray) is shown for spontaneous activity (black bars) and
visually driven activity (white bars). Asterisks indicate significant differences ($p < 0.05$) with respect to the activity
distant from the border of deafferentation. Note the peak of
excitability just outside the deafferented (gray) region and
the rising spontaneous and visually evoked activity inside
that indicates the ongoing reorganization.

weeks. Accordingly, the RFs of these reconnected cells change their retinotopy and shift to a new position located at the border of the retinal lesion (Eysel, Gonzalez-Aguilar, and Mayer 1980, 1981). This reorganization leads to a partial filling in of the scotoma on the subcortical level (Eysel, Gonzalez-Aguilar, and Mayer 1981) and is associated with a lateral spread of excitation in the dLGN by up to 300 μm (Eysel 1982). With the same type of lesion (combined with enucleation of the other eye), Kaas et al. (1990) observed a much more extended reorganization in cat visual cortex. Apart from the longer distances, the reorganization was exactly of the same kind as observed in the dLGN: originally silenced cells regained visual input that originated from the border of the retinal lesion, a retinal region that had not excited these cells before. The same kind of plasticity was found in monkey visual cortex (Heinen and Skavensky 1991). In cat and monkey, the reorganization followed a characteristic time course, filling in cortical regions that were depleted of retinal inputs by homonymous retinal lesions up to 10 mm across, equivalent to an intracortical lateral spread of excitation of 5 mm (Gilbert and Wiesel 1992). At the same time, a significant enlargement of RFs was observed that occurred quite early after lesioning (for reviews, see Chino 1995, 1997).

3.3.4 Cortical Immunohistochemistry after Chronic Retinal Lesions

When the immunohistochemistry (IHC) of the GABAergic system (glutamic acid decarboxylase IHC; Rosier et al. 1995) and of the glutamatergic system (glutamate IHC; Arckens at al. 2000) was investigated two weeks after homonymous lesions in the retina (central 10°), researchers discovered, inside and in the surround of the deafferented cortical region, a characteristric pattern of transmitter system immunoreactivity induced by the retinal lesions.

The glutamic acid decarboxylase (GAD) immunoreactivity, though downregulated inside the scotoma such that the number of positive profiles in the neuropil was extremely reduced, remained essentially unchanged in the cell somata (Rosien et al. 1995). The immunohistochemistry of the excitatory neurotransmitter glutamate revealed glutamate-positive cells in cortical layers II to VI of area 17. The retinal lesions caused a clear reduction (by 18–26%) in the number of glutamate-immunoreactive cells in the supra- and infragranular layers of the cortical area representing the lesioned retina, compared to normal cortex. Furthermore, the cortex just outside the deafferented region displayed a sharp increase (of 50–100%) in glutamate immunoreactivity throughout layers II to VI of area 17, with the largest peak, having a width of 600–800 μm, noted in layer VI (Arckens et al. 2000).

Both the changes in GAD and glutamate immunoreactivity diminished with time. When the central and the peripheral portions of area 17 in cats with postlesion survival times of longer than twelve weeks were compared, no significant differences in the number of glutamate immunoreactivity-positive cells and in the GAD immunoreactivity of the neuropil were observed, showing that the immunohistochemical reactions return back to normal once the functional reorganization is completed.

3.4 Cortical Lesions and Perilesional Cortical Reorganization

Retinal lesions that switch off the afferent input to the cortex are quite different from cortical lesions that destroy target cells for the retinal projection to the cortex; they also pose quite different problems for reorganizing, and restoring function to, the visual system. As described above, in the case of a retinal lesion, the system must reinnervate cortical cells that have lost their sensory input, using redundant information from the border of the scotoma. In the case of a cortical lesion, the retina and afferent pathways remain completely intact, but the cortical target cells used to represent a certain retinal topography are lost. The problem for reorganizing the system is completely different: surviving cells in the surround of the lesion must take over the topographical representation of their destroyed neighbor cells; accordingly, the functional outcome is fundamentally different because information is again made accessible for cortical processing from retinal regions no longer represented (reorganizing with nonredundant information). A chronic reorganization of this type has recently been described in cat striate cortex (Eysel and Schweigart 1999). Interestingly, the two completely different types of lesions seem to trigger common early effects leading to receptive field plasticity that appears useful for a certain recovery of function (Eysel et al. 1999).

The lesion-induced changes can be roughly subdivided into acute, subacute, and chronic effects. The pathology predominant in the acute phase (first postlesion day) is followed by events of neuronal plasticity in the subacute phase (two days to one week after a lesion) and the chronic phase (weeks to months after the lesion; Eysel 1997) that can be useful for minimizing the functional loss caused by the lesions. Here we will focus our interest on the properties of single cells and the functional reorganization following a cortical lesion that can again be related to cellular equivalents of perceptual learning in the primary visual cortex.

3.4.1 Acute Lesion-Induced Changes in Excitability

Acute and subacute effects were observed at small, round lesions of about 1.5 to 2 mm diameter induced either by surface photocoagulation (Eysel and Schmidt-Kastner 1991) or by ibotenic acid injections (Schweigart and Eysel 1998). The lesions were placed in one hemisphere of the cat visual cortex at a point some 3 mm lateral to the midline (area 17, sometimes extending into area 18). The typical lesion completely destroyed the supragranular layers and reached down into the infragranular layers (see figure 3.5A). The histological changes observed in the area surrounding these lesions are described in greater detail elsewhere (Eysel 1997; Schmidt-Kastner et al. 1993; Mittmann et al. 1994; Schroeter et al. 1995).

When we recorded single cells in anesthetized cats 1, 2, 7, and 30 days after cortical lesioning, we observed typical changes 1–2 days after the lesion. The spontaneous and visually driven activity of the cells was dependent on the distance from the border of the cortical lesions. Activity was suppressed close to the border of the lesion (up to 0.5 mm), increased at distances between 1 and 1.5 mm, and approached normal values farther away from the lesion (figure 3.5B). Seven to 30 days after the lesion, spontaneous excitability returned to normal values both for the depressed cells close to the lesion and for the hyperexcitable cells in the adjacent region.

In the acute and subacute phases, in vivo mapping of single cells using extracellular microelectrodes in cats with focal heat lesions of the visual cortex yielded activity in the surround of a lesion characterized by concentric rings of subnormal ($<$ 1 mm), hypernormal (1–2.5 mm), and normal spontaneous activity ($>$ 2.5 mm). The region of hyperactivity was also characterized by epileptiform discharge patterns in about one-third of the cells and by a typical loss of orientation specificity to visual stimulation. Although the early hyperexcitability of cells surrounding a lesion could lead to excitotoxic cell death, we have reasons to hypothesize that it could just as well support synaptic plasticity and reorganization by facilitating heterosynaptic LTP-like mechanisms.

A

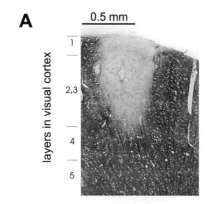

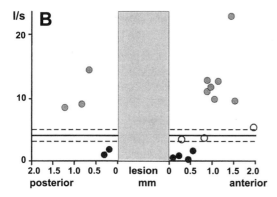

Figure 3.5
Focal ibotenic acid lesion in the visual cortex and the excitability at the borders of the lesion. (*A*) Immunocytochemical visualization of the neuronal loss with a monoclonal antibody against microtubuli-associated protein (MAP-2). The cortical layers are indicated on the left of the microphotograph. Tangential section of a lesion after 76 days survival time. (*B*) Mean spontaneous activity of 176 cells from 19 penetrations in the vicinity of cortical lesions (survival time: 1–2 days). The horizontal line depicts the mean spontaneous activity of 48 normal control neurons matched for eccentricity and layers; the gray area indicates the lesion. Spontaneous activity in impulses/sec is plotted on the ordinate; distance from the border of the lesion in mm, on the abscissa.

3.4.2 Changes in Receptive Field Size and Cortical Topography after Cortical Lesions

In patients with cortical lesions, the resulting visual field defects could be reduced in size by filling in from the border zone with time after the lesions occurred and by applying special training procedures (Zihl and von Cramon 1979, 1985; Kasten and Sabel 1995; Kasten et al. 1998). Two possible mechanisms for such a reduction in scotoma size might be (1) the activation of silent cells by their normal, topographically correct inputs in a partially surviving region at the border of the lesion and (2) the above-mentioned enlargement of RFs at the border of the lesion such that the lost cortical representation of the retina is regained by increasing the efficiency of divergent feedforward or feedback inputs from regions inside the scotoma to the cells bordering the cortical defect. In the somatosensory system, a similar change in receptive field sizes was observed for the hand representation several months after local surgical lesions in the monkey (Jenkins and Merzenich 1987). The adult visual cortex has a remarkable potential for plasticity, as has been shown by the extensive reorganization following retinal lesions in cat (Kaas et al. 1990) and monkey (Heinen and Skavenski 1991; Gilbert and Wiesel 1992). This functional reorganization is ascribed to the synapses of the long-range excitatory horizontal axonal system that are normally subthreshold but become more efficient during reorganization after lesioning (Das and Gilbert 1995a). By contrast, the cortical lesions destroy the cortical target cells and local intracortical fibers used in cortical reorganization after retinal lesions, whereas the subcortical input fibers remain unchanged. To gain more insight into these adaptive processes, we have recorded single cells at the border of chronic excitotoxic lesions in adult cat visual cortex (Eysel and Schweigart 1999).

Injection of ibotenic acid resulted in focal lesions characterized by a loss of all neurons 76 days after lesioning, with immunohistochemistry of micro-tubuli-associated protein (MAP) and neurofilaments as neuronal markers. Glial fibrillary acidic protein (GFAP) staining revealed a glial scar in the region free of neurons (panel A of figure 3.5). The average diameter of the lesions (determined from the Nissl stains) was 2.9 mm (range: 2.1–4.3 mm). The average depth of the lesions was 1.6 mm (range: 1.25–2.0 mm); they typically extended to the border between layers IV and V. RFs were mapped before lesioning, with penetrations spaced about 1 mm apart in both subacute and chronic phase experiments; their size and topography were carefully recorded. The RF position of cells in the visual cortex (area 17) migrated from the upper to the lower visual field when penetrations were displaced in the anteroposterior plane from posterior to anterior. Typical RF maps before and after an acute ibotenic acid lesion are shown in figure 3.6 as recorded with a linear array of five electrodes spaced 1 mm apart (panel A) and left in place throughout the 2- to 3-day experiment. When ibotenic acid was injected at one end of the electrode array, neuronal activity ceased at nearby recording sites after a period of strongly increased firing. After two days in total darkness, the RFs were mapped again at the electrode positions with surviving cells and no substantial changes in RF size or topography were observed (panel B). In two cases where the lesion was placed in the middle of the electrode array, 1° and 3° gaps of retinal representations were found in the RF map, indicating small cortical scotomas.

Chronic Changes in Receptive Field Size

Figure 3.7 summarizes a chronic phase experiment with a survival time of 76 days (76d) between lesion-

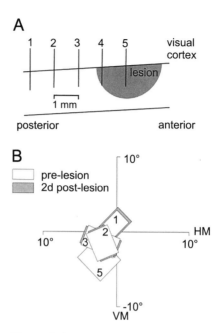

Figure 3.6
Ibotenic acid lesion of the visual cortex does not lead to acute changes in receptive field (RF) size. (*A*) Recording positions 1–5 in the visual cortex (anteroposterior section of right visual cortex shown schematically, with lesion in the upper left). The electrodes are positioned before lesioning and are left in place throughout the 2- to 3-day recording session. (*B*) Before lesioning, RF sizes were measured (white RF outlines) and drawn in the map of the contralateral visual field (1, 2, 3, 5). After lesioning and two days (2d) in total darkness, the RF sizes were carefully mapped again and showed only minimal changes in size (gray areas). (Adapted from Eysel and Schweigart 1999.)

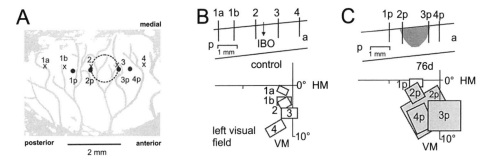

Figure 3.7
Significantly enlarged receptive fields (RFs) at the border of a chronic visual cortex lesion after two months. (*A*) Surface map with cortical vessels drawn from a macroscopic photograph. The positions of electrode penetrations (1p–4p) are indicated by crosses (prelesion recordings 1–4) and black circles (76-day postlesion recordings 1–4). (*B*) Control mapping at electrode positions 1 to 4 before lesioning. Anteroposterior positions of recording sites in the right hemisphere are shown schematically above and the location of the injection of 2% ibotenic acid (IBO; 500 nL). (*C*) Same cortical region is remapped after 76 days (76d). The electrode tracks (1p–4p) are shown above, the RF sizes below indicate a significant increase of RF sizes at the border of the lesion (penetrations 2p and 3p). (Adapted from Eysel and Schweigart 1999.)

ing and final experiment. The localization of penetrations was documented by photographing the cortical surface on the day of ibotenic acid injection, enabling us to retest the same cortical positions after the 76-day survival time: the recording sites and the lesion site were characterized by certain landmarks in the vascular pattern on the cortical surface (figure 3.7A). Panel B shows the RF locations and sizes as mapped before lesioning. Because the cells were vigorously responding, the location and outermost borders of the excitatory RFs could be exactly mapped. The largest RF found in each penetration is outlined and labeled with the number of the respective electrode penetration. The ibotenic acid injection was applied between the locations of the recording sites 2 and 3 (figure 3.7A,B). After the 76-day survival time, we recorded single cells with crisp responses, direction specificity, and sharp tuning for orientation in the supragranular cortical layers in penetrations anterior or posterior to the lesion site. The location and spatial extent of the RFs of these

cells could be determined with the same accuracy as the RFs during the initial lesioning experiment in the same animal. At recording sites 2p, 3p, and 4p, close to the posterior and anterior border of the lesion, individual cells displayed impressively increased RF sizes (figure 3.7C), although in the same penetrations we also encountered single cells with rather normal RF size (the smallest and largest fields obtained in penetration 2p). RFs showed normal (prelesion) sizes at the most posterior recording site (1p) and again decreasing RF size at the most anterior recording site (4p). This finding does not reflect the normal situation in the visual cortex where RF size increases with distance from the area centralis, and hence a continuous increase in average RF size should be present from the most posterior to the most anterior penetration. The cells with increased receptive field size were situated close to the border of the chronic lesions as evident from the position of the recording sites relative to the ibotenic acid injection site (figure 3.7A). This close vicinity was histologically verified in sections that both showed the lesion and identified the electrode tracks.

With an array of seven electrodes spaced 1 mm apart in the visual cortex and left in place from before to two days after the lesion, the mean size of 15 RFs stayed unchanged anterior and posterior to the lesion (mean: 101%; range: 75–156%). The scatter of absolute RF sizes also remained unchanged as can be seen in values before/after lesioning (mean: 3.6°/3.5°; median: 3.2°/3.2°; range: 2–6.4°/2–5.6°; standard deviation: 1.32°/1.06°), indicating, on average, no change in size within the first two days after lesioning. When RF sizes before lesioning ($n = 8$) were compared with those at the same topography in the visual field 55 and 76 days after lesioning ($n = 18$), the mean RF size was found to have increased to 182% (range: 64–385%). The larger scatter and increased mean RF size were due to the cell RFs within a distance of about 1 mm from the border of the lesion. Although RF width remained constant (close to 100% its size before lesioning) at 1 mm anterior as well as 1 and 2 mm posterior, there was a mean increase to 188% at the posterior border, and to 182% and 282%, respectively, at the anterior border and 0.5 mm away. Though close to the lesion, 13 out of 14 RFs were larger than the mean of all prelesion RFs by up to 7.8°; the RFs recorded 1–2 mm away were exactly in the range of the average prelesion RF sizes (−0.8° to +0.2°).

Reducing the Size of the Scotoma

Patients with visual field loss due to vascular or traumatic postgeniculate damage with homonymous defects were trained in the border regions of their residual visual fields by repeated stimulation to improve light difference thresholds (Zihl and von Cramon 1979) or by locating targets within the blind field region (Zihl and von Cramon 1985). Both types of training led to a reduction of the scotoma size and thus to an enlargement of the visual field in most patients. The recovery was specifically dependent on practice, which was also the case in a study where patients with homonymous visual field deficits were exposed to computer-based visual field training that specifically activated the border region of the visual field defect (Kasten and Sabel 1995; Kasten et al. 1998). It was hypothesized that this recovery might take place at the level of the striate cortex. The enlarged RFs of cells at the border of the cortical lesion represent a mechanism for functional recovery of primarily lost parts of the visual field and thus lead to a reduction of the size of a scotoma. This is a nonredundant, functionally useful reorganization because inputs that have lost their target cells are reconnected to surviving cortical cells. The absolute increase of RF size (figure 3.7C) would allow for a shift of the border of a scotoma by about 3–4° in the cat, which is in the range of the 4.9 ± 1.7° recently observed in patients treated with computer-based visual field training (Kasten et al. 1998). This finding suggests that the long-term plasticity of cells at the border of visual cortical lesions may represent a model in the mature visual system of the cat for the long-term reduction of visual field defects observed in human patients.

In light of determining that receptive fields can be changed in size and spatial substructure by repetitive visual stimulation, the next step was to test whether RFs in the cat cortical lesion model could be made to extend into the previously lost part of the visual field by visual training.

3.5 Fast Lesion- and Training-Induced Changes in Receptive Field Size near Subacute Lesions in Adult Cat Visual Cortex

Most studies of plasticity in sensory cortices have concentrated on the remarkable changes of the cortical topography (somatotopic or retinotopic organization, respectively) or on the extent of behavioral recovery (for example, by measuring the size of a scotoma). Comparatively little is known, however, of the extent to which individual neurons may change their response properties in the vicinity of a cortical lesion. Jenkins and Merzenich (1987) reported a complete filling in of the acutely lost representation of the palm after an experimental lesion in the primary somatosensory cortex of an adult owl monkey. This functional reorganization was due to strongly enlarged receptive fields of the cells surrounding the lesion after 129 days, a finding very similar to the increased RF sizes we observed in Eysel and Schweigart 1999 at the border of lesions in the adult cat visual cortex after two months, but not during the first two days of survival time.

In Schweigart and Eysel forthcoming, we concentrated on the first two-day period after the lesion. We recorded neurons in the most interesting border zone of 1–2 mm around the lesion to evaluate their RF sizes and their "on" and "off" subfields and to determine whether use is a necessary prerequisite to induce the RF size increase early after a lesion. Thus we kept the animals in total darkness for two days after lesioning before we applied a visual training procedure. The ibotenic acid lesions closely resembled those in the above-described chronic phase study: average lesion diameters were 2.9 mm anteroposterior (median: 2.5 mm; range: 2.1–5.4 mm); 2.8 mm mediolateral (median: 2.7 mm; range: 1.7–4.2 mm), and 2.0 mm dorsoventral (median: 1.7 mm; range: 1.2–3.6 mm). Histology supported the electrophysiological finding that as of postlesion day 2 no neurons had survived in the core of the lesion, although neurons that could be recorded in the surround were anatomically and functionally intact.

3.5.1 Lesion-Induced Changes in Receptive Field Size

Receptive fields were quantitatively mapped before lesioning and their topography and size were determined (Schweigart and Eysel forthcoming). From the most posterior to the most anterior electrode of the array in the visual cortex, the RF position of the cells migrated from the central visual field downward, and the average RF size increased with eccentricity.

RF sizes were, on average, no different before/after lesion (mean: 3.1°/3.0°; median: 2.8°/2.8°; range: 0.8–10.4°/0.4–7.2°). Although both the width and length of the receptive fields remained constant at most positions, data scatter was usually increased close to the lesions ($\leq \pm 1$ mm), and RF widths close to the anterior border of the lesions (within 1 mm) were slightly enlarged (width increase: 0.4–1.2°, $p < 0.05$; length increase: 0–2.4°, $p < 0.1$; paired one-tailed t-test). There was a significant positive correlation between change in neuronal activity and change in RF size.

In summary, we observed modest RF size changes in the immediate vicinity of the lesion, which correlate to lesion-induced changes in activity. Activity changes were inversely correlated to the distance from the lesion. RF changes were not found to depend on other parameters; in particular, they did not depend on horizontal or vertical eccentricity, RF type (simple or complex), and cortical area (area 17 or 18).

3.5.2 Effect of Visual Stimulation on Receptive Field Size

Two days after lesion, we tried to make single cells expand their RF width as a result of visual training. After visual costimulation (see above), the neurons could be affected both in an unspecific or specific way. Unspecific effects were characterized by an increase in RF size directed toward both sides, the costimulated and the opposite, nonstimulated side, together with an increase in spontaneous activity and visually evoked responses within the RFs. Where a RF expansion was induced in the formerly unresponsive region at the costimulated side of the RF, but not at the nonstimulated side, a specific increase of RF width was observed in roughly half of the tested neurons (6/10). Figure 3.8A,B shows a typical example, and figure 3.8C displays the statistical evaluation of the results from the neurons with specific effects. For statistical evaluation, we concentrated on five different positions: at the RF border of the nonstimulated side, (a) just outside the RF and (b) just inside the RF; on the stimulated side, (c) in the RF center and, at the RF border, (d) just inside the RF, and (e) just outside the RF. We made three observations. The values at the nonstimulated RF border, (a) and (b) in panel C, did not differ before and after visual costimulation. Moreover, the activity just outside the RF did not differ from the spontaneous activity after costimulation; thus the RF did not expand toward this side. At the costimulated sites, visual responses were increased at both the RF center, though the difference was not significant, and the stimulated RF border, see the position just inside the RF, (d) in panel C. In addition, after costimulation, the RF was expanded at the costimulated border; the activity just outside of the RF was significantly different from the spontaneous activity ($p < 0.05$); see (c) in panel C. RF increases ranged from $0.4°$ to $0.8°$ (although the visual costimulus often extended farther than $0.8°$ across the RF boundary).

The results compared well with those obtained from normal cats (Eysel, Eyding, and Schweigart 1998; see also above). Approximately half of the neurons showed specific expansion to the costimu-

lated side of the RF and no expansion to the other, nonstimulated side. RF expansions were only modest (on the order of $1°$); the effects could be seen after 20–60 min of visual costimulation, and the induced effect lasted for approximately one hour. Visual costimulation often induced, apart from a specific RF enlargement, a slight general increase in activity (both spontaneous and visually evoked activity) in the lesioned and in the normal cortex. Thus early visual training of cells close to the border of a cortical lesion can effectively be applied to increase RF sizes of single cells by about $1°$ within minutes to one hour of training and can thereby reduce the size of the scotoma; that is, the input to an enlarged part of the RF comes from retinal regions originally within the scotoma. Thus also formerly subthreshold synapses of the synaptic "integration field" (Pei et al. 1994; Frégnac et al. 1996) may be activated by a LTP-like mechanism (Eysel, Eyding, and Schweigart 1998).

3.6   Mechanisms for Modifying Visual Receptive Fields

3.6.1   *Changes in Activity and Imbalance of Transmitter Systems*

Several studies have shown an increase in activity at the surviving border of neocortical lesions. Heat lesions in cat visual cortex yielded subnormal activity in this region of less than 1 mm around the lesion, whereas hyperactivity was only seen at 1–2.5 mm from the border of the lesion; at more distant positions (> 2.5 mm) the activity was normal (Eysel and Schmidt-Kastner 1991; for reviews, see Eysel 1997; Eysel et al. 1999). This hyperactivity after heat lesions was already present one day after the lesion and was still visible (although no longer significant)

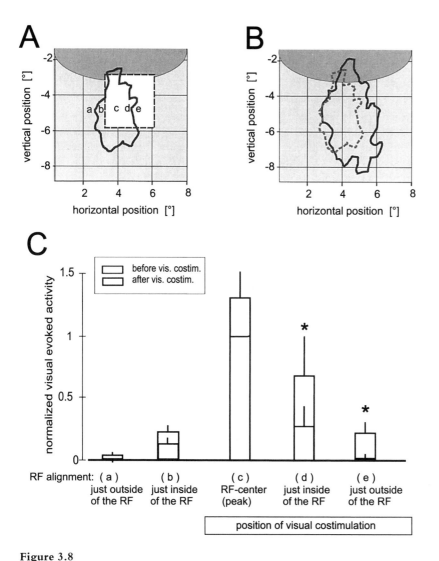

Figure 3.8

Training for receptive field (RF) size increment at the border of a 1-day (1d) visual cortical lesion. (*A*) RF size of a cell at the border of a cortical lesion after 2-day (2d) survival time (thick solid line). RF size comprises "on" and "off" response regions as obtained with the objective reverse correlation method. The cat was kept in darkness after lesioning. After the initial test, costimulation with a large field "on-off" stimulus (white square surrounded by dashed line) was applied for 60 min. (*B*) Resulting expansion of the RF is shown by the new solid line field boundaries as compared to the previous RF size (dotted line). Right visual field, with elevation (vertical position) plotted on the ordinate; horizontal position in degrees of visual angle, on the abscissa. The area of the scotoma is shown in darker gray. (*C*) In about half of the neurons investigated with the method described in panels A and B a modest but significant (* $p < 0.05$) and specific RF increase was observed. Note the significant increases of normalized activity at positions (d) and (e) on the RF side where the visual costimulation was applied. The activity after costimulation (gray columns) was significantly higher than the activity before costimulation (white columns). The average visual evoked activity (peak minus background activity) is normalized with respect to the maximal response in the RF center before costimulation (= 1) and shown for five different RF positions.

30 days after lesioning. Similar results were obtained in experiments photochemically inducing thrombosis in visual cortex (Eysel, Kretschmann, and Schmidt-Kastner 1993) and in somatosensory cortex (Domann et al. 1993; Schiene et al. 1996). Here mean discharge frequency was slightly higher in the immediate surround of the lesion (approximately 1 mm from the lesion border), but became considerably higher at a distance of 2–3.5 mm, whereas at distances greater than 4 mm lateral to the lesion border, the electrophysiological responses did not significantly differ from those of the controls. These alterations began on the first day after lesioning and were most pronounced 3–7 days after lesioning.

One possible mechanism for the increase of activity in the surround of lesions is an imbalance between GABAergic inhibition (loss) and glutamatergic excitation (increase). Mittmann et al. (1994) found that inhibitory postsynaptic potentials (IPSPs) were decreased; Schiene et al. (1996) found that GABA receptors were reduced in widespread brain areas surrounding the lesion. Changes in glutamatergic excitation were expressed in higher amplitudes and longer durations of excitatory postsynaptic potentials (EPSPs) mediated by N-methyl-D-aspartate (NMDA) receptors (Mittmann et al. 1994). The slice preparation allowed researchers to study the single-cell and network properties in the vicinity of a focal lesion in vitro. Field potentials were extracellularly recorded in the perilesional area at survival times between 1 and 6 days after lesioning (panel A of figure 3.9). Although potentials very close to the lesion were strongly depressed, as observed in vivo, in the adjacent region (1–1.5 mm from the border of the lesion), the field potentials were significantly larger than normal 1–5 days after lesioning. The enlarged potentials were blocked with d-amino-phosphono-valeric acid (APV), and thus are NMDA receptor dependent. The underlying single-cell responses

were recorded intracellularly with sharp electrodes, revealing EPSPs with longer durations and higher amplitudes in regions having increased field potentials. The upregulation of the glutamatergic responses was accompanied by a reduced GABA-mediated inhibition 1–5 days after lesion and 1–2 mm from the border of the lesions. Both the fast GABA$_A$-induced and the late GABA$_B$-induced IPSPs showed reduced amplitudes and peak currents. Although no spontaneously occurring bursts were observed, epileptiform burst activity could be evoked by strong stimuli applied to the white matter. Interestingly, after retinal lesions a quite similar hyperactive zone was found in the visual cortex at the border of the resulting cortical scotoma, where a simultaneous increase in glutamate immunoreactivity was observed (Arckens et al. 2000). On the other hand, downregulation of the GABAergic system within the cortical scotoma was demonstrated by decreased GAD immunohistochemistry (Rosier et al. 1995) and decreased GABA levels (Arckens et al. 2000).

The main lesion-induced effect may be the abovementioned increase of excitability (as indicated by increases in both spontaneous and visually evoked activity) in the surround of lesions; the changes in RF size may build on this changed excitability. A correlation of an increase in activity with an increase in RF size in visual cortical neurons was found after retinal lesions or when using the paradigm of the artificial scotoma (for review, see Gilbert 1998). When using bicuculline, a GABAergic antagonist that strongly enhances neuronal activity, RF expansion was found in the somatosensory cortex of cat and rat (Dykes et al. 1984; Kyriazi et al. 1996). These RF enlargements are discussed in terms of subthreshold inputs of intercolumnar connections that may be enhanced by the bicuculline application. Pernberg, Jirmann, and Eysel (1998) found a widening of RF subfields in cat visual cortex (A18) after local

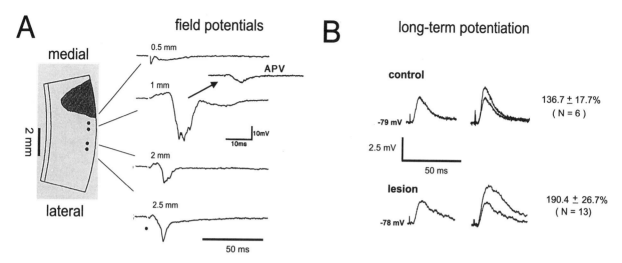

Figure 3.9
Increased field potentials and facilitated long-term potentiation in the surround of heat lesions in the rat cortex in vitro. (*A*)
Schematic drawing of the lesion with recording sites marked by black dots. The field potentials were recorded from the
cortex after electrical stimulation of the white matter. Note the depressed response very close to the border and the hyperexcitability in the adjacent recording site 1 mm from the border of the lesion. (Modified from Mittmann et al. 1994.) (*B*)
Long-term potentiation (LTP) was induced in age-matched sham-operated rats (control) and rats with 1–6 days survival
time after infrared laser lesions of the visual cortex (lesion). Postsynaptic potentials were recorded intracellularly; typical
example and statistical evaluation for 6 control and 13 lesion experiments are shown. Excitatory postsynaptic potentials
(EPSPs) had about 2.5 mV amplitudes before theta burst stimulation. During the first six days after lesioning, LTP was much
stronger in the surround of lesions (2–4 mm) than in control animals (190.4% versus 136.7%). (Adapted from Mittmann and
Eysel 1999.)

application of bicuculline. Sober et al. (1997) found
that, after subacute lesions, an increase in activity is
paralleled by an increase in RF size in macaque
middle temporal cortex (area MT, multiunit recordings). The factor of RF expansion was 1.1–7.0. As in
our work described here, the RF expansion of Sober
et al. (1997) was not consistently directed toward the
lesion. Because of the observed correlations between
RF size and excitability in these studies and our own
recent study (Schweigart and Eysel forthcoming), we
suggest that the early increase in RF size is at least
partially due to the increased excitability in individual
neurons and to already existing but primarily subthreshold synapses rising above threshold.

3.6.2 Growth Factors and Morphological Correlates of Receptive Field Plasticity

The neurotrophins brain-derived neurotrophic factor
(BDNF), neurotrophin-3 (NT-3), nerve growth factor (NGF), and insulin-like growth factor 1 (IGF-1)
have all been found to be elevated in visual cortex as
early as 3 days after binocular retinal lesions (Obata
et al. 1999); the related neurotrophin receptors were
elevated as well. This finding together with that of
increased transcription levels of calcium calmodulin–
dependent kinase II (CaMKII), microtubuli-associated protein 2 (MAP-2), and synapsins in visual
cortex after such lesions provide evidence for addi-

tional factors associated with cortical reorganization. The increased level of BDNF in turn may be related to the increased activity in regions with elevated BDNF expression (Prakash, Cohen-Cory, and Frostig 1996) and hence may combine with GABAergic and glutamatergic mechanisms to trigger the early unmasking of existing connections. Furthermore, BDNF may also represent a link to the late morphological changes involving axonal sprouting and synaptogenesis (Gilbert and Wiesel 1992; Darian-Smith and Gilbert 1994).

3.6.3 *Long-Term-Potentiation-like Effects and the Role of Learning and Training in the Visual Cortex*

The finding of enlarged receptive fields at the border of cortical lesions raised the question of how and under what special conditions cells can increase their receptive field size in the adult, completely wired visual cortex. We tested whether heterosynaptic LTP-like mechanisms might be a prime candidate for such RF changes (cf. chapter 7.1). Applying repetitive synchronous stimulation to the receptive field center of simple cells and regions just outside their receptive fields for 10 to 60 min, in many cases we were able to extend the area of the excitatory receptive field of the investigated cells specifically into the coactivated region (Eysel, Eyding, and Schweigart 1998). This effect showed a long-term recovery over hours. We interpreted this as a heterosynaptic LTP-like increase of the efficacy of formerly subthreshold inputs from the region just outside the classical excitatory receptive field. Because, according to in vitro observations (Hirsch and Gilbert 1993), lateral inhibition can suppress such LTP-like effects in cat visual cortex, reduction of lateral inhibition should facilitate LTP-like mechanisms. As mentioned above, both intracortical local inactivation (Eysel, Crook, and Machemer 1990; Crook,

Eysel, and Machemer 1991; Crook and Eysel 1992; Crook, Kisvárday and Eysel 1996) and lesions (Eysel and Schmidt-Kastner 1991; Domann et al. 1993; Mittmann et al. 1994) can reduce lateral inhibition.

A ring of increased excitability (high spontaneous activity, increased visually evoked activity) around the cortical lesion and the cortical region deafferented by a retinal lesion during the first days to weeks of survival time appears to occur in parallel to or as a consequence of increased extracellular glutamate levels in the surround of cortical lesions (Choi and Rothman 1990) and increased glutamate immunoreactivity in cells at the border of the deafferented cortex after retinal lesions (Arckens et al. 2000). A similar hyperexcitability was also present in slice preparations from animals with 1–6 days of survival time after cortical lesions in vitro. Under this condition, the NMDA receptor–mediated EPSPs were increased in the same region that was characterized by increased excitability in vivo (Mittmann et al. 1994). In addition, the fast $GABA_A$-mediated and the slower $GABA_B$-mediated IPSPs were strongly reduced (Mittmann et al. 1994) and $GABA_A$ receptors were downregulated (Schiene et al. 1996) in the region surrounding a cortical lesion. Related observations were the significantly reduced GAD immunoreactivity in the neuropil (Rosier et al. 1995) and the decreased GABA levels (Arckens et al. 2000) within the cortical scotoma resulting from retinal lesions.

The evidence to date indicates that an early shift toward locally increased excitability (both due to increased NMDA-mediated and decreased GABA-mediated transmission) accompanies or precedes neuronal reorganization in response to two quite different types of damage in the visual system: (1) retinal lesions in the eye and (2) cortical lesions in the brain. Transient local reactions of the inhibitory and excitatory cortical systems on the synaptic level are initially observed at the sites of lesion-induced reorganization irrespective of the kind of lesion. Increased excitability due to NMDA-mediated depolarization may be the most important trigger for synaptic plasticity. The reduced inhibition may play an additional important role because reduced GABAergic inhibition can lead to increased activation of NMDA receptors (Luhmann and Prince, 1991). Finally, the reduced activity in cells that are targets of synaptic reorganization may reduce the threshold for successful potentiation ("sliding threshold model"; Bienenstock et al. 1982). Based on the above-mentioned observations, we have predicted (Eysel 1997) the facilitation of LTP in the vicinity of visual cortical lesions.

Two mechanisms seem to prevail in lesion-induced and use-dependent reorganization of RF properties: a short-term mechanism acting within minutes to hours and a long-term mechanism taking weeks to months to develop (see Gilbert 1998 for review). Reorganization of the long-term mechanism, attributed to local sprouting (growth of axonal collaterals and synaptogenesis) of the long-range horizontal connections within the cortex (Darian-Smith and Gilbert 1994, 1995), ranges over some 6–8 mm in the visual cortex, although alternative pathways involving feedback projections from higher-order cortical areas have not yet been ruled out. In contrast, the short-term mechanism produces shifts of the cortical retinotopy within minutes to hours, ranging over only some 2 mm in the cortex. Because they are in the range of the spread of thalamocortical afferents and are fast, these shifts were attributed to the unmasking of formerly subthreshold thalamocortical synaptic inputs rather than to the forming of new connections (Gilbert 1998). In fact, the EPSP field area is about nine times larger than the spike discharge field (Pei et al. 1994; see also the synaptic "integration field" of Frégnac et al. 1996).

Parallel to changes in the retinotopic maps, the sizes of receptive fields in the visual cortex have also shown long-term and short-term changes in response to retinal lesions (Gilbert and Wiesel 1992; for reviews, see Chino 1997; Gilbert 1998) or artificial scotomas (Pettet and Gilbert 1992; Das and Gilbert 1995b). Moreover, RF expansion has been found after repetitive visual stimulation with stimuli covering the RF center and an unresponsive region outside the RF (Eysel, Eyding, and Schweigart 1998): the stimulus-induced RF expansion occurred in the region outside the RF that was costimulated with the RF center. At the border of focal excitotoxic lesions in the visual cortex of cats, the same repetitive stimulation protocol induced similar increases of RF size in the subacute phase (Schweigart and Eysel forthcoming).

Perceptual learning can play a key role in adult visual RF plasticity; LTP-like mechanisms are prime candidates for the underlying modifications of synaptic efficacy. Homosynaptic LTP and heterosynaptic LTP have been documented in vitro in slices of the visual cortex of adult rat (Artola and Singer 1987; Kossel, Bonhoeffer, and Bolz 1990; Kirkwood and Bear 1994) and cat (Hirsch and Gilbert 1993). Many in vivo studies have shown LTP-like changes of specific RF properties when repetitive stimulation was paired with postsynaptic depolarization in the visual cortex (Frégnac et al. 1988, 1992; Frégnac and Shulz 1999). Associative (heterosynaptic) LTP might also be the basis of the long-term effects elicited by synchronous costimulation of a nonresponsive RF region together with the excitatory center of the RF in the adult cat visual cortex in vivo (Eysel, Eyding, and Schweigart 1998). Intracortical lateral inhibition can suppress LTP in vitro (Hirsch and Gilbert 1993) and can also prevent receptive field plasticity in vivo, thus keeping the RF size and substructure stable and the subfields separated unless inhibition is reduced.

This was directly shown by the increase of RF size and loss of simple cell RF substructures when GABAergic inhibition was microiontophoretically blocked with bicuculline (Pernberg, Jirmann, and Eysel 1998). A similar shaping of RFs by inhibition was also shown by application of bicuculline in the primary somatosensory cortex of the cat (Dykes et al. 1984). Changes in the balance between excitation and inhibition were also held responsible for the fast changes in RF size observed after lesions in area MT of the macaque monkey (Sober et al. 1997). Intracortical local inactivation (Eysel, Muche, and Wörgötter 1988; Eysel, Crook, and Machemer 1990; Crook, Kisvárday, and Eysel 1998) and lesions (Eysel, Wörgötter, and Pape 1987; Eysel and Schmidt-Kastner 1991; Domann et al. 1993; Mittmann et al. 1994; Schiene et al. 1996) seem to reduce lateral inhibition. This reduction of lateral inhibition could facilitate LTP and LTP-like mechanisms. Lesions in the somatosensory cortex have been shown to induce LTP (Hagemann et al. 1998). In Mittmann and Eysel 2001, we induced LTP in vitro with repetitive stimulation of synaptic inputs combined with postsynaptic depolarization and have compared EPSPs of single cells in the normal adult rat visual cortex with those from age-matched rat cortices with focal infrared laser lesions having survival times of 1–6 days, and indeed found a significantly enhanced LTP in the surround of focal cortical lesions. Panel B of figure 3.9 exemplifies the nearly threefold facilitation of LTP in the surround of cortical lesions 1–6 days after lesioning. LTP amounted to more than 190% in the lesioned animals, whereas it amounted to less than 137% in the sham-operated controls.

On the other hand, increases in RF size were more pronounced after two months (Eysel and Schweigart 1999) than after short-term visual training (Eysel, Eyding, and Schweigart 1998; Eysel and Schweigart 1999), indicating that mechanisms of long-term recovery span larger distances and integrate across a larger cortical representation than do those of short-term recovery. The larger changes in RF size as observed in chronic phase cats seem to need longer training, longer time periods (over weeks to months), or both, and may additionally involve anatomical changes, such as axonal sprouting. This finding indicates that short-term recovery, even when using visual training, seems not sufficient for an extended recovery of lost visual function and that additional long-term mechanisms have to be effective over longer survival times. After retinal lesions, when the primary cortical reorganization has taken place on the basis of preexisting connections and functional strengthening of synaptic weights (Das and Gilbert 1995a,b), the functionally modified synaptic connections can become stabilized by terminal sprouting, as observed more than six months after retinal lesions in adult cat visual cortex (Darian-Smith and Gilbert 1994). Because these late effects after retinal lesions are preceded by early changes in RF size (Gilbert and Wiesel 1992), by a downregulation of the GABAergic system (Rosier et al. 1995), and by an upregulation of the glutamatergic system (Arckens et al. 2000), as observed at the border of cortical lesions (Mittmann et al. 1994), one can expect a similar long-term plasticity at the border of chronic lesions in adult cat visual cortex.

The above-mentioned psychophysical observations in human patients indicate that a scotoma resulting from central (postchiasmatic or postgeniculate) brain damage can be reduced in size by giving patients visual training in the border regions of their residual visual fields (Zihl and von Cramon 1979) or by locating targets within the blind field region (Zihl and von Cramon 1985; Kasten and Sabel 1995; Kasten et al. 1998). It was suggested that a correlate of this recovery of previously blind regions might be the RF expansion of surviving neurons at the border of the chronic visual cortex lesion. LTP-like mechanisms seem to be primarily involved in RF expansions in vivo, and LTP was increased early after visual cortex lesions in the surrounding tissue in vitro. Thus the effects of visual field training might be amplified, provided this training is applied in the right time window and to the cells in the right cortical locations during the early phase of postlesion recovery.

Neuronal Representation of Object Images and Effects of Learning

4

Keiji Tanaka

Abstract

Cells in the inferotemporal cortex of the monkey brain selectively respond to various moderately complex object features, with cells that respond to similar features clustering in a columnar region elongated vertically to the cortical surface. The stimulus selectivity of cells within a column is similar but not identical: there is a definite variation in the selectivity of cells within a column. The data of optical imaging have suggested that columns representing related features are located at neighboring positions with partial overlaps. The representation of a feature by multiple cells with largely overlapping but slightly differing stimulus selectivity can satisfy the two apparently conflicting requirements in visual object recognition: (1) the robustness to changes in input images due to changes in viewing condition; and (2) the preciseness of representation required in recognition at subordinate and individual levels. Because the stimulus selectivity of cells in inferotemporal cortex can be considerably changed by long-term discrimination training with new stimuli in the adult, it is clear that its neuronal machinery is kept tuned to the changing visual environment.

4.1 Introduction

Area TE, in the middle and inferior temporal gyri, represents the final purely visual stage of the occipitotemporal pathway, which is thought to be essential for visual object recognition. The occipitotemporal pathway starts at the primary visual cortex (area V1) and leads to TE after relays at areas V2, V4, and TEO (figure 4.1). Although skipping projections also exist, such as those from V2 to TEO (Nakamura et al. 1993) and those from V4 to the posterior part of TE (Desimone, Fleming, and Gross 1980), the step-by-step projections are more numerous. TE projects to various polymodal brain sites, including the perirhinal cortex, the prefrontal cortex, the amygdala, and the striatum of the basal ganglia. Because the projections to these targets are more numerous from TE, especially from the anterior part of TE, than from the areas at earlier stages (Ungerleider, Gaffan, and Pelak 1989; Barbas 1992; Yukie et al. 1990; Suzuki and Amaral 1995), there is a sequential cortical pathway from area V1 to TE, and outputs from the pathway mainly originate in TE. In monkeys, bilateral TE ablation or complete deafferentation resulted in severe and selective deficits in learning tasks that required the visual recognition of objects (Gross 1973; Dean 1976; Yaginuma et al. 1993).

4.2 Moderately Complex Features

An obstacle in the study of neuronal mechanisms of object vision has been the difficulty in determining the stimulus selectivity of individual cells. There is a great variety of object features in the natural world, and it remains to be determined how the brain scales down the variety. Although some studies (Schwartz et al. 1983; Richmond et al. 1987; Gallant, Braun, and Van Essen 1993; Gallant et al. 1996) have used mathematically perfect sets of shapes, the generality of these sets would hold only if the system were linear, which can hardly be expected in higher visual centers.

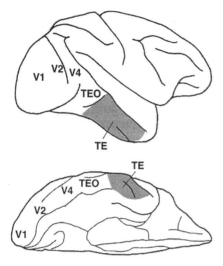

Figure 4.1
Lateral (*top*) and ventral (*bottom*) view of cortex, showing the visual cortical areas along the occipitotemporal pathway. The extent of TE is shaded.

We have developed a systematic reduction method that involves the use of a specially designed image-processing computer system (Fujita et al. 1992; Kobatake and Tanaka 1994; Ito et al. 1994, 1995; Wang, Tanifuji, and Tanaka 1998). After spike activities from a single cell were isolated, many three-dimensional animal and plant models were first presented manually to subjects to find the effective stimuli. Different aspects of the objects were then presented in different orientations. The images of several most effective stimuli were taken with a video camera and displayed on a TV monitor by the computer to determine the stimulus that evoked the maximal response. Finally, the image of the most effective stimulus was simplified step by step to determine which feature or combination of features contained in the image was essential for maximal activation. The minimal requirement for maximal activation was determined as the critical feature for

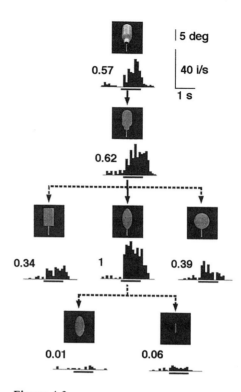

Figure 4.2
Example of the reduction process to determine the feature critical for the activation of individual cells. The responses were averaged over ten repetitions of the stimuli. Horizontal bars below histograms indicate the duration of stimulus presentation; numbers to the left, the magnitude of the maximum response. This cell was recorded from TE. (From Tanaka 1996.)

the cell. Figure 4.2 exemplifies the process for a cell, wherein the effective stimulus was reduced from the image of a water bottle to the combination of a vertical ellipse and a downward projection from the ellipse. The magnitude of responses often increased when the complexity of image was reduced, as it did for the cell illustrated in figure 4.2. This may be due to the adjustment of size, orientation, and shape as well as to the removal of other features that may

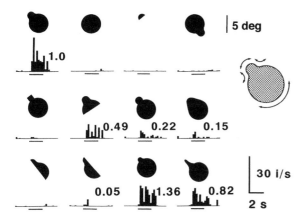

Figure 4.3
Example of further study of the selectivity after the reduction process was completed. This second cell, though different from the cell shown in figure 4.1, was also recorded from TE. Horizontal bars below histograms indicate the duration of the stimulus presentation; numbers to the right, the magnitude of the response normalized by that of the maximum response. (From Kobatake and Tanaka 1994.)

suppress the activation by the critical feature (Sato 1988, 1989, 1995; Missal, Vogels, and Orban 1997).

After the reduction was completed, the image was modified to examine the selectivity further. Figure 4.3 exemplifies this latter process for a second TE cell, one of the cases for which the domain of selectivity was most clearly determined. The cell responded maximally to the model of a pear among the routine set of object stimuli, and the critical feature was determined as "a rounded protrusion from a rounded body in the 10 o'clock direction with a concave smooth neck." The body or the head by itself did not evoke any responses. The head had to be rounded because the response disappeared when the rounded head was replaced by a square, and the body had to be rounded because the response decreased by 51% when the body was cut in half. The neck had to be smooth and concave because the

response decreased by 78% or by 85% when the neck was replaced by one with sharp corners or by a straight one, respectively. The critical feature was neither the right upper contour alone nor the left lower contour alone, because neither half of the stimulus evoked any response. The width and length of the projection were, however, not very critical, as long as the stimulus satisfied the above-described features. Thus the critical feature was defined not in the pictorial domain but in the more abstract, higher-feature domain. This point will be further supported by the data of the experiment in which the aspect ratio of the critical feature was systematically changed.

Additional examples of effective stimulus reduction for twelve other TE cells are shown in figure 4.4. The pictures to the left of the arrows are the original images of the most effective object stimuli and those to the right are the critical features determined after the reduction process. It should be noted that, even for the same object image, the directions of stimulus reduction and the final critical features were usually different from cell to cell. Some of the critical features were moderately complex shapes, whereas others were combinations of such shapes with color or texture. After determining the critical features for hundreds of cells in TE, we concluded that most cells in TE required moderately complex features for their maximal activation. The critical features for TE cells were more complex than just orientation, size, color, or simple texture, which are known to be extracted and represented by cells in area V1, but which are not complex enough to represent the image of a natural object through the activity of single cells. The combined activation of multiple cells, representing different features contained in the object image, was also necessary.

Although the critical features for the activation of TE cells are only moderately complex in general,

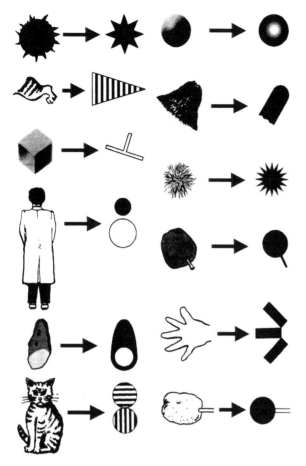

Figure 4.4
Further examples of the reduction for twelve other TE cells. Images to the left of the arrows represent the original images of the most effective object stimulus; those to the right, the critical features determined by the reduction.

there are cells that respond to faces and critically require nearly all the essential features of the face. Such cells were originally found deep in the superior temporal sulcus (Bruce, Desimone, and Gross 1981; Perrett, Rolls, and Caan 1982), but they have also been found in TE (Baylis, Rolls, and Leonard 1987). Thus there is more convergence of information onto single cells for the representation of faces than for that of nonface objects. This difference may be because discrimination of faces from other objects is not the final goal: further processing of facial images is needed to discriminate among individuals and expressions, although distinguishing a nonface object from other objects is close to the final goal.

4.3   Invariance of Responses

Our ability to recognize objects is retained even when these objects undergo many different kinds of translation in space. The invariances of recognition can, in part, be explained by invariant properties of single-cell responses in TE. By using a set of shape stimuli composed of the individually determined critical feature and several other shape stimuli obtained by modifying the critical feature, we have observed that the selectivity for shape is preserved over large receptive fields (Ito et al. 1995), although the magnitude of the response varies within the receptive field. The maximum response is usually obtained around the geometrical center of the receptive field, and the magnitude of response decreases toward the edges of the receptive field. The receptive fields of TE cells are larger than those of cells in areas in the earlier stages along the ventral visual pathway, but they are, in general, smaller than the largest receptive fields found in the dorsal visual pathway. The receptive fields of TE cells usually range from $10°$ to $30°$ in one-dimensional size.

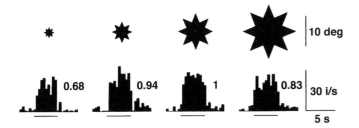

Figure 4.5
One TE cell responding to the critical feature in a wide range of size. Horizontal bars below histograms indicate the duration of the stimulus presentation; numbers to the right, the magnitude of the response normalized by that of the maximum response. (From Tanaka et al. 1991.)

The effects of changes in stimulus size, however, vary more among cells (Tanaka et al. 1991; Ito et al. 1995). Twenty-one percent of the TE cells tested responded to a size range of more than four octaves of the critical features with more than 50% maximum responses, whereas 43% of the cells responded to a size range of less than two octaves. The cell shown in figure 4.5 represents the former group. TE cells with considerable invariance for the location and size of stimuli have also been found by Lueschow, Miller, and Desimone (1994) and Logothetis, Pauls, and Poggio (1995), although these authors did not determine the critical features for individual cells. The tuned cells may be immature and those with various optimal sizes may converge to yield the size-invariant responses. Alternatively, both size-dependent and size-independent processing of images may occur in TE.

A definite number of TE cells tolerated reversal of the contrast polarity of the shapes. Contrast reversal of the critical feature evoked more than 50% of the maximum response to the critical feature in 40% of tested cells (Ito et al. 1994). Sary, Vogels, and Orban (1993) found that some TE cells responded similarly to shapes defined by difference in luminosity, direction of motion of texture components, and coarse-

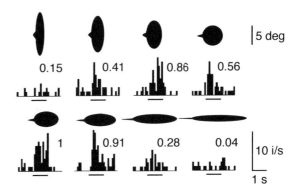

Figure 4.6
One TE cell tolerating a considerable change in the aspect ratio of the critical feature. Horizontal bars below histograms indicate the duration of the stimulus presentation; numbers to the right, the magnitude of the response normalized by that of the maximum response.

ness of texture, while maintaining their selectivity for shape.

Another kind of invariance of TE cells was found for the aspect ratio of shapes. The aspect ratio is the ratio of the size along one axis of the stimulus to that along the orthogonal axis. When an object rotates in depth, the features contained in the image change their shapes. Unless occlusion occurs, changes occur in the aspect ratio. For individual TE cells, we first

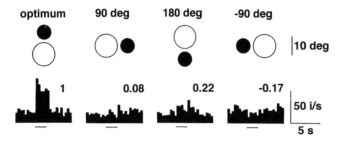

Figure 4.7
One TE cell selective for the orientation of the critical feature. Horizontal bars below histograms indicate the duration of the stimulus presentation; numbers to the right, the magnitude of the maximum response.

determined the critical feature using the reduction method, and then tested the effects of changes in the aspect ratio of the critical feature. We observed that 51% of cells responded to an aspect ratio range of more than three octaves with more than 50% of the maximum responses (Esteky and Tanaka 1998). Figure 4.6 shows an example of such cells.

Responses of TE cells are more selective for the orientation of stimuli in the frontoparallel plane (Tanaka et al. 1991). Figure 4.7 shows an example. Rotation of the critical feature by 90° decreased the response by more than 50% for most cells.

4.4   Columnar Organization in Area TE

We examined the spatial distribution of the cells responding to various critical features in area TE. By recording two TE cells simultaneously with a single electrode, we have found that cells located close together in the cortex have similar stimulus selectivities (Fujita et al. 1992). The critical feature of one isolated cell was determined by using the same procedure as described above, while the responses of another isolated cell, or nonisolated multiunits, were simultaneously recorded. In most cases, the second cell responded to the optimal and suboptimal stimuli

of the first cell. The selectivities of the two cells differed slightly, however, in that the maximal response was evoked by slightly different stimuli, or the mode of the decrease in response was different when the stimulus was changed from the optimal stimulus.

To determine the spatial extent of the clustering of cells with similar selectivities, we examined the responses of cells successively recorded along the length of long penetrations made vertically or obliquely to the cortical surface (Fujita et al. 1992). The critical feature for a cell located at the middle of the penetration was first determined. A set of stimuli, including the critical feature for the first cell, its rotated versions, and ineffective control stimuli, was constructed, and cells recorded at different positions along the penetration were tested with the fixed set of stimuli. As in the example shown in figure 4.8, cells recorded along the vertical penetrations commonly responded to the critical feature for the first cell or some related stimuli. The span of the commonly responsive cells covered nearly the entire thickness from layers II to VI. The situation, however, was different in the penetrations made obliquely to the cortical surface. The cells that were commonly responsive to the critical feature of the first cell or related stimuli were limited to within a short span

Effective stimuli

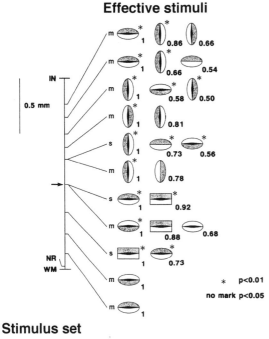

Stimulus set

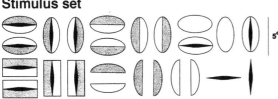

Figure 4.8
Responses of cells recorded along a vertical penetration in TE. The responsiveness of the cells was tested with the set of stimuli shown at the bottom, which were constructed in reference to the critical feature of the first cell indicated by the arrow. Effective stimuli are listed separately for individual recording sites, in the order of effectiveness; "m" indicates recording from multiunits, and "s" those from a single unit. (From Fujita et al. 1992.)

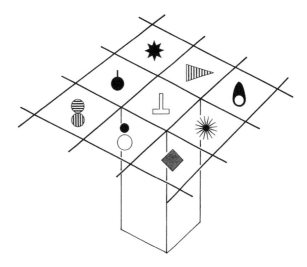

Figure 4.9
Schematic drawing of the columnar organization in TE. (From Tanaka 1996.)

around the first cell. The horizontal extent of the span was, on average, 400 μm. The cells outside the span were not responsive to any of the stimuli included in the set, or responded to some stimuli that were not effective at activating the first cell and included in the set as ineffective control stimuli. Based on these results, we proposed that TE is composed of columnar modules in each of which cells respond to similar features (figure 4.9).

4.5 Optical Imaging of the Columnar Organization

To further study the spatial properties of the columnar organization in TE, we used the technique of optical imaging with intrinsic signals (Wang, Tanaka, and Tanifuji 1996; Wang, Tanifuji, and Tanaka 1998). The cortical surface was exposed, illuminated with red light tuned to 605 nm. The reflected light image was taken by a video camera, and the reflected images for different visual stimuli compared.

At the wavelength of 605 nm, the differential components of signals mostly reflect the changes of the density of deoxidized hemoglobin in the capillaries. Activated neuronal tissue takes up more oxygen from hemoglobin, so that the density of deoxidized hemoglobin in the nearby capillaries increases. Because deoxidized hemoglobin absorbs more light than oxidized hemoglobin at the specified wavelength, the region of the cortex with elevated neuronal activities becomes darker in the reflected image; the absorption increase due to the swelling of glia cells may also make the region appear darker.

We first recorded the responses of single cells with a microelectrode to determine the critical feature, and then conducted the optical imaging. In the experiment shown in figure 4.10, the critical feature determined for a cell recorded at the cortical site indicated by the cross was the combination of a white and black horizontal bar. The post-stimulus-time histograms (PSTHs) in the left represent the cell's responses. The combination evoked a strong response in the cell, but a white bar alone or a black bar alone did not activate the cell. The images on the right were taken from the same 1 mm × 1.5 mm cortical region. A dark spot appeared around the penetration site when the monkey saw the combination of the two bars, whereas there were no dark spots around the site when the monkey saw the simpler features. Similar results were obtained in 11 out of 13 cases. Although the critical feature was determined for a single cell, a large proportion of cells in the region must be activated to produce observable metabolic change. The localized and specific occurrence of dark spots thus indicates a regional clustering of cells with similar stimulus selectivity.

On the other hand, when we observed a larger extent of the cortical surface, we found that the

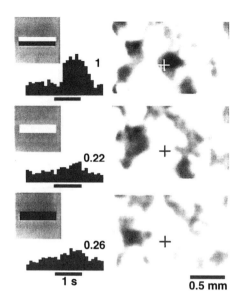

Figure 4.10
Correspondence of optical signals with neuronal activity. The histograms on the left show the responses of a cell recorded at the site indicated by the crosses in the optical images. The cell selectively responded to the combination of a white bar and black bar. The white bar alone or a black bar alone evoked much smaller responses. Correspondingly, the optical image showed a black spot covering the recording site while the monkey was seeing the combination shape, whereas there were no dark spots with the control stimuli. Horizontal bars below histograms indicate the duration of the stimulus presentation; numbers to the right, the magnitude of the response normalized by that of the maximum response. (From Wang, Tanaka, and Tanifuji 1996.)

presentation of a single feature activated multiple spots. In figure 4.11, the spots activated by eight moderately complex features are circumscribed with different kinds of lines and identified by feature number; features 1 through 4 in the upper half of the figure and features 5 through 8 in the lower half. For example, feature 1 evoked 6 spots, and feature 2 evoked 2 spots. A single feature is processed in multiple columns in TE.

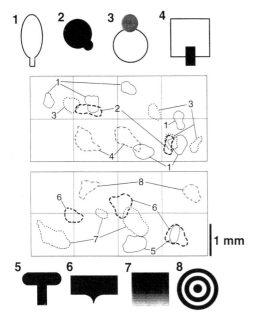

Figure 4.11
Activation maps evoked by the presentation of eight moderately complex features. To obtain the map, each image was subtracted by the reference image averaged over the images obtained for all the different stimuli combined in the experiment to remove the global darkening, the activation spots were delineated at $1/e$ of the maximum intensity in individual images. The contours of spots in the images for different stimuli are indicated by different line types.

Moreover, many of the activation spots evoked by different features overlap. Although some of the overlapping spots, which were activated by many stimuli, likely represent columns with nonselective cells, others, which were activated by only two of the stimuli, may represent specific overlaps. For many of these overlaps, we can find similarity between the two features, although the judgment of similarity is only subjective.

The partial overlapping of columns that responded to different but related features was most clearly

observed for faces presented in different views (figure 4.12). This experiment was also guided by a unit-recording experiment. We recorded five cells in one electrode penetration at around the center of the imaged region, and all of them selectively responded to faces. Three of the cells responded maximally to the front view of the face, whereas the remaining two responded to the profile, the lateral view of the face. In the optical imaging session, 5 different views of the same doll face were presented in combination with 14 nonface features. Although all of the faces evoked activation spots around the center of the illustrated 3.5×3.5 mm region, their center positions differed slightly. The contours of the dark spots are superimposed at the bottom of the figure. The activation spot moved in one direction as the face was rotated from the left profile to the right profile through the front view of the face. Individual spots were 400 to 600 μm in diameter and the overall region was 1500 μm. These regions were not activated by the 14 nonface features.

Similar results, namely, selective activation by faces and systematic shift of the activation spot with the rotation of the face, were obtained for three other monkeys, in which optical imaging was not guided by the unit recording. When the recording chamber with an inner diameter of 18 mm was placed in the same part of TE, the face-selective activation was found at roughly the same location (approximately, the posterior third of TE, on the lateral surface close to the lip of the superior temporal sulcus). The effects of rotating the face around a different axis (the chin up and down) and of changing the facial expression were also tested in some of the experiments, but neither of these caused a shift in the activation spot. Only two faces were tested: a human face and a doll's face. The two faces activated mostly overlapping regions. There are two possible interpretations for this result: either (1) the variations

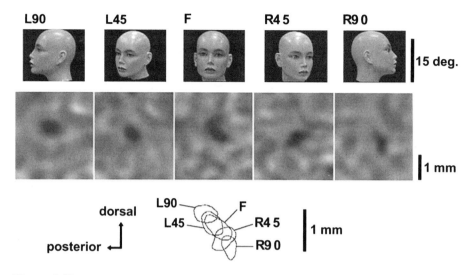

Figure 4.12
Systematic movement of the activation spot with rotation of the face. The images were obtained for five different views of the same doll face shown at top. The reference image obtained by averaging the five images has been subtracted. The contours circumscribing the pixels with *t*-values at $p < 0.05$, compared with the reference image, are superimposed at the bottom. (From Wang, Tanaka, and Tanifuji 1996.)

other than those with horizontal rotation are represented at different sites not covered by the recording chamber in the experiments or (2) only the variations along the horizontal rotation are explicitly mapped along the cortical surface as the first principal component, and other variations are imbedded in overlapping cell populations.

Although the data for the nonface features are more limited, I hypothesize that nonface and face features involve similar structures and propose a modified model of the columnar organization in TE in figure 4.13. The borders between neighboring columns are not necessarily distinctive. Instead, multiple columns that represent different but related features partially overlap with one another and as a whole compose a larger-scale unit. At least in some cases, some parameter of the features is continuously mapped along the cortical surface.

This systematic arrangement of related columns can be used for various kinds of computation necessary for object recognition. One simple possible computation is the generalization of activation by the horizontal excitatory connections (cf. chapter 1) to nearby columns representing related features, which we might call "selective blurring of activation." Another is the mutual inhibition among the nearby columns for winner-takes-all type selection.

The continuous mapping of different views of faces cannot be generalized to nonface objects. Because the critical features for TE cells are only moderately complex except in the case of faces, the image of a nonface object has to be represented by a combination of activations at multiple cortical sites. Rotation of a nonface object causes shifts of activation at multiple cortical sites, each of which corresponds to the partial change of a feature. To uncover

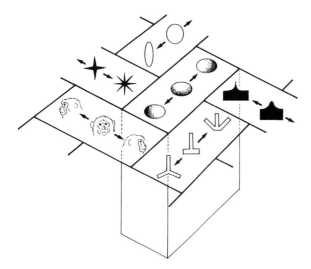

Figure 4.13
Revised schematic diagram of the columnar organization in TE. (From Tanaka 1996.)

the functional architecture in TE, we need to further examine the parameters along which the activation moves in nonface columns.

4.6 Changeability of the Selectivity in the Adult

The selectivity of inferotemporal cells can be changed in adult animals by long-term training. We found this by training two adult monkeys for the recognition of the twenty-eight moderately complex shapes shown on the left in figure 4.14 and recording from inferotemporal cells after the training (Kobatake, Wang, and Tanaka 1998). The training paradigm was a kind of delayed matching to sample shown on the right in figure 4.14. A stimulus, randomly selected from the set of twenty-eight stimuli, appeared on a television display as a sample, the monkey touched it, and the sample disappeared. After a delay period,

the sample appeared again on the display, together with four other stimuli randomly selected from the stimulus set. The monkey selected the sample and touched it to get a drop of juice as a reward. After an intertrial interval, the trial was repeated with a different sample. The monkey performed the task on a stand-alone apparatus placed in front of the home cage, coming to the apparatus and practicing the task whenever it wanted. The training was started with a 1 sec delay, and the delay was increased gradually to 16 sec. At the end of the training, the monkey performed 500 successful trials with greater than 80% correct responses.

After the training was completed, we prepared the monkeys for repeated recordings, and conducted recordings from TE under anesthesia, once a week for three to four months. Training was continued on the days when recordings were not conducted. From the same set of animal and plant models we used for the stimulus reduction experiment, we determined the most effective stimulus for individual cells, and the response to this best object stimulus was compared with the responses of the same cell to the training stimuli. In this experiment, we did not conduct the reduction process, but just took the images of several most effective object stimuli with a video camera and presented them under computer control in combination with the training stimuli.

Although the cell illustrated in figure 4.15 responded maximally to the sight of a watermelon among the object stimuli, it responded still more strongly to the cross shape, which was one of the training stimuli. There were also responses to several other training stimuli. Many cells recorded from the trained monkeys responded more strongly to some of the training stimuli than to the best object stimulus, as in this example.

To quantitatively compare the results obtained from the two trained monkeys with those obtained

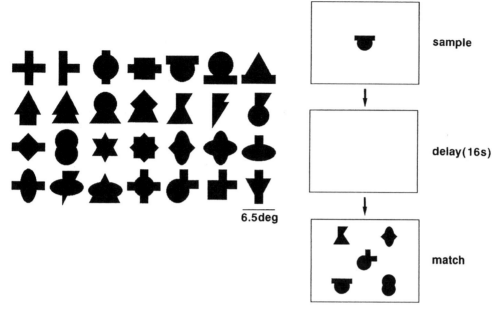

Figure 4.14
Twenty-eight shapes used for the training (*left*) and in paradigm (*right*).

from three untrained control monkeys, we calculated the ratio of the maximal response to the training stimuli to the cell's overall maximal response and compared its distribution between the two groups (figure 4.16). The *x*-axis in the figure is the ratio, and the *y*-axis the proportion of cells. The top histogram shows the distribution among 131 cells recorded in the trained monkeys, and the bottom histogram shows the distribution for the same number of cells recorded from the three control monkeys. One on the *x*-axis signifies that the cell was maximally activated by some of the training stimuli, and "0" signifies that the cell was not activated at all by any of the training stimuli. Twenty-five percent of the cells recorded from the trained monkeys responded maximally to some of the training stimuli, whereas only 5% of the cells recorded from the con-

trol monkeys responded maximally to some of the stimuli. These results indicate that the number of cells maximally responsive to training stimuli increased during the period of the discrimination training. Sakai and Miyashita (1991, 1994) and Logothetis, Pauls, and Poggio (1995; see also Sheinberg and Logothetis, chapter 6, this volume) had trained adult monkeys to discriminate among fractal patterns or wire-frame objects and found that many TE cells responded to the learned stimuli after the training. A unique contribution of our study is the demonstration that training increases the proportion of TE cells that respond to the learned stimuli, as measured against untrained controls.

The responses to the training stimuli, rather than being sharply tuned to a particular stimulus, were distributed for several different training stimuli; in-

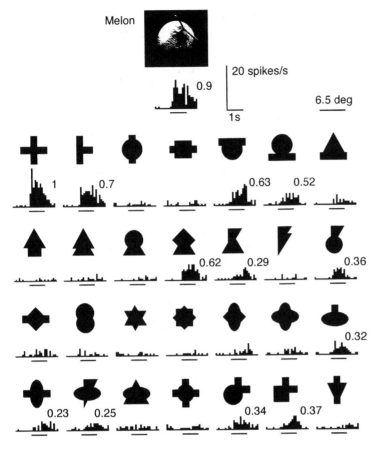

Figure 4.15
Responses of one TE cell to the image of the most effective object stimulus (*top*) and its responses to the twenty-eight stimuli used for the training. This cell was recorded from a monkey that had been trained with the twenty-eight stimuli. Statistically significant responses ($p < 0.05$) are labeled with their relative response magnitudes. Horizontal bars below histograms indicate the duration of the stimulus presentation; numbers to the right, the magnitude of the response normalized by that of the maximum response. (From Kobatake et al. 1998.)

deed, detectors of particular training stimuli did not appear. Such training effects were also found in responses of the cells to the eight stimuli shown in panel A of figure 4.17. These stimuli, referred to as "hidden stimuli," were not used during the training, but were presented for the single-cell recordings under anesthesia. Because they were composed of the same primitives as those of the training stimuli,

taken together, they covered the feature space occupied by the set of training stimuli. Cells recorded from the two trained monkeys responded to these hidden stimuli very well. The histogram at the middle of panel B shows the distribution of the normalized magnitude of individual responses to the hidden stimuli of TE cells recorded from the trained monkeys. It was nearly the same as the distribution of the

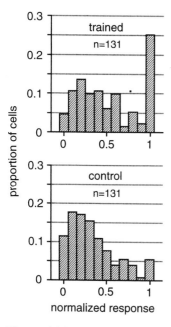

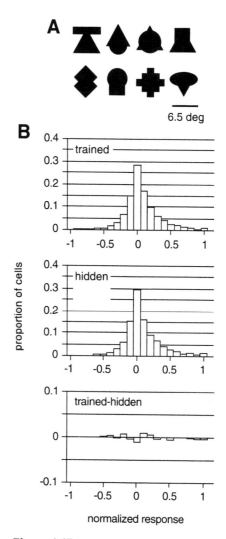

Figure 4.16
Distribution of the normalized magnitude of the strongest responses of individual cells to the training stimuli. Responses from 131 TE cells recorded from the two trained monkeys are shown at the top; those from 130 TE cells recorded from the three control monkeys are shown at bottom. The magnitude of the response was normalized with respect to the maximal response of the cell (the larger of the strongest responses of the cell to the reference object stimuli and to the training stimuli). (From Kobatake et al. 1998.)

normalized magnitude of the same cells to the training stimuli shown at the top of panel B. The difference between the two distributions, plotted at the bottom of the panel, was not significant. These results suggest that the training-induced changes in TE cells did not arise from individual cells becoming tuned to particular stimuli. Rather, these changes may have arisen owing to the feature space in which the training stimuli were distributed becoming more densely covered by TE cells.

Figure 4.17
Spread of training effects. (*A*) Eight stimuli not used for training but presented during the recordings under anesthesia. They are referred to as "hidden stimuli." (*B*) Distribution of the response magnitudes to the individual training stimuli of the cells recorded in the trained monkeys (*top*), distribution of the magnitudes of responses of the same cells to the individual hidden stimuli (*middle*), and the difference between the two distributions (*bottom*).

We investigated the properties of the distributed coding of the training stimuli by examining the correlation between the responses of two cells to the twenty-eight training stimuli. The correlation here is between the magnitude of responses (represented by the mean firing rate above the spontaneous firing level during the whole response period) to the same stimuli. The cell pairs were recorded at different times and in different penetrations. The correlations in four pairs are illustrated in the upper part of figure 4.18. The x-axis is the normalized response of cell 1, the y-axis the normalized response of cell 2, and there are 28 dots corresponding to the 28 training stimuli. In many pairs, including the two shown on the left in figure 4.18, the two cells responded to different sets of stimuli (thus there are no dots at the top right corners in the graphs). These pairs are not of interest for the purpose of analysis here. There were pairs whose responses overlapped partially, that is, the same stimuli evoked strong responses in both cells (as the two pairs shown on the right in figure 4.18). In these pairs, a group of stimuli evoked strong responses in both cells (indicated by the dots at the top right corners of the graphs), although there was always a second group of stimuli that evoked strong responses only in cell 1, and a third group that evoked strong responses only in cell 2. These results are consistent with the speculation that the responses of the cells were tuned to features contained in the stimuli, and not to the whole shape of the stimuli. Cell 1 responded to feature 1, whereas cell 2 responded to feature 2. Both cells responded to the first group of stimuli because the stimuli had feature 1 and feature 2. Only one cell responded to the second and third groups of stimuli because they had only one of the features. The correlation coefficient between the responses of the two cells tended to be very small and distributed around 0, as shown at the bottom of figure 4.18. Only a few pairs showed correlation coefficients larger than 0.5.

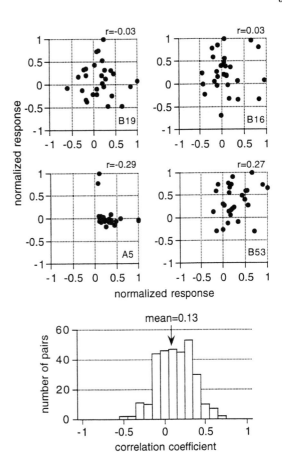

Figure 4.18
Independence of responsivity to different training stimuli among cells recorded in trained monkeys. (*Top*) Four examples of the scatter diagrams showing the correlation between the responses of two cells to the twenty-eight training stimuli. The x value of an individual dot represents the magnitude of the response elicited by one training stimulus in one cell of the pair, and the y value of the dot represents the magnitude of the response elicited by the same stimulus in the other cell of the pair. There are twenty-eight dots corresponding to the twenty-eight training stimuli. The values of r represent Pearson's correlation coefficient for the distribution. (*Bottom*) Distribution of Pearson's correlation coefficients among 309 cell pairs in which at least one training stimulus evoked responses exceeding 50% of the maximal response of either cell.

4.7   Functions of the Columnar Organization in Area TE

The finding of columnar organization in area TE has prompted investigation of the mechanism of object recognition based on the anatomical structure and physiological properties of neurons and networks. Representation by multiple cells in a columnar module, in which the selectivity varies from cell to cell, with effective stimuli largely overlapping, can satisfy two apparently conflicting requirements in visual recognition: the ability to disregard subtle changes in input images, on the one hand, and the preciseness of representation on the other. Although the image of an object projected onto the retina changes with changes in illumination, viewing angle, and pose of the object, the global organization of outputs from TE must change little. The clustering of cells with overlapping and slightly differing selectivities works as a buffer to absorb the changes. Although the responses of single cells in TE tolerate some changes in size, contrast polarity, and aspect ratio, these invariant properties at the single-cell level are not sufficient to explain the full range of flexibility exhibited by our object recognition. In particular, the responses of TE cells are generally selective for the orientation of the shape in the frontoparallel plane. Cells preferring different orientations and other parameters of the same three-dimensional shape may be packed in a column to provide invariant outputs. Whether signals from these selective cells converge to a group of single cells that show invariant responses is a matter for further discussion and investigation. Outputs of the cells preferring different orientations, sizes, aspect ratios, and contrast polarities of the same shape may overlap in the target structure to evoke the same effects. Indeed, one anatomical study (Cheng and Tanaka 1997), where

anterograde tracer was injected into a focal site in TE, suggested that the projections from TE to the ventrocaudal striatum of the basal ganglia have this property.

The representation by multiple cells with overlapping selectivities can be more precise than a mere summation of representations by individual cells. A subtle change in a particular feature, which does not markedly change the activity of individual cells, can be coded by the differences in the activities of cells with overlapping and slightly different selectivities. The projections from the ventroanterior part of TE to the perirhinal cortex have extensive divergence (Saleem and Tanaka 1996). The projection terminals from a single site of ventroanterior TE covers about 50% of the perirhinal cortex. This divergence in projections may distribute the subtle differences over a larger area of the perirhinal cortex so that objects recognized at individual levels can be distinctively associated with other kinds of information.

The function of the columnar organization in TE may go beyond the discrimination of input images. The results of the optical imaging experiments suggested that there is a continuous mapping of features within cortical units about 1.5 mm long across the cortical surface. The continuous mapping may be the structural basis for computing mapped features based on the local neuronal connections between the cells representing related but different features. Such computations may serve to transfer the image of an object for three-dimensional rotations, and to produce the image under different illumination conditions or different articulation poses. Thus the columnar organization of TE may enable overlapping and continuous representation of object features, on which various kinds of computations can be performed.

Electrophysiological Correlates of Perceptual Learning

5

Aniek Schoups

Abstract

In contrast to what is traditionally associated with memory, localized partly in the temporal lobe, some basic forms of learning probably involve much earlier stages of processing, even primary sensory cortex, and are associated with an improved ability to discriminate simple stimulus attributes, such as pitch, orientation, and texture. This chapter reviews studies investigating how neurons become better at coding for these simple stimulus attributes, how the brain codes for a particular stimulus attribute, and how this coding changes as a result of training. Researchers have only begun to understand these matters, and many possibilities remain to be studied. Are the changes to be found in the responses of the individual neurons, or should we look at them as a population? Are fewer neurons necessary for a particular task after extensive training? Are the same brain areas used when subjects are exposed to a stimulus for the first time as when they are extensively trained in identifying a particular attribute of that stimulus? Are other circuits being used? Because many indications of the "what" and "where" of the neurophysiological correlates of learning come from studies on cortical plasticity, the chapter turns first to studies of how cortical representation maps are modified and how neurons respond in a variety of conditions, from manipulations of the neuronal discharge, intracortical microstimulation, denervation, and digit amputation to enriched environments and enhanced use, before considering studies, my own included, of the most natural manifestation of plasticity: learning.

Over the last decade or two, it has become increasingly clear that sensory systems modify and reorganize in adult animals. The once predominant view of the adult brain as a static and fixed entity is long gone. All areas of cortex are capable of change, which can be induced by lesions, use, attention, and experience. Much of the interest in cortical plasticity stems from its potential relevance to learning. Are the same mechanisms applied by the brain during development, during recovery from a peripheral or central nervous system lesion, and during learning? The profound changes in adult cortical functioning and architecture observed in experiments where part of the cortex is deprived of its normal input most likely reflect how the brain recovers from lesions, just as use-induced changes most likely reflect how it reacts to stimulation and experience. But even more, these manifestations of cortical plasticity may reflect adaptive mechanisms associated with simple forms of learning such as perceptual learning. On the other hand, simply because the same kind of modifications are observed in learning and other conditions does not, in itself, mean that the mechanisms are the same.

When positing that a particular neuronal change is a manifestation of learning, there should be some behavioral index that attests to a particular instance of learning, and there should be a correlation between the changes in behavior and the changes in neurophysiology. Moreover, the processes underlying the observed "perceptual learning" should always be examined. Improved performance in a sensory discrimination task could reflect learning to perform the task, or it could reflect the development of an optimal attentional or performance strategy. The more interesting forms of perceptual learning involve improvement in sensory capacity per se, and thus should involve modifications of the sensory representations in the brain. The neurophysiological correlates of perceptual learning are to be found in that area of the brain where processing of a particular stimulus attribute occurs.

This brings us to another consideration about the neurophysiological correlates of perceptual learning: the link between neuronal activity and perception. The difficult task of understanding the neural mechanisms underlying improvements in sensory capacity is compounded by our failure to understand exactly how the cortex processes information. We expect to find changes in aspects or characteristics of the neuronal response responsible for coding a particular stimulus attribute that a subject is learning about. But very often, it is not clear what in a neuron's firing pattern determines the code for a particular stimulus attribute. Is it the size of the neuron's receptive field (RF)? Is it the sharpness of tuning, the strength of firing (cf. chapters 4, 6), or perhaps the variability of the neuron's firing rate, or even the latency of its response?

Traditionally, we start from the assumption that information is carried in the time-averaged firing rate. The alternative to this rate code is the temporal code, where temporal aspects such as interspike intervals and occurrence of bursts, rather than total spike count, carry the information.

The search for neurophysiological correlates of perceptual learning, especially when considering a visual task, is made even more difficult by the uncertainty of where the changes could occur. About 50% of our brain takes care of how we see things, and neurons in many areas, although specialized to a great extent, still show overlapping characteristics. Traditionally, the principal indicator for localizing the neurophysiological correlates of perceptual learning that involves changes in sensory capacity is

their specificity. Whereas "higher-order" learning generalizes to other tasks, some forms of perceptual learning are highly specific to the particular stimulus attributes used while training. Although these findings suggest an early cortical site of plasticity, where the physiological characteristics of the neurons and their spatial organization correspond to the psychophysical characteristics of the learning effect, we should be cautious: neurons in higher-order areas might exhibit the characteristics of neurons in lower-order areas as a consequence of training.

5.1   Lesion- and Use-Dependent Plasticity

Experimental manipulations such as nerve crush or transection, digit amputation, surgical syndactyly, skin translocation, or dorsal rhizotomy, on the one hand, and intracortical microstimulation or enhanced use, on the other, have been very important to demonstrate how primary cortical sensory areas remain under the influence of peripheral sensory activity throughout life (see Dinse and Merzenich, chapter 2, this volume). These studies demonstrated changes in the organization of the topographic maps in primary sensory cortex. Reorganizations were demonstrated not only for the somatosensory and barrel cortex, but also for the auditory cortex and the visual cortex (for review, see Buonomano and Merzenich 1998a). The timescale over which these changes occurred ranges from minutes to weeks. For example, in the visual cortex, within minutes after making a retinal lesion, cortical RFs near the boundary of the lesion expanded in size, and the area of cortex initially silenced to stimulation of the lesioned area recovered input from the surrounding area (see Eysel, chapter 3, this volume). These changes are most likely attributable to long-range intrinsic horizontal connections (Gilbert 1998, cf. also chapter 1).

5.2 Perceptual Learning and Physiological Correlates in Somatosensory and Auditory Cortex

However interesting, studies on lesion- or use-dependent plasticity still lack the behavioral index of learning. Dinse and Merzenich (chapter 2, this volume) describe a few innovating studies involving true perceptual learning, and the neuronal changes in somatosensory, motor, and auditory cortex that accompanied this form of learning. Of the electrophysiological changes observed in somatosensory cortical areas 3b and 3a (Recanzone, Jenkins et al. 1992; Recanzone, Merzenich, et al. 1992; Recanzone, Merzenich, and Jenkins 1992; Recanzone, Merzenich, and Schreiner 1992), the topographic reorganization in area 3b received the most attention: the representations of the restricted skin location trained in the behavioral task were significantly greater in area 3b than the representations of equivalent skin locations on control digits. Recanzone and coworkers also observed increases in receptive field size and response amplitude, as well as changes in the temporal response characteristics. When they tried to relate those neuronal changes with the behavioral performance, however, neither the strength of the responses, the RF size, nor the extent of the cortical representation was relevant in predicting the animal's behavior. We still do not know what percentage of neurons must exhibit selective changes for a map reorganization to occur. Indeed, not until Recanzone, Merzenich, and Schreiner (1992) examined a subpopulation of cortical neurons that consistently responded at an early time within the stimulus cycle was a good fit to the behavioral data obtained. Thus only changes in the timing of the response were found to correlate with the discrimination performance of the animals, specifically, an increase in the

temporal fidelity of the response evoked by stimulation of a trained digit. The response became more closely locked to the time course of the stimulus, leading to greater synchrony in the firing. In the normal adult, it is likely that temporal and not spatial response properties of these cortical neurons encode the required information for successfully discriminating tactile frequency differences (Mountcastle, Steinmetz, and Romo 1990). Changes in these temporal response properties may thus account for the animal's improved ability to make temporal distinctions about applied stimuli after extensive training.

Another experiment by Recanzone, Schreiner, and Merzenich (1993) used perceptual learning in tone frequency discrimination to study its effects on the tonotopic organization in area A1, primary auditory cortex. Monkeys were trained to discriminate small differences in the frequency of sequentially presented pairs of tone pips. The frequency of the first tone pip was constant in any given frequency discrimination task. For the comparison or S1 stimulus, both tone pips of the pair were equal in frequency (the standard frequency), and the monkey had to maintain contact with a mold bar. For the target or S2 stimulus, the frequency of the second tone pip was higher than the standard frequency, and the monkey had to release the bar to obtain a reward. At the end of the training period, monkeys were put under general anesthesia and the tonotopic organization of area A1 defined by recording multi-unit responses at 70–258 different locations. These responses were compared to those derived from normal (naïve) monkeys, and to those from monkeys receiving the same auditory stimuli but engaged in a different task. The results indicated that the total cortical area responding to the behaviorally relevant frequency was larger in trained monkeys than in control monkeys. Although sharper tuning curves and longer latencies were also observed after training, the cortical area of representation was the only parameter that correlated with behavioral performance.

The reorganization described here involved a dimension already present at the sensory periphery: selectivity for pure tone frequency. Moreover, the auditory cortex is organized in a tonotopic manner. Studies using associative training had previously shown a selective retuning at the frequency significant during training, a retuning that did not occur after pseudoconditioning. Associating a simple tone of a defined frequency with an aversive stimulus (foot shock) causes cells in primary auditory cortex to increase their response to tones of that frequency, even for cells whose pretraining best frequency is different from the conditioning frequency (Weinberger 1995; most experiments performed in guinea pig). Thus the cortical area responding to the trained frequency was found to be larger than that responding to other frequencies, a logical consequence of the neurons' having shifted their tuning to the trained (or CS) frequency.

In another study on auditory discrimination training in the unanesthetized Mongolian gerbils, the spectrotemporal characteristics of the responses of primary auditory cortex were examined by Ohl and Scheich (1997), who found both response increases and decreases, with the decreases occurring much earlier than the increases. Their findings suggest that the temporal organization of the neuronal discharges is more important than the spike rates in looking for the neuronal substrate of information processing during learning.

5.3   Experience–Dependent Plasticity and Perceptual Learning in the Visual System: Electrophysiological Correlates

In the visual cortex, much research on plasticity, mainly use-dependent plasticity, is based on observations obtained in the developing visual system. The primary visual cortex is organized in vertical columns, such as ocular dominance columns, which group together cells with a similar ocular dominance, and orientation columns, which group together cells with the same orientation preference (cf. chapter 1). Although the role of activity in modulating the formation of ocular dominance columns has been well established (Hubel and Wiesel 1962), its role in constructing higher-order receptive field properties, such as orientation selectivity, remains controversial. That some neurons seem to shift their orientation preference toward the experienced orientation upon enhanced exposure to a particular orientation is supported by studies of kittens reared with a biased orientation, such as those reared in striped cylinders (Blakemore and Cooper 1970; Stryker and Sherk 1975; Sengpiel, Stawinski, and Bonhoeffer 1999), those reared with goggles containing images of lines of a single orientation (Stryker et al. 1978), or those reared with strong cylindrical lenses that blur all but a narrow range of contour orientations (Freeman and Pettigrew 1973). On the other hand, cortical orientation maps are remarkably stable during the maturation period of orientation tuning, indicating that visual experience is certainly not the only determinant of cortical orientation selectivity during development (Frégnac and Imbert 1978; Godecke and Bonhoeffer 1996).

As described above, after the so-called critical period, once considered as the only period of plasticity, restricted to early postnatal development, there is ample evidence for lesion-induced plasticity in the adult primary visual cortex, as well. Retinal lesions were found to lead to remapping of the cortical topography, with a shrinkage of the representation of the retinal lesion and an expansion of that of the surrounding part of the retina (Kaas et al. 1990; Chino et al. 1992; Gilbert and Wiesel 1992; see Eysel, chapter 3, this volume).

Extensive use or experience also seems to shape our perception: when alphanumeric characters that are commonly tilted clockwise, such as displayed by digital clocks, are presented with a clockwise tilt, they are perceived as less tilted than the same characters horizontally inverted (Whitaker and McGraw 2000). This form of permanent adaptation must find a neurophysiological correlate in the visual neurons coding for orientation.

Cellular conditioning as a form of learning was also used in the visual system to demonstrate cortical plasticity. For example, Frégnac et al. (1988) used extracellular recordings from orientation-selective cells in kittens and cats and paired iontophoretically driven neuronal activity with presentation of bars of light of varying orientation. A significant proportion (32%) of the sampled neurons exhibited a shift in orientation preference to the orientation that was paired with neuronal activity.

Besides the study presented below, two other recent studies of perceptual learning in the visual system have linked behavioral improvement to an improved neuronal performance. In the middle temporal visual area (MT) and the medial superior temporal area (MST), neurons have large receptive fields and are typically direction selective. The first study (Zohary et al. 1994) found that improvement in direction discrimination at one position in the subject's visual field transferred to another location, indicating that the site of the learning effect most likely is at the level of area MT or MST. Within one training session, the increase in perceptual sensitivity was accompanied by an improvement in neuronal sensitivity that mirrored the perceptual effect both in magnitude and in time course, although the neuronal improvement proved to be transient: during long-term training, it was not consolidated into long-term gains in neuronal sensitivity (Zohary and Newsome 1994).

The second study (Rainer and Miller 2000) looked at the ability to recognize objects, and found a neuronal correlate in the prefrontal (PF) cortex, which receives input from the inferotemporal (IT) cortex, and plays a role in behaviors that involve discriminating and remembering visual stimuli. Although familiar objects were found to activate a smaller population of PF neurons than did novel objects, these fewer neurons were more narrowly tuned, and their object representation, more resistant to the effects of degradation after experience. Interestingly, the largest improvements in neuronal performance with familiarity were evident at the same stimulus levels for which there was also the largest improvement in behavioral performance.

The link between psychophysics and neurophysiology has also been the main interest of my coworkers and me. We have used orientation discrimination as a probe of early perceptual learning. Orientation is a simple stimulus attribute that is first and probably best coded for by neurons in primary visual cortex (area V1). Our main focus has been to find the neuronal changes responsible for better coding by the neuronal population and eventually for better behavioral performance. To study the electrophysiological correlates in the adult macaque monkey, we have used the following protocol: a monkey was intensively trained on an orientation discrimination task. By recording from single units while the monkey was awake and performing a fixation task, we could fully characterize the tuning properties of different populations of neurons. The purpose was to unravel changes in the firing pattern of trained neurons that not only appear as a result of training but, more importantly, could be responsible for the improvement in the sensory discrimination task.

The behavioral correlates of this type of perceptual learning were documented previously in humans

A

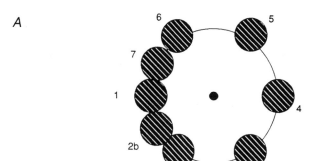

B

Subject A.S.

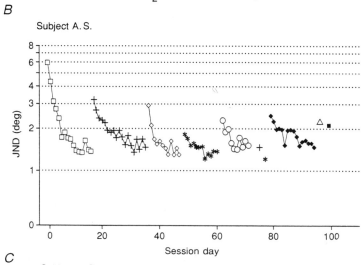

C

Subject A.C.

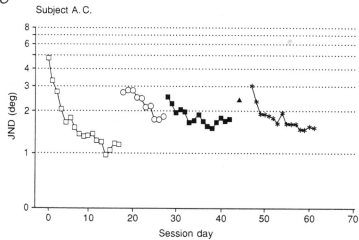

(Schoups, Vogels, and Orban 1995; Vogels and Orban 1985), and were then repeated in monkeys. Subjects were trained daily in identifying the oblique orientation of a small circular grating, always at the same position in their visual field. Only one orientation, tilted either clockwise or counterclockwise with respect to the oblique reference orientation, was shown on each trial, and the monkey had to indicate its decision by a saccade to a point above or below the stimulus position. The reference orientation was never shown. We strongly emphasized that any improvement observed had to originate at the sensory level and could not be attributed to a change in strategy. The phase was randomized so that the only cue that could be used to solve the task was the orientation of the bars in the grating. The monkeys, just like the human subjects, improved their performance, with a large improvement initially, and with smaller improvements as training continued. Improvement was most evident between sessions. The most interesting results were the specificity of the learning effect: the improvement was highly specific to the position of the stimulus during training. A mere displacement of the stimulus after training to an adjacent position caused a marked increase in threshold (figure 5.1). Similarly, no transfer was observed between orientations (figure 5.2). On the other hand, complete transfer was observed between the two eyes (cf. chapters 9.5, 14.3.1, but also 10.3.4, 11.6).

The specificity for the trained orientation and the highly precise specificity for position together sug-

gest that the neuronal correlates for this type of perceptual learning are likely to be found early in the visual processing pathway. Indeed, nowhere in the brain are receptive fields as small as they are in area V1. Moreover, early in the visual processing pathway, neurons with similar orientation preferences are grouped together, segregated in space from neurons with an orthogonal orientation preference. Instances of learning could thus be associated with neurons tuned to one orientation without development of an equivalent association with neurons tuned to an orthogonal orientation. Extremely well suited to code orientation, neurons in area V1 show a typical orientation tuning curve, characterized by the neurons' preferred orientation and by the selectivity of tuning or sharpness of the tuning curve (see figure 5.3).

This specificity for both position and orientation provided us with an interesting internal control: instead of comparing data from trained monkeys with those from naïve monkeys, we could use different populations of neurons within the same monkey. Indeed, neurons that have their RF at an untrained position in the monkey's visual field could serve as a naïve population of neurons. The trained population of neurons consisted of neurons that had their RF at the trained positions. Within this population of neurons, we specifically looked for changes in their responses to the trained orientation.

We introduced a second control population of neurons. During training, a second stimulus appeared

Figure 5.1
Position specificity of perceptual learning in orientation discrimination tested in two human subjects. (*A*) Overview of the different positions for the grating (2.5° diameter) in the subjects' visual field. The black dot in the center represents the subject's fixation point. (*B*) Learning curves for subject A.S. Just-noticeable differences (JND) represent the subject's thresholds. Orientation discrimination was first tested and trained at a central position, then different positions at 5° eccentricity were tested and further trained. □ = foveal position; + = position 1; ◇ = position 2; * = position 3; ○ = position 4; ◆ = position 5; △ = position 6; ■ = position 7. (*C*) Learning curves for subject A.C. □ = foveal position; ○ = position 6; ■ = position 2; * = position 4; ▲ = position 2b. (Schoups, Vogels, and Orban 1995, figure 4.)

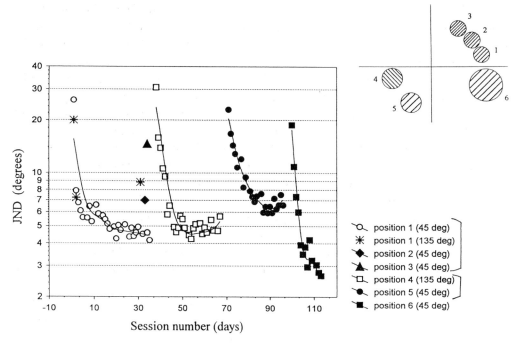

Figure 5.2
Specificity for stimulus position and orientation in a macaque monkey trained for orientation discrimination learning. Graph (*left*) shows the just noticeable differences (JND) that the monkey could discriminate; shaded circles (*upper right*) indicate stimulus positions and orientations of the grating tested. Orientation discrimination with the stimulus at position 1 was tested first for both oblique orientations, then training was continued for the 45° only. When threshold was reached, performance for the nontrained oblique was tested again and found to be worse than before training the 45°. Orientation discrimination with the stimulus at positions 2 and 3 in the same quadrant as position 1 were tested only once, without further training. Some transfer was found for these stimulus positions, probably due to the monkey's fixation errors during training. Untrained performance for the stimulus at positions 4, 5, and 6 in other quadrants were worse than for positions in the same quadrant.

at a different position in the monkey's visual field. Its orientation was randomly picked from a narrow range of orientations around the oblique reference orientation, orthogonal to the trained orientation. The monkey learned to ignore this stimulus, but at the same time, the neurons that responded to stimuli at that location were being exposed to the stimuli as many times as the trained neurons, only they did not learn the task.

These findings were always tested behaviorally: after the recordings, we tested the monkey's behavior for the stimulus at the trained position, for the trained as well as other orientations; we also tested the monkey's performance to identify these orientations for a stimulus shown at the two control positions, one completely naïve, and one passively stimulated. Only for the trained orientation, at the trained position, did the monkey perform well; its threshold for other

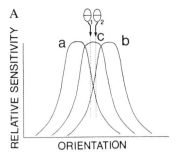

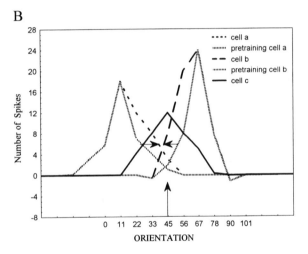

Figure 5.3

(*A*) When the orientation of a grating stimulus changes slightly from 1 to 2 (marked by arrows), the response of the most active of the hypothetical orientation-tuned neurons (neuron c) changes negligibly, but there is a substantial change in the relative activations of neurons a and b. (Regan and Beverley 1985, figure 5.) (*B*) Theoretical scheme for possible tuning function changes in area V1 neurons after perceptual learning in an orientation discrimination task (for training around 45°). Cell a, tuned around 11°, shows a broadening toward the trained orientation after training. Cell b, tuned around 67°, shows a broadening toward the trained orientation after training. Cell c is tuned around the trained orientation.

orientations and other stimulus positions was much higher.

Two monkeys were trained, and after intensive training which took several months, they achieved thresholds as low as 0.6° and 1.2°, respectively. Based on the well-documented studies by the Merzenich and other groups noted above showing expansion of representation areas in many instances of enhanced use and learning, we expected that cells would be recruited toward the trained orientation; we expected that some of these cells would have shifted their preferred orientation toward the orientation that was trained. What we found, however, was that the proportion of cells preferring the trained orientation was no larger than the proportion of cells preferring any other orientation.

At around the same time, we performed another experiment with one monkey that was also trained in orientation discrimination, followed by a double-labeled 2-deoxyglucose experiment. The monkey was trained to identify the 45° orientation at one position in its right visual field, followed by training until threshold to identify the 135° orientation at one position in its left visual field. Then, during the labeling experiment, the monkey fixated the center of a full screen grating. The bars of the grating had the 45° orientation while the first label was injected, and the 135° orientation while the second label was injected. This way, we radioactively labeled the populations of neurons activated by the two oblique reference orientations, respectively, over the whole operculum. If trained neurons would have shifted their preferred orientation toward the trained orientation, then the orientation columns made visible by the label injected while viewing the trained orientation (45°) would be broader at the position trained for identifying the 45° orientation. The columns representing activity evoked by the untrained orientation (135°), though not broader at this position, would be broader at the position in the other hemi-field trained for this orientation. Thus again, for each training, we had an internal control. Another control came from the orientation columns at positions away from the trained ones; these were naïve populations of neurons and should not have shown a broadening or narrowing of the orientation columns. The results from this experiment, however, confirmed the electrophysiological data: no broadening of the orientation columns was observed as a consequence of the perceptual learning, and thus no recruitment of cells responding to the trained orientation.

At this point, I would like to go back to the question what neuronal changes would be relevant. How do the responses of primary visual neurons reflect orientation differences? Even in area V1, orientation tuning curves are relatively broad, that is, 10 to 30°, with a large variability. One possible strategy could be that the experienced cortex has learned to select those neurons with the sharpest tuning curves, but even then, orientation differences of only 0.5° cannot be discriminated using the response of the most excited neurons only. Instead, as demonstrated in panel A of figure 5.3, using the difference signals between neurons that are tuned to orientations on either side of the trained orientation gives a much higher sensitivity to detect orientation differences (Westheimer, Shimamura, and McKee 1976; Regan and Beverley 1985). Thus the changes we really should be looking for are changes in the slope of the orientation tuning curves of the neurons that are tuned to orientations, close to and on either side of the trained orientation (Schoups et al. 2001).

When we examined the firing characteristics of the trained neurons obtained from the single-unit recordings, one change stood out sharply: in the population of trained neurons, those preferring the trained orientation exhibited a lower firing rate than the neurons preferring other orientations (Schoups,

Vogels, and Orban 1998). At first sight, this result seems counterintuitive. Indeed, why would less firing result in better performance in a sensory discrimination task?

Another change we observed in the population of trained neurons was that some neurons, tuned to orientations 30° away from the trained orientation, were broader than the analogous neurons from the naïve population. Theoretically, this could represent a recruitment of neurons responding to the trained orientation. For example, as shown in panel B of figure 5.3, if neurons b and c broaden their tuning curve, then the trained orientation, previously not included under the curve, now does evoke a response. The response of most of these neurons is lower than to some other behaviorally less relevant orientations. But the interest comes from the number of neurons responding. For a better coding, it may be more interesting that more neurons respond, all at the same, low firing rate, than that fewer neurons respond, with a high interneuron variability.

Building a model on perceptual learning in orientation discrimination, Qian and Matthews (1999) found that a lower firing rate by the neurons that prefer the trained orientation could lead to selective changes in the tuning patterns of neurons that prefer the orientations bordering the one trained, which then would lead to a better performance in the discrimination task.

5.4   Human Learning and Imaging Studies

Of the increases and decreases reported in imaging studies after learning a variety of tasks, I will especially focus on those reported in the visual system. First, a decrease is often associated with the task having become automatic. The circuitry used when performing a task can change as a consequence of practice (see also Walsh, Ashbridge, and Cowey 1998). Second, a decrease in the neuroimaging signal with learning may reflect learning-dependent improvements in neural coding efficiency (Földiák 1990; Barlow 1994; Scannell and Young 1999). It could also represent a more efficient "readout" of the information encoded at the sensory level.

Using positron-emission tomography (PET) to study activation of brain areas after perceptual learning in a visual discrimination task, researchers have reported large decreases in the visual areas. For example, regional cerebral blood flow (rCBF) was measured twice in humans: before and after training orientation discrimination. In accord with our electrophysiology findings, significant and orientation-specific decreases in activation were observed in striate and extrastriate visual cortex (Schiltz et al. 1999). Also testing the link between task difficulty and cerebral blood flow, Grady et al. (1996) found a negative correlation between accuracy and rCBF in striate cortex. They suggested that reduction in that area might improve performance on the task (a match-to-sample task of progressively degraded faces). Using fMRI, Vaina et al. (1998) found that brain activation specific to the discrimination of the direction of motion decreased in various areas after subjects had improved in this task.

Other research groups reported increases in the activation after learning a task. Karni et al. (1995) observed an expansion of the activation in primary visual cortex measured by fMRI, after training human subjects in a task to identify the orientation (horizontal or vertical) of a small target block (an array of three diagonal line elements differing only in their orientation from a background of identical elements) (cf. chapters 4, 6). They strongly suspected that the neuronal correlates for this type of perceptual learning would be found in primary visual cortex because of the specificity of the learning effect:

Karni and Sagi (1991) had reported learning to be specific for the target position in the subject's visual field, for the orientation, and for the eye (monocular). Our group (Schoups and Orban 1996) disputed the monocularity, however; it was difficult to imagine that learning could be both orientation and eye specific because monocular cells in striate cortex lack orientation specificity (cf., however, chapter 11) Finally, three research groups have reported that the fusiform gyrus shows an increase in activation when expertise is acquired in recognizing novel objects (Gauthier et al. 1999) or degraded faces (Dolan et al. 1997; Tovee, Rolls, and Ramachandran 1996).

The reported changes in rCBF with practice on a variety of tasks should be viewed with caution: they may reflect an automization of the task, a change in the involvement of attention, a familiarity effect, or a change in strategy. As we pursue perceptual learning studies, we must make sure that what is learned is under strict control—that learning represents a true sensorial improvement.

Perceptual Learning and the Development of Complex Visual Representations in Temporal Cortical Neurons

6

David L. Sheinberg and Nikos K. Logothetis

Abstract

At present, our understanding of the static properties of temporal cortical neurons, though more advanced than our knowledge of how the properties of these cells change over time, is still sorely lacking. In this chapter, we therefore review data from physiological studies that give some indication of what these cells might be doing, or at least what they might represent. If learning indeed modifies the properties of these neurons, then the snapshots of a cell's life provided by these standard single-unit studies can tell us something about *what* is learned. We present evidence that perceptual learning may provide a useful framework for understanding inferotemporal (IT) neurons. We argue that when novel patterns of sufficient complexity are regularly encountered, long-term changes occur in the connectivity of IT cells that implicitly incorporate these experiences. We do not suggest that the activity of these specialized cells ever replaces the activity of cells in earlier visual areas, but rather that it offers compact and reliable representations that can be used for rapid perceptual analysis and that can be associated with both actions and other neuronal representations. More important, we think that this experience-dependent modification is not a special process that is explicitly turned on and off, but is instead always operational during active (and perhaps even passive) visual processing. Thus object learning and object recognition may not be so easily distinguished.

6.1 Introduction

When we are faced with something visible for the first time, recognition is not a prerequisite for perception or awareness. But if the object is encountered regularly, its appearance does seem to change.

For example, the first time one visits a new city, perhaps viewing its sights from the back of a taxi, the scenery is novel, the buildings unfamiliar, and the streets confusing. However, after a number of visits things begin to look different. The initial impressions fade, and are instead replaced by concrete views of a place well known. At its peak, familiarity may even cause things to go unnoticed. Amazingly, this transformation from a primarily sensory experience to a recognized encounter usually happens effortlessly and without conscious intervention. Merely seeing something over and over can powerfully change how we see that same thing. In this view, every visual encounter has two related, but independent, consequences: one perceptual and one mnemonic. In the brain the same cells whose activity causes a perceptual experience are also possible participants in perceptual learning.

The problem of perceptual learning is not new. Philosophical interest in such learning dates back to at least Locke's empiricist theories, and psychophysicists have been studying such phenomena systematically for over a century. In the field of visual sensation, for example, Volkmann (1858) investigated how subjects' thresholds for two-point discrimination changed with experience. He found that a few hours of practice decreased the minimum detectable separation between two points of stimulation in these subjects by nearly 50%, and that continued practice, over days and weeks, further improved their performance. In light of such data, Gibson and Gibson (1955) asked what happens in the course of this type of learning. They forcefully resisted the notion that experience causes perception to become less a function of the stimulus and more a result of the observer's enrichment of that stimulus by internal processes. Instead, they proposed that the intrinsic properties of a well-learned stimulus become more closely associated with the percept, and that performance on discrimination tasks improves as a result of more specific *identifying responses.* "We suggest that the stimulation is complex, not simple, and that the observer continues to discover higher-order variables of stimulation in it. The percept becomes differentiated" (Gibson and Gibson 1955, 40). According to the Gibsons, there is no need to add information to an already rich stimulus. Instead, the brain becomes more capable of extracting the information that was there all along.

In a book on perceptual learning, it is reasonable to ask whether the problem of visual recognition qualifies as a form of perceptual learning at all. Basic treatments of vision often divide the problem into three distinct stages: sensation, perception, and recognition. In this view, sensation comprises the initial stage of sensory transduction, carried out by photoreceptors in the retina. The raw sensory signal, which we know is transmitted in large part to visual cortex through the thalamus, is then transformed into distinct percepts, probably as a result of complicated interactions between multiple visual areas. Finally, the completed percept may trigger a reaction (either physical or mental). In such a simplified view, learning to associate percepts with reactions (recognition) might well be considered a process separate from learning to perceive. A similar view is found in theories of computational vision, which often divide the problem of vision into early-level, middle-level, and high-level processes. Here again, perception would generally map onto middle-level vision, whereas recognition would be considered a high-level process.

We, however, find the processes underlying vision far more entangled than this. Where perception ends and recognition begins is almost certainly not so neatly defined. Traditional tasks in visual perception (orientation discrimination, contrast detection) generally require that the subject map a visual experience to a response, and this mapping requires that some internal representation of the stimulus be connected to explicit reactions (judgments, responses). On the other hand, classic paradigms in the domain of visual recognition, such as visual priming, are primarily aimed at probing the brain's internal representation of specific visual stimuli, and in these studies, the actual response is of only secondary interest. The addition of learning or memory into the equation further complicates the matter with regard to a simple parceling of visual function. Task demands and experience seem to play an important, and often overlooked, role in not only classification and categorization, but in perceptual analysis as well. One issue that remains paramount, though, is the question of representation. How does the brain represent a visual stimulus? In considering this, we can also ask how this representation changes with experience. From this perspective, we feel that a chapter devoted to learning of complex visual patterns and the neuronal correlates of this process does indeed belong in a book dedicated to the study of perceptual learning.

This view is not new. In arguing that perception is governed by the same processes as more conceptual activities like categorization, Bruner (1957, 124) wrote: "A theory of perception, we assert, needs a mechanism capable of inference and categorizing as much as one is needed in a theory of cognition.... [I]t seems to me foolish and unnecessary to assume that the sensory "stuff" on which higher order categorizations are based is, if you will, of a different sensory order than more evolved identities with which our perceptual world is normally peopled." He goes on to describe a simple experiment in which two 8-letter strings—YRULPZOC and VERNALIT—are briefly flashed and subjects are then asked to report the letters that were displayed. For the first string, which poorly approximates a real English word, subjects correctly reported, on average, 48% of the letters. For the latter, which could be but is not an English word, subjects correctly reported 93% of the letters. Why the difference in perceptibility? Bruner argues that English speakers, manifesting what has been described as the "word superiority effect," learn to code words in a way that accounts for the natural variation in the language, and that under "substandard" conditions (e.g., tachistoscopic presentation), words that conform to this model can activate pre-existing codes and thus be perceived more veridically than words that do not (see also Reicher 1969). Unlike the Gibsons, Bruner (1957, 127) argues that perceptual learning does indeed involve "learning" on the part of the perceiver: "I would propose that perceptual learning consists not of making finer and finer discriminations as the Gibsons ([Gibson and Gibson] 1955) would have us believe, but that it consists rather in the learning of appropriate modes of coding the environment in terms of its object character, connectedness, or redundancy, and then in allocating stimulus inputs to appropriate categorical coding systems."

In this chapter, we follow the direction spelled out by Bruner and address the question of how experience with visual patterns might lead to new "modes of coding the environment." Specifically, we consider how these codes may be evidenced in the physiological properties of neurons. We suggest that for the purposes of perceptual learning, the cortex of the lateral inferotemporal (IT) lobe roughly corresponding to Von Bonin and Bailey's area TE (1947), located in the middle and inferior temporal gyri, sits in a unique position within the visual system. On

one hand, neurons in this region are intimately connected with occipital brain regions that are thought to be essential for visual sensation. On the other hand, inferotemporal cortex has major reciprocal connections with medial temporal, limbic, and frontal brain areas known to be critical in mnemonic function (see Logothetis and Sheinberg 1996 for review). Physiological studies have shown time and again that single IT cells can be selective for complex patterns, but exactly how this selectivity comes about is still not clear, although there is increasing evidence that in the mature adult, visual experience continues to modify the synaptic connections (Buonomano and Merzenich 1998a; cf. chapters 2, 4). Within inferotemporal cortex, such modifications may create reliable and relatively sparse codes of encountered visual stimuli. At the same time, changes in the efficacy of divergent connections to limbic, frontal, and subcortical brain areas may provide a route for connecting visual encounters with appropriate reactions.

6.2 Features and Representations

What do cells in the inferotemporal cortex signal? Such a question is obviously impossible to answer unequivocally for this or any brain area. Even so, for neurons in early visual areas, neurophysiologists generally feel comfortable characterizing the kind of information transmitted by these cells using terms such as *contrast, orientation, color, disparity,* and *motion*. What about the activity of cells in inferotemporal cortex? The earliest published reports of the properties of such cells recount problems that to this day remain unresolved. Gross and his colleagues (Gross, Bender, and Rocha-Miranda 1969, 1305) remarked that "by largely confining the stimuli to bars, edges, rectangles, and circles we may never have found the 'best' stimulus for each unit. There were several units that responded most strongly to more compli- cated figures." What are these "complicated figures" and how could one ever hope to identify them systematically?

6.2.1 The Grandmother Cell

Konorski (1967) hypothesized that neurons in the visual system were organized in a hierarchical fashion, with low-level, elementary feature detectors at the base, and "gnostic units" at the most advanced stage. The gnostic units would be tuned to such complex feature combinations that they would, through their activation, implicitly "represent unitary perceptions." The most notable proponent of such a hierarchical scheme has been Barlow (1972, 1985, 1995). In the last three decades, his hypotheses about the relation- ship between single neurons and perceptual events have become almost synonymous with the most ex- treme version of this theory—the "grandmother cell" version—where a single cell is capable of responding to the sight of one's grandmother.[1] It is important to note, however, that Barlow (1972, 390) actually rejects this idea along with the notion that a single cell controls the whole of subjective experience:

The "grandmother cell" might respond to all views of grandmother's face, but how would that indicate that it shares features in common with other human faces, and that, on a particular occasion, it occurs in a specific posi- tion surrounded by other recognizable objects? Our per- ceptions simply do not have the property of being isolated unique events as one would expect if each corresponded to the firing of a unique neuron.

Important discoveries by neurophysiologists such as Hartline (1940), Barlow (1950), and Kuffler (1953) clearly pointed to the fact that the activity of indi- vidual neurons did convey useful information about stimuli in the external world, and the notion of a neuron's *receptive field* arose from such studies. In

particular, in the field of vision, these ideas seemed to apply well to cells in the retina, thalamus, and primary visual cortex. Hubel and Wiesel's landmark work (1962, 1968) in striate cortex also fit well with the notion of a hierarchical structure providing cells with increasingly complex representations of visual stimuli. More recent behavioral studies (see Parker and Newsome 1998 for review) have fueled interest in the information conveyed by single cells, sug- gesting that at least some perceptual decisions in the behaving animal can be predicted by the activity of single cells. But despite the intuitive appeal of en- capsulating so much information in a single neuron's activity, Konorski's gnostic units and Barlow's car- dinal cells have met mostly with ridicule and dis- belief in the three decades since they were introduced (see Gross 1992 for discussion). Hubel (1995, 223), for example, observed:

Do cells continue to become more and more specialized at more and more central levels, so that at some stage we can expect to find cells so specialized that they respond to one single person's face—say, one's grandmother's? This no- tion, called the *grandmother cell theory*, is hard to entertain seriously. Would we expect to find separate cells for grandmother smiling, grandmother weeping, or grand- mother sewing?

There is ample reason to resist the idea that a sin- gle cell is responsible for representing something as complicated as a whole object. It is true that we still know very little about how the activity of a single inferotemporal neuron participates in the generation of perceptual events. In Sheinberg and Logothetis 1997, we found that there are striking correlations between the activity of single temporal neurons and visual awareness. But we were also quick to point out that while such correlations may reveal impor- tant information about the perceptual organization of the visual system, they do not tell us that the activity of any one of these cells leads to the awareness or recognition of individual visual stimuli (see Crick and Koch 1998 for discussion on the neural basis of awareness). Furthermore, given the large number of successful studies of inferotemporal neurons in anesthetized animals, it would be hard to argue that activity of these cells alone caused awareness of anything. Indeed, from this perspective, the grandmother cell theory appears wrong. Even if there were cells that responded to specific objects, the activity of these cells may have little or nothing to do with the experience of "seeing" that object. It has been shown, for example, that in the human medial temporal lobe there are cells selective to responses to faces and expressions, and that some such cells respond differently to previously presented stimuli, even when the subjects denied having seen the stimulus before (Fried, MacDonald, and Wilson 1997).

6.2.2 Complexity, Selectivity, Generality, and Reduction

At the time Gross and his colleagues began investigating the properties of visual cells in the temporal lobe, they were "prepared to find IT cells that fired selectively to complex stimuli such as hands and faces" (Gross 1994, 465): they were fully aware of Konorski's hypothesis (1967) that inferotemporal cortex may be site of the controversial "gnostic units." The first published study on the physiological properties of IT cells (Gross, Bender, and Rocha-Miranda 1969), however, measured the response of IT neurons to relatively simple visual stimuli, such as diffuse light, bars, and edges. Only reluctantly, Gross (1994) recounts, did they include anecdotal information about a cell that seemed to respond best to a monkey hand. Almost an entire decade passed after the initial IT physiology studies before more reports of cells responsive to complex biological objects

started to appear. By far the most commonly reported cells of this type were the "face cells" first described by Perrett, Rolls, and Caan (1979, 1982) and by Bruce, Desimone, and Gross (1981). Since that time, cells responsive to faces have also been reported in areas outside inferotemporal cortex, such as in the amygdala (Rolls 1984) and the frontal lobes (O Scalaidhe, Wilson, and Goldman-Rakic 1997; Pigarev, Rizzolatti, and Scandolara 1979). Because the general properties of these cells have been reviewed in detail elsewhere (Desimone 1991; Gross 1992; Logothetis and Sheinberg 1996; Perrett, Mitslin, and Chitty 1987; Rolls 1994), our principal aim here is to address a subset of the outstanding issues that relate to the question of perceptual learning.

An important point to note is that the category of "face cells" is actually quite diverse and almost certainly comprises multiple subclasses (Perrett, Mitslin, and Chitlin 1987; Tovee 1995). The diversity of responses can, at least in part, be traced to the diversity of visual areas within which face cells have been found (Baylis, Rolls, and Leonard 1987). These visual areas include the superior temporal polysensory (STP) area, found within the upper bank and fundus of the superior temporal sulcus (STS), and inferotemporal cortex, in the lower bank and lip of the STS and the middle and inferior temporal gyri (area TE).

Specific testing of face selective cells has shown that the responses of some of these neurons are dependent on head orientation but less so than they are on the identity of the face (Desimone et al. 1984; Oram and Perret 1992; Perrett et al. 1985). Likewise, other cells seem tuned to particular facial expressions (Hasselmo, Rolls, and Baylis 1989). Figure 6.1 shows an example of a cell of the former kind, and it also illustrates a number of properties of many of the temporal cortical neurons we—and many others—have encountered (see figure caption

r052

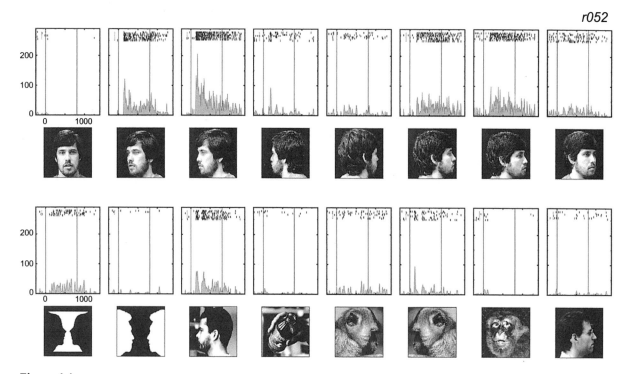

Figure 6.1
Response profile of a typical "face cell," which responded most vigorously to profiles, but was sensitive also to the subject in the profile. Note the large dynamic range in firing frequency between responses to preferred and nonpreferred (e.g., the frontal face views) stimuli. For all cells shown in this and the following figures (except figure 6.6), each neuron was tested with a series of briefly presented visual stimuli. The data in these figures were collected from two rhesus macaques, using surgical methods and chamber placement described in Sheinberg and Logothetis 1997. The activity of each cell was recorded while the monkey maintained fixation within a region approximately 2° square. Stimuli were approximately 4° on a side. None of the stimuli in this or the following figures (except for the wire objects in figure 6.6) was ever designated as special to the monkeys. Each graph represents the response of the neuron to the image shown beneath. Vertical ticks at the top of each plot denote a single, well-isolated, spike; the vertical lines show stimulus onset and offset times. The perfectly aligned horizontal ticks to the left of the stimulus onset line indicate a row corresponding to a single trial (useful for trials that contain no spikes). The firing rate for each stimulus condition is estimated as in Sheinberg and Logothetis 1997, and shown as the filled curve in each graph.

for a description of the basic methods).[2] First, the cell exhibits an enormous dynamic range of firing frequencies. Its spontaneous rate is quite low, firing, on average, below 1 Hz prior to the presentation of a visual stimulus. Although this rate leaves little room for inhibition, the cell's response to frontal views of either humans or monkeys appears to fully inhibit the cell: no spikes occurred from 120 msec after stimulus onset (the cell's latency) until stimulus offset, when these views were presented. The cell's most vigorous response was in excess of 100 Hz, achieved shortly after its onset latency. Note also that after effective stimuli, cells often continue to respond, even though the stimulus is no longer physically present.

Second, the cell's response modulation is quite consistent from trial to trial for at least some of the stimuli tested, although this reliability is limited to short epochs starting soon after the cell's overall onset latency. Tovee et al. (1993) have shown that a substantial portion of the information transmitted by IT cells can be extracted from intervals as short as 50 msec. Which parts of the spike train are most critical is clearly an important, but unresolved, issue. Richmond and his colleagues (Richmond and Optican 1987; Richmond et al. 1987) have argued that the temporal characteristics of the response must be taken into account to fully describe the information conveyed by single units (cf. chapter 5). We, however, would suggest that because most recognition problems can be solved on the order of hundreds of milliseconds, and because unconstrained fixation durations last, on average, about 250 msec, the critical information conveyed by IT neurons for the purposes of perception and recognition must be conveyed as early and as rapidly as possible (see also Oram and Perrett 1992).

Finally, for the cell in figure 6.1, there is a systematic relationship between head rotation and the cell's activity, with the maximal response elicited by the left profile, and a substantial response to the right profile. The response to the two views is not identical, however. This tuning demonstrates that while cells are "selective" with respect to the preferred set of stimuli, they also exhibit some generality for other dimensions. The details of other forms of generalization in IT cells has been investigated in numerous studies by systematically varying basic image attributes of the test stimuli, including both face and non-face objects (e.g., Fourier descriptors and wirelike objects). These variations include changes in contrast (Rolls and Baylis 1986) and position (Ito et al. 1995; Logothetis, Pauls, and Poggio 1995; Schwartz et al. 1983; Tovee et al. 1994), where generalization is quite robust, as well as in scale (Ashbridge et al. 2000; Ito et al. 1995; Logothetis, Pauls, and Poggio 1995; Schwartz, et al. 1983), spatial frequency content (Rolls, Baylis, and Leonard 1985), color (Perrett, Rolls, and Caan 1982), and lighting (Hietanen et al. 1992), variations that can lead to more dramatic changes in cell response.

Although the variation with head orientation seems to capture the *essence* of what the cell in figure 6.1 signals, dubbing it a "profile cell" does not seem entirely justified by its pattern of response. It certainly can contribute to a process of discriminating head orientation. But the response graphs and profiles shown in the bottom two rows show that the cell does distinguish between the various heads in profile. It may come as little surprise, then, that the most effective stimulus we found for this neuron was a profile of an individual who was well known to the animal (the scientist depicted in the top row of figure 6.1). It is commonly assumed that if and when high selectivity exists, it should be reserved for objects of extreme importance to the animal (such as the experimenter charged with its well being). Although such a view seems reasonable, we think it is probably not entirely correct. Figure 6.2 shows a cell that

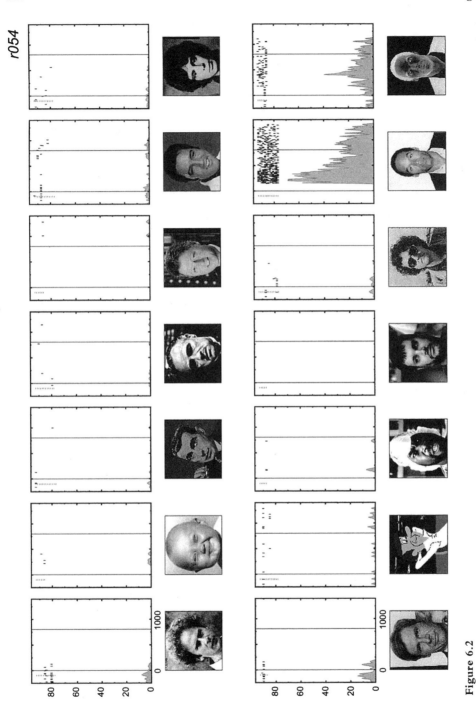

Figure 6.2
Highly selective inferotemporal (IT) neuron, which responded best to a single image from our test set. The contrast reversed image had never been seen before the trials depicted here. Note that the spontaneous activity of this cell, like many others we have encountered in IT cortex, was very low. There was generally no discernable response to nonpreferred faces. (See caption for figure 6.1.)

responded in a remarkably selective fashion to an image that was never singled out as important for the monkey. Like other cells of this sort, the spontaneous rate was very low—so low that there were periods during the recording when it was uncertain whether the cell was still there. The preferred stimulus in this example was an image that had been used in some twenty-five previous test sessions (along with the images of the other celebrities and scores of other test images). The contrast reversed image, a manipulation also reported in Perrett et al. 1984 evoked a significant, but reduced response, implying that high-order shape information is probably most critical for activating this cell. The cell's altered response to the contrast-reversed image is also evidence for limited generalization because this image had never been presented before this test session.

A common explanation for the kind of cell response depicted in figure 6.2 is that there must be some basic feature in the image that differentiates it from the others: perhaps it is the only elliptical stimulus, or perhaps it is lighter or darker than the others are. Perhaps the eyes, the nose, the ears, are somehow triggering the cell, as seemed to be the case for a subset of the cells reported by Perrett, Rolls, and Caan (1982). Such hypotheses must, of course, be taken seriously, and an entire approach to considering such issues has been developed by Tanaka's group in Japan (see Tanaka, chapter 4, this volume). In their "reduction method," the most effective stimulus for a cell is determined and then simplified, step by step, until the resulting image no longer activates the neuron (a similar approach was also used by Desimone et al. 1984). They characterize the simplest image that can effectively drive a cell as the cell's "critical feature." Using this technique, Kobotake and Tanaka (1994) found that the proportion of cells possessing complex critical features increases as one moves from area V4 into posterior, and then ante-

rior, inferotemporal cortex. Although a thorough dissection of the critical features for activating a cell is in principle a good idea, the method can be potentially misleading. Figure 6.3 illustrates a reduction attempt that underscores at least one problem with such an approach.

In panel a, we see that the cell responds best to either of two views of a monkey sitting on a rock. Similar cells, responding to pictures of whole human bodies, have been also been reported by Wachsmuth, Oram, and Perrett (1994). In line with the reduction technique, we found that if elements of the preferred image were shown in isolation—the head alone or the tail resting on the rock—the cell responded partway, still better than to other images, but less than its maximum (panel b). What is most interesting is that the subimage containing the tail (panel b, right), which activated the cell when shown alone, had almost no effect when it was shown as part of the complete image depicted in panel c.[3] In other words, we found that, though parts of an image can contribute to the response of a cell, the same parts placed in a different context may no longer be capable of eliciting a response. It is precisely this kind of behavior that has led many researchers to believe that faces are processed by specialized mechanisms, perhaps in specialized brain areas. The crux of this debate rests on the issue of how faces, as objects, are encoded. If faces are simply represented as a combination of features, then the processing of these features should proceed independently of whether the entire face is presented. On the other hand, if individual features are bound together in a unitary configuration, then faces as wholes may actually be processed differently than are the parts that compose them. Psychological data on this point seem to be converging on the view that faces are indeed processed as whole configurations and not just as combinations of parts (Tanaka and Farah 1993; Yin 1969).

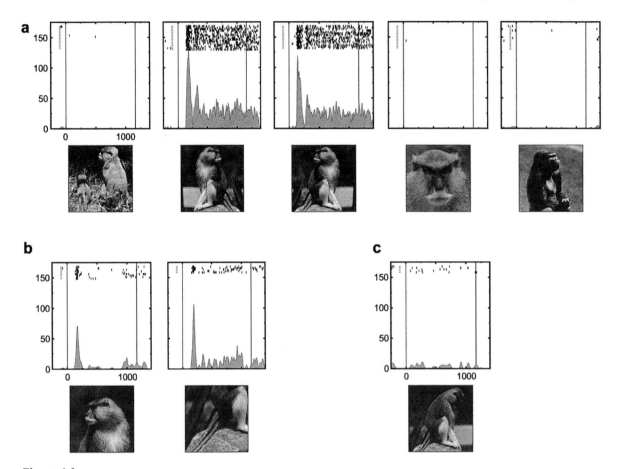

Figure 6.3

Difficulties with the reduction method. (*a*) This cell responded vigorously and reliably to a particular image of a monkey sitting on a rock, as well as its mirror image (both of which had been seen before this recording session). Response to other views of the same monkey elicited almost no detectable response. (*b*) Cropped images showing that individual parts—head and tail (at the same size as the original whole body image)—evoked a partial, but significant response from the cell. (*c*) Original image from which the tail in panel b was extracted had little excitatory effect on the cell's response, which shows that the essential features responsible for activating a cell cannot be reliably determined without placing those features in a different context. Here we would argue that the cell responded to the subparts shown in panel b as a result of its learned response to the images in panel a, and not that its response to the whole figure was a lucky consequence of various subparts appearing together. (See caption for figure 6.1.)

In any case, we believe that the notion of "critical features" found using the reduction technique is inappropriate for a cell that has developed its selectivity for a particular configural stimulus.

6.2.3   Biological Relevance

Although configural effects were originally thought to be unique to face processing, similar effects have now been found in expert dog breeders when recognizing dogs (Diamond and Carey 1986) and in other experts when processing a carefully controlled set of novel objects (Gauthier and Tarr 1997). Interestingly, our understanding of the physiological properties of IT neurons seems to be following a parallel path. Once the existence of face cells was finally accepted, the question arose of whether such cells constitute an exception in inferotemporal cortex or whether cells with similar selectivity for other objects also exist there but are simply more scarce (e.g., Desimone 1991). In considering this question, Gross (1992, 6) wrote:

With the exception of face- and hand-selective cells, there is no evidence for IT cells that are selective for visual objects such as fruit, tree-branches, monkey genitalia, features in the monkey's laboratory or natural environment or any other object. IT neurons may well discharge to these and other stimuli but they have not been shown to be particularly selective for them. Of course, it is possible that no one has presented the appropriate stimulus while recording from the appropriate cell.

Subsequent studies from our laboratory (Logothetis, Pauls, and Poggio 1995; Logothetis and Pauls 1995) have shown that selective responses in inferotemporal cortex are not limited to biological stimuli such as faces and hands. In these studies, discussed in greater detail below, monkeys learned to recognize entirely novel sets of objects. After training, a small percentage of IT cells were found to exhibit selec-

tivity for the specific objects that had been learned during training. More recently, we have found that even in the absence of extensive training, unusually high selectivity can still be found for images that have merely been observed in the past (see also Booth and Rolls 1998). It thus seems that extensive experience with configurally complex objects may alone account for the special processing and special cells originally ascribed to faces. Figure 6.4, for instance, illustrates two examples of cells selective for neither faces nor hands. Instead, arbitrary images taken from the large set of test stimuli activated these otherwise quiescent cells. Finding appropriate stimuli for such cells required presenting subjects with hundreds of images already shown in prior recording sessions, until at least one image had some systematic effect on the cell's response. Although novel images were also introduced on a regular basis (after which they were no longer novel), we never found selective responses for totally unfamiliar stimuli (a point to which we will return below). On a typical penetration during these explorations, anywhere from two to ten candidate cells had to be passed up simply because no appropriate stimulus could be found.[4] We will of course never know whether any appropriate stimulus actually existed for such cells.

6.2.4   Sparse and Distributed Representations

We are not suggesting that all cells in inferotemporal cortex are as selective as the ones described above. Many studies of IT neurons have concluded that these cells, though capable of distinguishing between general classes of stimuli (e.g., faces versus nonfaces), respond to many members of the preferred class (e.g., Baylis, Rolls, and Leonard 1985, 1987; Rolls and Tovee 1995; Young and Yamane 1992). Such conclusions are not incompatible with the view pre-

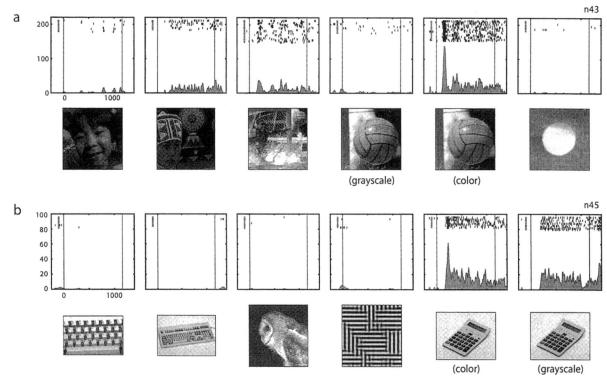

Figure 6.4

Response to nonbiological stimuli. Highly selective responses are not limited to biological stimuli such as faces or hands (Gross 1992). (*a, b*) Two neurons reliably activated by images of nonbiological objects likely to have never been seen by the monkey before our experiments began (although, by the time these cells were found, each of these images had already been presented during the basic fixation task many times). (See caption for figure 6.1.)

sented here, although we have chosen to emphasize the high selectivity of some cells as opposed to the mild selectivity of many others. Our purpose in doing so is not to mislead one into thinking that inferotemporal cortex is full of neurons responding to one and only one stimulus. Instead, we think the unusual selectivity of these neurons provides important clues that can guide our thinking about the population of IT cells as a whole. In figure 6.5, we present a cell that responds to the presentation of a small subset of images, but not at all to other, similar

images. Neither "faceness" nor head orientation can explain what makes one set of three stimuli excite the cell and another set not. There are no obvious visual features that distinguish the set of effective and noneffective objects. As far as useful generalization goes, the selectivity of this cell seems to have run amok. It is of course entirely possible that the same cell participates in the coding of multiple unrelated images, like bits in an ASCII code. We expect that a better understanding of the processes that underlie the development of selectivity may help explain the

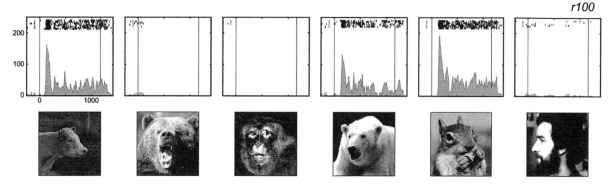

Figure 6.5

Robust responses to seemingly unrelated images. Here we show a cell that responded well to a subset of animals, and not at all to others. No obvious measure of similarity seems to link the effective stimuli and to exclude the ineffective stimuli. (Most cells did not respond to only a single object.) We see this as evidence that selectivities emerge for experienced images, and that the images ultimately activating a cell need not be especially similar to one another. (See caption for figure 6.1.)

variety of cell properties that exist within the temporal lobes.

From an information-theoretic perspective, there are important distinctions between very sparse and highly distributed representations (see, for example, Abbott, Rolls, and Tovee 1996; Barlow 1972, 1995; Rolls 1994; Rolls and Tovee 1995).[5] Here our purpose is not to settle the issue of which of these codes is most compatible with actual brain processing. Instead, we want to pursue the idea that whatever representations may exist can be attributed in large part to previous visual encounters experienced by the system under study. If single cells' synaptic interconnections can be biased in favor of multiple stimuli, then one would expect to find a whole range of selectivities across a population of cortical neurons. Many theories have been proposed regarding the development of selectivity and the stability of such processes (e.g., Bienenstock, Cooper, and Munro 1982; Kohonen 1982; Linsker 1988), some of which have received considerable neurophysiological support (Kirkwood, Rioult, and Bear 1996). One thing these theories have in common is their dependence on experience, even in the form of spontaneous neural activity (see Katz and Shatz 1996 for review).

6.3 Plasticity in Visual Cortex

The range of selectivities encountered in inferotemporal cortex makes one wonder exactly what forces are at work in the creation of these cells. What distinguishes the neural activity associated with novel objects from that associated with known objects? If one were able to simultaneously record from all visual areas of the brain, which areas or populations of cells would respond differently to an object once it became familiar? It seems unlikely that the pattern of retinal excitation elicited by a visual stimulus would differ as a result of familiarity, or that such differences would be detectable in the responses of cells in primary visual cortex (cf. chapter 5). Indeed, it is possible that no aspect of the visual representation of a stimulus would change as a result of stimulus familiarity. In such a scheme, memory and recognition would be completely separated from perceptual analysis. The latter could depend on a set of immutable, universal primitives that would be rich enough to represent all visual objects: although the particular combination of active cells would be novel for a stimulus encountered for the first time, subsequent encounters with the same stimulus would lead to nearly identical activation patterns. Just as combinations of letters of an alphabet can represent all words in a language, these visual primitives would be capable of representing any object, regardless of whether the object was novel or familiar.

6.3.1   Development of Representations

But what if the visual brain were less static and instead continued to create new visual primitives for representing visual stimuli? Such a process would be analogous to creating representations for words that were as "primitive" as representations of the letters that compose them. The "word superiority effect," briefly alluded to in section 6.1 (see, for example, Reicher 1969), in which letters imbedded in words are better recognized than letters in isolation or letters in nonwords, provides behavioral support for this notion. This kind of effect indicates that experience may play an important role in reorganizing perceptual processes. It is perhaps surprising, then, that numerous influential models of visual recognition are based on the idea of structurally constraining the space of all objects using a fixed set of primitives (e.g., Biederman 1987; Marr and Nishihara 1978). Recent treatments of the basic units of perceptual processing are clearly reconsidering the notion that primitives for vision, audition, language, and concepts are fixed or predetermined, arguing instead that they may develop throughout life (e.g., Schyns, Goldstone, and Thibaut 1998).

Using carefully designed experimental stimuli, researchers (Gauthier and Tarr 1997; Goldstone 1998;

Schyns and Rodet 1997) have recently been able to demonstrate that categorical judgments based on perceptual features critically depend on task demands and subjects' experience with the stimuli. For example, Schyns and Rodet (1997) devised a set of visual stimuli they called "Martian cells," which were circular backgrounds textured by amorphous blobs. Categories were determined by the presence of certain characteristic blobs. Two separate blobs (x and y), as well as a conjunction of the two (xy) were the defining features of three separate categories of cells (X, Y, and XY). The experimental question was whether learning to visually categorize XY cells before learning to categorize X or Y cells would effectively establish the combination xy as a "primitive" feature. The authors tested this hypothesis using objects that contained the individual features x and y presented as parts of the same object, but not conjoined (X-Y cells). Subjects who had learned the conjunction first (XY_X_Y) categorized the X-Y probe stimuli as either being an X or a Y, indicating that the feature xy was part of these subjects' feature vocabulary as a single unit that could not be broken apart. In contrast, subjects who had learned the individual features before learning the conjunction (X_Y_XY) categorized the X-Y probes as XY cells, suggesting the XY class was based on a second-order conjunction of the primitive x and y features. These data imply that categorical judgements can be systematically influenced by experience, and that perceptual analysis is clearly subject to learning effects (Schyns, Goldstone, and Thibault 1998).

The benefits of a flexible and dynamic set of feature primitives are rather obvious. First, it is not necessary to posit that the perceptual system is innately endowed with a set of primitives broad enough to represent all possible objects. And second, if such a broad set of primitives did exist, it would likely be wasteful because many feature dimensions might have representations that would never be used (Schyns, Goldstone, and Thibault 1998). On the other hand, it is entirely possible that the visual system has inherited a set of primitives that, without significant rewiring, may not be appropriate for solving the kinds of problems paramount to our survival. Because nature rarely scraps old hardware in favor of a totally new design, the primitives that we often place so much emphasis on (such as oriented line segments) may need to be modified before they can effectively solve more sophisticated visual needs. As an analogy, consider analyzing the individual pieces that make up a World War II aircraft. The components that went into building these planes may have been manufactured in a converted factory that originally built washing machines rather than flying machines. The parts may thus have properties that were optimized for a totally different class of products, but, when assembled appropriately, perhaps with ad hoc modifications, they may have been adequate for constructing the wings, bodies, and engines needed to build reliable airplanes.

Is such a dynamic, feature creation scheme consistent with the known physiological properties of the visual system? The "third dogma" of Barlow's neuron doctrine for perception (1972) addresses precisely this point. In it, he proposes that selectivity of individual cells adapts to the environment, both through genetic predispositions as well as through "plasticity of the neural structures involved" (p. 385). Referring to neuronal representations as words in a dictionary, Barlow asks:

Are the dictionary words there, only the ones experienced becoming permanently connected; or do the cells themselves determine that a frequently experienced pattern, such as lines of a particular range of orientations, are events for which words are desirable? The evidence favours modification, and the idea to which it leads of the successive hierarchical construction of a dictionary of meaningful neurons has enormous appeal. For the present we can only justify the third dogma by saying the evidence suggests such a dictionary may be built up, though we are far from being able to look into its pages by physiological methods. (p. 386)

6.3.2 Plasticity in Early Visual Areas

The importance of natural experience in the development of early visual areas was first studied in detail in the cat by Wiesel and Hubel (1963, 1965) and in the monkey by Hubel, Wiesel, and LeVay (1977). Demonstrating the importance of normal visual experience in the development of binocular representations in striate cortex, these visual deprivation experiments served as a springboard for literally hundreds of studies of cortical plasticity in both infant and adult animals, which have repeatedly shown how damage or surgical manipulation of the normal inputs to primary somatosensory, auditory, and visual cortices can lead to significant synaptic remodeling (see Buonomano and Merzenich 1998a, chapter 2). In visual cortex, such reorganization is most easily induced in early "sensitive periods" (Hubel, Wiesel, and LeVay 1977; Wiesel and Hubel 1965), during which both topographic representations and basic neurophysiological properties, such as eye dominance and orientation preference, can be altered (see Introduction). That these changes are more difficult to find in adult animals is not surprising if one accepts the tenet that the basic flow of visual information primarily feeds forward out of area V1 and into extrastriate areas. In such a hierarchical system, it is critical that reliable coding schemes at lower levels remain firmly in place. Otherwise, operations dependent on information derived in these areas would no longer make sense. (cf., however, chapter 20 for a possible solution).

Probably the most influential theory regarding the mechanism of synaptic modification is Hebb's postulate (1949), in which he states that that coactivation of an excitatory input and its postsynaptic target will lead to increased efficacy of that input. It should come as no surprise to many, though, that William James (1890/1950, 567) in his monumental *Principles of Psychology* proposed a similar theory in what he called the "elementary law of association": "*The amount of activity at any given point in the brain-cortex is the sum of the tendencies of all other points to discharge into it, such tendencies being proportionate (1) to the number of times the excitement of each other point may have accompanied that of the point in question; (2) to the intensity of such excitements; and (3) to the absence of any rival point functionally disconnected with the first point, into which discharges might be diverted*" (emphasis in original).

Hebb's postulate was framed using more modern anatomical references (axons, somas, dendrites, and synaptic knobs) and was sufficiently explicit to warrant naming synapses that exhibit modifiable connection strengths as "Hebbian." Experimental support for the existence of such synapses has come predominantly from slice studies in hippocampus, where, in a typical experiment, a brief conditioning stimulus delivered to a specific set of presynaptic fibers results in a specific strengthening of their postsynaptic connections (see Brown, Kairiss, and Keenan 1990; Katz and Shatz 1996 for reviews). It has been shown that this effect, called "long-term potentiation" (LTP) is both input specific and long lasting, and its molecular mechanisms have now been intensively studied (Roberson, English, and Sweatt 1996). LTP is not limited to the hippocampus, though, and has been recently demonstrated in visual cortex (Kirkwood and Bear 1994; Otsu, Kimura, and Tsumoto 1995, chapters 3, 7, this volume).

6.3.3   Plasticity in Higher Visual Areas

In one of the few direct studies of synaptic plasticity in extrastriate visual areas, Murayama, Fujita, and Kato (1997) compared activity-dependent plasticity in area V1 and inferotemporal cortex in an anesthetized adult monkey (*Macaca fuscata*). Interestingly, they found that an extracellular tetanic stimulus applied every 4 sec for 3–5 min had opposite effects in areas V1 and TEd (dorsolateral area TE). Stimulation in the supragranular layers of area V1 led to a decrease in the evoked extracellular field potential (EFP) that lasted at least 3 hours. In TEd, however, similar stimulation induced a gradual potentiation in the EFP's slope and amplitude that lasted for the duration of the recording session (up to 4 hours). Neurophysiological differences in synaptic modifiability between striate and temporal cortical areas are consistent with a reported neurochemical gradient in the same visual areas. Nelson et al. (1987) found a systematic increase in the phosphorylation of two protein kinase C (PKC) substrates between striate and temporal cortical visual areas. Phosphorylation of one of the PKC substrates, the homologue of the phosphoprotein F1 in the rat, is known to be critical in the induction of long-term potentiation (Roberson, English, and Sweatt 1996). Thus at least one line of neurochemical evidence suggests that there is greater opportunity for plasticity, possibly through the growth of presynaptic terminals, at higher stages in the ventral visual pathway (Nelson et al. 1987).

Although ablation studies in 1950s and 1960s established that inferior temporal cortex is essential for normal visual discrimination learning (see Dean 1976 for review), only recently have neurophysiological studies been able to demonstrate that changes associated with visual learning can also be found in the activity patterns of single IT neurons. Rolls and his colleagues (1989) were the first to look for such changes in the activity of face-selective cells as a result of experience. They found that the response patterns for 6 out of 22 neurons changed in the short period during which novel faces became familiar. In a second experiment, they found that 5 out of 26 neurons changed their response to familiar faces following the presentation of a single novel face. The results show that face-selective neurons are not static filters, and instead seem capable of adjusting their response selectivities as a result of experience. Because the effects reported were in the relative response of the neurons to the set of face stimuli, these changes seem to reflect a reorganization of ensemble codes in inferotemporal cortex, and not the creation of totally novel representations. Faces as objects were presumably well represented before the experiments began, and thus the incorporation of new exemplars into existing visual representations makes good theoretic sense.

But what happens when one is required to make visual judgments about a class of objects that has never been seen before? Logothetis and Pauls (1995) addressed exactly this issue by training monkeys to recognize wirelike and spheroidal objects, similar to objects used in previous psychophysical experiments in humans (Bülthoff and Edelman 1992; Rock and DiVita 1987). The monkeys' behavioral performance on these tasks was remarkably consistent with human results; it showed that initially recognition was viewpoint dependent, and that only after training could objects be recognized from all directions. The most striking result of these experiments, though, was that after training, individual neurons located in anterior inferotemporal cortex, near the anterior medial temporal sulcus (AMTS), were found to exhibit selective responses to test objects that the monkeys had previously learned. Figure 6.6 illustrates the responses of one such neuron, selective for a wirelike object. In the two top rows, the tuning of the cell is depicted, which shows a remarkable similarity to the view tuning of the face cell shown in figure 6.1. Note that, although the monkey was capable of recognizing all views of this wire, the cell responded to only a

subset of these views. The figure also demonstrates how selective these cells can be: none of the other wire objects, or other images, activated the cell significantly above its baseline rate. These results have important implications for models of object recognition because they provide neurophysiological evidence in support of view-based representations for visual objects (Logothetis and Pauls 1995; Logothetis, Pauls, and Poggio 1995; Perrett et al. 1984; Poggio 1990). In addition, they provide some of the strongest evidence to date for the modifiability of cell selectivity as a function of experience.

Further support for the idea that cells become selectively tuned for objects through learning comes from a study by Miyashita, Date, and Okuno (1993), who trained three adult monkeys in a matching task with a set of 97 fractal patterns, and then recorded the response of IT neurons to both the old set and a novel set of fractal stimuli. In 14 out of 15 cells fully tested, the maximum response of the cells was to learned stimuli, a result that could be attributed neither to chance nor to the nature of the stimuli because they were generated using exactly the same algorithm. In a subsequent study, Sakai and Miyashita (1994), having trained monkeys to recognize computer-generated Fourier descriptors in a paired-associate task, then tested neurons that exhibited any pattern-selective response to their stimuli, using the original stimuli and parametric transformations in the test patterns. They reasoned that if the activity of the cells they were recording from had been shaped by training with the specific patterns in the learning set, then alterations in the test patterns should lead to a decrease in cell response: the transformed stimulus would no longer match the learned pattern optimally. If, on the other hand, the pattern selective responses were simply a manifestation of selectivity that was always present in the connectivity of network of cells under study, then there would be no

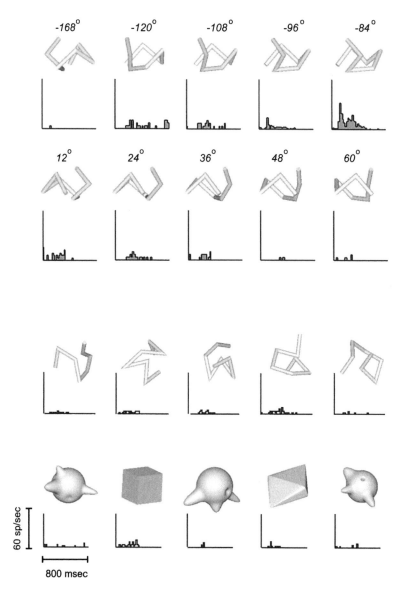

Figure 6.6
Example cell, taken from Logothetis, Pauls, and Poggio 1995, responsive to a particular view of a novel object. This cell provides convincing evidence that cell responses in inferotemporal (IT) cortex may be altered with experience. In contrast to the stimuli shown in the other figures, the top two rows of wire objects depicted here were behaviorally relevant to the monkey from whom the cell was recorded. He had learned to discriminate highly similar wirelike objects from each other, which may explain why almost 9% of the visually responsive cells from anterior IT cortex in this monkey responded to

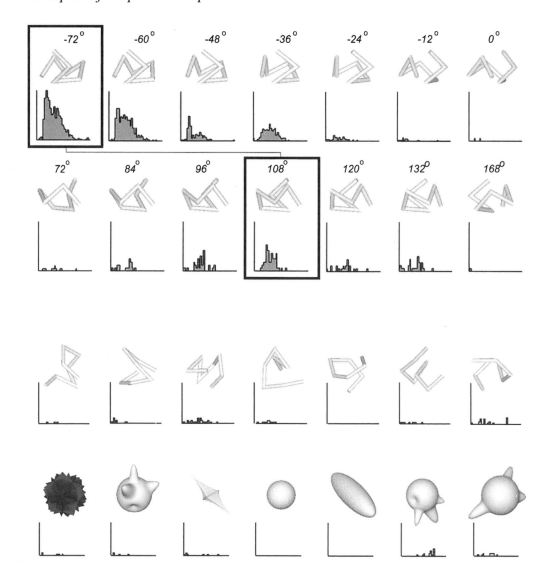

Figure 6.6 (continued)
images of wirelike objects. Note that the cell only responds to a very limited range of object views, supporting the idea that representations of three-dimensional objects may be constructed by combining the activity of a small number of cells selective to two-dimensional views.

reason to expect that the learned pattern should be a better stimulus than nearby transforms. The results clearly favored a model of selective tuning of cells: the altered forms always elicited a weaker response than the learned image. These data are also totally consistent with the findings of Logothetis and Pauls (1995), who reported that no selective cell was ever found to prefer an unfamiliar test stimulus.

Figure 6.7 depicts an example of our testing to show how a cell responds to digitally altered variants of its most effective stimulus. The top row shows the original image, along with five variants. Notice that no variant proved more effective than the original, although it is clear that the cell does continue to respond quite vigorously to a number of the altered images. Any time we have tried such a test, we, like Sakai and Miyashita (1994), have never been able to create on the fly a more effective stimulus than one that had been encountered before. If cells in inferotemporal cortex were elements of an elaborate, but fixed, coding system, then there would be no reason to expect that our randomly chosen test images would be more effectively represented than unencountered images.

In the initial studies on the coding of complex objects by Tanaka and his colleagues (1991; Kobotake and Tanaka 1994), because the monkeys were untrained and anesthetized during testing, it is not at all clear how much perceptual learning may have taken place during these experiments. Kobotake, Wang, and Tanaka (1998), however, have reported effects of learning on cell selectivity in inferotemporal cortex, comparing responses of IT neurons from control monkeys with cells recorded from monkeys trained to discriminate complex shapes. They found that the proportion of cells responsive to some of the training stimuli was greater in the trained monkeys than in the controls, suggesting that the characteristics of the population changed with experience. In gen-

eral, for the 28 out of 131 cells that responded best to the training stimuli, the response was not sharply tuned to only one of the training stimuli. On average, 3 out of the 28 training stimuli elicited at least a half-maximal response. This result, which can also be seen in the data shown in figure 6.5, strongly suggests that learning effects do not require that cells become selective for individual images. The details of selective tuning are not well understood, and many factors are likely to play a role in determining the distribution of cell selectivity. An informative aspect of the Kobotake, Wang, and Tanaka (1998) result is that the cells were recorded in anesthetized monkeys. The differences between the trained and control monkeys show that experience can lead to persistent biases within inferotemporal cortex that are not dependent on arousal, attention, or awareness. On the other hand, the conditions for inducing such changes may well depend on all three.

What conditions promote experience-based modification in IT cells? Discussions about the potential importance of past experience and training in determining the "adequacy" of a stimulus for activating these cells can be found in early theoretical hypotheses about IT function (Konorski 1967) and in the first neurophysiological reports of IT cells (Gross, Bender, and Rocha-Miranda 1969; Gross, Rocha-Miranda, and Bender 1972). It has further been argued that the extreme importance of faces in social communication, coupled with the need to identify individual faces within the class of all faces, may be a driving force behind the existence of face cells (e.g., Desimone 1991). To make fine discriminations that cannot be based on diagnostic features, the underlying representations may have to be more complex in nature. One prediction is that if monkeys are taught to make fine discriminations between objects other than faces, then configural selectivity for these items may be induced. Indeed, in experiments designed

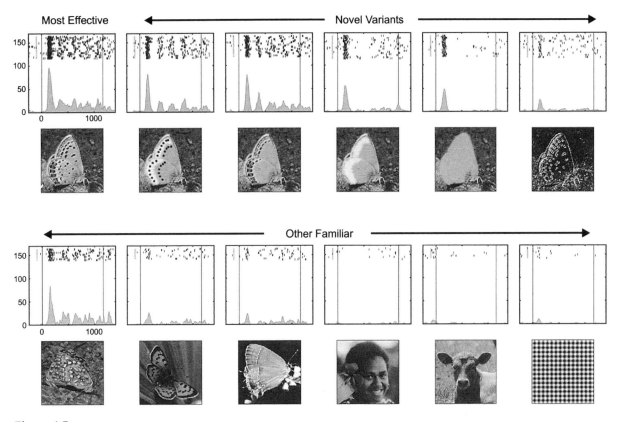

Figure 6.7

Generalization for images, never before seen, that are structurally similar to an effective image. The top row illustrates the response of this cell to the most effective stimulus we could find and to five altered views of that image created specifically for this cell. The response to each of these views was significantly better than the response to most other test objects. Note, though, that none of the variants elicited a stronger response than the original image. This finding is consistent with the idea that the learned, effective stimulus (along with other familiar stimuli, perhaps) had tuned the cell through prior experience to respond to its specific configuration, but that this tuning was sufficiently general so that similar images might still partially activate the cell (Sakai and Miyashita 1994). (See caption for figure 6.1.)

to test this, Logothetis and Pauls (1995) found cells responsive to images of individual objects that had been experienced during training. Although these results seem to show that very specific changes can occur in inferotemporal cortex, even at the level of single cells, they leave open the question of what served as the major force underlying the change. Is it the extensive training, the extensive exposure to particular objects, or both that leads to the neurophysiological changes?

A study by Vogels and Orban (1994) suggests that extensive training on its own is not sufficient to bias the properties of individual IT neurons. They trained monkeys to make fine orientation discriminations between successively presented gratings, and compared the response of IT neurons before and after training. The animals' performance clearly improved with practice, but no systematic changes were observed in the neurophysiological recordings (see chapter 5 for results in V1). An important implication of this study, especially in light of the positive effects obtained by Kobotake, Wang, and Tanaka (1998), is that the visual areas involved in various tasks are likely to be stimulus specific. For orientation discrimination, the cells in inferotemporal cortex may have little to contribute in such a task, and may therefore show little change with experience. On the other hand, in tasks where there may be large benefits to recoding complex configurations into perceptual wholes, these cells may play a much more active role.

One recent study has called into question the necessity for extensive training in biasing cell activity. In Booth and Rolls 1998, two monkeys were given a battery of ten objects to play with in their home cages. All neurophysiological testing was done using a fixation condition, and in no way depended on the monkeys' ability to recognize the test objects. Under these conditions, about 9% of the visual neurons not classified as face cells responded to multiple views of one or more of the cage objects. A larger proportion of the neurons responded in a view-dependent manner to one of the familiar objects or to another of the test stimuli. These results are consistent with a model of object representations built from combinations of multiple views (e.g., Perrett et al. 1984; Poggio 1990) and are very similar to data reported by Logothetis and Pauls (1995) for the novel objects used in that study. A major difference in Booth and Rolls 1998, though, is that view combination cells seem to have developed in the absence of extensive controlled training, suggesting that active interaction with visual objects alone may be sufficient to alter visual responsiveness in IT neurons. Inherent interest in exploring and coding the visual environment may provide sufficient exposure to particular stimuli to lead to detectable change in neural representations.

6.3.4   Time Course of Learning

Although the existing data indicate that cell properties are tuned through experience, the precise time course for these long-term changes is not known. When, for example, does plasticity begin? In their study of macaque IT and STP neurons, cells, Rodman, O Scalaidhe, and Gross (1993) found that visual cells in these areas are considerably less active, as a whole, in the infant than in the adult, and that the infant cells have longer and more variable visual latencies. But they also found that even by two months of age, single cells exhibit the same sorts of (varied) selectivity that adult IT cells do (see, for example, Rodman, O Scalaidhe, and Gross 1993, figure 13). Do these data imply that IT neurons selective for, say, faces, are genetically preprogrammed? Given that the neurophysiological properties of monkey striate cortex are quite functional at birth (Hubel, Wiesel, and LeVay 1977) and that monkeys' eyes open soon after, the opportunity for experience-based learning is clearly in place very early on. Further, anatomical data from Rodman and Consuelos (1994) indicate that the pattern of visual projections from earlier visual areas, including V4, TEO, and posterior inferotemporal cortex, is in place in monkeys as young as seven weeks. Thus the conjecture that the existence of face cells is not dependent on visual experience remains unsupported.

Interestingly, in our adult monkey recordings, we have also encountered a number of visual cells with long latency (greater than 200 msec), low magnitude, but selective responses—some of the same properties of "immature" neurons described by Rodman, O Scalaidhe, and Gross (1993). Three such examples are shown in figure 6.8. The responses of these cells were not tightly aligned with stimulus onset, and both their maximum and mean firings were considerably lower than most visually responsive cells in temporal cortex. Of particular interest are the data illustrated in panel a: the only effective stimulus we could find for this cell (the close-up image of the pill bottle) had first been introduced into the test set just five days prior. A comparison of the activity profile is quite similar to that of a cell recorded in a 39-day-old monkey (Rodman, O Scalaidhe, and Gross 1993, figure 13b), which responded to an adult monkey face, but not to another infant monkey's face or to other control stimuli. We wonder (but will of course never know) how the response patterns of the particular cells shown in figure 6.8 might have changed over the days and weeks after we recorded them.

The nature of the visual stimuli used in testing also seems to be an important factor in the development of representations in these cells. Even extended exposure to stimuli that do not contain combinations of visual features, such as sinusoidal gratings, seems to have little effect on learning in these areas (Vogels and Orban 1994). In studies using more complicated stimuli (Booth and Rolls 1998; Kobotake, Wang, and Tanaka 1998; Logothetis and Pauls 1995), the time between exposure and test ranged from several weeks to many months. At the other end of the time spectrum, Rolls et al. (1989) reported changes in the responses to their test stimuli in the first one or two presentations of a novel stimulus. One hypothesis holds that the time necessary to establish new representations will be a direct function of the preexisting representations at the time of exposure, coupled with the current task demands. We know from the extensive work on face cells that many cells do respond to a wide variety of faces, and are not specialized for a single face. If a novel face is encountered that can be adequately represented by the existing population of cells (unfortunately we cannot, at present, provide a solid definition of "adequately"), then there may be only slight modifications of existing connectivity to incorporate the new image, as reported by Rolls et al. (1989). A direct consequence of novelty may also be increased visual encounters, because monkeys, like human infants (Fantz 1964), have been shown to prefer looking at novel images compared with familiar ones (Gunderson and Sackett 1984).

For other novel objects, the importance of identifying individual exemplars may be critical. Most monkeys, for instance, may never feel compelled to distinguish between specific wirelike objects, just as most people do not generally distinguish between specific elephants (not counting Dumbo). In these instances, specific representations for individual exemplars may not exist. If, however, the need arises to differentiate one wire from another, or one elephant from another, then these representations may prove inadequate and the formation of new ones may be essential. Exactly what conditions may signal the need to create new representations is not at all clear, though, because we have repeatedly found selective responses for stimuli that were never

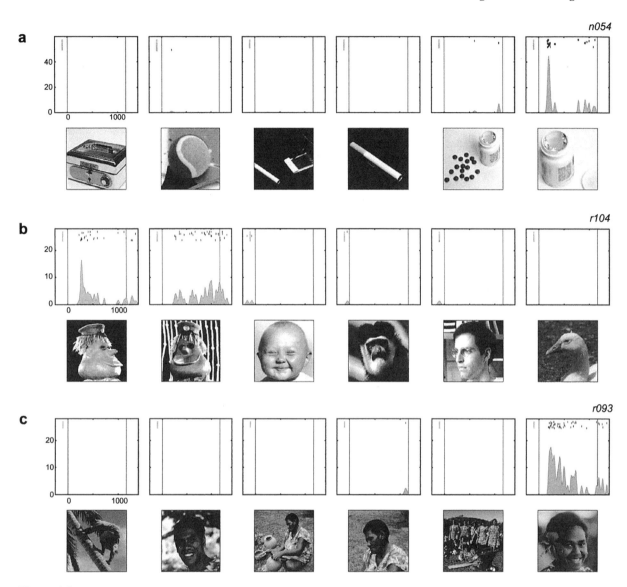

Figure 6.8
Adult inferotemporal (IT) cells with responses similar to those reported in infants. (*a, b, c*) The responses of the three cells shown are strikingly similar to the kinds of responses found in infant IT cortex (Rodman, O Scalaidhe, and Gross 1993). For each of these cells, the spontaneous firing rate was very near zero. The low overall responses and the long latency, relatively low magnitude, and variable stimulus evoked responses are clearly different from the brisk and reliable responses seen from many other cells. We hypothesize that these cells may have been recorded at a time when their connectivity was not firmly set. (See caption for figure 6.1.)

labeled as critical to the monkey. One possibility is that, though new representations at the level of single cells may come and go, once such a representation becomes critical, many others must also be recruited. This explanation would help explain why so many isolated, seemingly arbitrary, selective cells may be found alongside the more commonly encountered face-selective cells.

Another critical aspect to plasticity is neural stability. If synaptic modifications can adapt cells' responses based on visual experience, what will prevent cells from simply staying in a state of constant fluctuation? One possibility, inspired by a theoretical model, but now substantiated through neurophysiological experiments, is that thresholds for modification may not be fixed, but may instead vary as a function of the cells' history (Bienenstock, Cooper, and Munro 1982; Clothiaux, Bear, and Cooper 1991; Kirkwood, Rioult, and Bear 1996). In this model, cells that are rarely active will be more plastic than cells that are regularly active. This sliding modification threshold provides an internal source of stability, and has interesting implications for the development of cells not only in primary visual cortex, where it has been tested, but also in higher visual areas such as inferotemporal cortex. The requirements for plasticity in this theory are coincident pre- and postsynaptic activity, on the one hand, and a history of relatively low mean postsynaptic activity, on the other. Cells are candidates for plasticity provided they have not adapted to any other stimulus and can be reintegrated into the pool of candidate neurons if not exposed to any driving stimulus for a long period of time (because their history of activation would be low, and thus their threshold for modification would be also low). It is possible, therefore, that the cells depicted in figure 6.8, for example, may have been in the middle stages of a plastic process. They can clearly be activated by particular visual stimuli, satisfying the need for coincident pre- and postsynaptic activation, and they also have low overall activity, perhaps making them prime candidates for modification.

An exciting technique for answering some of these questions is the use of chronic recording electrodes, which are designed to record from the same set of cells for many days or weeks. Such electrodes have already been used to record from rat hippocampal cells and somatosensory cortex (Nicolelis et al. 1989), as well as from visual cortex in monkeys (Krüger 1989). Clearly, our understanding of the learning and changes in single-cell representations may change dramatically if we are not reliant on single snapshots of a cell's life.

6.3.5 Multiple Memory Systems

Acknowledging the growing body of evidence that there is no universal memory system in the brain (see Tulving and Schacter 1990), Desimone (1992) discussed four specific ways that memory can be expressed within the visual system: (1) by tuning, (2) by association, (3) by adaptive filtering, and (4) by sustained activity. All four ways have been found in inferotemporal neurons, but thus far we have concentrated mainly on one form of visual memory, tuning in visual cells (see Sakai, Naya, and Miyashita 1994). During tuning, the basic level of modification is the representation of a single stimulus, whereas during association, multiple representations are bound together, a process that appears critically dependent on the medial temporal lobe structures reciprocally interconnected with inferotemporal cortex (Suzuki and Amaral 1994; Saleem and Tanaka 1996; Van Hoesen and Pandya 1975). An elegant experiment by Miyashita and his colleagues (1996) serves to illustrate the distinction between tuning and association. In that study, monkeys were first trained to form arbitrary associations between a fixed set of fractal patterns. After this initial training, the anterior commissure was severed and the neurotoxin ibotenic acid was injected unilaterally into entorhinal and perirhinal cortical areas, thus removing a large source of neural backprojections into the inferotemporal cortex of one hemisphere. The authors then looked for any neurophysiological consequences of this missing projection, using the same paired-associate task, but now with both the old and new images. The unlesioned hemisphere served as a critical control. Consistent with previous results (Miyashita 1988), they found that in the control hemisphere, some cells responded to individual stimuli (both old and new), whereas others responded to both stimuli in a pair. In the lesioned hemisphere, however, the associated responses between paired stimuli were eliminated, whereas selectivity for individual stimuli remained intact. The results are in accord with the known behavioral deficits in visual associative learning after bilateral lesions to the perirhinal and entorhinal cortices, which include difficulties in forming new associations and recalling or relearning old ones (Murray, Gaffan, and Mishkin 1993). They also demonstrate that medial temporal lobe plays a critical role in the expression of associations between visual stimuli, and may be responsible for the view-invariant responses to entire objects that have been noted in inferotemporal cortex (Booth and Rolls 1998; Logothetis, Pauls, and Poggio 1995; Perrett, Mistlin, and Chitlin 1987). On the other hand, selectivity for particular views of objects seems not to rely on these structures, and instead to develop from repeated coactivation of earlier visual areas feeding into inferotemporal cortex and of the neurons within it.

Two other forms of visual memory, adaptive filtering and delay period activity, can also be distinguished from mechanisms of long-term tuning

and the development of selectivity. In adaptive filtering, information about stimulus properties is combined with temporal information about how recently a particular stimulus has been seen to change the response of visual neurons. Unlike tuning, adaptive filtering is almost always associated with a decrease in response to familiar objects (Miller, Li, and Desimone 1991; Riches, Wilson, and Brown 1991; Rolls et al. 1989). Early reports suggested that response decrements only appeared when stimulus repetition was separated by few stimuli and short time periods (e.g., Rolls et al. 1989), although Li, Miller, and Desimone (1993) have shown that reduced responses with familiarity can bridge even 150 presentations of other stimuli, suggesting that the decrease in response may induce attention systems to ignore recently encountered stimuli in favor of novel visual stimuli. Moreover, the short-term effects of adaptive filtering may be at least partly responsible for well-known visual priming phenomena, in which the repeated presentation of a stimulus leads to more accurate or more rapid responses to that stimulus (Schacter, Cooper, and Delaney 1990). Kersteen-Tucker (1991) found that repetition priming occurs even in the absence of preexisting memorial representations for visual shapes, although the effect is limited to very short lags. Priming effects are thus likely a combined consequence of both short-term adaptive mechanisms and their effects on preexisting representations that emerged through experience. This is in accord with the basic role of codability in priming (Schacter, Cooper, and Delaney 1990; Tulving and Schacter 1990), whereby experiences with objects that can be effectively coded by the visual system will be able to facilitate subsequent encounters with that object.

Sustained activity of visual cells, even in the absence of the physical stimulus, has often been thought to represent the short-term mnemonic process of keeping a stimulus "in mind" (Fuster and Jervey

1981; Miyashita 1993; Sakai and Miyashita 1991), and has generally been observed in the delay period between the presentation of a sample stimulus and a subsequent test presentation. Recent experiments have shown, however, that the sustained activity does not appear to depend on the need to explicitly remember a stimulus: this activity is found not only between sample and test, but also following the test and throughout the intertrial interval (Yakolev et al. 1998). Indeed, for most of the cells shown in the examples above, we see that even following the stimulus offset, cells continue to respond if the last presented stimulus was itself effective. Thus the importance of this sustained activity is still uncertain, although Yakolev et al. (1998) suggest that the ongoing activity presents an opportunity for association between neighboring views, and may have no perceptual consequence on a single trial. We know that the presentation of an ineffective masking stimulus that immediately follows an effective test stimulus can abruptly eliminate this sustained activity (Rolls and Tovee 1994). Because visually similar views of an effective stimulus shown in sequence do not seem to disrupt a cell's activity, it has been suggested that associations between neighboring views may occur as sustained activity bridges the slight changes in an objects' projection on the retina during visual exploration (Földiák 1991; Wallis and Rolls 1997). Such a model could form the basis for the development of view-invariant representations.

6.4 Conclusions

Although it is known that natural images contain statistical regularities that set them apart from random noise (Olshausen and Field 1996), the set of visual objects that can be found in these images is enormous. For an organism to both distinguish among these and,

at the same time, generalize across them, its visual system cannot depend on regularities that span the entire space of images. Instead, visual representations that emphasize important differences of individual objects, while ignoring insignificant variations, are a critical component of successful visual recognition. We have argued that one method of solving this problem is to build representations of visual objects by constantly incorporating experienced views of real objects into the neural connections that together make up the visual system.

Specifically, that complex representations may be created dynamically throughout life is consistent with the wide-ranging properties and selectivities of inferotemporal neurons. That neurons may respond to seemingly arbitrary stimuli, such as a particular view of a roller coaster, or a squirrel, or even one's grandmother, is not so shocking if one accepts the view that response properties can be molded by experiences with the very same stimuli. The activity of these neurons should not be mistaken for a representation of the actual object portrayed in the picture. Instead, it would seem more judicious to view such responses simply as a positive signal for the presence of configurations of visual patterns present in that image. The neurons are buried in the midst of an extensive network of cells, and only through interconnections with other cells can their activity have any influence on either behavior or cognition. We also think that the sparseness of a cell's response will, in large part, be a function of its history of plasticity and the organism's prior experience with similar stimuli. Because neither selectivity nor sparseness is a static property of an entire set of visual neurons, particular population tallies or general information-theoretic estimates may only give a small picture about what cells in these areas are doing.

As we pointed out in section 6.1, Gibson and Gibson (1955) argue that, in the course of perceptual learning, observers become more responsive to the details of a stimulus with practice, but that they do not add something to a stimulus not actually there. In no uncertain terms, they reject the idea that perceptual learning is contingent on memory:

There is no evidence in all of this literature on perceptual learning ... to *require* the theory that an accurate percept is one which is enriched by past experience, whereas a less accurate percept is one *not* enriched by past experience. Repetition or practice is necessary for the development of the improved percept, but there is no proof that it incorporates memories.... The observer sees and hears more, but this may be not because he imagines more, or infers more, or assumes more, but because he discriminates more. He is more sensitive to the variables of the stimulus array. (Gibson and Gibson 1955, 40)

On this issue, it is hard to conceive of a mechanism that would change the observer's sensitivity to a stimulus through repetition that does not depend on some long-term neural changes. Indeed, the data we have highlighted above suggest that perceivers' brains do seem to reorganize as a function of visual experience. It is quite possible, however, that this kind of memory is not directly related to imagination or inference, at least at a conscious level. Similarly, perhaps the current use of the term *memory*, especially with reference to its neural correlates, is far more general than the type of memory to which the Gibsons refer. Their major objection was clearly to the idea that perception improves by relying on information that is not directly available in the stimulus. We agree that the stimulus is information rich, and it is precisely through interaction with information-rich stimuli that we believe perceptual learning for recognition of complex objects occurs. One issue we have only barely addressed thus far is why the creation of these representations would be of any benefit to the perceiver.

Describing one such benefit, which he called "perceptual readiness," Bruner (1957) argued that

high-order representations reciprocally connecting with complex activity patterns in lower visual areas can later reactivate lower-order representations, even in the presence of degraded or otherwise suboptimal input. Models of this sort have been extensively studied (e.g., McClelland and Rumelhart 1981) and have been shown to account well for phenomena such as the word superiority effect described in section 6.1. Indeed, many of them contain "hidden units" that play a role quite similar to that we are proposing here for cells in inferotemporal cortex. The basic benefit is thus one of predicting, filling in, or augmenting visual information using previous experience as guide. Because interactive processes guided by both data and prediction can speed recognition and thus also response, this top-down modulation of perceptual processes may also affect responses to the visual stimulus. Incomplete inputs can also, with the help of top-down guidance, be induced to activate a response.

A related benefit stems directly from the need to respond to visual inputs. Vision is not just about sensing light from the environment. Appropriate and efficient reaction to this information is what makes the process so remarkable. Although the engineering behind high-end cameras is impressive, no one expects a camera to do anything with the data it so faithfully captures. On the other hand, living organisms must transform complex visual patterns into appropriate responses, and this mapping relies on connections between internal representations of the environment and the responding brain areas. Perhaps repeated visual encounters with a stimulus facilitate not only the process of seeing a stimulus in the future, but also the associating of an *action* with that stimulus.

Direct support for this idea comes from a study by Gibson and Walk (1956), who reared two sets of rats in controlled visual environments. The experimental rats were exposed to specific visual forms (circles and triangles) on the walls of their cages, whereas the walls of the control group's cages were covered only by white cardboard. After three months, both groups were trained in a standard discrimination task, using the forms present in the experimental group's cages as discriminanda. The results showed conclusively that the rats who had been preexposed to the visual forms were far more efficient at learning to discriminate the forms, as evidenced by their performance in a standard two-alternative forced-choice feeding paradigm. The experiment clearly suggests that even mere exposure to sensory stimuli can affect the process of connecting these stimuli to behavioral responses.

A common argument against the idea that cells may become selective for particular images in the world is that there are simply not enough cells to code for all the world's objects. If we believed that in order to recognize or react to visual objects one had to have at least one cell selective for that object, then we would be more concerned with this objection. However, our view is not that the development of selectivity in IT neurons is absolutely essential for all visual function. Indeed, TE lesions introduced early in life lead to only mild impairment in habit formation and visual short-term memory tasks (Malkova, Mishkin, and Bachevalier 1995), indicating that the role of these cells can either be fully compensated by other brain areas, or that the mild impairment that remains is a very specific form that does not disrupt all visual processing. Cooling studies (e.g., Horel et al. 1987), in which cryodes were surgically placed around the visual cortices of the temporal lobe, support the latter view. Deactivating anterior temporal cortical areas by cold affects discriminations of complex objects, such as faces, but not of simpler patterns, such as oriented lines. If we follow this logic, when objects can be recognized or reacted to on the

basis of individual diagnostic features, then the importance of a system for configural representations is minimized. Such deactivation may leave many forms of perceptual processing relatively intact, perhaps so intact that without careful scrutiny, these deficits may go unnoticed.

In humans, bilateral temporal lobe lesions have been implicated in the visual recognition disorder known as "visual agnosia." A number of researchers (Humphreys and Riddoch 1987; Zeki 1993) have postulated that visual agnosia is principally an integrative disorder. In patients with agnosia, the basic perceptual apparatus appears intact, meaning that low-level disturbances in acuity or contrast sensitivity cannot explain the higher-level recognition deficit. Humphreys and Riddoch (1987) conclude that Lissauer's original distinction (1890) between apperceptive agnosia and associative agnosia does not fit well with one of their most carefully studied agnosic patients, John. By Lissauer's definition, apperceptive agnosia results from problems in perceptual processing, whereas associative agnosics cannot appropriately connect perceptions to stored object memories. Humphreys and Riddoch argue that one of the major tests for intact perceptual processing—a patient's ability to accurately copy a visual image—is not necessarily a strong test for intact perceptual processing. John, for example, can copy quite reasonably, but he does so extremely slowly, and by paying focused attention to individual features of the source image. Similarly, when characterizing visual forms, John is also capable of differentiating objects, but he relies almost entirely on local features. He is unable to recognize familiar or famous faces, and even identified Winston Churchill as a woman simply because he was not wearing a tie in the picture (Humphreys and Riddoch 1987, 62). As strange as it may seem, though, Humphreys and Riddoch point out that John's deficits are not obvious to the casual observer because he has learned to rely on cues and features for solving problems that might be solved more efficiently by other means no longer available to him. We think these other means may be the formation and use of the kinds of complex representations that exist in the anterior temporal lobe.

If we are to understand how the visual system effectively deals with the complexity of the visual world, we must begin to account for its capacity to reshape itself to accommodate the details of the environment and each individual's particular needs. It has long been accepted that adaptability is fundamental for survival. What is new is the growing body of data that indicates that changes in representational capacity can be traced to properties of single cells throughout the visual system. The challenge now is to find ways to systematically examine these single neurons as they cooperate with their neighbors and as they react and adapt to stimuli that more accurately reflect the richness of the real world.

Acknowledgments

The authors wish to thank the Max Planck Society for their generous support. David Sheinberg was also supported by National Institutes of Health grant NRSA 1F32EY06624. We are also grateful to Natasha Sigala for her helpful comments, suggestions, and assistance in preparing this manuscript.

Notes

1. Lettvin describes in a letter, reprinted by Barlow 1950, appendix), how he came up with the idea of the grandmother cell as part of a lecture he used for introducing MIT undergraduates to the topic of the biological basis of perception and knowledge.

2. Although many of these observations have been made before by various investigators, because of the general skepticism often associated with such data, we present a number of examples of cells we have recorded.

3. Note that because all the test images were intermixed at the same time, the effects of short-term learning should be minimal. Indeed, for most cells, such as those presented here, we found very little persistent change in the response properties over the course of a 1- to 3-hour recording session.

4. Neither we nor our monkeys had the "dogged persistence" described by Hubel and Wiesel (1998, 403) that kept them going for nine hours with a single cell.

5. Note that by "distributed" we mean the type of representation that cannot be properly decoded without access to a large number of contributing cells. Even a sparse code, where only a few, relatively tuned neurons are used to detect a stimulus, will be distributed across a brain area, but access to any one of these neurons will, on its own, offer a reasonable description of an encountered stimulus.

7

Functional Reorganization of Human Cerebral Cortex and Its Perceptual Concomitants

Annette Sterr, Thomas Elbert, and Brigitte Rockstroh

Abstract

This chapter describes the plastic modeling of cortex in response to both deafferentation and increased use for different modalities. Such brain plasticity is a functionally relevant phenomenon; its perceptual and behavioral consequences are adaptive in most cases. On the other hand, brain reorganization is linked to symptoms such as phantom pain, tinnitus, and focal hand dystonia. By revealing the principles underlying representational alterations of the adult brain, research in the last decade has made possible the development of clinical interventions for the treatment of symptoms linked to altered representation, and given rise to treatment for musicians suffering from focal hand dystonia. The many mechanisms that seem to be involved in neuroplasticity include the unmasking of inhibited connections, rearrangement of the synaptic inhibitory-excitatory equilibrium, arborization of thalamocortical neurons, and the sprouting of new projections. Although it is still not clear just how these mechanisms are involved, there is general agreement about the functional significance of cortical reorganization: the ability to reorganize allows the brain to deal with the organism's special needs throughout its life.

7.1 Introduction

Perception and processing of stimuli depends on the functional organization of the respective neural network. The brain has the potential to reorganize this functional organization and even to alter its structure in response to experience. Perception will vary with these changes. On a microscopic scale, structural changes include alterations in synaptic efficacy, syn-apse formation, synaptic plasticity, spine density, and alterations in dendritic length. As a consequence, supportive tissue elements such as astrocytes and blood vessels are also changed (for review, see Kolb and Wishaw 1998).

The cortical representations of sensory perception relate in an orderly way to the spatial arrangements of receptors in the periphery forming so-called organotopic maps. The most prominent example of this organizational principle is the homunculus of the somatosensory system. Not only are representational maps highly plastic during "critical periods" in the development of cortical structures, but they maintain limited ability to respond to alterations in afferent input throughout life. For example, the cortex can allocate an enlarged area to represent peripheral input sources that are of particular behavioral relevance and that are most used. Reviewing both fields of synaptic and cortical reorganization, Buonomano and Merzenich (1998) reinforce the hypothesis that synaptic plasticity underlies even large-scale cortical reorganization. Dinse and Merzenich (chapter 2, this volume) provide a detailed description of functional plasticity on a microscopic scale and summarize the results of invasive experiments carried out in animals. This chapter focuses on functional plasticity and its perceptual correlates in humans, on maladaptive consequences of neuroplasticity, and on the methods that allow the noninvasive investigation of functional cortical organization in humans.

The construction and maintenance of the functional brain organization relies on the mechanisms of synaptic interactions postulated by Donald Hebb as early as 1949. Hebb elaborated that synaptic contacts are plastic and are modified as a consequence of simultaneous activation of the pre- and postsynaptic neuron. More precisely, when the presynaptic action potential precedes the firing of the postsynaptic cell, the synaptic response will increase (long-term potentiation, or LTP; see chapter 3.6.1); when the order is reversed, the synaptic response will decrease (long-term depression, or LTD). A typical temporal window for synaptic plasticity to occur varies around 100 msec. For pyramidal neurons in neocortical slices, Markram et al. (1997) observed that a difference in spike timing of 10 msec near coincidence switched the plasticity from LTP to LTD. That is, every spike in a pyramidal cell could potentially affect every excitatory synapse of a cell that was active within 100 msec. However, there are reasons to believe that synaptic plasticity is regulated in distinct ways. A general form of activity-dependent regulation of synaptic transmission called "synaptic scaling," recently described by Turrigiano et al. (1998), enhances or suppresses *all* synaptic inputs of a neuron as a function of activity. The mechanism of multiplicative synaptic strength scaling preserves the relative differences between inputs and allows the neuron to adjust the total amount of synaptic excitation it receives. Synaptic scaling may thus contribute to stabilization in firing rates during development and in the adult brain; moreover, it may help to counterbalance the destabilizing effects of Hebbian-type synaptic modifications within the neural network. According to Fregnac (1998, 845), synaptic scaling can be seen "as a demonstration of basic homeostasis, designed to return the integrative function of the cell to within a reference working range." Synaptic plasticity underlies alterations of complex neural networks like the cortical representation of the body surface in the primary somato-

sensory cortex (Brodmann area 3b; Finnerty, Roberts, and Connors 1999; Prescott et al. 1998) and is related to learning and memory processes (Baudry 1998; Kleim et al. 1999).

Animal studies by Merzenich and colleagues demonstrated as early as 1984 that the deafferentation of digits (fingers) results in an altered representation of the hand in cortical area 3b. Pons et al. (1991) investigated the organization of the primary somatosensory cortex in owl monkeys that had been deprived from somatosensory input of an upper limb twelve years earlier. The authors found that the deafferented area, which usually comprises the representation of the hand, contained neurons that were responsive to the stimulation of neighboring representations, such as those of the trunk and the face. This large-scale reorganization encompassed a cortical space across more than 10 mm in response to the long-term deafferentation. In magnetoencephalographic (MEG) studies, Elbert et al. (1994) observed the same type and corresponding magnitude of map alterations in human amputees. Subsequent work revealed that the amount of cortical reorganization was strongly correlated with the amount of phantom limb pain (Flor et al. 1995). Thus the loss of somatosensory input does not result in silence and degeneration of the respective cortical neurons but is followed by a functional reorganization of the homuncular representation of the body surface in the cortex. In addition, increased use of a body part also alters the homunculus, leading to an expansion of the representational cortical zones (Elbert et al. 1995) and also to changes of perception such as the ability to localize different receptive fields to light tactile stimuli (Sterr et al. 1998). These observations indicate that the capacity of the human brain for plastic reorganization in response to either injury or altered use of a body part is retained into adulthood and is accompanied by changes in perception.

7.2 Noninvasive Techniques to Investigate Functional Cortical Organization in Humans

Cortical maps like that of the body surface or of the tone frequencies in Heschl's gyrus can be individually determined in humans by a number of brain imaging techniques, such as electric and magnetic source imaging (MSI), functional magnetic resonance (fMRI), and positron emission tomography (PET). These noninvasive techniques can also be used to map motor areas along the central sulcus and areas of the frontal lobe. As an alternative, transcranial magnetic stimulation (TMS) may be employed to stimulate output from motor cortex or to disrupt ongoing activity, resulting, for instance, in transient speech arrest.

7.2.1 Electromagnetic Source Imaging

Biomagnetic signals in the brain are generated by neuronal excitation and originate from an intracellular current flow having a relatively high current density. Pathways through extracellular body tissue close this current flow. Because some of the current penetrates the skull and scalp, bioelectric potentials can be measured on the scalp as the electroencephalogram (EEG), which measures the voltage derived from two electrodes attached to the surface of the scalp. The magnetoencephalogram (MEG), on the other hand, measures the magnetic field generated by intracellular current flow in the brain (Elbert 1998). Brain magnetic fields have a very low amplitude: the evoked cortical magnetic fields, that is the transient brain response to a sensory stimulation, have an approximate strength of 100 fT (100 femto-tesla $= 10^{-13}$ tesla). An example of an evoked magnetic field is plotted in figure 7.1.

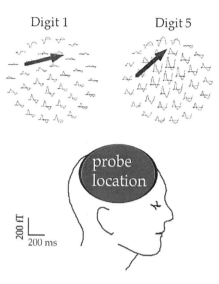

Figure 7.1
Examples for evoked magnetic fields elicited by tactile stimulation of the thumb ("digit 1") and little finger ("digit 5") in a normal control subject.

Measuring biomagnetic activity is completely noninvasive and free of contact with the subject. Because conductivities for scalp, skull, cerebrospinal fluid, and brain vary greatly with their complex geometries, neuronal sources can be modeled only to a very limited extent using the EEG alone. By contrast, biomagnetic measurements most often allow us to determine the source of biological activity with a greater spatial resolution than do measurements of bioelectric potentials. This is particularly true for the source of magnetic fields evoked by various sensory modalities within the primary representational zones of the cerebral cortex. In many instances, this activity can be modeled as a single current dipole. The simplest and still most powerful constraint is the assumption of a focal source which can then be modeled with good approximation by one such dipole regardless of the real shape of neuronal fields. The location of the equivalent current dipole (ECD) is allowed to move with time. A high goodness of fit of the field produced by the modeled ECD to the real measurement provides a reasonable justification for the application of the model. More sophisticated approaches incorporate the knowledge of anatomical structures. It is known, for instance, that regions occupied by ventricles or white matter lack active structures. More explicitly, for most of the neuromagnetic data, only current dipoles with an orientation perpendicular to the surface of gray matter contribute to electromagnetic activity on a macroscopic scale (for a review of MSI and MEG, see Elbert 1998).

Equivalent current dipoles (ECD) can be localized to within millimeters (Lütkenhöner 1996; Lütkenhöner, Hoke, and Pantev 1990). The accuracy of source localization is not identical with the accuracy of separating different, simultaneously active sources, however. Whereas we can localize isolated ECDs to within a few millimeters, we can separate several simultaneously active sources only to within a range about one order of magnitude smaller.

Currents flowing perpendicularly to the surface of the head produce only a small signal strength in conventional MEG: they are magnetically silent, so to speak, although they create a pronounced electrical potential on the scalp. Because magnetic fields and electric potentials contain complementary information with respect to their sources (Eulitz, Eulitz, and Elbert 1997), the simultaneous measurement of both signals provides additional constraints on source localization that are not available using one type of signal alone.

Magnetic source imaging (MSI) integrates MEG and fMRI information into one data set. Whereas the location of a single ECD determined from MEG data was superimposed on the corresponding fMRT section in earlier attempts, current techniques use

fMRI information to constrain source configurations to the gray matter of the cortex. This has proven to be useful in reconstructing the cortical sheet by surface rendering and in displaying anatomy, pathological tissue, and functional activation in a single image.

Biomagnetic responses to stimuli such as event-related electric potentials (ERPs) and event-related magnetic fields (ERFs) benefit from signal averaging to enhance their signal-to-noise ratio (SNR). Data are generally digitized at a fixed rate to fill a data array, while a stimulus or other synchronizing event defines the time epoch of interest within this array. The event is repeated and a time-locked signal average calculated. Signal averaging improves the SNR provided the signal is invariant across trials and the background EEG represents random noise. This is not always true (Makeig 1993). Moving visual stimuli, for example, reliably produce increases in spectral power in the 40 Hz band (Müller et al. 1996, 1997). But because the oscillations elicited during stimulation are not phase locked to the stimulus, they are lost by averaging in the time domain.

Alterations of Somatosensory Representation in Braille Readers

Braille reading is an impressive example for a specialized perceptual capability of the tactile sense. Braille, a tactile language, is based on dot patterns that can be recognized by moving the fingertips slowly across the surface. For efficient reading, the tactile discrimination of the characters has to be fast and correct. Experienced Braille readers can read up to 200 words per minute (Foulke 1991), whereas Braille-naive persons find it difficult to distinguish different Braille patterns and require intensive training to learn to read Braille even at average level. Most likely, perceptual learning is involved in this process, and the question arises whether the improved tactual skills go along with (1) an alteration of the cortical somatosensory hand representation and (2) changed tactual capacity of the fingers. We examined two groups of blind subjects (experienced multifinger and one-finger readers) and one sighted control group. Multifinger and one-finger readers differed in their way of reading: one-finger readers used one index finger to read Braille, multifinger readers employed three adjacent fingers simultaneously to decode the dot pattern. Sighted control subjects had no experience in Braille reading.

The sensory capacity of the fingers was explored by measuring the threshold for passive touch and the frequency of mislocalizations. A light tactile stimulus was used to determine the sensory threshold; it was also applied to different fingers in pseudorandomized order, and the subjects were asked to indicate the finger being touched. Mislocalizations occurred when subjects named a nonstimulated finger.

The hand representation in multifinger readers encompassed a larger area than in sighted controls. In one-finger readers the expansion was restricted to the reading finger. Furthermore, MSI of the hand representation in area SI revealed a disordered somatotopical arrangement of the finger representations in multifinger readers but not in one-finger readers nor in sighted controls (indicated schematically in figure 7.2). These results demonstrate that different reading habits, associated with different stimulation conditions, modulate the cortical representations differently. This finding is mirrored by the perceptual data. In both groups of blind subjects, the threshold for passive touch was lower than in the sighted controls. Moreover, multifinger readers expressed mislocalizations. Within threshold range, blind subjects attributed the tactile stimulus to a nonstimulated finger. These perceptual errors did not occur in control subjects. The disarrangement of the digital representations in the multifinger readers results from simultaneous stimulation during read-

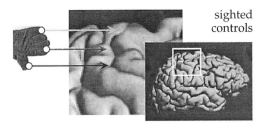

sighted controls

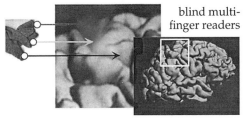

blind multi-finger readers

Figure 7.2
Schematic illustration of the hand organization in sighted controls and multifinger readers. In sighted controls (*top*), the finger representations are arranged in order along the central sulcus. In blind multifinger readers (*bottom*), the typical arrangement of the finger representations is disordered. (Data from Sterr et al. 1998.)

ing. As a result of this disarrangement, it is more difficult for multifinger readers to localize a light tactile stimulus within threshold range, thus the mislocalizations.

7.2.2 Metabolic Imaging Procedures: Positron Emission Tomography

Positron emission tomography (PET) studies are based on radioactive isotopes that decay within a short time by emitting a positron (the positive antiparticle of the electron). Nearly any organic molecule can be labeled with such a radioactive isotope. For instance, carbon dioxide can be labeled with ^{15}O; when the gas is inhaled, blood volume can be recorded by measuring the distribution of the radioactive decay. Once a positron is emitted, it will collide with an electron after traveling only one or a few millimeters. When particle and antiparticle collide, they are annihilated, and two gamma ray photons are emitted at an angle of 180° to one another (impulse preservation). If detectors for the gamma ray photons are connected in a way that only temporal coincidence of the two photons is recorded, the density of the decaying substance can be reconstructed by means of computer tomography. As noted above, $^{15}O=C=O$ is used to measure blood volume. For the investigation of regional cerebral blood flow (rCBF), ^{15}O-labeled H_2O is used: the oxygen consumption can be imaged with $^{15}O_2$. ^{15}O as a tracer with a short half-life of about 2 min allows repeated measurements within one session. The brain mapping of a subject relies on the subtraction of blood flow patterns between two conditions, often an active task condition and a resting condition. This approach has been subject to various criticisms. Considering these, correlational techniques have been suggested as an alternative (see below).

Many of the techniques that have been developed for PET-based imaging have also been implemented for fMRI. To allow group comparisons, many investigators use a normalization of the brain anatomy (mostly, the atlas by Talairach and Tournoux 1988). Alternatively, individual filters, averages, and scores may be extracted. One persistent problem is that global alterations in blood flow (within a subject or across a group of patients) are superimposed on task-specific changes in rCBF. Introducing global flow into an analysis of covariance may offer a solution, assuming that the effect is linear. The assumption of linearity is not always justified, however, making interpretations sometimes difficult. For instance, it is unlikely that twice the stimulus intensity will simply double the intensity of the blood flow without also changing the particular spatial distribution as a consequence.

Neural Networks for Braille Reading and the Role of Primary Visual Areas in the Blind

In congenitally blind persons, the visual system cannot develop or adapt to visual processing. Empirical data suggest that the occipital cortex is active in blind individuals when somatosensory and auditory information is processed (Kujala et al. 1997; Röder et al. 1996). Sadato and coworkers (1998) employed PET to explore the functional role of primary visual areas in congenitally blind persons and the neural network used for Braille reading. Regional cerebral blood flow (rCBF) was measured in a Braille reading and a non-Braille reading task. In the Braille reading task, only experienced Braille readers but no sighted controls were tested, whereas the non-Braille reading task was performed by all subjects.[1] Thus brain activation to tactile tasks could be compared directly between groups. rCBF images were obtained by integrating the activity occurring during the 60-sec periods after tracer injection. Subtraction of task from rest condition images was used to reproduce task-related focal activity. In the blind the primary visual cortex was active in both the Braille reading and the non-Braille reading task. The non-Braille reading tasks elicited different patterns of activation in sighted and blind subjects. In the blind, the ventral occipital cortex (including the primary visual cortex and the fusiform gyri) was activated, whereas the secondary somatosensory area was deactivated during the non-Braille discrimination tasks. The reverse pattern was found in sighted subjects: the secondary somatosensory area was activated, whereas the ventral occipital regions were deactivated. These results suggest that the tactile processing pathways usually linked to the secondary somatosensory cortex are rerouted in blind subjects to ventral occipital cortical regions that are engaged in visual shape discrimination in sighted persons.

7.2.3 *Functional Magnetic Resonance Imaging*

Every atomic nucleus has a small magnetic moment (nuclear spin). For the hydrogen nucleus (proton) it is largest. The orientation of these tiny magnets is random such that there is no net magnetic field. When the body is exposed to a very strong magnetic field (1.5 tesla or more) the protons gyrate around a stable orientation (B_0). In nuclear magnetic resonance, a secondary transient field pulse, radio frequency (RF) pulse,[2] flips the atomic nuclei toward a different orientation (B_1). In a fraction of a second, the strong permanent field will draw the nuclei back towards their original orientation. As long as the proton spin has not reached its original orientation (relaxation time), it will gyrate or spin around the axis in direction of B_0 and emit electromagnetic radiation. The intensity of the latter provides information about the density of protons. The signal of this detectable signal provides us information about the density of protons. Because the frequency of electromagnetic radiation depends on B_0, we can code the location of the protons by varying B_0 across a section of the head. Depending on the direction of the excitation, there will be two different relaxation times, T1 parallel to and T2 perpendicular to B_0. These magnetic resonance signals are transient (30–50 msec up to 2–3 sec for a standard T2 spin echo sequence) and refractory. Functional magnetic resonance imaging (fMRI) exploits the fact that oxygenated and deoxygenated hemoglobin have different magnetic properties. Hemoglobin carries oxygen and becomes deoxygenated when the oxygen is absorbed. Because active brain regions have a higher ratio of oxygenated to deoxygenated hemoglobin and fMRI is sensitive to changes of this ratio, it creates a map of changes of regional cerebral blood flow that are coupled to local neuronal activity.

Blood Oxygenation Level Dependent Technique

The regional cerebral blood flow (rCBF) increases in brain regions with higher metabolism, that is, with greater neural activity. As a net effect, the relative concentration of oxyhemoglobin increases. This effect (based on the different magnetic properties of oxy- and deoxyhemoglobin) is measured in most fMRI techniques. Because the hemodynamic parameters change much more slowly than neural activity, the blood oxygenation level dependent (BOLD) technique does not take full advantage of the technically possible temporal resolution of fMRI. Furthermore, the measured changes in rCBF are small (2–5% when a 1.5 T-scanner is used). In the same tasks, PET would detect changes of 10–40%. Larger signals can be obtained with stronger magnets (measuring up to 15% changes in rCBF with a 4T-scanner). However, the biological noise (blood flow changes not related to the stimulus or task) also increase as does the sensitivity to movement artifacts.

Motor Reorganization in Phantom Limb Pain

Exploring the cerebral activation when movements with the amputated arm were imagined, Lotze and coworkers (1999) used fMRI to determine the relationship between phantom limb pain and the reorganization of the sensorimotor cortex. As a control condition, the pattern of activation for imagined and executed movements with the intact arm was measured in the amputees as well as in controls. Fourteen amputees, seven with and seven without phantom limb pain, and ten control subjects participated in the study. In the executed movement condition, movements of the lips, intact arm, and amputated arm had to be imagined. Each movement had to be executed or imagined for four seconds. This study revealed that in phantom pain patients the cortical activation

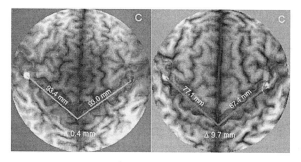

Figure 7.3
Two individual examples of altered cortical motor reorganization in upper limb amputees. (*Left*) Patient with no phantom pain. (*Right*) Patient with acute phantom pain. Precentral gyrus (area M1) is top shaded area, postcentral cortex (area S1) is lower shaded area. Distances from activation maxima during lip movement to the crossing of the interhemispheric fissure–central sulcus are measured for ipsi- and contralateral hemispheres to estimate displacement of the face representation. In both pictures, the deafferented hemisphere is on the right (marked with "C" in the top right corner). Although for the patient with nonphantom pain, distances are nearly the same for deafferented and intact hemisphere, as is the case in control subjects, in the phantom pain subject, the distance is much smaller contralateral to the amputation, indicating a displacement of the lip representation into the former hand region. (Reprinted from Lotze et al. 1999 with kind permission)

during imagined movement was displaced, and the amputated hand was displaced from the face to the hand region in the sensorimotor cortex contralateral to amputation (figure 7.3). No such changes were present in the no-phantom pain group and in controls. Furthermore, no differences between groups were found for cerebellar activation. These findings suggest that cortical reorganization in phantom pain is not restricted to somatosensory areas but can extend to motor areas as well.

7.2.4 *Transcranial Magnetic Stimulation*

A pulsed magnetic field that is generated by a conduction coil in the vicinity of the scalp penetrates the scalp and skull and affects neuroelectric activity within the brain. This technique is called "transcranial magnetic stimulation" (TMS) or, when delivered at regular intervals, "repetitive transcranial magnetic stimulation" (rTMS). Recently developed devices are capable of alternating very strong magnetic fields at rates up to 25 Hz (high-frequency rTMS). Transcranial magnetic stimulation can affect various brain functions, including movement, visual perception, memory, reaction time, speed, and mood. To map the motor cortex, the TMS probe is placed serially over various points on the subject's scalp. At each point of stimulation the electromyogram (EMG) responses from the muscles to a TMS pulse are recorded. A given muscle responds vigorously when the TMS is located over or in the vicinity of its cortical representation, but shows no response when distant sites are stimulated. In this way, it is possible to determine the cortical representational zone for a given muscle.

Consecutive Alterations of Motor Representations Following Upper Limb Amputation

Transcranial magnetic stimulation was used to map cortical motor outputs to various muscles of the body. Pascual-Leone et al. (1996) investigated the time course of functional cortical reorganization of the motor cortex in a twenty-two-year-old male student subject who had lost his arm in an accident.[3] Prior to the accident, the patient participated in two of the mapping experiments as a normal volunteer. Therefore, the preaccidental (normal) organization

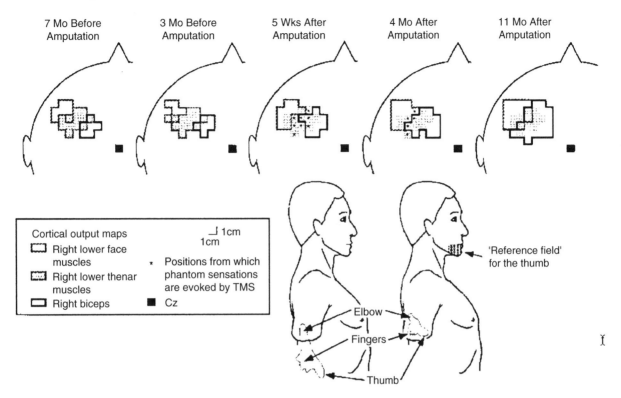

Figure 7.4
Cortical output maps to focal right lower face muscles, right thenar muscles, and right biceps. Transcranial magnetic stimulation (TMS) was applied to scalp positions arranged in a 1 × 1 cm grid. Grid position on the scalp can be inferred from the location of the Cz electrode position from the international 10–20 system for EEG electrodes. Asterisks mark the positions which, when stimulated, evoked phantom sensations in at least 60% of the trials. The schematic drawings of the lateral view of the body depict the subject's own drawing of the phantom limb at five weeks (wks) and four months (mo) following the traumatic amputation. The area of the thumb "reference field" that evoked phantom sensations when stimulated by vigorous rubbing is depicted in the second body scheme, four months after the amputation. (Reprinted from Pascual-Leone et al. 1996 with kind permission.)

of facial and upper extremity muscles was known. Both the progression of sensorimotor reorganization and the development of phantom sensations were measured during an eleven-month period. The results are illustrated in figure 7.4. Within this period, the organization of the sensorimotor cortex ipsilateral to the amputation underwent marked alterations. Before the amputation, a typical arrangement of muscle representations and normal thresholds for the EMG response were found for the face, biceps, and thenar muscles. Five weeks after the amputation, TMS of the denervated area elicited phantom sensations in the amputated limb but no contractions of face and arm muscles. Face and muscle contractions elicited by stimulation of the deafferented hemisphere were not observed until four months after amputation. By then, stimulation of the deafferented area elicited reduced muscle contractions of biceps and face muscles, and the subject reported weaker phantom sensations, which might indicate the beginning of an injury-induced invasion of neighboring representations. After eleven months, TMS of the deafferented area revealed a total invasion by adjacent muscle representations.

7.3 Basic Aspects of Cortical Reorganization

As proposed by Merzenich and Jenkins (1993, 100), cortical representations are "dynamic time-based constructs," formed by coincident temporal activation. Animal experiments demonstrated that different input conditions lead to discernible alterations of cortical representations. Five principles aspects of cortical reorganization can be deduced from current research: (1) injury- and use-related reorganization; (2) synchronicity; (3) behavioral relevance; (4) multiple maps; and (5) critical periods (cf. also chapter 1).

7.3.1 Injury- and Use-Related Reorganization

Damage to either the peripheral or the central nervous system can cause deafferentation to cortical neurons, which then change their original receptive field properties and adopt the representational properties of neighboring neurons. Adjacent representations "invade" the deafferented field; this form of reorganization is thus also known as "injury-related invasion" (cf. chapters 2, 3). Such an invasion has been demonstrated in amputees (Elbert et al. 1994) after unilateral hearing loss (Vasama et al. 1995), and spinal cord injury (Lotze et al. 1999).

Enhanced use of a limb—and enhanced afferent input condition—induces enlargement of the respective representation in the primary sensory cortex, a form of cortical plasticity called "use-dependent expansion." An important prerequisite for use-dependent expansion is the behavioral relevance of the stimulation or task. Use-related expansion has been demonstrated, for instance, for players of string instruments (Elbert et al. 1995), and in Braille readers (Pascal-Leone et al. 1993 a, b; Sterr et al. 1998).

Injury and use-related changes of cortical representations can coexist within the same sensory system, as demonstrated in upper-limb amputees, in whom the two hemispheres are subject to different stimulation conditions. The hemisphere contralateral to the deafferented limb is subject to a loss of sensory afferent input, whereas increased use of the remaining hand increases sensory stimulation to the intact hemisphere. These "hemisphere-specific input conditions" are mirrored in distinct alterations of the deafferented versus the intact hemisphere (Elbert et al. 1997). Tactile stimulation applied to the lower lip evoked responses not only in the face area, but also in the region that would normally respond to stimulation of the (amputated) hand. Ipsilateral to the amputation, the hand representation was found to increase significantly with increased use of the hand as a consequence of the dependence imposed on that hand by the loss of the contralateral extremity.

Cortical reorganization following injury may reflect an extreme manifestation of mechanisms involved in the use-related formation and alteration of cortical representations (Irving and Rojan 1996). Although this hypothesis remains to be confirmed, it is supported by evidence for the crucial influence of behaviorally relevant and massive sensory input on the self-organization of cortical representations (see below; Dinse and Merzenich, chapter 2, this volume).

7.3.2 Synchronicity

Use-related alterations of cortical representations depend on the temporal arrangement of the afferent input flow. As emphasized by Clark and coworkers (1988), representations of neighboring fingers constitute "separate entities." The receptive fields overlap along the distal-proximal axis of a single finger but not in rostrocaudal direction. This separation may be due to the fact that neighboring fingers are rarely stimulated synchronously. When synchronous stimulation is enforced, as by surgically connecting two neighboring fingers, their distinct representations can be fused. In individuals having fused fingers (syndactyly) representations of the webbed fingers share a common representation, whereas after surgical separation of the webbed fingers, the respective representations become separated (Mogilner et al. 1993). Presumably, segregated finger representations develop because individual fingers are stimulated asynchronously after surgery. Synchronous temporal input has been found to induce a disarranged soma-

totopic organization (in the example of multifinger Braille readers presented above; Sterr et al. 1998; Wang et al. 1995) or to result in a fusion of representational zones (as in the case in musicians suffering from focal hand dystonia; Elbert et al. 1998; Byl personal communication).

7.3.3 Behavioral Relevance

Use-dependent reorganization requires sensory stimulation within a behaviorally relevant setting. Recanzone and coworkers (1992) compared the effect of enhanced input conditions on cortical representations for active and passive stimulation conditions in adult owl monkeys. Tactile stimuli (vibration with different frequencies) were applied to a small part of the fingertip. One group of monkeys ("active" group A) was rewarded for learning to detect differences in the frequency of a tactile vibration stimulus. A second group of monkeys ("passive" group B) had to accomplish an auditory task while the tactile stimuli (identical to those in group A) were applied. Thus, for group B monkeys, the tactile stimulation was not behaviorally relevant. Cortical mapping of the somatosensory cortex (area 3b) disclosed an enlarged representation of the stimulated finger in the "active" group (A), whereas no expansion of the finger representation was found in the "passive" group (B). The cortical reorganization of string instrument players and Braille readers constitutes further examples of the relevance—the rewarding effect—of the stimulation and behavioral response.

The statistics of sensory inputs (i.e., the amount of stimulation, temporal concurrence) may not be sufficient to guide changes in cortical representations because the behavioral importance of the input is not necessarily related to their frequency of occurrence.

As is well known, learning is controlled by the behavioral relevance of the stimulus and behavioral relevance has been shown to directly modulate cortical plasticity in cortical learning models. In a series of experiments, Weinberger and Bakin (1998 for review) provided evidence that associative learning involves systematic changes in the frequency tuning of cells in the auditory cortex (area A1) of adult animals. Animals were trained in a classical conditioning task in which a tone (CS) was immediately followed by a mild food shock (UCS; aversive conditioning). Before and after the conditioning procedure, tuning curves of specific cortical neurons in area A1 were assessed via chronically implanted microelectrodes. For training, CS frequencies other than the best frequency of the neuron were chosen. After 10 to 30 paired CS-UCS presentations, the best frequency of the monitored neurons had shifted toward the CS frequency, indicating learning-induced reorganization of receptive fields. The model suggested by Weinberger and colleagues to explain CS-specific plasticity is presented in figure 7.5.

There are two prerequisites for functional reorganization of the cortex in the adult organism: (1) cortical capacity has to be optimized and adapted to the organism's special needs throughout its life; (2) stable functioning of the cortex has to be ensured to prevent maladaptation. Plasticity in the adult brain is supposedly determined by a higher order process that allows sufficient both adaptation and homoestasis of brain function. Stimulus relevance is a good candidate to provide this "supervisor process." A possible neural substrate for the mediation of behavioral relevance of particular stimuli is the nucleus basalis, a subcortical structure uniquely positioned in the brain, receiving input from limbic and paralimbic structures and sending projections to the entire brain. In addition, this nucleus is known to be involved in the modulation of learning. Recent evidence

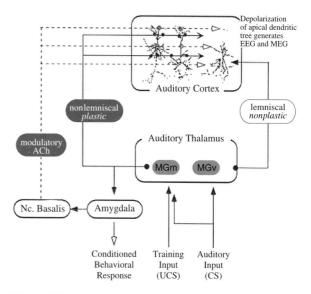

Figure 7.5
Schematic model of the anatomical projections of three systems that act synergistically within the auditory cortex to produce and maintain tone (CS) specific receptive field plasticity and conditioned behavior. Together, the three systems (1) provide detailed frequency information to the auditory cortex (via the lemniscal nonplastic pathway originating in the ventral medial geniculatum (MGv), (2) indicate the behavioral significance of the acoustic stimulus (via the nonlemniscal plastic pathway originating in the magnocellular medial geniculatum (MGm), and (3) produce neuromodulation proportional to the importance of the auditory stimulus (by the modulatory cholinergic projection originating in the nucleus basalis). Auditory and nonauditory inputs converge in auditory thalamus. Learning produces increased responses in the MGm, which are projected to the nucleus basalis and the auditory cortex. Increased activity in the nucleus basalis produces increased cholinergic release in the auditory cortex, which, combined with increased synaptic drive from the auditory thalamus, produces long-lasting plasticity in the auditory cortex. (Adapted from Weinberger and Bakin, 1998.)

indicates that the activation of the nucleus basalis is essential for cortical reorganization (Kilgard and Merzenich 1998). That is, use-related changes do not occur when activity of the nucleus basalis is blocked.

7.3.4 Multiple Maps

Although evidence is still limited, results indicate the possibility that multiple maps can share the same circumscribed cortical area in the visual and motor systems. Using fMRI, Karni et al. (1995, 1998) showed that two different keyboard tasks that required the same muscle activation but differed only in their pattern of activation evoked responses in different areas of the primary motor cortex (see also Ungerleider 1995). Evidence for multiple maps in the somatosensory domain is provided by Braun et al. 1999, in which five subjects were trained to discriminate tactile directional stimuli on a daily basis for four weeks. Brain mapping analysis of high-resolution EEGs revealed that a single type of prolonged repetitive simultaneous stimulation of two digits produced two different and opposite use-dependent effects on the spatial relationship of the representations of the digits in the somatosensory cortex, depending on the nature of the discrimination condition used during the neuroimaging sessions. The results suggest that the two maps share the same somatosensory neural network specific to different modes of discrimination within the somatosensory modality. The particular context may determine which map dominates processing.

7.3.5 Critical Periods

Many findings suggest that there are critical periods for when a certain brain organization and a certain ability develops (for review see Nelson 1999; Nelson

and Bloom 1997). For one example, ocular dominance columns become elaborated by experience during a critical period that coincides with rapid overproduction of synapses in the visual cortex. For another, the ability to readily discriminate phonemes from languages to which an infant is not exposed is present only between the ages of 6 and 12 months, but is lost later in life. Although some abilities can be regained by intensive training (Merzenich et al. 1996; Tallal et al. 1996), it seems unlikely that they can be fully recovered. For example, in Elbert et al. 1995, there was a tendency for greater cortical representation in the somatosensory cortex of players of string instruments who had begun their musical training before the age of 10 years, an advantage that was not overridden by more intense or longer practice later on. Pantev et al. (1998) report similar observations for the auditory system in humans.

7.4 Time Course of Cortical Reorganization

The evidence of use-dependent cortical reorganization should eventually affect neurological rehabilitation procedures. Relevant questions in this respect concern the length of training and the amount of stimulation necessary to induce cortical reorganization that results in recovery of lost abilities. Evidence from animal studies suggests that two phases of reorganization can be distinguished. Short-term reorganization is highly reversible and may occur hours to days after somatosensory deafferentation (Kelahan and Doetsch 1984; cf. chapter 3). It is assumed that such short-term changes of receptive field characteristics reflect the loss of inhibition provided by the fibers before deafferentation (Alloway and Aaron 1996; Calford and Tweedale 1988, 1990, 1991). Long-term reorganization occurs after weeks to months. In rats, complete invasion of the deafferented area of the forepaw by neighboring representations was found seven to eight months after deafferentation (Cusick, Wall, and Wiley 1990). Comparable results have been reported for owl monkeys (Churchill et al. 1998; Jain, Catania, and Kaas 1997; Kaas, Jain, and Florence 1998) and in a human (Pascual-Leone et al. 1996; see above).

Alterations of cortical representations are progressive in nature, so that short- and long-term representations most likely depict distinctive stages on that continuum. Both stages in the reorganizational process are presumably based on neural interactions that are also involved in perceptual learning (Kelahan and Doetsch 1984; Irvine and Rajan 1996).

In humans, empirical evidence for the time course of reorganization is limited. Short-term reorganization within minutes to hours has been demonstrated in transient deafferentation studies where local anesthesia procedures are applied. Birbaumer et al. (1997) employed axillary brachial plexus anesthesia in upper limb amputees to induce transient deafferentation of the stump. Cortical reorganization and phantom sensations were recorded before, during, and after the anesthesia. Within minutes, the axillary brachial plexus anesthesia virtually eliminated cortical reorganization as well as phantom limb pain. Rossini and coworkers (1994) reported reversible alteration of finger representations following ischemic anesthesia. This transient deafferentation induced an expansion in neighboring unanesthetized finger representations that reversed to the normal organization after the effects of anesthesia wore off.

The phenomenon of short-term plasticity is not restricted to transient sensory input cutoff. However, state-dependent alterations of cortical representations are further observed following increased use or practice of trained skills, as demonstrated in professional blind Braille readers working full-time as proofreaders. Pascual-Leone et al. (1995) examined

alterations in the representation of reading finger muscles[4] after (1) one day of Braille reading under workday conditions[5] and (2) after a three-day "Braille-free" period. On both days, motor output maps (to TMS) were obtained in the morning before measurement and in the evening after measurement. No significant differences in the sensorimotor representations of the reading fingers were found before measurement between "workday" and "holiday" conditions. However, after one day of Braille reading, the representation of the reading finger was markedly larger than it was before measurement or in the "holiday" condition. This demonstrates reversible use-related changes within the short time period of a day. It seems interesting in this respect, that Braille readers often report that they find reading much more difficult after "Braille-free" periods, that is, after weekends or vacations. It is possible that the cortical representation of the reading finger muscles has to be adapted over the short term, so that fast and efficient Braille reading is possible. Thus a "state-dependent" representation may exist within the neural network of the sensorimotor map that can be reestablished under special circumstances. This "switching" of the map could explain why professional Braille readers say they need a "warm-up phase" after a break.

Similarly, training-induced alterations of cortical representations were demonstrated in the above-mentioned study (Braun et al. 1999), which depicted the cortical organization (1) after the first week of training (five training sessions); (2) after another seven sessions (middle of the third week of training); and (3) at the end of the fourth week of training. A significant enlargement of the hand representation was found at the end of the training, but no difference in size between the hand representation after the first and that in the third week, which suggests that two weeks of training are just not sufficient to induce measurable changes in the cortical representation of the hand. In this study, the subjects trained in the task daily for one hour. In Braun et al. 1999, the subjects trained in the task for one hour; our laboratory is currently investigating whether the same results can be obtained by a two-week training schedule with daily two-hour sessions.

From these results, we may infer different time courses for injury-related and training-related reorganization. Injury-related changes are progressive in nature. After deafferentation, the brain continues to adapt its cortical representations; this process continues for approximately one year. Use-related changes can be obtained within the range of weeks, although early and thus more subtle alterations in cortical reorganization may not be uncovered with the available imaging procedures.

7.5 Experimental Evidence for Intramodal Cortical Reorganization in Humans and the Perceptual Consequences

Functional plasticity can be divided into *intramodal reorganization*, alterations of brain functions within one perceptual modality, and *cross-modal reorganization*, alterations across different modalities. If cross-modal alterations are of interest, it is typically asked to what extent the loss of one sense, say hearing or vision, alters the cortical processing of the unimpaired senses. Because it primarily affects the developing brain, we will briefly summarize findings on cross-modal plasticity and then examine evidence for intramodal reorganization in greater detail.

7.5.1 *Cross-Modal Plasticity*

According to the "compensation hypothesis" (Galton 1883), the loss of a sensory modality leads to compensatory gain in the perceptual capacities of the remaining senses. Although data on perceptual compensation are poor, in recent years the investigation of the cortical aspect of cross-modal plasticity has attracted new interest.

The most prominent example in studying cross-modal reorganization is blindness. The visual cortex in persons blind from birth is not functionally silent, but rather is employed in the processing of auditory and tactile tasks (Franzen et al. 1991; Rösler et al. 1993; Uhl et al. 1993, 1994; Kujala et al. 1995; Röder et al. 1999). If blind subjects are asked to perform a tactile delayed matching-to-sample task, enhanced EEG activity can be measured over occipital areas, indicating the coactivation of the visual cortex (Röder et al. 1996). As reported before, the visual cortex is also active during Braille reading (Sadato et al. 1996, 1998), and the pattern of activity differs in persons who are blind from birth and those who became blind as adults (Büchel et al. 1998).

Deafness constitutes another example of cross-modal plasticity. Auditory areas are activated by tactual vibration stimuli in deaf persons, indicating additional functionality of the deprived auditory cortex (Levänen, Jousmäki, and Hari 1998).

In sum, the literature suggests that gross functional adaptations of the remaining senses can be detected following near-complete sensory deprivation of one modality. In addition, a different functional connectivity of the deprived area itself occurs, which allows the activation of the deprived zones. Because basic functional organization of the mammalian brain is achieved during prenatal development and is very much controlled by genes, it seems unlikely that rewiring leads to a total reallocation of the respective primary cortical areas. Nevertheless, there is no doubt that additional functional capacities are assigned to the deprived areas, most likely via unspecific thalamocortical projections and associative cortical structures.

7.5.2 *Somatosensory System*

Cortical reorganization has been extensively studied in the somatosensory system. Evidence has already been mentioned for amputees, for players of string instruments, and for blind Braille readers. Altered homuncular representations can also be found in humans suffering from chronic back pain and focal dystonia of the hand.

The ongoing painful stimulation in *chronic pain* patients was assumed to result in cortical reorganization due to excessive nociceptive input entering the nervous system. Accordingly, an expansion of the somatosensory representation that is specific to the site of pain should be observed. When this hypothesis was tested by Flor and coworkers (1997) in patients suffering from chronic back pain, they indeed found enhanced cortical reactivity to tactile stimuli applied to the painful area, particularly in states of chronic pain. The intensity of the cortical response to tactile stimulation correlated with the chronicity of the pain. Furthermore, in the group with chronic back pain cortical representation of the back had shifted toward a more medial position, indicating an enlargement of the back representation. Assuming such an enlargement gives rise to reactivity, it may contribute to and even maintain the continuing experience of pain in chronic patients.

Another clinical phenomenon related to reorganization of the primary somatosensory cortex is *phantom limb pain* (Flor et al. 1995). Nonpainful phantom phenomena, such as referred sensations and telescoping, may be related to changes in posterior or secondary somatosensory cortex or both (Flor et al. 1998c). Individuals born with a missing limb (congenital aplasia) never suffer from phantom limb pain. Interestingly, in these individuals, the reorganization of primary somatosensory areas found in amputees is not present (Flor et al. 1998a). Doetsch

(1998) advances two distinct hypotheses on the functional significance of injury-related cortical reorganization. According to the functional respecification hypothesis, sets of partially deafferented cortical neurons, as they start to respond to new peripheral inputs, acquire new receptive fields and thus undergo corresponding changes in perceptual meaning. Excitation of these neurons should change the referral of sensation from the original (now denervated) skin fields to the newly acquired skin fields. According to the conservation hypothesis, however, even though deafferented neurons can be activated by novel peripheral inputs, they still retain their original perceptual meaning. Excitation of these neurons should evoke sensations in the missing limb. Evidence of phantom limb pain supports the second hypothesis.

Focal dystonia of the hand often affects professions that require repetitive forceful movements of the fingers, and often results in occupational disability. This condition involves manual discoordination; its causes are still under investigation. Focal dystonias, also known as "writer's cramp," "musician's cramp," "occupational cramp," are characterized by a loss of motor control over one or more digits and uncontrollable cocontractions of the dystonic fingers. Typically, the symptoms occur under circumscribed situations: for example, pianists who cannot play a piano properly any more can use a typewriter without symptoms. Byl and coworkers (1997) associate the deficit in motor control with an altered representation of the hand resulting from the repetitive, synchronous, fast, and powerful movements of the digits that are executed during training and practice for hours over periods of years. In an animal model for focal dystonia, they have demonstrated that fast movements produced an almost synchronous input for afferent somatosensory neurons, which induced a degradation and dedifferentation of the hand representation in area 3b. Thus use-related fusion of digit representations may be involved in the etiology of focal dystonia. Indeed, when Elbert and coworkers (1998), using MSI, mapped the cortical hand representation of the affected hand in musicians suffering from unilateral focal dystonia, they found it to be smaller than that of the corresponding unaffected hand and smaller than that in nonmusician control subjects. This abnormal somatosensory organization was also found in patients with writer's cramp and in patients in whom the dystonic symptoms were associated with several different tasks (Bara-Jimenez et al. 1998). According to the Byl et al. (1997) model, the abated representation of the dystonic hand may indicate a fusion of dystonic fingers. Another plausible interpretation is that the perturbed motor control in patients suffering from focal dystonia of the hand is due to fused finger representations, as in the model for multifinger Braille readers (Sterr et al. 1998). If this interpretation is valid, the segregation of the finger representations by asynchronous stimulation may be a promising approach to treatment. Indeed, Candia et al. (1999, 2000) have developed a successful therapy for focal dystonia of the hand using just such an approach. Their subjects were eleven professional musicians, six pianists, two guitarists, and three players on wind instruments with long-standing symptoms who had previously received a variety of treatments. One or more of the unaffected digits were immobilized with splints; the focal dystonic finger was required to carry out repetitive exercises in coordination with one or more of the other digits for $1\frac{1}{2}$–$2\frac{1}{2}$ hours a day over eight consecutive days under a therapist's supervision. The subjects were instructed to continue the exercises using the splint at home for 1 hour every day for one year after supervised treatment. The three players of wind instruments did not improve substantially, whereas each of the pianists and guitarists showed marked and significant improvement in spontaneous repertoire performance without the splint at the end of the treatment, two into the normal range. Subsequently, four subjects showed further improvement, one additional subject into the normal range. Three subjects retained the improvement they had previously made. Neuroimaging results indicate normalization of the cortical representational maps in successfully treated subjects. The outcome demonstrates that learning-induced alterations in the functional architecture of the brain can be maladaptive, and that resulting pathology can be treated using behavioral techniques based on learning principles derived from recent research on neuroplasticity.

7.5.3 Sensorimotor and Motor Function

Studies of deafferentation and use-related reorganization in patients suffering from spinal cord injuries (Levy et al. 1990; Topka et al. 1991; Streletz et al. 1995; Green et al. 1998; Lotze et al. 1999), from cortical lesions (Cohen, Bandinelli, and Sato 1991b; Weiller et al. 1992), and from amputations (Hall et al. 1990; Cohen, Bandinelli, and Findley 1991a; Fuhr et al. 1992; Kew et al. 1994; Seitz et al. 1995; Ridding and Rothwell 1995; Chen et al. 1998) have consistently found that the lesion-bound muscle representations expand into the deafferented area. Transient forearm deafferentation is not restricted to the somatosensory domain but leads to significant reversible short-term changes of motor representations (Brasil-Neto et al. 1992, 1993). The amplitudes of motor evoked potentials induced by transcranial magnetic stimulation from muscles proximal to the temporarily anesthetized forearm increased within minutes after the onset of anesthesia and returned to preanesthesia values after the anesthesia subsided. Further investigation of this phenomenon recently revealed that plastic changes in the transient deafferented cortex can be modulated noninvasively (Ziemann, Corwell, and Cohen 1998). Transcranial magnetic stimulation of the deafferented hemisphere induces an upregulation of reorganizational processes. A downregulation is achieved by applying TMS to the intact hemisphere. The short-term alterations of cortical output maps in Braille readers observed by Pascal-Leone et al. (1995) and described before (see section 7.4) are an example for the correlation of enlarged representations and highly skilled perceptual capacities in the motor domain.

7.5.4 Auditory System

Reorganization in the auditory domain has been studied less extensively than in the somatosensory system. Examples demonstrating reorganization of the primary auditory cortex include expanded representations of tones in highly skilled musicians (Pantev et al. 1998) or a structural enlargement of the planum temporale in musicians, as indicated by fMRI (Schlaug et al. 1995). In skilled musicians, the enhancement of the representations tended to be more pronounced in musicians who started musical training early in life (Pantev et al. 1998). Use-related reorganization of the auditory cortex was also found in blind persons, who rely to a greater extent on auditory information than sighted persons do. Sounds that are typically neglected by sighted persons may be relevant for blind people, thereby imposing a greater demand on the capacity of the auditory system. Unilateral hearing loss represents another example of adaptive cortical reorganization in the auditory system. Scheffler et al. (1998) report smaller response amplitudes for monaural than for binaural stimulation in individuals with normal hearing. However, in unilaterally deaf persons, cortical activation to monaural stimulation of the intact ear equals the response to binaural stimulation in

individuals with normal hearing, which indicates adaptation of the auditory system in these individuals.

By contrast, subjective tinnitus, or "ringing in the ears," characterized by the perception of auditory signals in the absence of any external stimulation, is an example of maladaptive cortical reorganization. Cortical plasticity may account for tinnitus and its associated symptoms (Lockwood et al. 1998). Mühlnickel and coworkers (1998) demonstrated the similarity between tinnitus and phantom pain phenomena vis-à-vis brain plasticity. Their MSI-based mapping of the tonotopic organization of the auditory cortex revealed an altered representation for the tinnitus frequency, the expansion of the tonotopic map being correlated with the subjective intensity of the tinnitus. It is still unclear whether the observed reorganization arose from a loss of peripheral input that may subsequently have been recovered. Nevertheless, the positive correlation between the subjective strength of the perceptual phenomenon and the amount of cortical reorganization in tinnitus as well as in phantom pain strongly emphasizes the functional role of altered brain organization.

7.6 Cortical and Behavioral Plasticity Following Brain Lesions

Brain damage resulting from cerebrovascular accidents can lead to complete destruction of a given brain structure, combined with total loss of activity in this area; to a decrease in brain activity with no loss of structural integrity; or to disintegration of distributed cooperative activities, that is, alteration of spatiotemporal patterning of brain activity secondary to focal damage. To assess focal brain damage, we must measure the extent of the necrotic center versus the surrounding area of reduced perfusion (penumbra) and the outer edematous zones using fMRI, and we must learn what we can about the status of function of the particular area. Using MSI and fMRI we can assess the functionality of areas directly affected by a stroke and their neighboring regions using somatosensory magnetic fields evoked sensory alterations (Maclin et al. 1994).

Alexander Luria (1963) postulated that recovery after brain injury depends largely on the reorganization of complex neuropsychological systems. Cortical plasticity and functional reorganization following brain lesions are thus of particular interest in neurological rehabilitation. Systematic investigation of functional plasticity following brain injury in animal models strongly support this early assumption. Good recovery is always correlated with enhanced connectivity, whereas poor recovery is always correlated with the absence of altered neuronal reorganization. Furthermore, factors that stimulate functional recovery, such as neurotrophins or experience, stimulate synaptic changes and dendritic growth, whereas factors that retard functional recovery, such as depletion of neuromodulators, block synaptic change (Kolb 1999). These results support the hypothesis that neuronal plasticity underlies behavioral and cognitive changes and thus is the key mechanism of functional recovery after brain injury. It was shown in stroke patients, for example, that successive alterations in the motor cortex occurring within the first four months after the stroke were significantly related to clinical improvements (Traversa et al. 1997).

Although we do not know whether rehabilitation treatments and functional reorganization interfere with each other, and if they do, how, it appears reasonable to expect that recovery after brain injuries can be greatly enhanced with treatment that supports use-dependent adaptation of the damaged and of the related intact brain structures. Constraint-induced movement therapy (CIMT, Taub 1994; Taub, Uswatte, and Elbert 2001), for example, helps to improve functional capabilities of the affected upper extremity in chronic hemiplegic patients (Taub et al. 1993; Taub, Crago, and Uswatte 1998; Wolf et al. 1989). CIMT involves constraining the unaffected extremity and intensively shaping the movements of the affected extremity, thus inducing patients to greatly increase the use of the affected extremity. Such treatment provides massively enhanced and behaviorally relevant stimulus conditions that are known to induce use-related reorganization. Kopp et al. (1999) reported substantial cortical reorganization of motor areas in the unaffected hemisphere in six stroke patients after CIMT. EEG measurement revealed that activity (readiness potential) evoked in the ipsilateral primary motor cortex by moving the affected arm was greater after than before treatment. Most likely these results reflect the recruitment of intact primary motor areas to control motor function of the affected hand. Using TMS, Liepert and coworkers (1998) reported increased excitability of damaged motor areas after treatment, indicating reorganization of adjacent motor areas. In both studies, therapy-induced changes in motor organization were accompanied by substantial improvements of motor function in daily life situations. It is important to note that such improvements are rarely, if ever, achieved by other therapeutic interventions such as the Bobath approach or proprioceptive neuromuscular facilitation (Duncan 1997).

Acknowledgments

This work was supported by the German Research Foundation. We are grateful to Herta Flor, Stefan Knecht, Christo Pantev, and Edward Taub for many stimulating discussions and to Lisa Green for editorial assistance.

Notes

1. The Braille-reading task included three conditions: (1) rest; (2) nonword reading; and (3) word reading. In the nonword reading condition, subjects had to detect three words (targets) randomly embedded in a string of forty-one nonwords. In the word reading condition, they had to detect three nonwords (targets) randomly embedded in a series of forty-one words. Subjects were instructed to articulate "num" when they detected the targets. The non-Braille-reading task comprised five conditions: (1) rest; (2) sweep over a rough surface with Braille dots; (3) discrimination of the rotation angle of two simultaneously presented grooves as same or different; (4) discrimination of the width of two simultaneously presented grooves as same or different; (5) discrimination of three strings of characters consisting of either identical characters or two identical characters and a different middle character. In all conditions, subjects were instructed to articulate "num" when the difference was detected.

2. The radio frequency corresponding to the resonance frequency of the rotating nuclei, hence, the nuclear magnetic resonance (NMR) frequency.

3. The subject fell over railroad tracks and was run over by a passing train, sustaining the amputation of his right arm just above the elbow, but no further injuries.

4. First dorsal interosseous and abductor digiti minimi.

5. All subjects were employed as professional proofreaders working six hours per day. Thus, in the workday condition, measurements were taken after six hours of reading.

Low-Level Psychophysics

II

Learning to Understand Speech with the Cochlear Implant

8

Graeme M. Clark

Abstract

Training of deaf children having cochlear implants was carried out to achieve discrimination of vowel pairs, first, where the formant frequencies were most widely separated and, then, where they were more closely separated. Two of the four children trained improved in their abilities to distinguish vowel pairs; in one child, gains of minimal vowel pair recognition carried over to improved speech recognition. These results suggest that training to distinguish vowels first with widely, then with more closely, separated formant frequencies can be effective: the benefits are retained and carry over to the perception of speech. Improved knowledge of the effect of developmental and postdevelopmental plasticity on the perception of simple and complex signals should lead to better training procedures and improved speech perception with the cochlear implant.

8.1 Introduction

8.1.1 Indications for the Cochlear Implant

Persons classified as "severely" to "profoundly deaf" (with 71–90dB or greater hearing loss in the better ear for the frequencies 500, 1,000, and 2,000 Hz) can derive more benefit from a cochlear implant, a device for electrically stimulating residual auditory nerves to produce hearing sensations (see figure 8.1), than from a hearing aid. The most important indicator for an implant is the aided-speech test result: if the open-set Central Institute for the Deaf (CID) word-in-sentence score or its equivalent is less than 40% in the better ear the operation is justified. The cochlear implant is particularly helpful to adults who have lost their hearing after learning language (the postlinguistically deaf), although adults who have lost their hearing *before* learning language (the prelinguistically deaf) may also gain some benefit, especially awareness of sound. Prelinguistically deaf teenagers may also get help if they have had a slow onset in hearing loss or have received an auditory-oral education. If the implant occurs before the end of the critical period for speech and language development, up to approximately five years of age, speech perception is comparable to that for postlinguistically deaf children and adults (figure 8.2). These data were for the initial speech processing

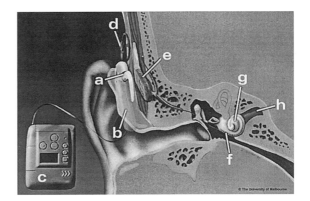

Figure 8.1
Diagram of the Cochlear Limited multiple-channel cochlear prosthesis, showing microphone (a), behind-the-ear speech processor (b), body-worn speech processor (c), transmitter coil (d), receiver stimulator (e), electrode array (f), cochlea (g), and auditory nerve (h). (From Clark 1996.)

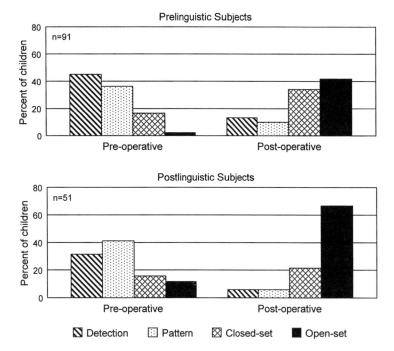

Figure 8.2
Speech perception abilities of two groups of children for electrical stimulation alone: those born without hearing or becoming deaf before language has developed (prelinguistic subjects, top panel) and those becoming deaf after developing language to sound (postlinguistic subjects, bottom panel). Their best perception skills preoperatively and postoperatively ranged from mere detection of sound to recognition of open sets of words and sentences that were age appropriate.

strategies F0/F2 and F0/F1/F2, and although speech perception was comparable between the two groups, speech understanding of open sets of words in sentences was better for the postlinguistically deaf children. The benefits are also greater the younger the child when implanted (figure 8.3).

8.1.2 Principles

Coding of Frequency and Intensity
The multiple-channel (multiple-electrode) cochlear implant gives better speech perception than single-channel (single-electrode) electrical stimulation of

the residual auditory nerve fibers (Clark 1986). With multiple-channel stimulation, the speech frequencies are filtered into a number of frequency bands. The peaks of energy or formants in the speech signal can be used to stimulate appropriate electrodes in the cochlea through place coding, where frequency is recognized according to the site of stimulation in the brain. Sound is first filtered by the inner ear (cochlea), with high frequencies at the basal end and low frequencies at the apical end (figure 8.4); the nerve impulses (action potentials) generated from the different frequency regions of the inner ear are then conveyed to the neurons in the auditory brain cen-

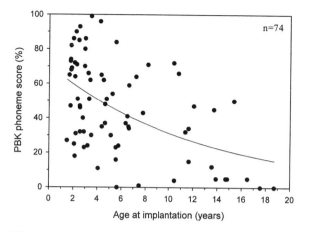

Figure 8.3
Phonetically balanced (PBK) phoneme-in-word scores for electrical stimulation alone versus age at implantation on seventy-four children born deaf with a profound hearing loss. Data from the Cochlear Implant Clinic of the Royal Victorian Eye and Ear Hospital, plotted with the curve of best fit. (From Personal communication with R. Dowell.)

ters. These neurons have different frequencies of best response, and are arrayed anatomically so that a frequency scale is preserved. To reproduce the place coding of sound with electrical stimuli, the current should be localized to separate groups of auditory nerve fibers.

Frequency can also be coded by the timing or rate of stimulation. With sound, such temporal coding, which depends on the fine time structure of the responses in a small group of fibers (figure 8.5), can be achieved up to approximately 3,000 Hz (Clark 1996), although it is difficult to achieve using the electrical stimuli currently available.

For cochlear implant patients, psychophysical studies have shown that place of electrical stimulation produces a sound percept that conveys timbre, which refers to the quality of the perceived sound, rather than to its pitch per se. The sound percept for each stimulated electrode varies in timbre from sharp

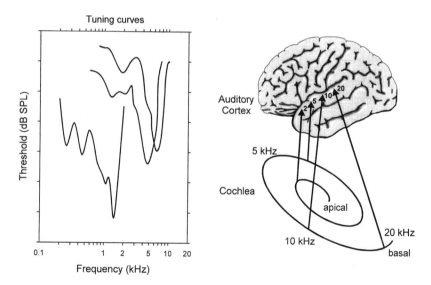

Figure 8.4
Tuning curves (left) show how the cochlea filters sound through the place coding of frequency, with high frequencies in the basal turn and low frequencies in the apical turn. Diagram of auditory cortex (top right) and cochlea (bottom right) shows how frequencies of best response of the neurons are ordered anatomically for a frequency scale to occur. SPL, sound pressure level.

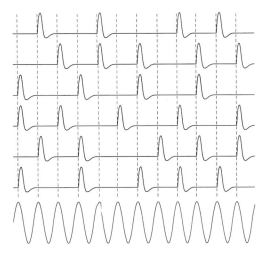

Figure 8.5
Temporal pattern of action potentials in an ensemble of nerve fibers in response to a sound wave, the basis for the temporal or rate coding of frequency. Note that the neural responses occur at the same phase on the sine wave, and that, even though the individual fibers do not fire every cycle, the population does.

to dull as the stimulus shifts from the high-frequency (basal) to the low-frequency (apical) end of the cochlea. On the other hand, rate of stimulation produces a pitch sensation, although, at rates above 300 pulses/sec, pitch cannot be discriminated, thus such rates are not so useful for speech processing.

Speech Processing
The main challenge with cochlear implantation is to present appropriate acoustic signals to the auditory central nervous pathways so that the patient can achieve maximum speech understanding. The limitations of reproducing the rate and place coding of frequency made it necessary to process speech for electrical stimulation by selecting the signals that conveyed most information, and by decoding these in the appropriate way. The first important clue

to the development of such a strategy came when stimulating different electrodes in our first patient. It was discovered that he perceived vowels, which varied according to the electrode being stimulated. Further analysis of the data revealed that the vowels for each electrode stimulated corresponded to the single formant vowels perceived for excitation of a similar site in the cochlea with acoustic stimulation in subjects having normal hearing (Tong et al. 1979, 1980). For example, stimulating the high-frequency basal end of the cochlea produced the vowel /i/, as in "seat," whereas stimulating a more low-frequency or apical region produced the vowel /ɔ/, as in "cord."

Formants are concentrations of frequency energy important for speech understanding; the second formant, which is in a higher frequency range than the first, is particularly important for speech intelligibility (see figure 8.6). Our initial speech-processing strategy extracted the second formant frequency (F2) and stimulated electrodes through place coding (perceived as timbre). The voicing frequency (F0) in the low range of approximately 100–300 Hz, was conveyed by rate of stimulation on each individual electrode (pitch); the amplitude of the speech signal was conveyed by current level (loudness). This F2/F0 strategy resulted in patients' gaining considerable benefit when using the speech-processing strategy combined with lipreading; they obtained some open-set speech understanding, where words could be selected from any within the vocabulary of the subject, using electrical stimulation alone (figure 8.7).

With more research, a speech processor was developed that extracted the first formant (F1) as well as the second (F2); their amplitude levels were used to stimulate two electrodes nonsimultaneously. Voicing information (F0) was still conveyed by rate of stimulation, simultaneously on each electrode. This strategy (F0/F1/F2) further improved the ability of the profoundly deaf adults with a postlinguistic hearing

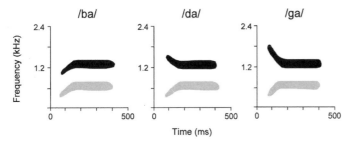

Figure 8.6
First (*bottom*) and second (*top*) formant frequencies for the syllables /ba/ (*left*), /da/ (*middle*), and /ga/ (*right*), highlighting the change in the second formant frequencies.

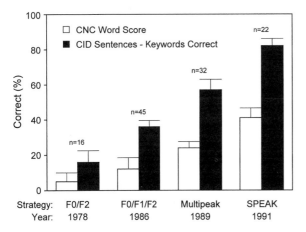

Figure 8.7
Average open-set word in sentence and word scores for multiple-electrode speech processing strategies using electrical stimulation alone. Each improvement presented more frequency information on a place-coding basis. The results are on unselected adult postlinguistically deaf implant patients presenting to the Cochlear Implant Clinic of the Royal Victorian Eye and Ear Hospital; the strategies are F0/F2, F0/F1/F2, Multipeak, and Speak. The error bars are one standard deviation; CNC words are phonetically balanced monosyllables, consisting of a consonant-vowel-consonant.

loss to understand speech both by lipreading and by using electrical stimulation alone (figure 8.7).

Additional improvements have been obtained by extracting more speech information and presenting this as place of stimulation. The strategy referred to as "Multipeak," which also extracted the filter outputs for the frequencies in the ranges of 2,000–2,800 Hz, 2,800–4,000 Hz, and 4,000 Hz and above, further improved speech understanding (figure 8.7). Some of this frequency energy is in the region of the third formant. The most recent strategy, called "Speak," does not pick the peaks of sound energy as the former strategies do, but selects six or more maximal outputs from a 16- to 20-band-pass filter bank, and uses the outputs for place of stimulation. In this case, however, rate of stimulation is not used to convey voicing; because a constant rate of stimulation is produced, voicing is conveyed through the amplitude variations in the signal. Constant rate of stimulation helps overcome the difficulties of providing channel separation when the electrodes are too close together (figure 8.7).

Alternative strategies adopted elsewhere for multiple-channel electrical stimulation have been to extract the outputs from 6- to 8-band-pass filters. Symbion (Ineraid; Eddington 1980) and Storz/

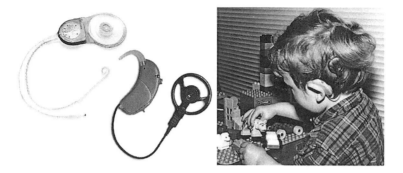

Figure 8.8
(*Left*) Nucleus 24 ESPrit behind-the-ear speech processor, which activates the implanted Nucleus CI-24 Contour receiver-stimulator; (*right*) child wearing the behind-the-ear speech processor.

Richards (Minimed; Merzenich and White 1980) systems provide respectively, analog and pulsatile stimulation to the auditory nerve fibers. More successful than Ineraid and Minimed has been the continuous interleaved stimuli (CIS) strategy (Advanced Bionics; Medel), which not only extracts the outputs of 6- to 8-band-pass filters, but uses, as does the Speak strategy, a constant rate of stimulation (Wilson et al. 1991). Results with the CIS strategy are more similar to those of Speak than to those of other multiple-channel strategies.

8.1.3 Engineering Implementation

The cochlear implant, as illustrated in figure 8.1, consists of an external wearable component and an internal implanted section. In the external component, a directional microphone placed in a unit above and behind the ear converts sound into electrical energy, which is transmitted to a speech processor worn on a belt or in a bag hung from the neck. Alternatively, Cochlear Limited has developed a behind-the-ear speech processor worn like a behind-the-ear hearing aid (see figures 8.1 and 8.8).

In both cases, the speech processor extracts the appropriate signals, refers the extracted message to a map where the thresholds and dynamic ranges for stimulating each electrode for that particular patient are recorded. The appropriate electrical outputs for each electrode are then determined and converted into a digital signal for transmission through the skin by inductively coupling (radio waves) to the antenna of the implanted device. Power to operate the implanted section is also transmitted inductively through the skin. The implanted receiver-stimulator then decodes the signal and transmits a pattern of stimuli through the 22 electrodes to stimulate up to 21 separate groups of auditory nerve fibers. This temporal and spatial pattern of stimulation conveys the speech information required for its understanding in the higher centers.

The Nucleus 24 system also has telemetry (figure 8.9) that enables the voltages on the electrodes in the cochlea to be transmitted externally, and the pathological changes in the cochlea affecting the electrode-tissue impedance determined. In addition, neural responses from the auditory nerve, brain stem, and auditory cortex can be recorded to help deter-

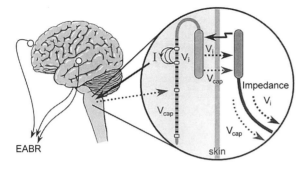

Figure 8.9
Diagram of the Nucleus 24 telemetry system (*right*) shows the transmission of voltages from the cochlea and the auditory nerve through the skin to the external device. The electrical auditory brain stem and cortical responses (*left*) can also be recorded by the system. EABR, field potentials from the brain stem and auditory cortex; I, stimulating current; V_i, voltage between electrodes in the cochlea allowing the tissue impedance to be calculated; V_{cap}, compound voltage from the auditory nerve and brain stem.

mine the thresholds and comfortable listening levels for children too young to say what they experience.

8.2 Mapping the Patient's Range of Stimulus Parameters into the Speech Processor before Training

When a person has a cochlear implant, it is necessary to determine the thresholds and comfortable levels of stimulation for each electrode. The threshold will vary depending on the number of residual nerve fibers in the area of the electrical field, the distance of the electrode from the nerve fibers, and the nature of the intervening tissue. The comfortable level of hearing also depends on these factors. In adults, determining this level is a relatively straightforward procedure. The thresholds are determined by a rising

or falling routine, whereas the maximum comfortable levels are based on obtaining a level just below discomfort. To achieve these results, the electrical current output from the device is varied. Not only can the current levels be changed, but the intensity can be increased by prolonging the pulse duration, there being a relationship between pulse duration and current amplitude. Furthermore, increased sensation levels can be achieved when high thresholds are present by increasing the spread of the current so that, instead of bipolar stimulation between an active electrode and a neighboring one, the current passes from an active electrode to a more distant one.

Training children in the use of the cochlear implant for the perception of speech and environmental sounds requires that the speech processor be correctly programmed—that thresholds and maximum comfortable levels be very carefully set for each electrode: the audiologist needs to observe the behavioral responses to the stimuli, particularly an aversive or withdrawal reaction, because discomfort will impair the child's learning. When this information is recorded on a "map" in the speech processor, the latter is ready for use, although changing pathology in the inner ear after implantation, especially during the early postoperative phase, requires that the audiologist make repeated measurements of thresholds and comfortable levels.

8.3 Auditory Central Nervous System Plasticity: Application to Cochlear Implantation

Learning to use the perceptual information provided by the cochlear implant will depend in part on the plasticity of the responses in the central auditory nervous system.

8.3.1 Plasticity in Experimental Animals

There are two types of plasticity in the central auditory nervous system: the first, called "developmental plasticity," results from the development of neural connections within a critical period after birth; the second, called "postdevelopmental plasticity," results from a change in the central representation of neurons in the mature animal after neural connectivity has been established. Evidence for developmental plasticity in the gerbil is the increase in the number of projections from the cochlear nucleus to the ipsilateral inferior colliculus when the cochlea on the opposite side is destroyed in the neonate (Nordern, Killackoy, and Kitzes 1983). A similar phenomenon was demonstrated in the ferret (Moore and Kowalchuk 1988), where the critical period for this neural modeling was observed to extend to postnatal days 40–90. In the mature animal, when an area of the cochlea is destroyed, the corresponding area of the brain, in particular, the cortex, has increased representation from the neighboring frequency areas that are still functional (Robertson and Irvine 1989), similar to somatosensory and visual cortex (cf. chapters 2, 3). This postdevelopmental plasticity probably occurs because there is loss of inhibition, which normally suppresses the input from neighboring frequency areas. In the cat, lesioning has been shown to result in reorganization of the topographical map in the primary auditory cortex contralateral to the lesioned side, whereas the cortical field remains normal for ipsilateral excitation from the unlesioned cochlea (Rajan et al. 1993). In addition, behavioral training has been found to modify the tonotopic organization of the primary auditory cortex in the primate. Recanzone, Scheiner, and Merzenich (1993) report an increase in cortical representation for frequencies where there was improved discrimination (cf. chapter 3).

8.3.2 Cochlear Implants and Developmental Plasticity

Developmental and postdevelopmental plasticity are assumed to have important implications for learning with the cochlear implant in young children and in older children and adults, respectively. Developmental plasticity in children with cochlear implants is being studied to determine whether there is a critical period for speech perception. In figure 8.3, the phonetically balanced (PBK) phoneme-in-word scores for children born with a profound hearing loss are plotted against age at implantation. The scores were obtained two or more years after implantation. Although there is considerable variation in results, scores clearly decrease as age at implantation increases: speech perception is significantly better, the younger the child. The data do not, however, indicate a specific critical period for speech perception.

Developmental plasticity in implanted children is also being studied to see whether the ability to discriminate both electrode place of stimulation and perceived place pitch show a similar change with age at implantation. Plotting electrode place discrimination against age, figure 8.10 shows the mean discrimination scores for three electrodes along the array from 14 children, 11 of whom were born deaf and 3 of whom lost hearing early in life from meningitis. The finding that the discrimination of electrodes is better, the younger the child suggests there is a limited time over which the neural connectivity for place discrimination can occur, which may be important for the development of speech perception.

To see whether there is a correlation between electrode place discrimination and speech perception, a comparison has been made using a closed-set speech test. The findings in figure 8.11 from the same group of children show that the smaller the

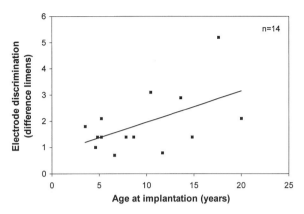

Figure 8.10
Electrode place discrimination versus age at implantation in fourteen prelinguistically deaf children. Results show a positive correlation between discrimination of electrodes and age at implant. (From Busby and Clark 2000.)

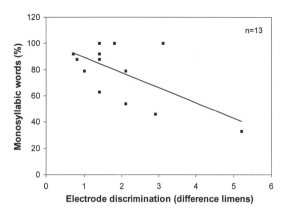

Figure 8.11
Place discrimination versus speech perception tested using closed sets of words. (From Busby and Clark 2000.)

separation between electrodes that can be detected, the better the speech perception, which supports the view that if developmental plasticity is responsible for creating the neural connections required for place coding, then speech perception will be enhanced as well.

On the other hand, when the ability of children to rank pitch tonotopically (i.e., according to place of stimulation) rather than simply to discriminate electrode place, is compared with their speech perception scores, as shown in figure 8.12, it can be seen that not all children who can rank pitch have good speech perception results. Although 75% of the sixteen children in the study were able to order pitch percepts tonotopically, only 58% of these children had satisfactory speech perception of 30% or more. This finding suggests that the effect of developmental plasticity on the neural connectivity required for place discrimination is not the only factor for learn-

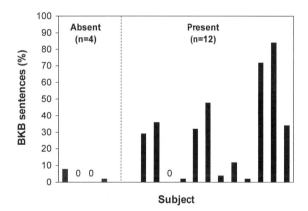

Figure 8.12
Place pitch ranking versus word scores for the Bench-Kowal-Bamford (BKB) open-set sentences for electrical stimulation alone on sixteen children using cochlear implants. (From Busby and Clark 2000.)

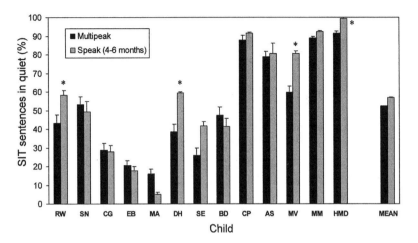

Figure 8.13
Word scores for open-set Sentence Intelligibility Test (SIT) for thirteen children comparing the Multipeak strategy with the Speak strategy at 0–3 months and 4–6 months after changeover. (*Top*) Sentences in quiet; (*bottom*) sentences in noise at a +15 dB signal-to-noise ratio. (From Cowan et al. 1995.) Speak scores significantly higher than Multipeak scores, according to a one-way analysis of variance at $p < 0.0.5$, are asterisked.

ing speech. At least one other factor is required for speech perception, namely, language.

8.3.3 Cochlear Implants and Postdevelopmental Plasticity

Postdevelopmental plasticity in older children has been studied by comparing the results of changing children from the Multipeak to the Speak speech-processing strategies. It was not clear whether the pattern of stimulation in the brain for one speech-processing strategy could prevent the learning of another one that provided more information. The Multipeak strategy selects up to five spectral peaks and stimulates at a rate proportional to the voicing frequency. On the other hand, the Speak strategy selects six or more spectral maxima and stimulates at a constant rate with amplitude variations conveying voicing information. Results in figure 8.13 reveal a

significant improvement at six months after changing strategies for four out of thirteen children taking the Sentence Intelligibility Test (SIT; developed by the Clarke School for the Deaf) sentences in quiet. However, the performance for M.A. deteriorated. Note that, for one child (B.D.), there was a decrease in scores within the initial three months after changeover, but scores returned to similar levels for the Multipeak strategy by six months. This trend was seen for other children, but was not statistically significant. It suggests that a period of learning is required to effectively use the new strategy. Note also that the results were similar when the children were presented speech material in quiet and in noise.

The need for learning is illustrated in figure 8.14, which shows that six out of seven children tested were able to gain significant improvement with longer use of the Speak strategy. These findings suggest that, although children have learned to asso-

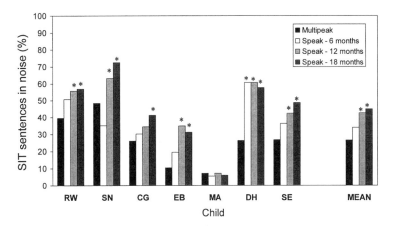

Figure 8.14

Word scores for open-set Sentence Intelligibility Test (SIT) in noise at +15 dB signal-to-noise ratio for seven children comparing the Multipeak strategy with the Speak strategy at 6, 12, and 18 months after changeover. (From Cowan et al. 1995.) Speak scores significantly higher than Multipeak scores, according to a one-way analysis of variance at $p < 0.0.5$, are asterisked.

ciate certain spectral and temporal patterns of cortical stimulation with words, they can readjust to the new strategy, presumably because of perceptual learning.

Further evidence for postdevelopmental plasticity has been seen in a pilot study of an adult cochlear implant patient, where the perceptual vowel spaces were mapped at different intervals after implantation. With the normal two-formant vowel spaces, there is a limited range or grouping of frequencies required for the perception of each vowel (figure 8.15). With electrical stimulation at first, as shown in figure 8.15, there was a wider range of electrodes contributing to the perception of each vowel, and a greater variability in the results. After learning to use the implant, however, the range of electrodes contributing to the perception of the vowels became more restricted, and the vowel spaces came to more closely resemble those for normal hearing.

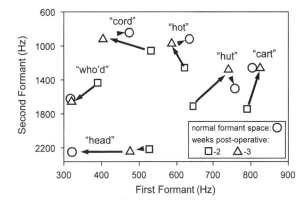

Figure 8.15

Two-formant vowel spaces for the vowels /ɔ/, /ɒ/, /ʌ/, /ɑ/, /u/, and /ɛ/, (as in "cord," "hot," "hut," "cart," "who'd," and "head," respectively) and the shift in the electrodes representing these vowels from two to three weeks post-operatively. (From personal communication with Blamey and Dooley.)

8.3.4   Learning to Perceive Speech with Cochlear Implants

Factors Affecting the Perceptual Learning of Speech

The factors correlated with learning to perceive speech in adults have been evaluated in a number of studies (Dowell et al. 1985; Hochmair-Desoyer and Burian 1985; Blamey et al. 1992, 1996), which have shown that a long duration of deafness and elderly patients are associated with poorer results. Although a longer duration of deafness may result in a greater loss of neurons or their connections, loss of ganglion cells does not appear to be the reason that duration of deafness leads to poorer results (Blamey et al. 1996; Nadol 1989). On the other hand, the duration of deafness is correlated with age, which is the more probable explanation because learning is more difficult for the elderly with a number of perceptual tasks.

When stimulating the auditory nerve as a whole with an electrode placed on the inner wall of the middle ear, there was also a positive correlation between preoperative tests of temporal processing and speech scores. The ability to detect changes in rate of stimulation and gaps between stimuli appears to be a central function: it is important for segmenting speech and processing the slow frequency changes that occur in voicing. In addition, a positive relationship was seen between the number of electrodes in use and speech perception, which highlights the importance of multiple-electrode stimulation needed for the spectral information in speech. Finally, there was a positive correlation between the dynamic range and speech score. The greater the dynamic range (between the threshold and maximum comfortable level), the more steps in loudness that are likely for presenting speech information.

Thus the data suggest that, to learn speech, the essential sensory information must be transmitted, and that skills at a higher processing level are required for speech perception. In studies of children using the initial speech-processing strategies, the open-set scores were poorer for children who were born deaf or who lost hearing before learning language than for those who were postlinguistically deaf. The final result also depended on a number of other factors: age at implantation, length of deafness, mode of education, and duration of implantation.

Rate of Perceptual Learning in Children and Adults

In presenting speech through electrical stimulation of the auditory nerve in both children and adults, learning is required for maximum understanding. The degree of learning over a period of twelve months for adults who had lost their hearing well after birth and who used the inaugural F0/F2 strategy is shown in figure 8.16. As can be seen, the mean open-set CID sentence score for electrical stimulation alone increased 150% from three to twelve months postoperatively (Dowell et al. 1985).

On the other hand, the Speak strategy reached higher levels and a plateau within one to two months. By contrast, the F0/F2 strategy, which provides less information, had not reached a plateau by twelve months of implant use, which indicates that, given more information with the Speak strategy, the adults learn more quickly than for the F0/F2 strategy, and reach a plateau at an earlier stage.

The rate of learning for speech perception in children, as evaluated by Dowell, Dettman, and Barker (1998), shows some interesting changes, depending on the age of the child at implantation. In a study of the children at the University of Melbourne's Cochlear Implant Clinic at the Royal

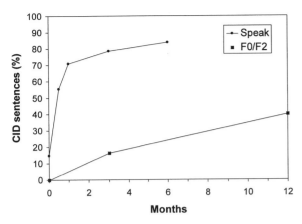

Figure 8.16
Open-set Central Institute for the Deaf (CID) speech scores for electrical stimulation alone over time for adults using the inaugural F0/F2 and the recent Speak cochlear implant strategies.

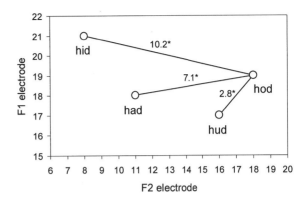

Figure 8.18
First and second formant frequencies for four short Australian vowels presented to appropriate electrodes in the inner ear through place coding in patient 3. Formant (F1–F2) electrode separation indices are asterisked.

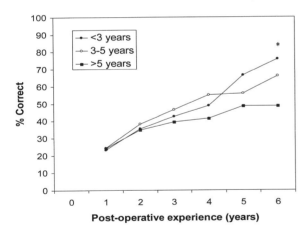

Figure 8.17
Postoperative changes in open-set word scores for electrical stimulation alone in children divided according to the age at implantation. Subjects with less than three years' postoperative experience scored significantly higher than those with more than five years' experience, according to a one-way analysis of variance at $p < 0.05$.

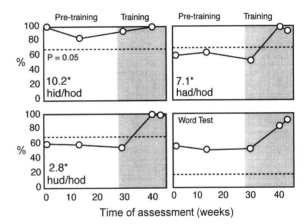

Figure 8.19
Scores for patient 3 on the discrimination of minimal vowel pairs of similar short durations pretraining (unshaded zones) and posttraining (shaded zones). Formant electrode separation indices are asterisked. (From Dawson and Clark 1997.)

Victorian Eye and Ear Hospital (figure 8.17), the children who were implanted before five years of age tended to have a greater increase in speech scores over time than those children who were implanted after five years of age, which may suggest that changes in the perceptual pathways appropriate for effective learning failed to develop in children implanted after the age of five years.

Specific Training of Synthetic and Natural Vowel Perception and Perceptual Learning

Our research on implanted children, referred to in section 8.3, shows a positive correlation between the ability to discriminate electrodes and speech perception. In a group of children where vowel perception was poor, we undertook a study (Dawson and Clark 1997) to see whether their ability to discriminate electrodes corresponded with the spatial separation of the formant frequencies presented as a place code for vowel recognition. Four out of five of the children in the group could discriminate the percepts from different places of electrode stimulation that were close enough to distinguish the formant frequencies important for vowel discrimination. Through place coding, the first and second formant frequencies for six short Australian vowels were presented to appropriate electrodes in the inner ear of patient 3 (figure 8.18). The formant-electrode separation index was calculated as the lengths of vectors in a Euclidean space, the distance between a pair of vowels being the square root of the sum of squares of the first and second formant electrode separations. Patient 3 could discriminate 1.8 electrodes apart, which was sufficient for vowel discrimination down to a separation index of 2.8 (figure 8.19), and the patient was able to discriminate between "head/hood," "had/hod," "had/hud," and "hud/hod" after training.

Acknowledgments

I would especially like to thank Peter Busby, Peter Blamey, and Richard Dowell for providing data and their helpful comments, and David Lawrence for assistance in the preparation of the figures.

9

Adaptation and Learning in the Visual Perception of Gratings

Adriana Fiorentini and Nicoletta Berardi

Abstract

This chapter describes phenomena of perceptual plasticity in vision demonstrated with a particular class of visual stimuli: simple and complex gratings. Historically used to quantify the basic spatiotemporal characteristics of visual perception, gratings were subsequently used to draw correlations between perceptual phenomena and properties of single cells or assemblies of cells at various levels in the visual system. After briefly introducing these stimuli and their historic role, we present evidence for (1) the short-term aftereffects in visual perception demonstrated with gratings; (2) the selectivity of these effects with respect to various stimulus parameters; and (3) possible correlations between such short-term aftereffects and those demonstrated electrophysiologically for the response of single visual cells. We describe long-term improvements with practice in the ability to discriminate between gratings with different waveforms. These effects and improvements represent a perceptual learning process. The use of gratings allows us to hypothesize the involvement in this process of certain visual areas or populations of neurons with specific functional properties.

9.1 Simple and Complex Gratings in the Study of the Visual System

Sinusoidal gratings are one-dimensional patterns where luminance varies sinusoidally along one direction and is constant along the orthogonal direction (figure 9.1, panel A). A sinusoidal grating is defined by four variables: contrast, spatial frequency, orientation, and spatial phase. By analogy with sound (where, according to the Fourier theorem, every complex sound wave can be expressed as the sum of an infinite number of sinusoidal waves), every complex one-dimensional or two-dimensional visual scene can be decomposed in an infinite number of sinusoidal gratings differing for the values of these four variables.

Contrast is defined as

$$m = (L_{max} - L_{min})/(L_{max} + L_{min}),$$

where L_{max} and L_{min} are the maximum and minimum luminances, respectively; it varies between 0 and 1. *Spatial frequency* is the reciprocal of the visual angle subtended by one grating period (cycle), and is expressed in cycles/degree, indicating the number of cycles that fall within one degree of visual angle. The *orientation* of a one-dimensional grating may vary within $\pm 90°$ from vertical. *Spatial phase* refers to the position of the grating with respect to a fixed reference in space and is expressed in terms of a fraction of the stimulus period (either in radians or in degrees of visual angle), with distance measured perpendicularly to the grating bars.

The sinusoidal one-dimensional luminance distribution can be expressed by

$$L(x) = L_0\{1 + m \cos(2\pi f_s x - \phi)\},$$

where $L_0 = (L_{max} + L_{min})/2$ is the average luminance, m is contrast, f_s is spatial frequency, and ϕ is spatial phase.

A complex (or compound) grating would result from the sum of two or more sinusoidal gratings of different spatial frequencies. The component of lowest spatial frequency is called "fundamental component." Harmonic components have spatial

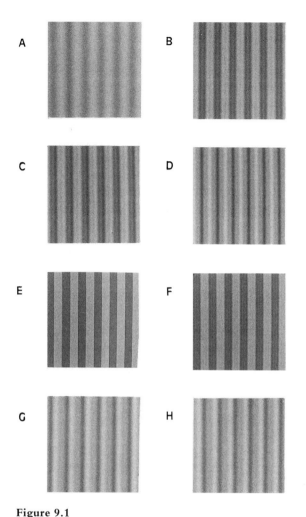

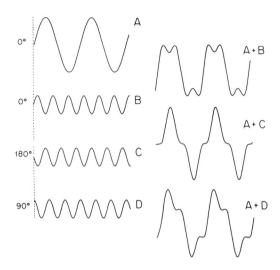

Figure 9.2
(*A*, *B*, *C*, *D*) Sinusoidal luminance profiles (left) of spatial frequency f (panel A) and $3f$ with relative phase $0°$ (panel B), $180°$ (panel C), and $90°$ (panel D). (*A + B*, *A + C*, *A + D*) Luminance profiles (right) of complex gratings, sum of f and $3f$ sine waves, with relative phase $0°$ (panel A + B), $180°$ (panel A + C) and $90°$ (panel A + D).

Figure 9.1
(*A*) Sinusoidal grating. (*B*, *C*, *D*, *F*) Complex gratings, consisting of the sum of first and third harmonic of a square wave, with relative phase $0°$ (panel B), $90°$ (panel C), and $180°$ (panel D); or of the sum of first, third, and fifth harmonic of a square wave (panel F). (*E*) Square-wave grating. (*G*, *H*) Complex gratings consisting of the sum of a fundamental and its second harmonic with relative phase $+90°$ (panel G) or $-90°$ (panel H).

frequencies that are multiples of the fundamental. Figure 9.1 shows examples of complex gratings obtained by superimposing either two components (fundamental plus second harmonic or plus third harmonic) with various spatial phases, or three components (fundamental, plus third, plus fifth harmonic). Adding the same components with different spatial phases yields complex gratings with different luminance profiles.

A square-wave grating (consisting of bright and dark bars of the same width and with sharp edges) results from an infinite number of odd harmonics and is approximated by the sum of a number of odd harmonics with decreasing amplitude and alternating (peak-subtract and peak-add) phases (figure 9.1, panels B and F; figure 9.2, panel A+B). A triangular wave is approximated by the sum of a number of odd harmonics with decreasing amplitude and peak-add phases (figure 9.1, panel D; figure 9.2, panel A+C). Two-dimensional gratings are obtained by adding sinusoidal components of different orientations.

Ideal gratings have unlimited extension, whereas real gratings, such as those generated on a computer screen, are obviously limited. For some visual tests, it is desirable to avoid sharp edges; the grating contrast is spatially smoothed with a Gaussian function (either one-dimensional or two-dimensional) to generate a so-called Gabor pattern.

The minimum contrast required to detect a sinusoidal grating and to discriminate it from a uniform field of the same mean luminance is the contrast detection threshold, and its reciprocal is contrast sensitivity. The contrast sensitivity function describes how contrast sensitivity depends on grating spatial frequency (figure 9.3). The shape of this function and in particular the maximum contrast sensitivity and the highest resolvable spatial frequency (visual acuity) depend among other things on the mean luminance. The top curve of figure 9.3 represents the psychophysical contrast sensitivity function at photopic levels. At lower mean luminances (mesopic and scotopic levels), the maximum sensitivity, the maximum resolvable frequency, and the spatial frequency at which sensitivity is highest all decrease. The loss in sensitivity with decreasing mean luminance is comparatively greater for higher spatial frequencies (figure 9.3, bottom curve).

The contrast sensitivity function also varies with stimulus eccentricity. If the length and width of the test grating are scaled according to the peripheral visual acuity, the shape of the contrast sensitivity function remains approximately constant, but is shifted along the spatial frequency axis by the same amount as visual acuity at increasing distances from

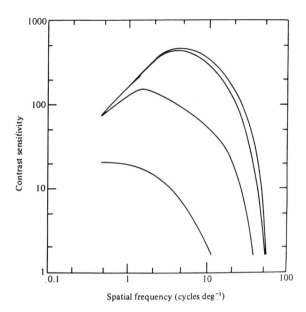

Figure 9.3
Contrast sensitivity for sinusoidal gratings as a function of spatial frequency, at four different mean retinal illuminances: photopic (top two curves), mesopic (middle curve), and scotopic (bottom curve). (Adapted from Van Nes and Bouman 1967 with permission.)

the fovea (Rovamo and Virsu 1979; see Drasdo 1991 for review).

Detectability of a complex grating depends on the detectability of its sinusoidal components. If these differ sufficiently in spatial frequency (e.g., fundamental and third harmonic) and have contrasts in a fixed ratio, the detectability of the complex grating is determined by the contrast sensitivity for either the fundamental or the third harmonic component, depending on which is higher.

The gratings described thus far consist of a spatial modulation of luminance. Chromatic gratings result from a spatial modulation of the spectral properties of the stimulus. For instance, a red-green chromatic grating can be obtained by superimposing in anti-

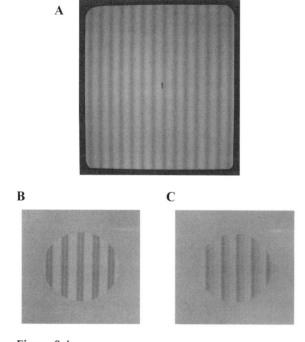

Figure 9.4

(*A*) Equiluminant red-green sinusoidal grating, obtained by superimposing a red and a green grating of the same spatial frequency and mean luminance in antiphase. (*B, C*) Equiluminant blue-yellow complex gratings, consisting of a fundamental plus third harmonic, with relative phase 0° (panel B) and a fundamental plus second harmonic with relative phase 90° (panel C).

phase two sinusoidal gratings generated on the red and the green electron guns of a color television screen and having the same orientation, spatial frequency and contrast (figure 9.4, panel A). If the mean luminances L_R and L_G of the red (R) and the green (G) gratings are matched, the resulting grating is equiluminant (or isoluminant) and has a pure chromatic contrast, but no luminance contrast. (Red-green gratings that are not equiluminant have both luminance and chromatic contrast.) The color

ratio (ratio of the mean luminance of the red grating, L_R, to the total luminance, $L_R + L_G$) is by definition 0.5 for the equiluminant red-green grating. Color ratios of 0 and 1 correspond to green and red gratings, respectively, with pure luminance contrast (green-black and red-black). Gratings with color ratios between 0 and 0.5 or between 0.5 and 1 have both luminance contrast and chromatic contrast. A yellow-black grating with pure luminance contrast can be obtained by adding in phase the red and green gratings of equal spatial frequency and contrast.

Chromatic gratings have been used to study the spatial properties of color-opponent mechanisms; a red-green mechanism, receiving inputs of opposite signs from the cones for middle (M) and long (L) wavelength cones (M−L), and a blue-yellow mechanism, with signals from the short-wavelength (S) cones opposing those from the L and M cones $\{S - (L + M)\}$. Spectrally broadband retinal neurons, responsible for the luminance response, are fed by nonopposing signals $(L + M)$ from L and M cones. The effective color contrast of chromatic gratings is less than the physical chromatic contrast because of the partial overlap of the spectral sensitivity curves of the cones. It is preferable to express chromatic contrast in terms of cone contrast, which is evaluated taking into account the spectral sensitivity curves of the cones and the spectral properties of the stimulus (Smith and Pokorny 1975; Mullen 1985).

Contrast sensitivity for equiluminant chromatic gratings is the reciprocal of the minimum detectable chromatic contrast. The contrast sensitivity function for equiluminant red-green (figure 9.5) and blue-yellow gratings is low pass (Mullen 1985). For stimuli chosen to optimize cone contrast, color contrast sensitivity exceeds luminance contrast sensitivity at low spatial frequencies, whereas visual acuity is lower for chromatic equiluminant than for lumi-

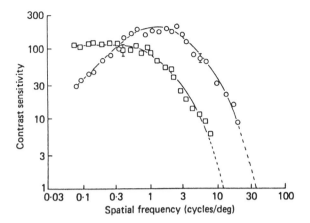

Figure 9.5
Contrast sensitivity function for an equiluminant red-green sinusoidal grating (squares) and for a green monochromatic grating (circles), as a function of spatial frequency. (Adapted from Mullen 1985 with permission.) Similar results are obtained for blue-yellow equiluminant and yellow monochromatic gratings, respectively.

nance gratings, reaching at most 10–12 cycles/degree, in comparison to about 50 cycles/degree for luminance contrast.

9.2   Adaptation to Sinusoidal Gratings: Psychophysical Findings

Looking for a sufficiently long time (one minute or so) at a sinusoidal grating of high contrast affects the contrast sensitivity for gratings having the same spatial frequency and orientation as the adapting grating: the contrast sensitivity decreases, so that a grating of low contrast that was visible before adaptation may become invisible for a few seconds after adaptation (Blakemore and Campbell 1969). This aftereffect of adaptation is selective for both the spatial frequency and the orientation of the sinusoidal grating: no threshold elevation is observed for grat-

ings of spatial frequency, orientation, or both, substantially different from the adapting grating (figure 9.6).

The selective adaptation to gratings observed in psychophysical experiments in humans has been interpreted to imply that gratings of different spatial frequencies and orientations activate different spatial frequency and orientation "channels" in the brain (see Braddick, Campbell, and Atkinson 1978 for review). The bandwidth of spatial frequency channels and the tuning of orientation channels are estimated by measuring the increase of contrast threshold for gratings of spatial frequencies or orientations near that of the adapting grating. The spatial frequency bandwidth resulting from psychophysical threshold elevation in adaptation experiments is about 1.2 octaves (width at half-height), the range of orientation tuning is about $\pm 10°$ (Blakemore and Campbell 1969; Blakemore and Nachmias 1971; Movshon and Blakemore 1973).

A further aftereffect of adaptation to a high-contrast grating is a shift in the perceived spatial frequency of gratings of somewhat different spatial frequency: gratings of spatial frequency slightly lower than the adapting grating appear to have an even lower spatial frequency, and vice versa for gratings of slightly higher spatial frequency (Blakemore and Sutton 1969; Blakemore, Nachmias, and Sutton 1970).

A perceptual phenomenon in some ways similar to the aftereffect on apparent spatial frequency just described, but related to a shift in the perceived orientation of a grating, is the well-known tilt aftereffect. After prolonged observation of a high–contrast grating oriented obliquely (e.g., 30° clockwise from vertical), a vertical line or grating appears tilted counterclockwise (Campbell and Maffei 1971; see Braddick, Campbell, and Atkinson 1978 for review).

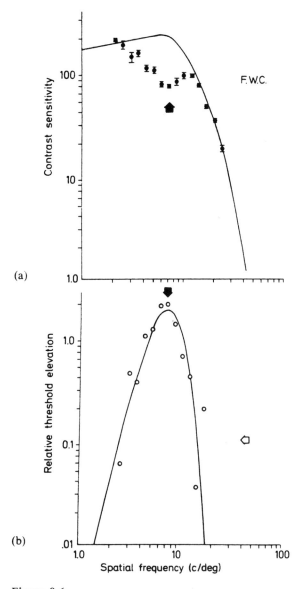

(a)

(b)

Adaptation to a high-contrast chromatic grating (e.g., a red-green equiluminant grating) of a given spatial frequency temporarily elevates the contrast threshold for chromatic gratings of the same or similar spatial frequency and orientation; the effects are similar to those described above for luminance gratings. On the other hand, the chromatic tuning functions for spatial frequency and orientation are somewhat broader than the luminance functions (Bradley, Switkes, and De Valois 1988; Losada and Mullen 1994).

9.3   Adaptation to Sinusoidal Gratings: Electrophysiological Experiments

In the visual system of mammals, from retina to visual cortex, there are neurons selectively sensitive to a limited range of spatial frequencies and in the visual cortex the majority of neurons are also selective for the orientation of the stimulus (line, edge, grating). Electrophysiological experiments in cats and monkeys show that neurons at various levels in the visual system undergo plastic changes of their response properties under stimulation with high-contrast patterns (of a spatial frequency at which the cell is sensitive). Retinal ganglion cells of the cat and a class of ganglion cells (M cells) of the monkey (Benardete and Kaplan 1999) show contrast gain control: the amplitude of their response to a fixed contrast modulation depends on the average contrast of the stimulus pattern, and is relatively attenuated when the mean contrast is high (see Shapley and Enroth-Cugell 1984 for review). Neurons of the primary visual cortex also exibit a fast-acting contrast gain control (Ohzawa, Schlar, and Freeman 1982; Geisler and Albrecht 1992; Carandini, Heeger, and Movshon 1997). In addition, when subjected to prolonged stimulation with a high-contrast grating,

Figure 9.6
(*a*) Change in contrast sensitivity following adaptation to a grating of 7.1 cycles/degree (filled circles). The solid line represents the contrast sensitivity function in absence of adaptation. (*b*) Relative threshold elevation caused by adaptation. (Adapted from Blakemore and Campbell 1969 with permission.)

most of these neurons undergo adaptation after-effects, resulting in a decrease of contrast sensitivity for stimuli of the same spatial frequency and orientation as those of the adapting stimulus (Maffei, Fiorentini, and Bisti 1973; Movshon and Lennie 1979; Albrecht, Farrar, and Hamilton 1984). The aftereffects of adaptation typically last several seconds after one-minute exposure to the adapting stimulus, a time course similar to that observed psychophysically in humans. No similar decrease of contrast sensitivity after high-contrast stimulation is observed in neurons at subcortical levels.

The attenuation in contrast sensitivity following adaptation and the contrast gain control of single neurons are two aspects of plastic changes taking place in the visual system. Perceptual aftereffects of adaptation can be interpreted in terms of changes of response properties of a class of neurons selectively tuned to the adapting stimulus. This interpretation requires us to assume that, although a grating stimulus may excite neurons tuned to somewhat different spatial frequencies, the psychophysical contrast sensitivity is determined by the amplitude of the response of the neurons whose sensitivity peaks at the spatial frequency of the stimulus. The change in apparent frequency for stimuli of lower or higher spatial frequency than the adapting stimulus requires that the perceived spatial frequency results from the balance of response amplitude between populations of neurons tuned to different spatial frequencies. Following adaptation to a given spatial frequency, the response of the neurons tuned to that spatial frequency is mostly depressed, and the peak of activity in response to a somewhat lower (or higher) spatial frequency is shifted toward lower (or higher) frequencies (see Braddick, Campbell, and Atkinson 1978 for review). The cellular mechanisms underlying adaptation to high-contrast patterns in cortical neurons have long been debated; both reduction in

excitation and increase in inhibition have been proposed as possible substrates for cortical adaptation (see Barlow 1990a for discussion). Carandini and Ferster (1997) have suggested that the most likely explanation is the presence in cortical cells of a particular tonic excitatory input (or excitatory current) that is reduced following adaptation and that slowly recovers, mirroring the recovery of the response amplitude. The presence of this particular current could explain why only cortical neurons adapt to contrast, whereas retinal and lateral geniculate nucleus (LGN) neurons do not.

Thus adaptation to gratings is a striking example of short-term modification in visual perception that can be interpreted in terms of short-term plasticity in the response of single cells or of small cell assemblies. The presence of plasticity at such a basic level of visual function (detection) responds to the necessity of continuously adapting the working point of the visual system to the most recent history of inputs to its neural components.

9.4 Discrimination of Simple and Complex Gratings

Before introducing perceptual learning in the discrimination of complex gratings, let us briefly describe the limits of the ability to discriminate simple and complex gratings. Simple (sinusoidal) gratings can be discriminated in terms of differences in spatial frequency, contrast, or orientation. Under optimal conditions, all three tasks can be performed quite accurately. For spatial frequencies below about 12 cycles/degree and for contrast three times the detection threshold, sinusoidal gratings differing in spatial frequency by only 8% can be discriminated (Campbell, Nachmias, and Hukes 1970). On the other hand, for pairs of gratings with spatial frequencies differing by a factor of 3, discrimination is limited only by detectability: the gratings are discriminated provided the contrast is sufficient for detection (Nachmias and Weber 1975). Just-noticeable differences (JNDs) in contrast between two gratings of the same spatial frequency are less than 1%; for reference (pedestal) contrast, they are less than about 5%; and for very low pedestal contrast, the discrimination threshold is lower than the detection threshold (Nachmias and Sansbury 1974). Orientation difference thresholds for gratings of high contrast are of the order of 1° or less, depending on spatial frequency and mean orientation (Burr and Wijesundra 1991).

The psychophysical thresholds for contrast and spatial frequency discrimination seem to reflect the properties of those neurons in the primary visual cortex that are most sensitive to changes in contrast and spatial frequency, respectively (Geisler and Albrecht 1997). Orientation discrimination is also related to properties of single cortical neurons, and in particular to the slope of the neuron orientation tuning function (Burr and Wijesundra 1991). Thus the limits in simple grating discrimination are likely to be set at a relatively early level of visual processing, probably in the primary visual cortex. Orientation and spatial frequency discrimination thresholds for chromatic equiluminant gratings are about 1.5 times larger than the thresholds for comparable luminance gratings (Webster, De Valois, and Switkes 1990).

Discrimination of complex gratings consisting of the sum of two harmonics (e.g., a fundamental and its third harmonic with different phases; see figure 9.1, panels B and C) depends on the difference in relative spatial phase of the harmonics as well as on contrast. For short presentations, it also depends on the duration of the stimulus. For gratings consisting of the sum of a fundamental spatial frequency (f)

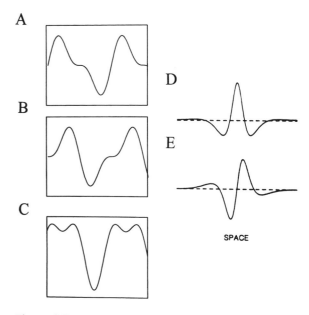

Figure 9.7
(*A*, *B*, *C*) Luminance profiles of complex gratings consisting of the sum of a first plus second harmonic, with relative phases +90° (panel A), −90° (panel B), and 180° (panel C). (*D*, *E*) Sensitivity profiles of cortical receptive fields with even (panel D) and odd (panel E) symmetry.

and its third harmonic ($3f$), with $3f$ contrast being one-third of the fundamental contrast, the minimum discriminable relative phase is of the order of 30°, provided the $3f$ contrast exceeds threshold. Sensitivity to phase differences is best when one grating of the discrimination pair has the harmonics added in the "square-wave" (peak-subtract) phase (Burr 1980).

For gratings consisting of a fundamental plus its second harmonic, two phase relationships have been extensively investigated: those in which the phase of $2f$ is either 0° or 180° (figure 9.7, panel C), and those where the $2f$ phase is +90° or −90°. The latter (figure 9.1, panels G and H) have mirror-symmetric luminance profiles (figure 9.7, panels A and B). The discrimination of these patterns has been interpreted in terms of the activity of broadband channels with different sensitivity profiles, either even symmetric or odd symmetric (Field and Nachmias 1984; Bennett and Banks 1987) with properties similar to those of single neurons with sine or cosine sensitivity profiles observed in the visual cortex of animals (figure 9.7, panels D and E; Pollen and Ronner 1981). This interpretation holds in general for other types of complex gratings that involve the sum of two harmonics with different phases; the findings of experiments with stimuli resulting from the sum of a large number of harmonics are also consistent with the hypothesis that phase discrimination is mediated by two types of detectors with even and odd symmetry (Burr, Morrone, and Spinelli 1989; Martini et al. 1996).

For stimuli consisting of two harmonics, phase discrimination may be worse in peripheral than in central vision; for eccentric patterns, it also depends on the orientation of the grating: gratings oriented along a retinal meridian (i.e., pointing to the fovea) are better discriminated than orthogonal gratings (Berardi and Fiorentini 1991). For gratings that consist of a large number of harmonics, however, phase sensitivity is the same for central and peripheral vision, provided contrast is scaled according to detection threshold (Morrone, Burr, and Spinelli 1989).

Complex chromatic gratings can be obtained by superimposing in antiphase two complex gratings of different colors (e.g., red and green) having the same harmonic content. Sensitivity to spatial phase for equiluminant chromatic gratings is similar to phase sensitivity for luminance gratings of the same profile, provided that contrast is scaled according to detection threshold (Martini et al. 1996). Only chromatic gratings consisting of a fundamental plus third harmonic seem to be an exception to this rule: phase sensitivity for these chromatic gratings is worse than for luminance gratings, even if the contrast is scaled to compensate for difference in detection threshold (Troscianko and Harris 1988; Martini et al. 1996).

9.5 Perceptual Learning in the Discrimination of Complex Gratings Defined by Luminance Contrast

The discovery of the presence of perceptual learning in the discrimination of gratings was rather serendipitous. In the course of an experiment on pattern discrimination, two observers who had done thousands of forced-choice discriminations using vertical complex gratings with luminance profiles such as those in figure 9.1, panels B and C, were surprised to find that when the grating orientation was turned from vertical to horizontal, they were unable not only to discriminate the gratings, but even to see the details of the patterns. Turning the grating orientation back to vertical immediately restored the discrimination performance (Fiorentini and Berardi 1980). What might have happened? That grating discriminability was known to be as good with vertical as with horizontal gratings led us to interpret the decline in performance as a failure to transfer the experience acquired in the discrimination of vertical patterns to the newly presented horizontal patterns. And, indeed, the performance of both observers progressively improved during further training with horizontal gratings until it reached a level equal to that for vertical gratings. Because the use of a forced-choice procedure ensured that the observers' improvement did not result from a change in criterion, we interpreted it as an example of perceptual learning (Gibson 1969).

The discovery of perceptual learning in grating waveform discrimination allowed us to infer that the neural mechanisms selective for stimulus orientation and spatial frequency described in the previous sections were involved in the learning process (Fiorentini and Berardi 1981). Examples of improvement in performance with practice in the forced-choice discrimination of complex gratings defined by luminance contrast are shown in figure 9.8. The pairs of gratings to be discriminated differed in their waveform: one grating was the sum of two sinusoids of spatial frequency f and $3f$, with relative spatial phases 0° and contrast in the ratio 1/3 (like the first two harmonics of the square-wave grating in panel B of figure 9.1), and it had to be discriminated from a grating consisting of the sum of f plus $3f$, but with the phase of $3f$ shifted by 90° (grating C in figure 9.1). It is evident from the top graph of figure 9.8 that performance improves steadily with practice, starting from near threshold and reaching values around 95–100% correct within 50–60 trials. The effect of practice is retained almost completely when the subject is tested the next day after the first learning session; performance then remains constant (figure 9.8, middle and bottom graphs) and is retained for weeks or months. Similar results are obtained for the discrimination of different pairs of gratings among those shown in figure 9.1. The only difference is in the rate of increase of performance in the first session, which differs from one discrimination task to the other, although the number of trials required to improve from threshold to almost perfect performance in the discrimination of complex gratings is at most a few hundred. It may seem surprising that such a long-lasting memory trace is obtained after a relatively short learning period. Other examples of perceptual learning, such as improvement in vernier acuity or figure-ground discrimination, require thousands of trials and several training sessions to reach optimal performance (see, for example, chapter 11, this book).

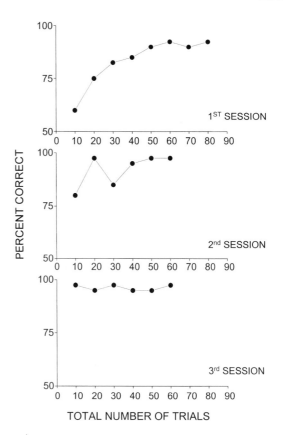

Figure 9.8

Learning curves for the forced-choice discrimination of complex gratings. The gratings to be discriminated differed for the relative phase of the two harmonic components (see text). Mean of six subjects. Each point is the percentage of correct responses in a block of ten two-alternative forced-choice trials. (*Top*) First training session. (*Middle, bottom*) The second and third sessions were run in subsequent days after the first day session and show partial (middle curve) and complete (bottom curve) retention of learning. Vertical gratings, fundamental spatial frequency 1 cycle/degree, contrast of fundamental component 1 log unit above detection threshold. (Adapted from Fiorentini and Berardi 1981.)

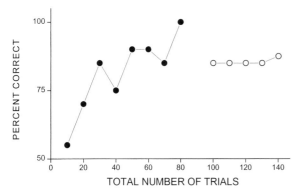

Figure 9.9
Interocular transfer of the effects of practice in the discrimination of complex gratings. Improvement in performance during training with one eye (filled circles) and subsequent testing with the other eye (open circles). Stimuli and discrimination task as for figure 9.8.

The results shown in figure 9.9 suggest that the plastic changes underlying the buildup and retention of the learning effects occur at or beyond the level of integration of monocular information, namely, the visual cortex. Indeed, it is evident from this figure that the effects of practice acquired in monocular viewing are completely transferred to the untrained eye (cf. chapters 5.3, 14.3.1; however, 10.3.4, 11.6).

9.6 Specificity of Perceptual Learning for Orientation, Spatial Frequency, and Position in the Visual Field

The perceptual learning demonstrated for the discrimination of complex gratings turned out to be selective not only for the stimulus orientation, as noted in section 9.5, but also for the stimulus spatial frequency and position in the visual field (Fiorentini and Berardi 1981). A demonstration of the lack of transfer when the stimulus orientation is changed

by 90° is given in figure 9.10, panel A. It is clear that the level of performance reached with the vertical gratings is not maintained when orientation is changed to horizontal: indeed, performance drops from 95% correct to levels at or below threshold; it then takes the same number of trials to again reach an optimal performance. Figure 9.10, panel B, shows the results of an experiment aimed at estimating the degree of selectivity for stimulus orientation of the learning transfer. Learning was first completed and consolidated for the discrimination of vertical gratings; when the stimulus orientation was turned 30° clockwise, there was complete transfer of previous learning, whereas, when the stimulus orientation was turned 45° counterclockwise, there was an obvious lack of transfer. This finding suggests that the selectivity for orientation of the process is between 30° and 45°, a range considerably broader than the bandwidth of orientation channels estimated from adaptation experiments (see section 9.2). It should be noted that adaptation experiments are based on contrast measurements at threshold and are thus likely to involve most of all the neural channels most precisely tuned to the orientation of the adapting stimulus. Perceptual learning, which implies discrimination of suprathreshold stimuli, probably involves a greater variety of channels tuned to slightly different orientations. It is even possible that phase discrimination may require the recruitment of a number of channels of different orientations. Although examples of perceptual learning in various visual tasks have been shown not to transfer when the orientation of the stimulus is changed by 90° (Ramachandran and Braddick 1973; Karni and Sagi 1991; Fahle 1994; Schoups, Vogels, and Orban 1995; Ahissar and Hochstein 1996b), because the degree of selectivity for orientation of the learning transfer has not been measured in most of these

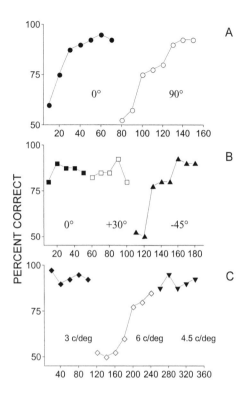

Figure 9.10

Selectivity of the learning process in the discrimination of complex gratings for the orientation (*A*, *B*) and for the spatial frequency (*C*) of the stimulus. The points are percentages of correct responses in subsequent blocks of 10 (panels A and B) or 20 (panel C) trials per subject, in a single experimental session devoted to the discrimination of complex gratings, both sum of a first plus third harmonic, and differing for the spatial phase of the third harmonic (0° versus 90°). Different symbols indicate gratings of different orientation (panels A and B) or different spatial frequency (panel C). Points in panel A represent means of six subjects. The filled squares and diamonds represent the average performance of three (panel B) or two (panel C) subjects already trained in the discrimination of vertical gratings of fundamental spatial frequency 3 cycles/degree. The other symbols refer to gratings rotated either clock-

experiments, it is impossible to know whether it depends on the particular task. One hint that it may comes from Fahle 1998, which reports that the orientation selectivity of learning in a vernier acuity task is 10° or less (see chapter 11.11).

Selectivity of the learning process for the spatial frequency of the stimulus was tested with the same procedure employed for orientation: learning was first consolidated for gratings of a given fundamental spatial frequency and then spatial frequency was either increased or decreased by one octave and successively decreased or increased by one-half octave (see figure 9.10, panel C). Increasing the spatial frequency from 3 to 6 cycles/degree was found to result in a complete lack of transfer; decreasing the spatial frequency from 3 to 1.5 cycles/degree was found to produce the same result (data not shown); changing spatial frequency from 6 to 4.5 cycles/degree resulted in a complete transfer. In this case, the estimated selectivity for spatial frequency (between one-half and one octave) is, if anything, better than that measured with adaptation. This finding would suggest that recruiting several channels tuned to different spatial frequency is not necessary for phase discrimination.

Unexpectedly, the effects of the learning process turned out to be selective for the location of the stimulus in the visual field (figure 9.11, panel A). Learning the discrimination of two complex gratings located in the upper visual hemifield took about 140 trials to be completed, leveling off at nearly 100% correct; these learning effects were not transferred when the fixation point was moved from 1° below to 1° above the stimulus, so that the stimulus was

wise 30° from vertical or anticlockwise 45° from vertical (panel A) or to vertical gratings of fundamental spatial frequency 6 or 4.5 cycles/degree (panel B). (Adapted from Fiorentini and Berardi 1981.)

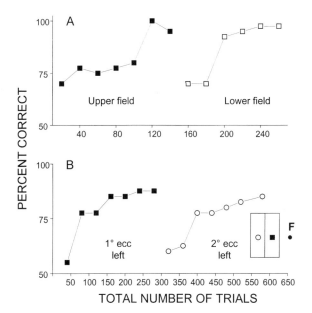

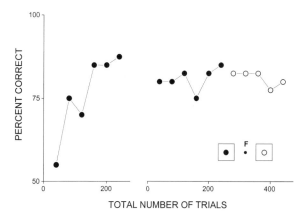

Figure 9.11
Selectivity of the learning process for the retinal location of the stimuli. (*A*) Learning the discrimination of complex horizontal gratings presented 1° above a fixation point does not transfer to the discrimination of the same gratings presented 1° below the fixation point. (Adapted from Fiorentini and Berardi 1981.) (*B*) Learning the discrimination of horizontal complex gratings 4° high and 1° wide, extending 1–2° from the vertical meridian in the left visual field, does not transfer to the discrimination of the same gratings located in the adjacent region, 2–3° on the left of the meridian. F = fixation point. (From Berardi and Fiorentini 1987.)

Figure 9.12
Interhemispheric transfer of learning the discrimination of complex gratings. Learning with gratings presented at 1° eccentricity in the left hemifield (solid circles, 240 trials each in the first session and in the second session on the following day) and transfer to the discrimination of stimuli presented at the same eccentricity in the right hemifield (open circles). The stimuli were horizontal complex gratings (*f* plus 3*f*, as in figure 9.1, panels B and C), 5° × 5° size, with their inner edge at 1° on the right or left of a fixation point. (Adapted from Berardi and Fiorentini 1987.)

now located in the lower hemifield. Practicing in this new situation brought performance back to nearly 100% correct in 120 trials. The same lack of transfer was obtained for stimuli initially located in the left (right) visual hemifield (at 5° eccentricity) and then moved, upon completion of learning, in the opposite visual hemifield at the same eccentricity (Fiorentini and Berardi 1981). The selectivity for the stimulus location is even stricter than suggested by

the examples above, where the stimuli were separated by at least 2°. As shown in figure 9.11, panel B, there is no transfer of the practice effects between stimuli located in the same hemifield and adjacent to each other. The specificity of perceptual learning for the location in the visual field has subsequently been confirmed in many other visual tasks (see chapters 10–12).

There is an exception, however, as illustrated in figure 9.12. Learning is completely transferred from a location on one side of the vertical meridian to the mirror-symmetric position when the distance from the meridian is small (1°). The selectivity for stimulus orientation and spatial frequency is preserved in the interhemispheric transfer of learning effects (Berardi and Fiorentini 1987). The limitation of the transfer to mirror-symmetric regions close to the vertical meridian and the selectivity for the orientation suggested that this interhemispheric transfer is mediated by callosal fibers, which are known to connect cortical regions representing strips on opposite sides of the vertical meridian. These findings might also be explained in terms of a bilateral representation of the central retina, although this would require that the ipsilateral projection of either retina extend up to more than 1° from the vertical midline, which seems unlikely on the basis of monkey data (e.g., Tootell et al. 1988). In addition, measurement of reaction times (RTs) for the discrimination of complex gratings at various distances from the vertical meridian has shown that RTs are longer in the left than in the right visual field, even for stimuli of low spatial frequency at close distance from the vertical meridian. This finding indicates that a functional dissociation of the hemispheres is present for this task, even near the vertical meridian (Berardi, Fiorentini, and Gravina 1988). On the whole, a bilateral representation of the foveal region seems not to account for the observed interhemispheric transfer of learning (see Berardi and Fiorentini 1997 for full discussion).

9.7   Perceptual Learning in the Discrimination of Chromatic Complex Gratings

To complete our study of the selectivity of perceptual learning processes for the characteristics of the stimuli, we checked whether the effects of practicing in the discrimination of a pair of complex gratings of a given waveform defined by luminance contrast (e.g., the pair in figure 9.1, panels B and C) would transfer to the discrimination of a pair of gratings with the same waveforms, but defined by chromatic

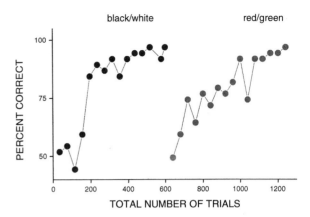

Figure 9.13
Learning the discrimination of black-white complex gratings with pure luminance contrast and lack of transfer to the discrimination of red-green equiluminant gratings with pure chromatic contrast. The gratings consisted of the sum of first (1 cycle/degree) plus third harmonic, with spatial phase +90° and −90°. The contrast of the luminance and chromatic gratings was equated in terms of cone contrast. (From Berardi and Fiorentini in preparation.)

contrast (figure 9.4, panels B and C). It is clear from figure 9.13 that this is not the case. Here the performance of around 90% correct after many previous trials with luminance gratings drops to 50% correct when the task requires discrimination of red-green equiluminant gratings. This result not simply due to the new task's being more difficult because the performance starts increasing with practice and reaches 90% level after 400 trials. The same result is obtained when the initial training is made with red-green gratings and the transfer is tested with luminance gratings. The important point in determining the lack of transfer is not the change in the chromatic appearance of the gratings but the change from luminance contrast to chromatic contrast; indeed, the mere change from a black-and-white grating to a black-and-red (or black-and-green) grating does not prevent learning transfer. It is clear, then, that the

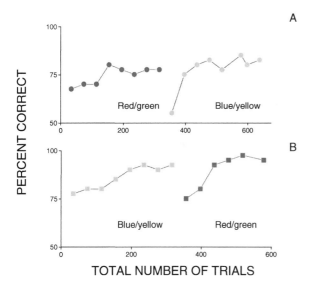

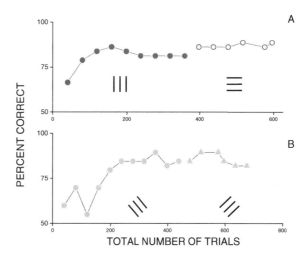

Figure 9.14

(*Left*) Learning the discrimination of equiluminant red-green (panel A) and blue-yellow (panel B) complex gratings differing for the relative spatial phase of the harmonics (first plus third harmonic, as for figure 9.13); (*right*) lack of transfer to equiluminant gratings of the same waveform but different chromaticity (panels A and B). (From Berardi and Fiorentini in preparation.)

Figure 9.15

Lack of selectivity for stimulus orientation of the effects of learning the discrimination of gratings with chromatic contrast. (*A*) Learning with equiluminant red-green gratings oriented vertically (filled circles) and transfer to the discrimination of the same gratings oriented horizontally (open circles). Stimuli as for figure 9.14. (*B*) Learning with blue-yellow gratings oriented at −45° (circles) and transfer to the discrimination of the same gratings oriented at +45° (triangles). Stimuli: first (1 cycle/degree) plus second harmonic, phases +90° and −90°, presented in the lower field, with 1° eccentricity. (From Berardi and Fiorentini 1997.)

processing of luminance and chromatic contrast implies separate neural mechanisms that can be affected independently by practice.

The next question is whether changing the chromaticity of the isoluminant gratings from red-green to blue-yellow (or vice versa) impairs the transfer of learning effects. As shown in figure 9.14, where two typical examples are reported, there is a substantial lack of transfer from red-green to blue-yellow and vice versa. This selectivity for the chromatic channel is in accordance with the properties of color-opponent neural channels as observed in the primate visual system.

A rather intriguing finding in perceptual learning of chromatic grating discrimination is illustrated in

figure 9.15. It is clear that there is complete transfer of learning effects when the orientation of the gratings is rotated by 90° both for red-green and blue-yellow equiluminant gratings, contrary to what we found for luminance gratings. This would imply, on the one hand, that non-orientation-selective neural mechanisms are involved in the discrimination of chromatic gratings; yet the discrimination processing must nonetheless be located cortically because there is complete interocular transfer of learning for chromatic gratings as well. On the other hand, the discrimination of symmetrical gratings differing for the spatial phase of their higher harmonic should require orientation-selective neural mechanisms, which seems to rule out simply explaining the orientation transfer in chromatic grating discrimination in terms of color-opponent nonorientational receptive fields such as those found in primary visual areas of primates. One could conceive the simultaneous use of neural mechanisms that are singularly orientation selective and the convergence of many of them on higher-order processing stages that lack orientation selectivity. A similar hypothesis of convergence of first-order, selective units on second-order collectors has been put forward by Morgan and Baldassi (1997) to explain the encoding of a defined texture orientation.

9.8   Conclusions

The choice of studying a process such as perceptual learning with stimuli thitherto used to study basic properties of the visual system proved to be particularly fruitful, enabling us, first, to demonstrate selectivity of the learning process for each parameter of a grating: orientation, spatial frequency, location, and luminance or chromatic contrast, and, second, to compare the degree of selectivity found with the selectivity for the same stimulus parameters found for the neural channels present in the mammalian visual system. That the selectivity of the learning process was very similar to the selectivity of the adaptation aftereffects suggested initially that the plastic changes underlying perceptual learning might occur at an early stage of visual processing, that is, in areas where neurons have small receptive fields and are selective for the stimulus orientation and spatial frequency. This hypothesis was reinforced by the findings on the interhemispheric transfer of learning, which exhibited limits similar to those found for the callosal transfer at the border between areas V1 and V2. In

addition, the transfer of learning effects between regions connected by callosal fibers, which is the only exception to the selectivity for stimulus location of this learning process, suggests that an essential requirement for different groups of neurons to share the same plastic changes is the simultaneous activation of these groups of cells by the afferent activity. This simultaneous activation does not occur for groups of neurons with different preferred orientations or separate receptive fields, but is present between neurons with similar preferred orientations and overlapping receptive fields, as is the case for callosally connected neurons.

The initial hypothesis of an exclusive involvement of early visual areas in this perceptual learning, put forward on the basis of the selectivity of the learning process, is probably too naive. First of all, the use of a temporal forced-choice paradigm and of a same-different discrimination task requires a short time retention of the information. This may imply some kind of working memory and therefore the additional involvement of association cortical areas.

Moreover, as discussed elsewhere in this book (see especially Ahissar and Hochstein, chapters 14 and 20), locating the plastic modifications in early sensory areas does not exclude a contribution from higher cortical areas. Rather, most models attempting to account for perceptual learning explicitly include a top-down control exerted by higher cortical areas. More recently, the possibility that the plastic changes may take place exclusively at central sites has been proposed by Mollon and Danilova (1996). They explain the selectivity of the learning process by asserting that what subjects learn is to select, among the many inputs to a nonselective stage, the incoming sets of neural signals that are most adequate to make a final decision and that are selective for the stimulus parameters.

Plasticity of Low-Level Visual Networks

10

Barbara Zenger and Dov Sagi

Abstract

Although it is our everyday experience that we improve in tasks we perform repeatedly, it is in most cases unknown where in the brain the practice is manifested. What parts of the brain have been changed during or after practice? Perhaps the most important method for answering this question is testing how specific the practice effects are to the practiced condition and to what other tasks the practice effects generalize. This chapter describes studies that document practice effects in contrast-masking experiments (where observers have to detect a defined target stimulus in the presence of defined mask stimuli) and texture segmentation tasks (where observers have to discern a foreground region made up of one type of element from a background region made up of another). The observed transfer of learning between tasks shows that practice is in some cases highly specific, and in others rather general. We examine how the observed practice effects and the pattern of transfer between tasks can be explained by assuming specific synaptic changes in neural network models of the primary visual cortex.

10.1 Introduction

During the first stages of visual processing, local image properties, such as intensity, orientation, color, and spatial frequency, are extracted in processes that operate in parallel over the whole visual field. The different feature detectors can be viewed as operating independently only to a first approximation; as a result of the significant interactions observed, some features are enhanced, whereas others are suppressed. These mechanisms can be interpreted as a means by which the visual system mediates simple context

effects, with context representing either remote image parts or visual memory. Several studies (Sagi and Tanne 1994; Ahissar and Hochstein 1999; Karni and Bertini 1997) have shown that these (early) context effects can be modified by practice, suggesting plasticity in low-level visual networks (cf. also chapters 9, 11, 12).

We introduce here a combined experimental-theoretical approach to study context effects and their plasticity. Specifically, we are trying to relate behavioral learning phenomena to changes in the synaptic efficacy of simple neural networks. Such studies are useful from two different perspectives: they can reveal new information, first, about the type of processing that underlies the visual system, and second, about the rules that govern plasticity of this system.

1. *Learning data constrain models of neuronal processing.* Recording data from observers at different stages of practice is like obtaining information about different states of the same perceptual system. A neuronal model with a certain architecture that accounts only for one state of practice but not for another can be rejected. Thus, even for the researcher whose primary interest is not to understand how practicing a certain task can lead to a performance improvement, it may be worthwhile to study learning, as a way to create "behavioral variants." The goal is to develop a model that naturally accounts (by simple parameter change) for all stages of practice while being at the same time biologically plausible and as simple as possible.

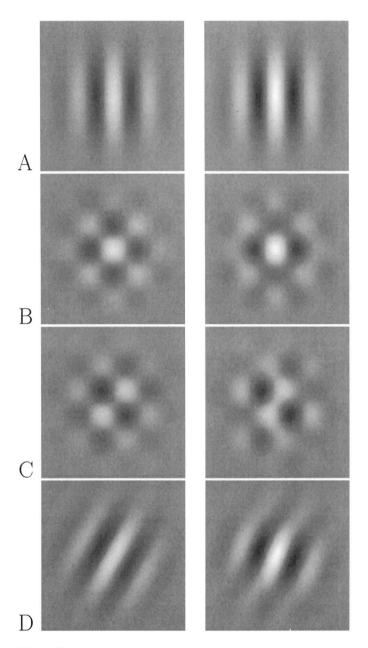

Figure 10.1
Stimuli patterns used in the experiments reviewed here were presented for 90 msec at the center of a computer screen, which was otherwise gray. These contrast modulation patterns were generated by modulating the amplitude of a sine wave grating with a two-dimensional Gaussian window (Gabor 1946). Each mask configuration was shown twice: once without

2. *Learning data can suggest mechanisms that govern synaptic plasticity.* Why have the changes in network connectivity occurred in precisely the way they have? Why have the efficacies of some connections increased, whereas others remained constant or decreased? The goal is to discover a set of learning rules that can successfully predict how performance changes after practice of a specific task and how other tasks will be affected by these synaptic modifications. For our approach to be successful, our behavioral paradigm should be simple and well understood in terms of cortical processing. A good candidate for a simple model system of neuronal processing is the primary visual cortex (area V1), where cells are rather stimulus specific (e.g., location, orientation, scale), interconnected by a rich local network (Gilbert 1993).

10.1.1 Psychophysics

Experimentally, these local circuits can be studied with a variety of psychophysical paradigms, such as selective adaptation (Blakemore and Campbell 1969), subthreshold summation (Kulikowski, Abadi, and King-Smith 1973), and contrast masking (Campbell and Kulikowski 1966, Legge and Foley 1980; Wilson and Humanski 1993). Here we use results from contrast-masking experiments (Zenger and Sagi 1996; Dorais and Sagi 1997) to study properties of the primary network units, their interactions and plasticity. In these experiments, observers are required to detect a briefly presented target stimulus. The target is a Gabor patch (see figure 10.1, panel A), a stimulus that is designed to selectively excite a

specific unit in the primary visual network. (Such a unit is thought to correspond to several neurons in the cortex.) By measuring the contrast of the signal that is required for the observer to detect the stimulus, one obtains an indirect measure of this unit's sensitivity. In subsequent experiments, the detection threshold of the target is measured in the presence of other stimuli (composed of Gabor patches) called "masks," which will usually either enhance or suppress detection of the target (depending on mask configuration and mask contrast). These sensitivity changes in the target unit can then be explained by assuming specific types of interactions between mask and target units. Facilitation points to excitatory interactions from the mask unit to the target unit, whereas suppression points to inhibitory interactions. Both suppression and facilitation are affected by perceptual learning.

10.1.2 Modeling

The model emerging from these studies is one that consists of *perceptual filters*, which interact with each other via plastic excitatory and inhibitory interactions. Each of the perceptual filters assumes a receptive field covering a small portion of the visual field, selective for orientation and size (spatial frequency; Wilson and Wilkinson 1997). Excitatory or inhibitory interactions, or both, take place between filters with spatially overlapping receptive fields that are tuned to different spatial frequencies (Tolhurst and Barfield 1978) and different orientations (Foley 1994; Zenger and Sagi 1996). In addition, there are interactions between filters with similar orientation

target (*left*), once with a vertical target added (*right*). (*A*) Just-noticeable difference (JND): vertical mask. (*B*) 45(++): two mask components tilted by 45° clockwise and counterclockwise, respectively; both components had "positive phase" (they were white in the center). (*C*) 45(−+): mask components were as in panel B, only one component had "negative phase" (it was black in the center). (*D*) 30(○+): a single mask component tilted clockwise by 30°.

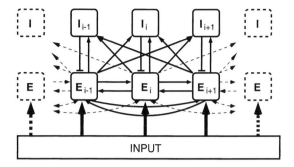

Figure 10.2
Schematic diagram of a model that consists of *E* subunits that form excitatory connections and *I* subunits that form inhibitory connections. The *E* subunits receive the input and also represent the output layer. Connectivity is restricted: *I* subunits only project to the corresponding *E* subunit.

and spatial frequency tuning but corresponding to different retinal locations (Polat and Sagi 1993; Polat and Sagi 1994a). These interactions may allow context to spread across remote image parts; their plasticity may further allow the context effects to change in an experience-dependent manner.

Some of the computational models put forward to account for psychophysical data assume a feedforward architecture, where information is passed progressively from lower to higher processing stages (Foley 1994; Zenger and Sagi 1996); others use a feedback architecture (Wilson and Humanski 1993; Adini, Sagi, and Tsodyks 1997; cf. chapter 20). Although feedforward models are easier to analyze, the results considered in the following sections strongly suggest a feedback architecture, which in any event seems to be the more plausible option in terms of brain anatomy. In the specific model we consider here, each unit consists of two subunits, *E* and *I*, with the *E* subunits forming excitatory connections and the *I* subunits forming inhibitory connections. The *E* subunits represent the input layer as well as

the output layer. The complexity of the connectivity pattern is simplified by assuming that each *I* subunit projects only to its corresponding *E* subunit, but not to other *E* or *I* subunits (figure 10.2).

10.1.3 Learning Accounts

Facilitatory as well as suppressive mask effects were found to be affected by perceptual learning (Polat and Sagi 1994b; Zenger and Sagi 1996; Dorais and Sagi 1997). Models of perceptual learning generally fall into two categories: high-level and low-level models.

A *high-level* model would assume that the network (such as the one presented above) is not modified due to experience, but that observers "merely" learn to better discriminate between different "perceptions" (Gibson 1969), that is, patterns of activity in the low-level network, and to optimize their decision strategies.

A *low-level* model explains the performance improvement by assuming specific modifications in the low-level network. Moreover, these changes are explained by learning rules that depend on network activity only, preferably on the activity in the connected units (local rules), and not on variables external to the network (e.g., stimulus and task, though both may affect network activity). A famous example of such a local rule, the Hebb learning rule (1949) suggests that changes in the efficacy of a specific synapse depend on correlations between the pre- and postsynaptic activities (*associative learning*).

Purely high-level models cannot account for the high stimulus specificity (e.g., for stimulus orientation, visual field position, and eye) that has been observed in many perceptual learning studies (Sagi and Tanne 1994), whereas purely low-level models cannot explain that performance improvement depends not only on the stimulus that is viewed during practice, but also on the task that was attended by the observer (Ahissar and Hochstein 1999; cf. chapter 14). That learning (with the same stimulus) can go in different directions depending on the task employed means that the task effect on learning cannot simply be seen as a switch that is set into "on" position when the task is attended and into "off" position when the task is not attended. In texture learning (Karni and Bertini 1997), where a target consisting of several oriented lines is to be detected in an array of lines having a different orientation, performance improvement for a specific target was found to depend on the relevance that this specific target had in the practice sessions. Post-learning performance may show (1) improvement when the tested target is the one practiced (Karni and Sagi 1991), (2) no change in performance relative to the initial value when the tested target presented during practice has no relevance to the task (Karni and Sagi 1995), and (3) reduced performance when the tested target served as a distractor during practice (Tanne and Sagi 1995). Such results imply that *simply looking at the stimulus* does not lead to learning: for learning to take effect, we need to act on the stimulus, and the way we act determines the learning path.

10.1.4 Working Hypothesis

Changes made in the low-level visual network to account for stimulus-specific learning effects are presumably task specific, and would not occur when stimuli were viewed only passively, indicating involvement of high-level processes. We assume here that these high-level processes affect only learning (i.e., how the system moves from one practice state to another), but not the performance level at any given state of practice. Although attentional processes may modulate network activity (Ishai and Sagi

1995; Tanaka and Sagi 1998; Lee, Koch, and Braun 1997) and its "readout," these operations are expected to be acquired on a short time scale of a few trials (Karni and Sagi 1993; Karni and Bertini 1997). In other words, we assume that performance in the tasks considered here is limited exclusively by the low-level visual network, irrespective of whether observers are naive or practiced. (Of course, whether observers reach these limits or not may depend on whether they fully attend the task or not.)

10.2 Short-Range Interactions

We first describe experiments where the target was masked with Gabor patches presented at the target location, but with varying orientations. These masks presumably excite units which are located within the same hypercolumn as the target unit, and they thus probe cortical short-range connectivity.

Our masks typically consist of two components: one tilted counterclockwise and the other clockwise with respect to the target. Each component can either have positive polarity (i.e., the center of the even-symmetric Gabor patch is white) or negative polarity (where the center of the even-symmetric Gabor patch is black). In the experiments described here, target polarity was always positive, and target orientation was either horizontal or vertical.

To describe a specific mask configuration, we use the following terminology: the tilt angle (with respect to the target) is followed by the polarities of the two components. The notation "30(++)," for instance, refers to a mask configuration where both mask components are of positive polarity, and they are tilted with respect to the target by $+30°$ and $-30°$. The notation "45(+−)" describes a mask configuration where the component that is tilted counterclockwise (by 45°) has positive polarity, whereas the component tilted clockwise (also by 45°) has negative polarity. In some conditions, only one mask component was used, tilted either counterclockwise, referred to as "$(+\bigcirc)$", or clockwise, referred to as "$(\bigcirc+)$". When the mask orientation corresponds to the target orientation, the task becomes a simple contrast discrimination task. The corresponding masking curve is called the "just-noticeable difference" (JND) curve. (For examples of different mask configurations with and without target see figure 10.1.)

10.2.1   The Dipper Function

In typical masking experiments, the target's detection threshold is plotted as a function of mask contrast, with mask contrast referring to the sum of the contrasts of the different mask components. (All other mask parameters such as orientation, size, and the like are kept constant.) The classical finding is that, with increasing mask contrast, thresholds first decrease, reach a minimum, and then increase, resulting in a dipper-shaped function (Legge and Foley 1980). The two parts of the dipper function seem to reflect two different types of interactions. The initial performance improvement is attributed to excitatory input from the mask to the target unit, whereas the performance decay for further increasing mask contrast is attributed to inhibitory interactions. Figures 10.3 and 10.4 depict several examples of masking curves. Dipper functions for different mask configurations (i.e., masks with different orientations and polarities) differ in location and magnitude of the dipper, but the slopes of the two sections are usually stable (when plotted on a log-log scale; see also Zenger and Sagi 1996).

Performance Improvement with Increasing Mask Contrast

The explanation of performance improvement with increasing mask contrast is strongly related to the concept of a response threshold. The basic idea is

that the target unit does not respond to low-contrast stimuli, but responds only if the stimulation exceeds a defined threshold (but see Pelli 1985 for an alternative explanation using uncertainty concepts). If the mask provides excitatory input to the target unit it brings this unit closer to threshold, and thus increases its sensitivity. The magnitude of excitatory input from a specific mask can be estimated from the location (on the log mask contrast axis) of the dipper section with negative slope.

Note that one can distinguish two kinds of excitatory input from the mask to the target unit: when the mask is presented within the receptive field of the target it provides *direct input*, whereas, when the mask stimulates a unit that in turn stimulates the target unit it provides *indirect input*.

Performance Decay with Increasing Mask Contrast

This regime corresponds to the Weber-Fechner law, which describes human sensitivity to changes of sensory input ($\Delta I / I$ = constant, where I is the sensory input magnitude and ΔI is the JND), predicting a slope of one on log-log coordinates. Contrast masking produces slopes smaller than 1 (see figures 10.3 and 10.4), thus presenting a deviation from the classical sensory law. Performance decay may be the result of response saturation (Wilson 1980), inhibitory network interactions (Heeger 1992; Foley 1994), or both (Wilson and Humanski 1993). Network interactions can be implemented as divisive inhibition from units that surround the target unit. Such a mechanism normalizes a unit's response with respect to the average activity in this region, and may thus be an important means to avoid response saturation (Heeger 1992). The divisive input reduces the gain of the target unit and thus decreases its sensitivity. With increasing mask contrast, the inhibitory input becomes stronger and stronger, and performance deteriorates more and more. The magnitude of in-

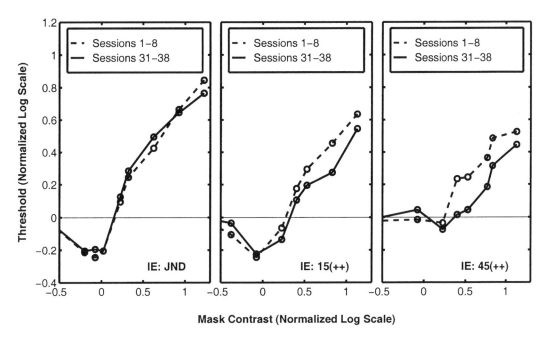

Figure 10.3
Masking curves for observer I. E. in conditions with different mask configurations, before and after practice. The mask contrast as well as the detection thresholds are presented on a normalized log scale, that is, the values shown represent the logarithm of the ratio of specific contrast values and the detection threshold; hence zero denotes identical contrast values of both stimuli—a ratio of 1. Masking curves differ in the magnitude and mask contrast value of the maximal dip (sometimes there may be no dip at all). After practice, there was a notable decrease in suppression in the 45(++) condition (*right*); the practice effect was smaller in the 15(++) condition (*middle*); and there was no effect on the just-noticeable difference (JND) curve (*left*), even though long-term practice lasted for almost forty sessions in each of the conditions.

hibitory input from a specific mask configuration can be estimated from the location (on the mask contrast axis) of the dipper section with positive slope.

10.2.2 Practice Effects

When an observer repeats this type of masking experiments for several sessions, the dipper function changes in a characteristic way. The most obvious change is a decrease in suppression, that is, the masking curve section with positive slope is shifted to the right (along the mask contrast axis), whereas the slope is unchanged. The absolute threshold (i.e., the

detection threshold in the absence of masks) and the initial section of the dipper function are only slightly affected by practice, if at all (Zenger and Sagi 1996). Examples are shown in figures 10.3 and 10.4. To characterize the effect quantitatively, we estimate the *suppression threshold*, which is the mask contrast at which masks start to have a negative effect on target detection (i.e., the point where the dipper crosses the baseline) normalized by the target's detection threshold. An interesting observation is that even though for almost all masking conditions suppression thresholds increased with practice, such a practice effect was never observed when the mask and target

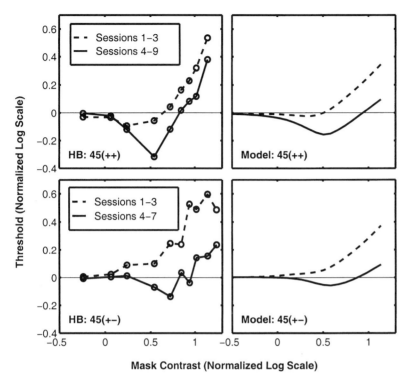

Figure 10.4
Masking curves for observer H. B. in conditions with different mask configurations, before (solid curves) and after (broken curves) practice, actual (*left*) and modeled (*right*). Mask contrasts as well as detection thresholds are presented on a normalized log scale. A strong decrease in suppression was observed in both conditions. In some cases, masks that led to a suppression in the naive state produced facilitation after practice. (See section 10.2 for a description of the model.)

parameters were the same, that is, when the pattern discrimination task reduced to a contrast discrimination task (see figure 10.3; Dorais and Sagi 1997).

How can we explain the decrease in suppression with the proposed neural network model? The region with positive slope is affected primarily by the inhibitory interactions, suggesting that the inhibitory input from the mask on the target unit decreases during practice. Within the framework of the neural network model considered here, the inhibition from the mask on the target is not determined by a single

synapse, but there are several synaptic modifications which all lead to in a decrease in inhibition. In the following, three simple models are briefly described where learning is attributed to change in the efficacy of a single synapse (see figure 10.5). Each of these models makes distinctive predictions on how practice would transfer between different conditions. Clearly, learning might be more complex, and several synapses might change their efficacy simultaneously, but it seems worthwhile to first explore the simple cases. In the following, units tuned to the

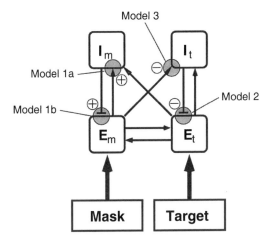

Figure 10.5
Monosynaptic changes that may account for a decrease in suppression. Model 1 suggests that mask activity is reduced after practice due to increased self-inhibition of the mask. Model 2 assumes a general reduction of inhibition on the target filter. Model 3 attributes the decrease in suppression to a reduction in inhibition from the mask unit to the target unit. The different models may be distinguished based on the practice transfer pattern between different tasks.

mask stimulus are indexed with "m," whereas units tuned to the target stimulus are indexed with "t."

Model 1: Decrease in the E_m Activity Learning may lead to a decrease in the activity in the mask units, which could, for instance, be mediated by increased self-inhibition of the mask (increase in the weight of the $E_m \to I_m$ connection, in the weight of the $I_m \to E_m$ connection, or in both). If so, we would expect that *learning is specific to the practiced mask, but generalizes to new targets.*

Model 2: Decrease in the $I_t \to E_t$ Efficacy Continuous practice may make the inhibition of the target unit less and less effective. If inhibition is reduced in a very general way, one would expect

that *learning is specific to the target, but generalizes to new masks.*

Model 3: Decrease in the $E_m \to I_t$ Efficacy A third obvious possibility is that interactions between mask and target are modified. When inhibition from the specific mask component on a specific target unit is reduced, practice is expected to be very specific. Transfer would be observed only when the same target is used and when, in addition, at least one of the mask components is identical to the practice mask. If so, one would expect that *learning is specific to the combination of mask (component) and target.*

Note that the three models correspond to three different "strategies" that an observer can adopt to deal with the masking problem: (1) ignore the maskers (model 1); (2) improve on target discrimination (model 2); and (3) isolate the target from the mask (model 3).

10.2.3 Transfer of Learning

Results of critical transfer experiments carried out by Dorais and Sagi (1997) are summarized in table 10.1. As can be seen, none of the three models suggested above accurately describes the experimental observations.

In the first four conditions, the target orientation was the same during practice and transfer conditions, whereas in the last condition, the 45(++) mask was fixed and the target was rotated. Model 1 predicts that learning transfers to a new target when the mask is kept constant, but this prediction is inconsistent with the experimental data: practice with a horizontal target and a 45(++) mask did not transfer to a vertical target. Model 2 is also inadequate because learning does not always transfer to new masks: practice with a 30(++) mask, for instance, does not

Table 10.1
Transfer pattern found by Dorais and Sagi (1997), compared with predictions of three simple models

Practice		Transfer	Result	Model 1	Model 2	Model 3
30(++)	→	30(+○)	No	Yes	Yes	Yes
45(++)	→	45(+−)	No	Partial	Yes	Partial
45(+−)	→	45(−+)	Yes	No	Yes	No
30(+○)	→	30(○+)	Yes	No	Yes	No
H target	→	V target	No	Yes	No	No

transfer to a $30(+○)$ mask, and transfer is further not observed from the $45(++)$ to the $45(+−)$ mask.

Model 3, which states that practice is specific to the combination of target and mask components, cannot account for the data either. In fact, this third model predicts in most cases the exact opposite of the behavior observed in the experiments: in cases where the practice and transfer masks do not share a mask component, the model predicts that there is no transfer of learning. When practicing the $45(+−)$ condition, for instance, no transfer is expected to the $45(−+)$ condition. The same holds for the transfer from the $30(+○)$ condition to the $30(○+)$ condition. In both cases, complete transfer was found in the experimental data. In conditions where practice and transfer masks do share a component, the model predicts (at least a partial) transfer. Thus improvement in the $(++)$ condition should lead to an improvement in the $(+−)$ and $(+○)$ conditions. In the psychophysical data, however, no transfer was found in these conditions.

Here we show that the observed pattern of transfer can be explained by assuming redistribution of gain control during practice, that is, we suggest that after practice, the target unit is inhibited (controlled) mainly by the target unit, whereas the mask components are inhibited mainly by the mask units. In

addition, we assume that the response of each unit to the isolated target and the isolated mask stays the same during practice, that is, the magnitude of gain control does not change, but only the cell pool from which this gain control is recruited.

How can this account for the observed transfer pattern? Let us first consider the effects of redistribution of target gain control. Inhibitory synapses from the target units would strengthen somewhat, without affecting the response to the isolated target because of a counterbalanced weakening of inhibitory effects from other units (which have some spurious activity even in the absence of masks and thus contribute to the gain control). As a result, the contrast discrimination functions for the isolated target (just-noticeable difference or JND curve) are not affected much, whereas the effects of tilted masks are considerably reduced. The expected transfer pattern due to redistribution of target and mask gain control during practice is shown in table 10.2.

Whereas distribution of target gain control leads to a target-specific performance, redistribution of mask gain control leads to a negative transfer when the transfer mask shares a component of the practice mask: such redistribution consists of a strengthening of inhibitory interactions between units that belong to different mask components. This increase in gain control, however, is balanced by a decrease of self-inhibition, such that the overall level of inhibition does not change during practice. When, in the transfer test, only one component of the previously practiced mask is presented, the unit's activity will explode because this unit is controlled to a large degree by the units corresponding to the other mask component, which is now missing. The highly active mask unit provides considerable inhibition to the target unit, and thus causes a performance detriment. Such a detriment (negative transfer) is expected whenever the transfer mask contains only one (of

Table 10.2
Transfer pattern found by Dorais and Sagi (1997) and effects of redistributing gain control during practice

Practice Task	Transfer Task	Redistribution of Target Gain Control	Redistribution of Mask Gain Control	Net Effect
30(++)	30(+○)	+	−	0 (no)
45(++)	45(+−)	+	−	0 (no)
45(+−)	45(−+)	+	0	+ (yes)
30(+○)	30(○+)	+	0	+ (yes)
H target	V target	0	0	0 (no)

several) components of the practice mask, whereas no effect is expected when practice mask and transfer mask are the same or do not share a component.

If the two processes are balanced in a specific manner, their net effect is compatible with the experimental observations (see table 10.2). The summary in the table represents, of course, merely a qualitative account of the data. To demonstrate that such a hypothesized principle really works, model implementations are crucial.

The model we consider has twenty-four units, each of which consists of a E subunit that forms excitatory connections and an I subunit that forms inhibitiory connections. The E subunits represent the input layer as well as the output layer. To compute the input to a specific unit E, we assume linear receptive fields with an orientation bandwidth of 15°. The different units differ in their preferred orientation (sampling distance 15°) and preferred polarity (positive or negative). Each unit's activity is described by a differential equation, that is, the responses of each unit change in time, depending on the input it receives from the stimulus, and other excitatory and inhibitory units. To assess the model's

performance, we assume that two stimuli can be discriminated when they produce at steady state a response difference of 1 in the E unit that is tuned to the target. (Details can be found at ⟨http://www.weizmann.ac.il/masagi/zs00.pdf⟩.) Simulation results of this model are shown next to the psychophysical results in figure 10.6. As one can see, a fairly good fit is obtained.

10.2.4   Constraints on Architecture

As outlined in section 10.1, learning data can be useful in two ways. First, they can provide constraints for possible model architectures, and second, they can reveal the nature of learning rules. Disregarding for a moment the issue of learning rules (i.e., why the system moves from one state to another), we would like to illustrate how data obtained by one observer at different stages of practice can constrain models.

One of the most critical findings in this context is that practicing detection of a horizontal target in the presence of a compound mask with two components tilted by +30° and −30° with respect to the target did not transfer to either of the two components (see figure 10.6, panel A). This finding clearly demonstrates that one can in general not predict performance with a compound object (mask) based on the performance with the individual components: one can apparently manipulate performance in the compound task (by practice) without affecting performance with the components.

Independent variation of performance with compound masks and its components implies that we cannot simply view the compound as a sum of its components but that there is some process that is specific to the combination of two specific mask components. Perhaps the simplest assumption is that the *interactions between the mask components* are

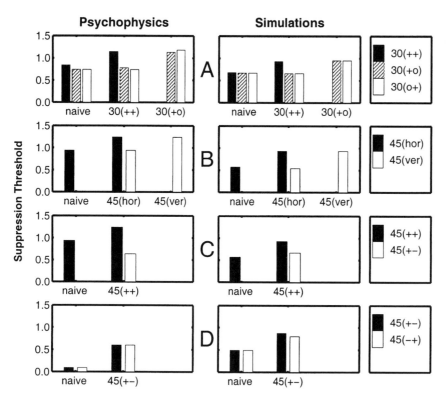

Figure 10.6

Psychophysical suppression thresholds (*left*) estimated from the data of Dorais and Sagi (1997), together with model simulations (*right*). (Note that the higher bars correspond to the weaker masking effects.) The labels on the x-axis denote which task was practiced before a specific data set was obtained. (*A*) Practice of the 30(++) condition followed by practice of the 30(+o) condition. Practice with the compound mask did not transfer to the individual components, but consequent practice with one component transferred to the other component. (*B*) Practice of the 45(++) condition with a horizontal target, followed by practice with a vertical target. When switching target orientation, the suppression threshold returns to the naive level, indicating no transfer. (*C*) Practice of the 45(++) did not lead to a good performance in the 45(+−) condition, being suggestive of a no-transfer situation. (Unfortunately prepractice data are missing for the 45(+−) condition.) (*D*) Practice in the 45(+−) condition led to an improvement in both the 45(+−) and 45(−+) conditions.

relevant and that these interactions change during practice. Such effects of mask interactions on target detection cannot be incorporated into simple feedforward models. The lack of transfer from practice of the compound to its components was one of the major motivations to adopt a feedback architecture.

There is a second transfer result that has direct consequences for possible architectures. Dorais and Sagi (1997) describe one observer who practiced detection of a horizontal target in the presence of a mask consisting of two components. The polarities of all three Gabor stimuli (target component and two mask components) were positive (white in the center). After practice, transfer was tested in a task where the polarities of all three stimuli were reversed. The absence of transfer implies that the model cannot contain only phase-insensitive units (mimicking typical complex cells) but that there have to be phase-sensitive units (mimicking typical simple cells). Otherwise, performance in the two tasks (detection of negative target in the presence of negative mask versus detection of positive target in the presence of positive mask) would be mediated by the very same units, which are blind to the difference between the two tasks, and the observed "independent variation" of the two performance levels would not be understandable. Furthermore, it is implied that the modifications that occur during practice affect these phase-sensitive cells; otherwise, an independent variation of the performance levels in the two tasks would not occur. Note that it would be comparably difficult to obtain such strong architectural constraints without the analysis of learning data.

10.3   Long-Range Spatial Interactions

In section 10.2, we presented a framework for analyzing orientation masking data, using spatially

overlapping oriented filters with excitatory and inhibitory interactions. Similar interactions were found between spatially nonoverlapping filters (Polat and Sagi 1993; Polat and Sagi 1994a; Wilson and Wilkinson 1997). These experiments involve detection of a Gabor signal in the presence of flanking high contrast masks (figure 10.7, panel A).

10.3.1   Spatial Interactions

When the target-to-mask distance is varied, two effects can be observed: increased threshold (suppression) with small separations, and decreased thresholds (facilitation) with larger separation (figure 10.7, panel B). When using high-contrast masks, the location of the transition between suppression and facilitation changes with the Gabor scale used (wavelength, λ) and is at about 2λ (Polat and Sagi 1993). Interactions within the range of 2λ can be viewed as short-range interactions, mainly within the size of a receptive field (see section 10.2), with effects being contrast and phase dependent (Zenger and Sagi 1996). The short-range lateral effects reflect a balance between lateral inhibitory interactions and excitatory interactions, with inhibition taking over at high contrast levels (Sagi and Hochstein 1985; Stemmler, Usher, and Niebur 1995; Polat et al. 1998; Somers et al. 1998; Bonneh and Sagi 1999). Because we assume that the external input to a network subunit can be represented as linear integration over some retinal receptive field (linear filters), and connections between subunits as nonlinear interactions, we expect processes within the subunit integration area (receptive field) to have a spatial phase–dependent component, whereas long-range interactions may show phase independence (Zenger and Sagi 1996; Bonneh and Sagi 1998).

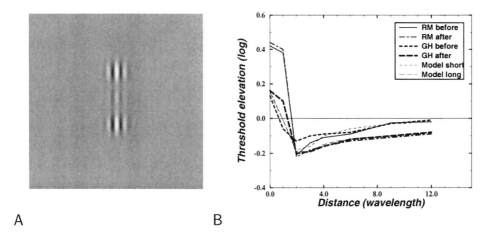

A   B

Figure 10.7

(*A*) Stimulus used for exploring lateral interactions, with two high-contrast masks (Gabor signals) flanking a low-contrast target. (*B*) Data from the lateral masking experiments, before and after practice. (Redrawn from Polat and Sagi 1994b.) Observers detected a Gabor target flanked by two high-contrast colinear Gabor signals at different distances. Contrast detection thresholds relative to absolute threshold (no mask) are plotted as a function of target to mask distance, using Gabor wavelength units. Data are shown for two observers (R. M. and G. H.) and for a model network assuming activity propagation through lateral excitatory connections with local normalization. (From Sagi 1996.) Observers show an increased range of enhancement after extensive practice. The model emulates practice by increasing excitatory synaptic efficacy and thus increasing the range of signal propagation through the excitatory lateral connections. Note that suppression is not affected by practice in these experiments and simulations.

10.3.2   Network Architecture

Long-range spatial interactions are configuration dependent (figure 10.8; largest facilitation is obtained with cooriented and coaxial target and masks or with cooriented but parallel target and masks; Polat and Sagi 1994a). In terms of the model network presented here (figure 10.2), these results indicate that excitatory connections ($E_i \rightarrow E_j$) take place between excitatory subunits corresponding to neighboring spatial locations, only in directions along, and orthogonal, to the subunit's preferred orientation. Inhibitory connections ($E_i \rightarrow I_j$) are isotropic (but see section: 10.3.3 on nonisotropic modulation of connections' efficacies). This result imposes a strong constraint on possible interactions that can take place

in these low-level networks, and limits the "learnable."

10.3.3   Learning

Long-range spatial interactions are experience dependent. Both excitatory and inhibitory effects may change with practice, depending on stimuli used. As a general rule, it seems that frequently activated connections increase their efficacy with practice (though depending on some task-dependent gating; see section 10.1).

Learning Excitatory Effects

Observers practicing the lateral masking task, with target flanked by two high-contrast masks at varied

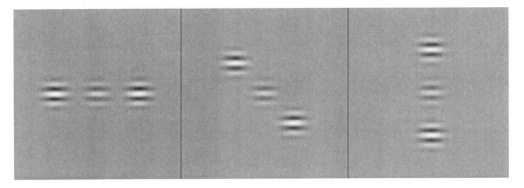

Figure 10.8
Stimuli used for exploring performance limits imposed by network connectivity. (From Polat and Sagi 1994a.) Lateral facilitation is greatest with colinear configurations, independent of local or global orientation. Parallel configurations (i.e., local orientation orthogonal to global orientation) produced lateral facilitation, whereas locally tilted configurations (i.e., local orientation diagonal to global orientation) failed to produce facilitation even after extensive practice (Polat and Sagi 1994b); lateral inhibition affected all configurations (Polat and Sagi 1994a).

distances, show an increased range of facilitatory effects. Depending on the range that is practiced the interaction range can reach up to seven times the receptive field size (Polat and Sagi 1994b). This learning is highly specific for basic visual features such as orientation, location, spatial frequency, and eye (Polat and Sagi 1995). To account for the increased facilitatory range, there seem to be two plausible alternatives: practice causes a selective increase either in the efficacy of direct long-range interactions between mask unit and target unit ($E_m \rightarrow E_t$) or in the efficacy of synaptic transmission between neighboring subunits ($E_i \rightarrow E_{i+1}$), positioned between mask and target units. Experimental evidence supports the latter, pointing to the existence of a feedback network in which local interactions enable an efficient propagation of neuronal activity.

Propagation is not isotropic (see section 10.3.2), but is constrained by existing connections. Learning studies have shown learning effects of facilitatory interactions along two cardinal directions (coaxial and parallel relative to local orientation; see figure

10.8), but not along other directions (Polat and Sagi 1994b).

Learning Inhibitory Effects
Whereas masks at distances of 3λ and more seem to probe mainly excitatory interactions, masks presented at distances of 2λ and less appear to involve also inhibitory interactions (see contrast and range effects in section 10.3.1). Practicing a lateral masking task with multiple high-contrast flankers placed at 2λ intervals (see figure 10.9) was found to increase the range and efficacy of these inhibitory interactions (Adini, Sagi, and Tsodyks 1997). Results from these experiments are presented in figure 10.10 for chains of colinear Gabor signals (figure 10.9, panel B). For unpracticed observers, increasing the number of flankers beyond two or four (one or two on each side) has no effect on contrast threshold. For practiced observers, increasing the number of flankers has a nonmonotonic effect on threshold: adding flankers cancels the facilitation, and adding still more flankers restores some of the facilitation.

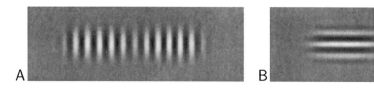

Figure 10.9

(*A*, *B*) Stimuli used in chain lateral masking experiments: parallel configuration (panel A); colinear configuration (panel B). (From Adini, Sagi, and Tsodyks 1997.) Target is flanked by a total of ten Gabor signals: five on each side, spaced 2λ apart.

These results indicate the development of lateral inhibition between neighboring units that respond to the high-contrast flankers, possibly involving redistribution of mask gain control (section 10.2). These effects were found to be configuration specific: colinear stimuli (figure 10.9, panel B) showed little indication for inhibition at the initial phase of practice (figure 10.10), whereas parallel stimuli (figure 10.9, panel A) seemed to successfully utilize existing strong inhibitory interactions. Practice had the effect of equalizing inhibitory effects along these two cardinal directions.

In addition to the increase in lateral inhibition, a second practice effect was observed in these experiments: practice increased facilitation of target detection by neighboring flankers (figure 10.10), probably the result of decreased inhibitory effects from masks to target (see section 10.2 on redistribution of target gain control).

10.3.4 Applications to Texture Learning

In texture segmentation tasks, observers detect an image region (target, foreground) that is different from the background. When target and background differ in some distinctive basic feature (e.g., orientation), segmentation is said to be "effortless" and preattentive (Julesz 1981), and performance is limited by the low-level visual network (Rubenstein and Sagi 1990). Performance on texture discrimina-

tion tasks improves with increasing texture density (Nothdurft 1985; Sagi and Julesz 1987; Sagi 1990), pointing to a performance limit set by network connectivity range. Karni and Sagi (1991), using dense textures composed of line elements with three tilted lines serving as a target and 357 horizontal lines as the background (figure 10.11), found large performance improvement with practice. In a later study (Karni and Sagi 1993), they found that some fast performance improvement occurs within the first practice session, followed by a slower learning that takes a few sessions to converge; that, once learning reaches an asymptotic level, it can last for a long time without further practice, at least for two years; and that these different time scales do not seem to reflect a time-dependent decrease in effectiveness of a unique mechanism, but rather correspond to distinct mechanisms, operating at different levels of brain processing, as implied by the different selectivity properties of these two temporal regimes. During slow learning, memory traces may take a few hours to consolidate, with consolidation being enhanced during night sleep, with the different sleep stages having selective effects (Karni et al. 1994; Stickgold et al. 2000) on the memory traces.

The main finding of Karni and Sagi (1991) is that learning is specific for some basic visual features, such as orientation, location, and eye. Monocularity of learning implies an anatomical learning site below or at the site where the images from the two eyes

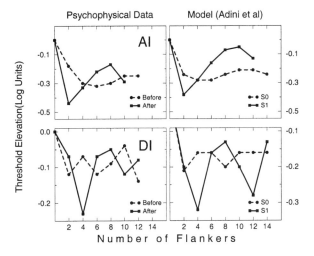

Psychophysical Data   Model (Adini et al)

Figure 10.10

Results from experiments using multiple maskers. (From Adini, Sagi, and Tsodyks 1997.) (*Left*) Psychophysical data are presented from psychophysical experiments where the two observers (A. I. and D. I.) detected the presence of a Gabor target flanked by a variable number of colinear Gabor masks, before and after practice. The initial performance level (broken curves) was affected by only the closest masks, with masks 6λ apart having no effect on performance. After practice (solid curves), these remote masks inhibited performance, with masks placed farther away restoring some facilitation (showing disinhibition). (*Right*) Simulating the two observers with two different sets of parameters, the model (Adini, Sagi, and Tsodyks 1997) assumes a network like that in figure 10.2, with lateral inhibition and excitation. Practice is simulated as increased range and efficacy of lateral inhibition, with inhibition between mask units being more prominent after practice. In addition, lateral inhibition on the target is reduced, to account for the increased short-range facilitation with practice.

converge (i.e., monocular synapses onto binocular or monocular cells; see chapter 11.6, but also 5.3, 9.5, 14.3.1). Locality and orientation specificity also support plasticity at an early stage of visual processing. Perhaps the most puzzling result, however, is that slow learning was found to be very specific to the background orientation, but not specific to the target orientation. Which is to say, target specificity holds only for the first session (fast learning).

Many different network units respond to the different background elements; all these units are thought to interact with each other through lateral inhibitory processes and can thus be expected to go through a redistribution process. Units responding to background elements will develop stronger inhibition between them and may reduce background visibility. However, decrease in self-inhibition within these units would make their response unchanged in the presence of neighboring background elements. In other words, the unit responding to an individual background element would reduce its self-control and would instead "hand over" some control to the units that respond to the neighboring background elements. In this way, the background would be imprinted into the system as a pattern (rather than as many individual lines). When one of the neighboring background elements is missing, as when the background element has been replaced by a target, the unit gets slightly "out of control" and will respond more strongly. This increase in the response may mediate the performance improvement.

Although we do not attempt here to present a detailed model for texture and popout learning, we do wish to point out that such a redistribution mechanism seems an attractive way to naturally account for a number of findings. First, the redistribution implies that the activity of background units that are surrounded by background do not change as a result of practice, that is, background visibility

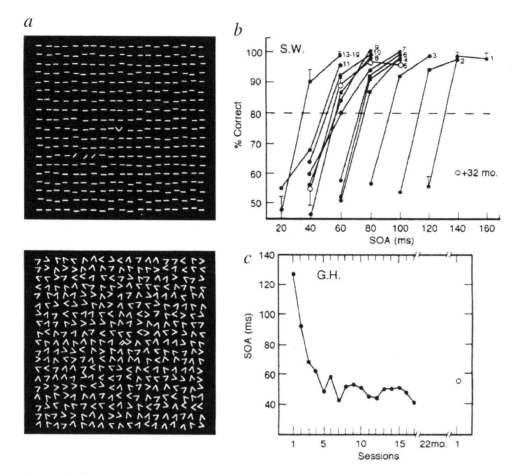

Figure 10.11

Computer-generated displays used in texture-learning experiments. (*a*) For small target texture (three diagonal bars) embedded within a background of horizontal bars (*top*), target position was varied randomly from trial to trial but always within a specific display quadrant and within 2.5°–5° visual angle from center of display. A fixation target was also presented at the stimulus center (T or L). For mask pattern made of randomly oriented V-shaped micropatterns and a central compound pattern of superimposed T and L (*bottom*), a stimulus sequence consisted of a texture pattern (10 msec) followed by a blank period (stimulus onset asynchrony, or SOA), followed by a mask pattern (100 msec). Observers had to identify the fixation target and the global orientation of the texture target. (*b*) Psychometric curves from one observer (S. W.) depict mean percentage correct for performance on texture target discrimination (whether target elements are arranged vertically or horizontally) on consecutive sessions (spaced 1–3 days apart). Each data point represents mean (± one standard deviation) percent correct responses from 3–5 blocks (150–250 trials) for a specific SOA. Initial performance curve is on the right; as learning occurs, the curves are displaced to the left (shorter SOA needed for task performance). The leftmost curve represents asymptotic performance. Tests carried out 32 months after the last session (open circles) show almost no forgetting. Note that curve shape does not change from curve to curve—indicating a genuine change in sensitivity. (*c*) Learning curves for one observer (G. H.), obtained by plotting the daily SOA thresholds (80% correct), show convergence of performance after 5 sessions, with no forgetting after 22 months. This learning does not transfer to conditions where target is presented in a different stimulus quadrant or when background orientation is changed (i.e., performance returns to its initial level and observers need to relearn the task). (From Karni and Sagi 1993.)

remains constant. Only those background units that surround the target become more active. This prediction is supported by recent recordings from monkey visual cortex (Bertini et al. 1995, 1996) showing constant response through practice of single units that respond to texture background elements, but increased response in units that respond to background elements in the neighborhood of a target. Second, the mechanism seems consistent with the finding that (slow) texture learning is specific for background orientation but not for target orientation (Karni and Sagi 1991). It would further be consistent with the finding that conditions involving different background orientations can be learned independently of each other (Ahissar et al. 1998; Karni and Sagi 1991), that is, when observers practice several tasks, these practice effects do not need to interfere with each other. Of particular interest here are conditions where target and background orientations are swapped, thus creating an apparent conflict between two learned conditions. Our network, after practicing these two conditions, produces equally good performance in these two conditions.

10.4   Conclusions

Perceptual learning appears to produce significant changes in networks of early vision, changes that modify the effective connectivity of the network. The type of modification taking place presumably depends on stimulus and task. We suggest some simple, certainly simplified, rules that were developed to account for contrast detection data, but have, in addition, some more general flavor.

When practicing visual tasks that include several objects—some of them targets—inhibitory effects are redistributed to achieve independent gain control within functional groups: inhibitory interactions increase within groups and decrease between groups. Although network states at different stages of practice can be characterized by the suggested segmentation process, the rules governing the transitions between the different network states are not obvious. One question left open here is how the system knows which units correspond to the target and which units correspond to the mask (or, in general, which unit corresponds to which functional group). There may be several plausible answers to this question; two possibilities are briefly described.

1. *The system may use high-level information.* In the experiments described here, observers are well informed about what is the target they are supposed to detect, and what is the mask (and even if they were not told, they might still be able to figure out on a cognitive level what is the task). This type of high-level information might be used to direct synaptic modifications that result in an effective segregation of the two patterns.

2. *The system may use low-level information.* The activity of units belonging to different functional groups have (at least to some degree) uncorrelated activities, whereas the activities in different units belonging to the same functional group are highly correlated. Knowing, for instance, the activity in one of the mask units completely determines the activity in other mask units, but does not say much about the activity in the target unit (i.e., whether the target is present or absent). Note that these correlations cannot be estimated within a single trial, but require that information be integrated across many trials or several blocks. Presence or absence of correlations may allow the system to determine the units that belong to different functional groups.

These learning rules are not necessarily specific for low-level vision, but may apply also to other domains where objects need to be segmented. The redistribution of inhibitory effects within functional neuronal groups responding to external objects may serve to keep constant relative activity within groups (object normalization). Without this process, different object parts would be normalized to the local activity, being different at different parts. Parts of an object that are presented on a salient background would be more suppressed than those parts presented on a "quiet" background, introducing distortions into the recognition process.

Acknowledgments

This work was supported by a grant from the Grodetsky Center for Research of Higher Brain Functions at the Weizmann Institute of Science. We thank Yael Adini, Jochen Braun, and Daniella Meeker for comments on an earlier version of the manuscript.

Learning to Perceive Features below the Foveal Photoreceptor Spacing

11

Manfred Fahle

Abstract

Minute visual features, smaller than the diameter and spacing of foveal photoreceptors, have been used as extremely sensitive probes to monitor improvement through training in visual discrimination tasks. This chapter discusses the neuronal mechanisms allowing such fine spatial discriminations and presents the results of recent investigations of perceptual learning that demonstrate a surprising specificity of improvement through training for stimulus attributes such as orientation, position, and exact type of task, as well as for the eye used during training. Control experiments ruled out a significant contribution by motor components of learning, for example, by improving the quality of fixation, accommodation, or both. The specificity of learning and the occurrence of short latency changes in cortically evoked responses over the human occipital cortex argue strongly in favor of an involvement of primary visual cortex in perceptual learning, as does perceptual learning in amnesic patients. On the other hand, perceptual learning also involves strong top-down influences from higher cortical areas: attention and error feedback exert strong influences on learning speed, and there is no transfer between different tasks that all use the same type of early orientation-specific neuronal filter.

11.1 Visual Hyperacuity as a Probe of Perceptual Learning

As outlined in the introduction to this volume, learning is understood to mean a lasting change of behavior as a result of previous experience. Perceptual learning, therefore, is a lasting change of perception and of perception-related behavior such as

pressing a response button in the course of training. Although it has long been known that perception can be refined and thresholds lowered by—sometimes extended—experience with a perceptual task, this improvement was generally ascribed to cognitive processes in the brain. The primary sensory cortices, on the other hand, were believed to be "hardwired" in the adult monkey and human. For example, Marr (1982, 185) noted that "the human visual system incorporates a permanent 'hard-wired' table of similarities," a belief that agrees well with the finding by Wiesel (1982, 583) that "neural connections present early in life can be modified by visual experience. Such neural plasticity was not observed in the adult. . . ."

For our investigations into the improvement of visual performance as a function of training, we chose a class of perceptual tasks known as "hyperacuity" (Westheimer 1976). What these perceptual tasks, such as stereoscopic depth perception and vernier discrimination, have in common is that experienced observers regularly achieve thresholds far below a foveal photoreceptor diameter, discriminating between stimuli that differ from each other by far less than the spacing between adjacent photoreceptors in the fovea. For readers unfamiliar with photoreceptor sizes, another example might be more instructive. If a midsize car is placed on a mountaintop that can be seen from a great distance, with a long straight vertical bar fixed above one of the car's headlights and another very long vertical bar underneath the other headlight, then an average trained observer will be able to detect this horizontal offset of approximately 1.5 m from an observation distance of 100 km, and a very good observer will still be able to detect it from a distance of 160 km. At this distance, the offset between the two bars will correspond to an angle of 3 arc sec, resp. 2 arc sec, corresponding to the best discrimination thresholds of around 2 arc sec obtained by some well-trained observers.

The amazing precision of these judgments misled Wülfing (1892), who performed some quantitative measurements on vernier discriminations, to the opinion that foveal photoreceptors had to be much smaller than his anatomist colleagues thought. In this instance, however, the psychophysicist was wrong and the anatomists were right. The photoreceptors are indeed larger in diameter than the vernier thresholds of trained observers, by a factor of at least 2 to 3, and still more for a few especially gifted observers. Thus Hering (1861), accepting the values given for photoreceptor spacing, postulated that vernier acuity is achieved by spatial sampling over a large number, perhaps hundreds of photoreceptors, that are all stimulated by the two lines composing a vernier stimulus (see figure 11.1, panel a). This elegant explanation was falsified, however, by Ludvigh (1953), who showed in a clever experiment that the explanation given by Hering could not be correct. Ludvigh presented three dots that were arranged almost exactly on an imaginary line (figure 11.1, panel b). The midpoint was, however, offset to the left or to the right relative to the imaginary line between the endpoints, and observers had to indicate the direction of offset: left versus right. At the optimal distance between the endpoints, observers were able to achieve thresholds that were hardly at all higher than the ones obtained with vernier lines. Because the points only stimulated a very small number of photoreceptors, Hering's hypothesis of averaging over long rows of photoreceptors could not be the

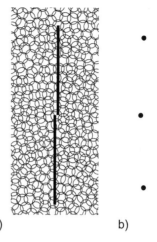

a)   b)

Figure 11.1
(*a*) Hering's explanation (1861) for the achievement of visual hyperacuity, that is, thresholds far below the diameter of foveal photoreceptors, by interpolation over many dozens of photoreceptors. (*b*) Ludvigh's falsification (1953) of Hering's explanation by means of three-dot vernier discrimination. Thresholds for lateral displacement of the middle dot are below a foveal photoreceptor diameter.

correct answer to the problem of how to achieve hyperacuity.

11.2   The Computational Mechanisms of Visual Hyperacuity

How, then, can the human visual brain achieve such a high spatial accuracy? Curiously, the answer partly relies on the limited resolution of the eye's optics. If a small dot in the outer world, such as a bright star, could be projected onto the retina with extremely high resolution, such that all the light coming from this dot would hit only one photoreceptor, any stationary eye would be unable to signal the location of this star as projected onto its retina with a resolution better than the photoreceptor spacing. Positions on

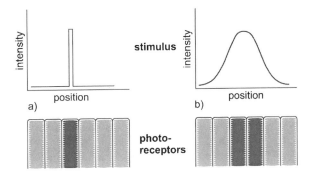

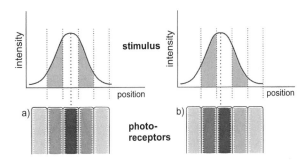

Figure 11.2
Stimulus (*top*) and schematic photoreceptors (*bottom*) for projection of a point light source in the outer world onto the retina. (*a*) Optics of unlimited resolution stimulates only one photoreceptor. (*b*) Optics with a point spread function similar to the human eye's optics, stimulates several photoreceptors.

Figure 11.3
Stimulus (*top*) and photoreceptors (*bottom*) for projection of a point or line situated at marginally differing positions in the outer world onto the foveal receptor mosaic. (*a*) Position exactly above the middle of the photoreceptor, where the middle photoreceptor is stimulated most strongly (darkest shading) and both its neighbors equally less stimulated (medium gray). (*b*) Position shifted slightly to the left, where the neighbors are stimulated asymmetrically.

the middle of the receptor would be equivalent and indiscriminate to others somewhat to the left or right (figure 11.2, panel a). But resolution of the human optics is not all that good. Even a point in the outer world would produce an airy disk on the retina with a half-width of around 40 arc sec, that is, slightly more than one photoreceptor diameter (e.g., Campbell and Gubisch 1966). Each stimulus of sufficient energy will thus activate a cluster of photoreceptors: those in the center of the projection most strongly, with decreasing activation toward the sides (figure 11.2, panel b). This limited resolution allows the visual system to compute the position of a bright object in the outer world with a precision that is only limited by the signal-to-noise ratio. As you can see in figure 11.3, panel a, a star whose projection is centered exactly over the middle of a photoreceptor will activate this photoreceptor most strongly. Neighboring photoreceptors to the right and left receive less activation, but the decrease is symmetrical. If, one the other hand, the star is shifted by, say, one-

fifth of a photoreceptor diameter to the left, then the same photoreceptor will still be most strongly activated (figure 11.3, panel b). However, its neighbor to the left will receive more activation than its neighbor to the right. Hence, by comparing the relative amount of activation of a few neighboring photoreceptors, the visual system can in principle locate the position of the stimulus in the outer world with arbitrary precision. This argument can be made more formal by referring to the sampling theorem (Shannon 1948). In mathematical terms, the sampling theorem states

$$X(t) = \sum_{n-\infty}^{\infty} X\left(\frac{n}{2B}\right) \frac{\sin[\pi(2Bt - n)]}{\pi(2Bt - n)},$$

which is to say, an arbitrary function (curve) can be reconstructed from a sequence of samples taken at regular intervals as long as the density of sampling points is high enough to collect slightly more than two samples from each period of the highest fre-

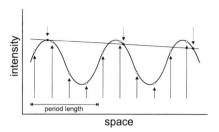

Figure 11.4
Schematic reconstruction of an arbitrary function according to the sampling theorem. The function (here a sine-wave) is sampled either more than twice per period (arrows from below), allowing perfect reconstruction, or about once per period (dotted arrows from above), not allowing correct reconstruction.

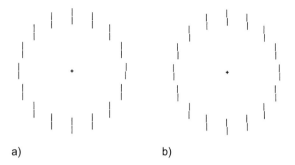

a)   b)

Figure 11.5
Parallel versus serial detection of vernier offsets. (*a*) Vernier offset to the left is immediately perceived among straight distractors: it "pops out." (*b*) Vernier offset to the left is not easily found among verniers offset to the right but requires time-consuming, serial search.

quency contained in the signal (figure 11.4). The requirements of the sampling theorem are fulfilled in the human visual system. The resolution of the eye, as mentioned above, is limited: the highest spatial frequency reaching the retina contains around 60 cycles per degree. Because, however, the spacing of foveal photoreceptors is around 35 arc sec, all but the highest spatial frequencies present in the retinal image are sampled twice per period. Thus the limited resolution of the eye's optics ensures that the neuronal part of the visual system receives the information necessary to determine the exact localization of visual features beyond the grain of foveal photoreceptors.

11.3   What Is Hyperacuity Good For?

On the other hand, perhaps vernier acuity is an unnatural ability of human observers, present only under laboratory conditions for highly trained observers, and having no bearing on normal life. A first argument against this view is the observation that even untrained observers will usually achieve dis-

crimination thresholds that are below a photoreceptor diameter: hyperacuity is thus not just an achievement of highly trained observers. A second argument is that no scrutiny is required for vernier judgments (i.e., discriminations between aligned versus misaligned vernier elements): they can be made in parallel over the visual field. If sixteen vernier stimuli are presented simultaneously, as in figure 11.5, panel a, we immediately spot the one that is offset. This feat is by no means trivial; it requires detectors in the hyperacuity range to be present for a great number of visual field positions, so that the visual field can be processed in parallel regarding the feature "offset" versus "straight."

Consider, in this regard, figure 11.5, panel b. Again, we have to find the vernier whose lower element is offset to the left. However, opposite to panel a, all the distractors are not straight, but offset to the right. Obviously, our visual system does not have parallel detectors in the entire visual field that allow us to discriminate between offsets to the left versus offsets to the right, so we have to perform a serial search and look through all the stimuli se-

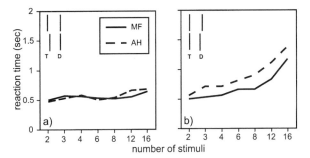

Figure 11.6
Reaction times for detection of (*a*) vernier target (T) offset to the left among different numbers of straight distractors (D) and (*b*) straight target among distractors offset to the left. Results of two observers (M. F. and A. H.). (After Fahle 1991.)

quentially until we find the target—at least if orientation cues are masked (Fahle 1991). And, indeed, search times for detecting an offset target among straight distractors do not strongly increase with the number of elements displayed simultaneously (figure 11.6, panel a), even if the vertical gaps between the upper and lower vernier elements are randomly varied in size. But finding a target offset to the left among distractors offset to the right and even to find a straight target among offset distractors requires search times that increase almost linearly with the number of elements displayed simultaneously (panel b). Similar results were obtained for the search for a target curved to the left among distractors that were straight versus among distractors curved to the right. The reaction times in the first case were virtually independent of set size, whereas they increased steadily with the number of elements in the second.

The human visual system thus obviously devotes a large number of detector neurons to the task of discriminating between straight and nonstraight line elements. This discrimination must be an important one, while the discrimination between the directions of offset is less important. And, indeed, detection of corners and discontinuities in lines may be an important prerequisite for discriminating between objects and their surrounds, especially in complex visual surroundings. We can therefore safely assume that, by investigating vernier acuity and perceptual learning in visual hyperacuity, we choose a relatively simple, well-defined, and extremely sensitive measure, one that is relevant not only under artificial conditions but also for the everyday function of the visual system.

11.4 Possible Neuronal Mechanisms Underlying Hyperacuity

Hyperacuity is an important ability of the brain used for analyzing the visual world, for example, in making stereoscopic depth estimates from the minute differences between the images of the same object cast into the two eyes. But how can the brain improve its ability to discriminate between vernier offsets? One possible way that springs to mind is by adjusting receptive field size, as shown in figure 11.7. Many receptive fields in the visual cortex consist of elongated regions, stimulation of which leads to an activation of the cell, with side bands whose activation leads to inhibition of the same neuron (see figure 11.7). These receptive fields have all kinds of orientations and cover the visual fields with a fine-grained layer. As can be seen in figure 11.7, a cell with a receptive field oriented vertically will not be able to discriminate between a straight and an offset vernier stimulus, as long as the vernier is centered on the cell's receptive field. But nearby cells, whose receptive field centers are shifted somewhat to the side compared to the first neuron, will be able to discriminate between these two stimuli: the offset stimulus will activate part of the inhibitory surround.

Before

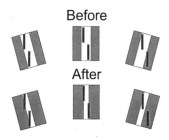

After

Figure 11.7
Orientation-specific receptive fields of the visual cortex with antagonistic center (excitatory = bright)-surround (inhibitory = dark) zones may change their dimensions after perceptual learning, and thus increase hyperacuity performance by better discriminating beween minute spatial offsets. (*Top*) Original size before training; (*bottom*) hypothetical size after training. With smaller centers and wider surrounds, the offset verniers will activate more of the inhibitory surround in the example given here than the straight stimulus will.

The same is true for receptive fields that are somewhat slanted relative to the orientation of the vernier. Cells with receptive fields of this orientation will be best suited to discriminate between straight and offset verniers. Indeed, Waugh, Levi, and Carney (1993) have shown that a grating mask has strongest masking effects if its not oriented parallel to the vernier stimulus, but at an angle around 10° relative to the vernier's axis.

Perceptual learning may lead to a narrowing of the receptive field centers. As can be seen in figure 11.7, panel b, narrowing the receptive fields will better enable the neurons to discriminate between straight and offset verniers. Indeed, the most straightforward explanation for possible modifications as early as the primary visual cortex, and one initially favored by many researchers, is based on the assumption of a narrowing of receptive field centers. But we are getting ahead of ourselves. At this point, we can still assume that the reason the brain im-

proves through practice on vernier discrimination tasks is that it just makes better use of the information brought to it through the eyes and afferent visual pathways and filtered by some hardwired primary sensory cortices. This assumption does not require plasticity in the primary visual cortex. To examine the assumption of purely cognitive improvement, let us review the evidence that points to such plasticity of the primary visual cortex.

11.5 Improvement through Training of Vernier Acuity Is Highly Orientation Specific

One bit of evidence, and one that this author is most familiar with, stems from experiments on vernier stimuli trained at one orientation and presented subsequently at different orientations. To test improvement in vernier acuity discriminations by training, we presented vernier stimuli to twelve observers. One group of six observers was trained to discriminate with horizontal orientation of the stimuli, whereas the second group of six observers started to train the vernier oriented vertically. Within a one-hour session, nineteen blocks of forty stimulus presentations each were performed. The results for each block were averaged over all observers of both groups and plotted in figure 11.8, panel a. As can be seen, average performance improved from around 74% correct responses to around 85% correct responses. Improvement was fastest during the first 20 minutes and slowed down thereafter. (Informal experiments with a few observers indicate that improvement through training continues over many weeks to asymptotically approach an optimal threshold.) Usually on the next day, training continued at first with the old stimulus orientation (last data point to the left of thin vertical line). Thereafter, the stimulus was rotated by 90° so that the group

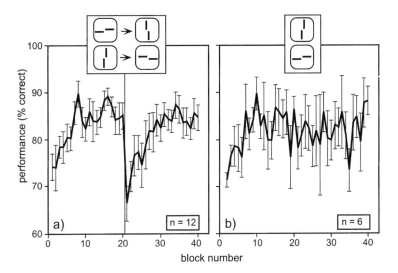

Figure 11.8
Improvement through training in a vernier discrimination task. (*Left*) Mean number of correct responses by twelve observers increased over the training period of twenty blocks with constant stimulus orientation, but improvement did not transfer to the new orientation when the stimulus was rotated by 90°. (*Right*) For six control observers, stimulus orientation was constant, and no drop in their performance occurred. (After Poggio, Fahle, and Edelman 1992.) Vertical bars indicate standard errors of means.

who had trained with horizontal stimulus orientation now saw vertical stimuli, and vice versa.

Although there were large interindividual differences, mean performance of all observers fell off sharply at the time of stimulus rotation. Initial performance for the new orientation was even below the baseline level of the same observers at the start of the experiment, that is, for the first orientation. During the following hour, average performance of all observers improved steadily, especially during the first half hour, up to the level obtained for the first orientation. For a control group of another six observers, stimulus orientation remained constant throughout the experiment (figure 11.8, panel b). There was no dip in performance for this group of observers.

This result clearly indicates that the improvement in vernier discrimination obtained through training is specific for stimulus orientation, at least for the relatively fast component of perceptual learning that takes place within the first half hour or so of training. To assess whether this orientation specificity is due to some form of fast switching processes or whether it also occurs for long-term learning, we performed a similar experiment with another group of twelve observers.

In this control experiment, discrimination thresholds, defined as the offset size yielding 75% correct responses, were measured rather than percentages of correct responses as in the previous experiment. The results are plotted in figure 11.9 and show that this group of twelve unexperienced observers yielded

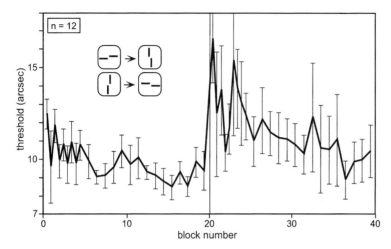

Figure 11.9
Orientation specificity of perceptual learning with vernier stimuli. Average thresholds of twelve observers improved over the five-hour period of learning, but increased sharply when the stimulus was rotated by 90°. (After Fahle and Edelman 1993.) Vertical bars indicate standard errors.

thresholds around 13 arc sec initially, roughly corresponding to one-third of a foveal photoreceptor diameter. Again, six observers initially trained with horizontal stimulus orientation, whereas the remaining six started with vertical orientation of the stimulus. Training continued in one-hour sessions usually on subsequent days, for five hours altogether. Thereafter, stimuli were rotated by 90°, as in the first experiment. As a result, thresholds rose dramatically, to more than 15 arc sec. Thus the rebound overshoots: initial performance for the second stimulus orientation is clearly inferior to that for naive observers as tested with the first orientation. In other words, training a vernier discrimination with a stimulus in one orientation improves performance for that orientation, while clearly impairing performance for stimuli at right angles to that orientation.

Over the next five hours of training, observers gradually improved performance and finally obtained levels of performance comparable to the final levels

reached with the first orientation. Thus we can establish that improvement of performance in a vernier discrimination task is highly specific for stimulus orientation and that both the fast and the slow phase of learning are specific for the orientation of the vernier stimulus, as is the case for grating stimuli (cf. chapters 9, 10).

11.6   Position and Eye Specificity of Perceptual Learning

In the next experiment, we tested whether improvement in the vernier discrimination task achieved at one visual field position would transfer to another visual field position. Another group of eight naive observers performed a vernier discrimination task at 10° eccentricity (figure 11.10). The eight positions to be tested were arranged, at constant distances from one another, on an imaginary

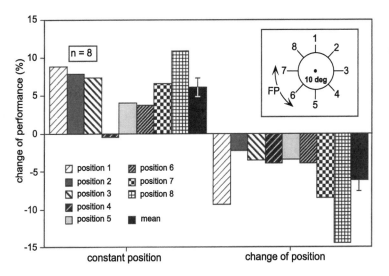

Figure 11.10
Improvement in mean performance through training at eight different positions in the visual field for eight observers. (*Left*) Mean improvement at each of the visual field positions; (*right*) decrease of performance at transition from one position to the next. (After Fahle, Edelman, and Poggio 1995.) FP, fixation point. Vertical bars indicate standard errors of means.

circle around the fovea with a radius of 10°. The sequence of testing these positions was counterbalanced between observers. Within the one-hour sessions spent with each visual field position, observers improved their performance on average by about 6–7% (upward columns in figure 11.10). When, however, they moved their gaze to the new position, there was a significant falloff in performance (downward columns) that matched in size the improvement obtained at the previous position. Which is to say, observers, on average, started learning completely anew at each visual field position. In contrast to the results on orientation specificity, there was no overshoot, that is, performance deteriorated, but just to the baseline, not below it. Thus we can safely conclude that perceptual learning is specific for visual field position, at least if the positions are more than 5° apart (Fahle, Edelman, and Poggio 1995; cf., however, Beard, Levi, and Reich, 1995).

The next question was whether the specificity of perceptual learning would also be true for the eye used during training. To answer this question, we tested another group of twelve naive observers regarding eye specificity on a vernier discrimination task: six observers started with the left eye patched; the remaining six, with the right eye patched. Performance increased fastly during the first 20 minutes of training, corresponding to the first six to eight blocks of stimulus presentations, and more slowly thereafter (figure 11.11). The last block of presentations to the eye trained first, taking place usually after one night's rest, yielded the best performance, indicated by the last data point before the vertical line that symbolizes transition between presentations to the two eyes. After the transition, performance fell off sharply, but the rebound was faster than in the case of orientation change. The data indicate a certain specificity for the eye used during training,

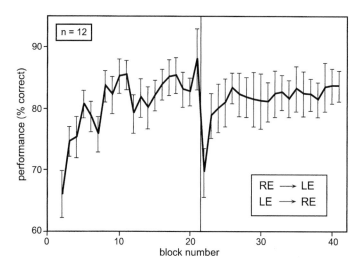

Figure 11.11
Monocular training of a vernier discrimination task in twelve observers leads to improvement in mean performance followed by a moderate drop of performance when the other eye is used for testing (vertical dividing line corresponds to time of transition between eyes). (After Fahle, Edelman, and Poggio 1995.) RE, right eye; LE, left eye. Vertical bars indicate standard errors of means.

but are not completely convincing in this respect, because the falloff in performance is pronounced for only one datapoint (cf., however, chapters 5.3, 9.5, 14.3.1).

We therefore repeated this experiment with a new group of six observers, measuring thresholds during five hours of training. Initial performance in this group of observers was around 16 arc sec, improving to around 10 arc sec within the training period. At the transition from testing one eye to the other, thresholds increased sharply, again to values above the initial level. This increase was again less pronounced than in the case of changing orientation, but nevertheless highly significant (figure 11.12). Obviously, observers had to relearn the task of vernier discrimination when the trained eye was covered and they had to perform the discrimination with the eye covered during training. After another five hours of training, performance in the second eye

was about as good as it was in the first eye at the end of training (cf. chapter 10.3.4).

11.7 Possible Cortical Localization of the Neuronal Changes Underlying Perceptual Learning

Thus far, we found that the improvement in vernier discrimination achieved through training is highly significant for the orientation of the stimulus, for its position in the visual field, and for the eye used during training. This combined specificity allows us to hypothesize about a possible localization, in the visual system, of the neuronal changes underlying the improvement in perceptual discrimination. Hubel and Wiesel have shown (1959) that the majority of neurons in the primary visual cortex (area 17, or V1) of the cat and monkey have elongated

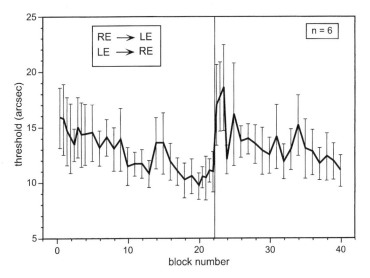

Figure 11.12
Monocular thresholds for vernier discrimination improve over a five-hour period in six observers. Continuation of testing with the other eye leads to an overshooting increase of thresholds, followed by a gradual relearning. RE, right eye; LE, left eye. Vertical bars indicate standard errors of means.

receptive fields of the type displayed in figure 11.7. On the other hand, ganglion cells in the retina and neurons in the lateral geniculate nucleus, that is, in the structures peripheral to the primary visual cortex, have circular symmetric receptive field characteristics. Because neurons on levels below the visual cortex cannot discriminate between different orientations, given the somewhat unstable visual fixation of humans, it would be difficult to realize an improvement of performance specific for stimulus orientation by modifying these neurons. Because they would be activated by all possible stimulus orientations, changing the properties of neurons coding for one stimulus orientation would tend to influence the processing of all other stimuli projected on these neurons. And because we certainly would expect use-dependent long-term changes in the primary visual cortex before postulating them for the human retina, ganglion cells and cells in the lateral geniculate body are even less probable candidates for adult plasticity than the primary visual cortex is (cf. chapter 1.6.1).

On the other hand, the primary visual cortex seems to be the last structure—in the course of visual information processing—where information coming from the two eyes is separated, namely, within the so-called ocular dominance columns, first described by Hubel and Wiesel (1968). Though binocularly activated in all extrastriate areas, many cortical neurons are monocularly activated in the primary visual cortex. Thus the eye specificity of vernier learning indicates that the learning takes place in the primary visual cortex, which seems able to improve function through training even in adults, contrary to the view of a "hardwired" primary cortex cited above (cf. chapter 10.3.4, but see Mollon and Danilova 1996 for another view). This hypothesis of adult cortical plasticity is in agreement with recent electrophysio-

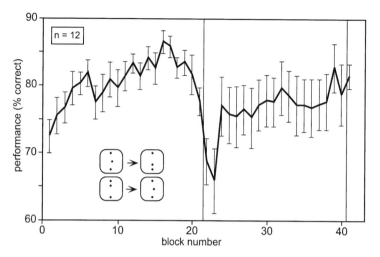

Figure 11.13
Improvement of performance (percent correct responses) through training in a three-dot bisection and a three-dot vernier task. Six observers started with the bisection task; six others with the vernier task. Average percentages of correct responses improved for both groups of observers in the first task, but there was no transfer of improvement to the second task (results right of vertical dividing line). Rightmost data point shows results for retest of the first task. The insets show the differences between stimuli of the two tasks. (After Fahle and Morgan 1996.) Standard errors (vertical bars) were somewhat larger for the second task, indicating larger interindividual differences. Actual displacements of the central dots were far smaller than shown here.

logical (chapters 2–4, 6–7) and anatomical results (chapter 1).

11.8 Possible Motor Artifacts in Perceptual Learning

But is all this improvement really due to sensory learning, rather than to improvement of some motor component? One could argue that observers learn, during the course of the experiment, to improve fixation or accommodation of the stimuli on the monitor, or both. According to this argument, the falloff in performance observed after the change of stimulus would be caused by a loss of applicability for a motor ability learned during the first part of the experiment, for example, fixation would have to be

relearned for a changed stimulus orientation. To test this possibility, we performed an experiment with two extremely similar stimuli: a three-dot vernier task and a three-dot bisection task (see inset of figure 11.13). Six new observers performed a three-dot vernier task, indicating whether the middle of three points was offset to the right or to the left relative to an imaginary line through the endpoints. The other six observers performed a three-dot bisection task, indicating whether the middle point (which was perfectly aligned on the imaginary line between the endpoints) was closer to the upper or to the lower dot.

Thresholds in these tasks were usually around 20 arc sec, corresponding to half a foveal photoreceptor diameter. In the vernier tasks, the middle dot was offset by half a receptor diameter to the right or left, whereas in the bisection task, it was offset by half a photoreceptor diameter toward the upper or lower dot. The two bisection stimuli differed from each other by more than they differed from either of the two vernier stimuli (see inset of figure 11.13). Moreover, the vernier stimulus offset to one side was more similar to both bisection stimuli (regarding Euclidean distance) than to the opposite vernier stimulus. Thus the physical stimuli in the two types of tasks were physically very similar indeed, and any motor adaptation to one type of task should certainly also apply to the other type of task. Observers' performance showed highly significant improvement during the one-hour training, falling off slightly for the retest of the old task on the second day. The transition to the new task was marked by a sharp falloff in performance, once again below baseline level, which gradually improved afterward through training on the new task. At the end of the experiment, we retested observers on the first task. The result is indicated by the rightmost data point in figure 11.13, showing that performance did not fall off when returning to the first task.

This experiment has two important implications: (1) improvement of vernier detection is indeed based on sensory rather than motor factors; (2) training on the second task does not interfere with performance on the first, ruling out a possible neuronal mechanism to explain perceptual learning. One may have supposed that, through training, a pool of neurons is recruited for the task trained, at the expense of other tasks or other preferred stimulus orientations. This hypothesis would predict that by training vertical verniers, more cells would be devoted to analyzing these vertical stimuli, at the expense of the cell pool analyzing horizontal stimuli. Such a mechanism would explain the undershoot of performance at the time of change in task or orientation. There would be fewer neurons available for the task or orientation

not trained than available at the start of the experiment. But such a mechanism, if implemented, would cause a sharp falloff in performance when the first task or orientation was retested after the second one had been learned. Because this is not what we found when we tested different tasks or different orientations, another neuronal mechanism must underlie perceptual learning.

11.9 Perceptual Learning in Amnesic Patients

If perceptual learning at least partly relies on changes at an early level of visual information processing, without much cognitive involvement, then even amnesic patients might be able to improve performance through perceptual learning. To test this possibility, we examined six patients suffering from organic amnesia due either to Korsakoff syndrome or to ischemic damage to the anterior thalamus (Fahle and Daum in press). Because it was far more difficult to explain the task to these observers, only five blocks of eighty vernier presentations each could be measured within each one-hour session. And because the two sessions were separated by a gap of one week, the patients had completely forgotten about the setup, the task, and the experimenter after the one week interval. Nevertheless, three of the patients showed clear improvement in performance through training, two of them even highly significant improvement (figure 11.14). Improvement was less clear in one additional patient, whereas there was no improvement in the remaining two patients. Although it comes as no suprise that the interobserver differences in these patients were even larger than the already high variation in normal observers, a clear message of this experiment is that even patients suffering from severe amnesia, with no recollection of having performed the task previously, can strongly

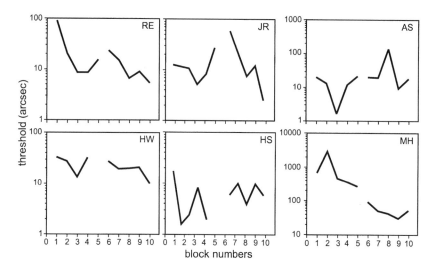

Figure 11.14
Vernier discrimination thresholds as a function of training in six patients (R. E., J. R., A. S., H. W., H. S., M. H.) suffering from amnesic syndromes. At least some of these patients (R. E., M. H., J. R., H. W.) improved performance. (After Fahle and Daum in press.)

improve their vernier discrimination through training of the task.

11.10 A Sum-Potential Correlate of Perceptual Learning

The hypothesis that perceptual learning involves relatively early parts of the visual cortex also suggests that the potentials evoked over the occipital cortex might change as a result of perceptual learning. To test this possibility in an electrophysiological experiment, we presented five verniers, each consisting of three elements that were first perfectly aligned, but whose middle segments were displaced slightly to one side at a defined time. The appearance of the offsets evoked cortical potentials especially over the occipital pole of the brain; we recorded these evoked potentials by an array of sixteen electrodes (see Fahle and Skrandies 1994). To increase the attention of

the observers, we asked them to silently count the number of presentations with verniers offset to the left during part of the experiments. These offsets represented a clear minority, with the large majority of presentations displaying offsets to the right. The potentials were averaged over six hundred presentations and subsequently analyzed.

The latency of the main component of the evoked response in ten observers decreased by around 10 msec, from 118 to 105 msec over the course of the learning. Subsequently, the stimuli were rotated by 90°. Latencies for this orientation were around 125 msec after the transition, decreasing to around 114 msec over half an hour of training. The combined effect was significant on the 5% level.

We statistically compared the distributions of potentials over the occipital pole for the first versus second 600 presentations of the stimulus. The differences between pre- and posttraining distributions

First presentations

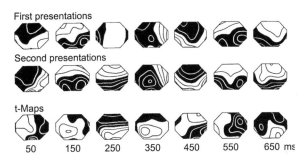

Second presentations

t-Maps

50   150   250   350   450   550   650 ms

Figure 11.15
Potentials evoked by introduction of a vernier offset in five parallel vertical vernier targets. (*Top row*) Potential distributions for the first block of 600 stimulus presentations at 50 msec, 150 msec, and so on after offset introduction. The eyes are located above the upper pole of each head, the occipital pole at the lower end. (*Middle row*) Potential distributions for the second block. (*Bottom row*) T-maps (statistical comparisons) of the first and second block of presentations. (After Fahle and Skrandies 1994.)

for early potentials, that is, short latencies around 50 msec after the transition between the stimuli (figure 11.15), were highly significant: they were localized predominantly over the occipital pole and were most likely produced by the primary visual cortex. Other significant potential differences occurred around 250 msec after stimulation, localized much farther frontally. Overall, the pre- versus posttraining potential distributions differed significantly on the 5% level for 223 of the 512 time slots compared (Fahle and Skrandies 1994). Thus the recordings of sum potentials over the occipital pole in normal observers yield results that correspond well with our hypothesis that perceptual learning partly relies on changes in the primary visual cortex. This electrophysiological correlate of perceptual learning is another indication of plasticity in adult primary visual cortex (area V1) in humans, well in line with animal studies (chapters 1–3).

These sum potential results also agree well with the training-induced changes found in recent single-

cell recordings in the visual cortex of cat and monkey, for example, by Gilbert and Wiesel (1992) and by Eysel (chapter 3, this volume).

11.11   Perceptual Learning Is Not Due to Sharpening of Early Orientation-Specific Filters

As mentioned in 11.4, a possible explanation for the improvement of performance in a vernier discrimination task as a result of training would be that the receptive fields of neurons in the primary visual cortex sharpen (decrease the width of) their excitatory central region. This sharpening would lead to a better signal-to-noise ratio and hence to a better performance in vernier discriminations. Unfortunately, there are a number of findings that are not easily reconciled with this simple and straightforward explanation. Starting from the finding that the improvement obtained through training does not transfer to a stimulus rotated by 90°, we stepwise decreased the amount of stimulus rotation to determine the critical orientation bandwidth. For a first group of observers, we changed the stimulus orientation after one hour from 22.5° clockwise to 22.5° counterclockwise from the vertical, or vice versa, which resulted in a sharp falloff in performance. For the next group of six observers, we changed the orientation from 10° clockwise to 10° counterclockwise from the vertical, or vice versa, which resulted in only a moderate falloff in performance. Changing the orientation from 5° clockwise to 5° counterclockwise from the vertical, or vice versa, in a new group of observers, again resulted in a sharp falloff in performance. Only when the difference between orientations was as small as 2° or 4°, did the improvement caused by learning transfer completely from one orientation to the other. Figure 11.16 indicates the orientation bandwidth of perceptual

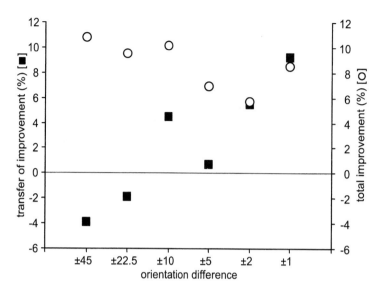

Figure 11.16
Orientation bandwith of perceptual learning. Change in stimulus orientation for different groups of observers, from 90°
down to 2°, plotted along abscissa; resulting amount of transfer of improvement (squares) and improvement obtained with
the first stimulus orientation (circles), plotted along ordinate.

learning by plotting the differences in start levels for
the first versus second stimulus orientations, plus the
improvement of performance during training with
the first orientation. Complete transfer has been
achieved only if the difference between the start levels
equals the improvement obtained at the first level.

These findings indicate that orientation specificity
of perceptual learning is on the order of less than
10°, probably around 5°. Which is to say, the neuronal mechanisms underlying perceptual learning
must have a half-width that is even lower. This high
specificity for orientation contrasts quite sharply with
the orientation specificities of single neurons in the
primary visual cortex of, for example, monkeys. De
Valois, Yund, and Hepler (1982) found the half-
width of single neurons to have a median around 20°
(with a few cells showing bandwidths of only 3°
half-width). Adaptation and masking studies in hu-

man observers yielded similar values (e.g., Campbell
and Kulikowski 1966; Movshon and Blakemore
1973). Because the orientation specificity of perceptual learning is thus far more pronounced than that
of single neurons or neuronal populations as measured by adaptation techniques, it is probably not the
receptive field of primary visual cortex neurons that
is modified as a result of perceptual learning, and we
have to dismiss the speculative explanation put forward in 11.4.

Another argument against the hypothesis of adapting early filters comes from a study investigating
transfer between three hyperacuity tasks, namely
vernier discrimination, orientation discrimination,
and curvature detection. Eighteen observers were
sequentially trained on each of these three hyperacuity tasks for one hour in counterbalanced order.
The results, as shown in figure 11.17, panel b, show

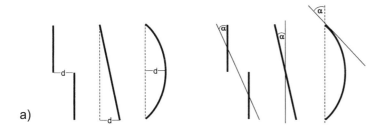

a)

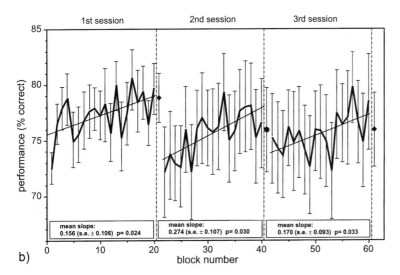

b)

Figure 11.17
Training of three hyperacuity tasks: vernier (*left*), orientation (*middle*), and curvature (*right*) discrimination. The six groups of observers trained these tasks in counterbalanced order, without indication of transfer between the tasks (at the times indicated by vertical dividing lines). (*a*) Orientation cues inherent in the three types of stimuli; (*b*) mean performances and standard errors of all observers for the three tasks in chronological order. (After Fahle 1997.)

a clear improvement of performance during the first session. In each of the sessions, the same number of observers were trained on each of the three hyperacuity tasks. The first measurement on the second day of testing (nearest point to the right of the dotted vertical line) proved that there was no change of performance during the night. When subsequently the next hyperacuity task was tested, performance fell off to pretraining levels, improving gradually during the one-hour training phase of the second task. Basically, the same was true for the transition to the third task. Perceptual learning thus displays a high specifity for the exact type of hyperacuity task. If, on the other hand, perceptual learning sharpened the tuning characteristics of the early orientation selective filters, such as simple cells in the primary visual cortex, then, because all three hyperacuity tasks can be solved by using orientation information, we would have expected some form of transfer of improvement (see figure 11.17, panel a).

11.12   Perceptual Learning Is Based Partly on Top-Down Influences: Feedback

We have seen that a simple, straightforward assumption regarding the neuronal mechanisms underlying perceptual improvement through learning and training cannot be true. Moreover, important theoretical considerations would contradict the assumption of early filter adaptation. If these early filters were indeed permanently modified as a result of training, then these modifications would influence the future processing of all previously learned visual patterns, which in turn might be detrimental for the detection of those earlier patterns. To avoid massive cross-interference between the processing of different patterns, the visual system should keep the early filters constant, as was already clearly stated by Marr (1982). How, then, can perceptual learning be so highly stimulus specific? How can it indicate a neuronal site at a relatively early level of visual information processing—being specific even for the eye used during training—yet avoid modifying the early orientation-specific filtering mechanisms?

The only resolution to this dilemma, in my opinion, is to suppose the influence of strong feedback signals stemming from higher levels of visual information processing and acting on the primary visual cortex (see Herzog and Fahle 1997 and chapter 20, this volume). We performed a number of experiments to determine whether higher cortical levels actually influence perceptual learning. The first class of experiments concerned error feedback. Although it had been shown previously (McKee and Westheimer 1978; Fendick and Westheimer 1983) that improvement through training in hyperacuity tasks is

possible even without error feedback, these experiments employed stimuli well above discrimination threshold. Thus some form of backpropagation may have taken place, that is, correct perception of some of the clearly identifiable stimuli may have been used to identify less clear presentations. We therefore performed an experiment with vernier offsets of only 10 arc sec, below the perceptual thresholds of most observers. As can be seen from figure 11.18, the initial level of performance was around 60% correct responses, not far above the chance level of 50%. The six observers who received error feedback (panel b) improved rapidly, within less than ten blocks, and slowly thereafter. But observers not receiving error feedback were also able to improve performance, even if more slowly than the ones receiving feedback (panel a) (cf. chapter 13.3). At the end of the one-hour training period, both groups of observers yielded about the same level of correct responses. Thus it seems that perceptual learning is indeed possible without feedback, even close to threshold, but that feedback increases the speed of learning.

How might feedback signals achieve this speeding up of perceptual learning? One straightforward hypothesis is that feedback acts as a teacher, helping in the classification of each vernier as offset to the right or to the left by providing observers all the information they need to correctly classify—after the response—the vernier's offset direction. In the next experiment, we therefore omitted half the error signals, that is, half the stimulus presentations incorrectly identified by the observer did not receive error feedback. Thus these stimuli would not only be incorrectly classified at first, but this incorrect classification would be confirmed because the lack of error feedback would indicate a correct classification. Any learning strategy based on a teacher signal would suffer from severe misclassifications of the

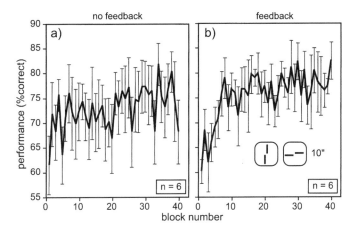

Figure 11.18
Effect of training with subthreshold vernier stimuli, plotted as mean performances of six observers. (*a*) Without error feedback; (*b*) with error feedback. Performance improves significantly under both conditions. (After Fahle, Edelman, and Poggio 1995.) Vertical bars indicate standard errors of means.

stimuli under such a regime of error feedback, leading to a much slower learning speed or even to a lack of perceptual learning through training. But as can be seen in figure 11.19, the number of correct responses as a function of training in this new group of six naive observers increases by about the same amount as it did with error feedback, generating some doubts that a system relying on a teacher signal underlies perceptual learning.

In our next experiment, feedback was even sparser. There was no immediate error feedback at all, but after each block of 80 presentations, observers were informed about the percentage of correct responses they had attained for the entire block. Surprisingly, they improved quite vigorously through training with this type of feedback, even though they had certainly received no teacher signal that told them to which class any individual vernier presentation belonged.

Thus perhaps feedback does not matter in perceptual learning after all. If it does not, uncorrelated

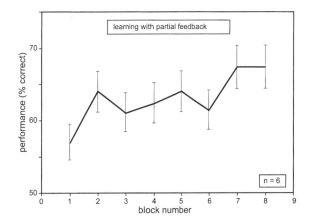

Figure 11.19
Perceptual learning with partial feedback, where half of the error messages were omitted, plotted as mean performances of six observers over time. Whereas a mechanism based an a teacher signal would suffer badly, improvement through training is quite robust under this condition. (After Herzog and Fahle 1997.) Vertical bars indicate standard errors of means.

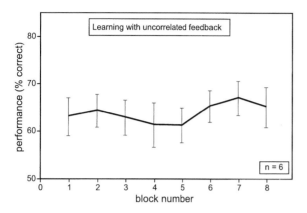

Figure 11.20
Perceptual learning with uncorrelated feedback, plotted as mean performances of six observers. On average, no improvement of performance was achieved under this condition. (After Herzog and Fahle 1997.) Vertical bars indicate standard errors of means.

feedback should not impair performance either. Therefore, in the next experiment, another group of observers received completely uncorrelated feedback, that is, error feedback was given completely randomly, without any correlation to the correctness of the observers' responses. As is evident from figure 11.20, this regime abolishes any significant improvement. Observers are unable to increase the amount of correct responses through training, even when the uncorrelated feedback is given in the block condition. Uncorrelated *block* feedback means that the score given to the observers after each block of eighty presentations was uncorrelated to their actual performance. We used a false number of 62 ± 3; thus observers lived under the impression that their performance varied between 59% and 65% correct, irrespective of their actual level of performance. This manipulated block feedback completley abolished improvement through training, with results very similar to the ones shown in figure 11.20.

In summary, our experimental findings show that feedback does indeed have a strong influence on perceptual learning: it may completely disrupt improvement if given in an uncorrelated way, or else it may increase the speed of improvement if given in a consistent way. This effect of feedback indicates an influence from higher cortical levels, where error feedback is evaluated, on the early sensory cortices where neurons have stimulus specificity. Thus perceptual learning involves cortical processing both at a more cognitive level and probably also at a quite early level of the visual cortex. (See also Rubin et al., chapter 13. For a more detailed account of the possible computational mechanisms of perceptual learning, see Herzog and Fahle, chapter 20, and Ahissar and Hochstein, chapter 14, both this volume.)

11.13 Another Top-Down Influence: Attention

A last experiment tested another form of top-down influence on perceptual learning, namely, visual attention. In this experiment, two vernier stimuli were presented simultaneously, one oriented vertically and the other horizontally. The eight observers were separated into two groups, the first of which started by responding to the offset of the vertical vernier, indicated by solid bars in figure 11.21. The second group started by attending and responding to the horizontal vernier. Physically, the stimuli for both groups were identical, only the instruction to the observers differed. Performance improved through training, first rapidly and then more slowly during the one-hour period of training.

In the second part of the experiment, unlike in all our previous experiments, we did not change the stimulus, but only the instructions to the observers. Observers were now required only to attend and

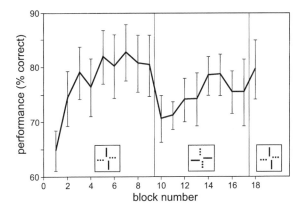

Figure 11.21
Influence of attention on perceptual learning with a stimulus containing two orthogonal vernier stimuli, plotted as mean performances of eight observers. (After Weiss, Edelman, and Fahle 1993.) For the first eight blocks, the vertical stimulus was attended to, then the horizontal one, or vice versa. Switching attention without changing the stimulus led to a drop in performance. Vertical bars indicate standard errors of means.

respond in the second part of the experiment to the vernier oriented 90° to the one they had responded to during the first part of the experiment, with the same number of presentations of verniers in the new orientation they had experienced in the old orientation. Following this change of instruction, the falloff in performance was pronounced and highly significant although the stimuli were constant. Observers had to relearn the second orientation as they had with a physical change of stimulus orientation. The experiment thus shows that mere exposure to a stimulus, if the stimulus is not attended to, does not lead to a distinct improvement of performance for this stimulus. If perceptual learning were a pure exposure-dependent type of process, mere exposure to a stimulus would be sufficient. But clearly, this is not the case: improvement through training—learning—is not due just to sharpening of orientation-

sensitive units (which can be performed automatically), but has to incorporate top-down influences.

11.14 Conclusions

Hyperacuity is a highly sensitive measure of visual performance, yielding thresholds that are far below the diameter and spacing of foveal photoreceptors. It is made possible by the limited optical resolution of the eye and by appropriate cortical mechanisms that are able to extract the information present in the retina in implicit form only. We find two phases of hyperacuity learning, a fast one that takes place in about twenty minutes or less, and a slower one that continues over five and more hours, possibly over months. The improvement through training is very specific for relatively basic features of the stimulus such as orientation, the position in the visual field, the exact type of task trained, and even for the eye that was used during training. This stimulus specificity strongly supports the hypothesis that neuronal mechanisms involved in perceptual learning operate at a relatively early level in the visual system. In accordance with this hypothesis, even amnesic patients improve performance through training; at least some patients yield significantly better results after training even though they cannot remember having ever performed the task. Also in accordance with this hypothesis, perceptual learning has a correlate in visual evoked potentials, especially over the occipital pole and for rather short latencies. Moreover, animals studies suggest that the adult primary visual cortex shows more plasticity than was hitherto believed. Thus we can assume that perceptual learning involves changes in neuronal connectivity taking place as early as the first levels of cortical visual information processing. These changes cannot rely (exclusively) on sharpening orientation-selective early filters. Several experiments and theoretical considerations indicate that the changes have to be governed by top-down influences from higher cortical areas, and that error feedback and visual selective attention play important roles. The exact neuronal mechanisms underlying perceptual learning and its possible role not only in learning new tasks in normal observers, but also in recovery of function after brain lesions remain to be investigated.

Specificity versus Invariance of Perceptual Learning: The Example of Position

12

Marcus Dill

Abstract

Many studies on perception have found learning to be specific to the stimulus position in the visual field. In summarizing a variety of findings, this chapter explains why some perceptual learning phenomena are position invariant, whereas others are not. Although the positional specificity of learning suggests that early stages of the visual pathways may be involved in perceptual learning, the lack of position invariance may also come from complex decision processes on higher levels of processing. Perceptual learning at different locations may be an important prerequisite for the position invariance of visual pattern recognition.

A consistently reproduced characteristic of perceptual learning is its specificity to the experimental conditions and to the stimuli employed during training. These findings have been discussed in detail in chapters 9 and 11 of this volume. I will focus on the role of stimulus position in the visual field. After discussing why transfer of learning to new spatial locations has been widely used to identify both the processing and the anatomical levels of perceptual learning, I will summarize what experimental results tell us about the locus of plasticity—and what they do not. Finally, I will relate positional specificity of perceptual learning to position invariance of visual pattern recognition.

12.1   Organization of Visual Field and Retinal Image

One of the fundamental concepts of human spatial vision is the *visual field*, roughly defined as that part of the surrounding space actually seen at each moment in time. Locations and distances within the visual field are generally given in angular degrees with the zero reference of the coordinate system being defined as the line of sight. In normal human adults, the visual field covers only about one-third of the overall space (about $\pm 60°$ in the vertical and slightly more in the horizontal direction). Many researchers divide the visual field into four quadrants separated by the vertical and horizontal meridians, respectively (figure 12.1).

The optical apparatus of the eye transforms incoming visual data to ensure that every sensory receptor in the human retina is stimulated only by light from a particular direction of the visual field. Neighboring receptors receive inputs from adjacent sections of the visual field. The center of the visual field is always viewed by receptors in the fovea, that is, the retinal area with highest receptor density and best spatial resolution. Stimuli farther away from the line of sight are said to be "parafoveal" if located less than about 5° away from the fovea and "peripheral" if located 5° or farther away. Each receptor is responsible for light detection at a very specific location within only a small fraction of the visual field.

Likewise, in most visual areas of the brain, a cell is responsive to stimulation in only one part of the visual field, an area called the cell's "receptive field." According to a characteristic of the visual system known as "retinotopy," the spatial order of the visual field is preserved at least to some extent throughout the system: neighboring sections of the retinal image are represented by neighboring cells and cell groups

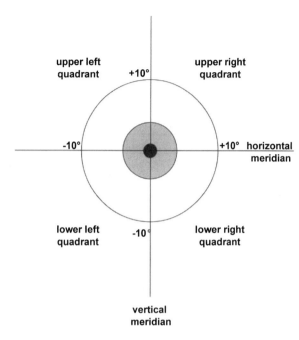

Figure 12.1
Schematic drawing of the central portion of the visual field. Vision is sharpest in the center of the fovea (symbolized by the black circle), but acuity progressively drops off toward the periphery (gray and white concentric rings). The distance from the fovea is measured in degrees of visual angle.

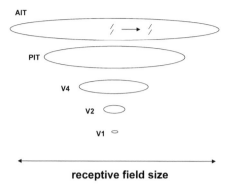

Figure 12.2
Schematic illustration of the correlation between receptive field size and the anatomical level of the visual hierarchy (not drawn to scale). With each level of processing, the mean receptive field size (ellipses) of neurons becomes larger. V1, V2, V4, PIT (posterior inferotemporal) cortex, and AIT (anterior inferotemporal) cortex are areas within the visual pathways of the brain. Many cells in higher areas respond to the same stimulus in ways largely independent of its location within the visual field.

in the visual brain. A functional consequence of this organization is that, depending on the position of a stimulus in the visual field, the image of the stimulus is projected on different parts of the retina and stimulates different cell populations in primary visual cortex (area V1) and higher brain areas.

It is a remarkable ability of the human brain that it can—at least in principle—identify objects regardless of where they are presented in the visual field. Apparently, the brain achieves position invariance of recognition in several steps. With each level of visual processing, the mean size of receptive fields becomes larger and larger (figure 12.2). Cells in the primary

visual cortex (area V1), the major input stage for visual information to the brain, have relatively small receptive field centers of about 1° diameter—at least in the central parts of the visual field. Cells in areas V2 and V4 have progressively larger receptive fields, normally subtending over several degrees of the visual field. Finally, cells in anterior inferotemporal (AIT) cortex often respond to stimuli within 20° or more. Indeed, AIT cells can cover nearly the whole visual field; the anterior inferotemporal cortex is generally considered to be responsible for high-level pattern and object recognition.

12.2 The Rationale of Position Transfer Experiments

The correlation of receptive field size and level of processing offers an elegant way to investigate

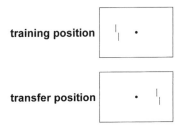

Figure 12.3
Typical position shift experiment. Subjects fixate a special sign on the screen (here a black dot). (*Top*) During training, they are presented stimuli only at a particular location (here left of the fixation mark). (*Bottom*) After successful learning, they are presented stimuli shifted to a new location to test for transfer.

where in the visual processing hierarchy perceptual learning actually occurs: by measuring behavior, one can determine the perceptive field size of the site of plasticity, that is, the spatial extent of perceptual learning. Because cells on higher levels of visual processing have larger receptive fields than cells on lower levels (figure 12.2), testing positional specificity of perceptual learning can suggest whether the site of plasticity is at later or earlier stages of processing, or at both.

Most perceptual learning experiments that test for positional specificity follow the same basic design. Human observers sitting in front of a computer monitor or a projection screen are instructed to continuously fixate on a special fixation mark (e.g., a dot as in figure 12.3). After some time, a stimulus is displayed very shortly at a specific location relative to this fixation spot. If the presentation time is short enough (less than 180 msec), eye movements toward this stimulus cannot be initiated (Saslow 1967). Stimulation is thus restricted to a relatively small area. If one wants to ensure that subjects really follow instructions and do not move their eyes away from the fixation spot, it is possible to control steady

fixation by means of eye-tracking devices. An alternative would be to force subjects to solve a control task at the fixation location, for example, a letter identification test. This procedure, however, can interfere with the perceptual learning task itself, which quite often requires full attention for learning to occur.

During training, the stimulus to be learned is normally presented at only one location relative to the line of sight. Performance improves over minutes, hours, days, or weeks—depending on the specific paradigm. After successful training, stimuli are displayed at a different location (figure 12.3). Theoretically, three different outcomes of such a transfer experiment are possible (figure 12.4). First, performance after position shift may stay on the level acquired during training—as if nothing had changed (bottom panel). This complete transfer to new locations would indicate that the locus of plasticity is on higher levels only, whether visual or in part even nonvisual. Second, at the other extreme, performance may fall back to the base level at the beginning of the training (top panel). Complete positional specificity would indicate that learning predominantly occurs at lower levels or at their output synapses projecting to higher levels. And third, performance may fall off after position shift, with partial transfer compared to the base level (middle panel). Or, alternatively, in an intermediate result not shown, performance may fall back to the base level, but recover quickly so that high performance levels are reached faster than during the previous training period. Thus, in the case of partial transfer, learning may happen at different processing stages at the same time.

Most everyday forms of learning—such as studying vocabulary or getting acquainted with streets and places after moving to a different city—are generally considered to be cognitive processes occurring on higher brain levels, far beyond the sensory areas. For

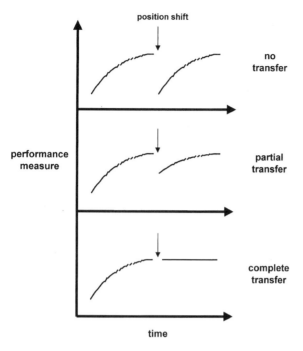

Figure 12.4
Typical results from position shift experiments. In a first training period, performance (measured by some arbitrary value) improves due to perceptual learning. After a predefined time or when reaching a criterion level the position is changed (position shift, indicated by arrow), resulting in no, partial, or complete transfer.

that reason, many researchers investigating stimulus specificity of perceptual learning did not rule out high-level learning, but were only interested to find out whether there was any contribution from position-specific levels at all. They therefore tended to ignore the distinction between partial transfer and no transfer, quite often not comparing performance after position shift with that at a reasonable baseline; transfer tests were often too short to test whether relearning at the new location might be faster indicating partial transfer of the second type.

12.3 Positional Specificity in Perceptual Learning Tasks

12.3.1 Overview

Transfer of learning to new locations in the visual field has been tested for a variety of perceptual tasks (see table 12.1). These experiments differ not only in visual stimuli and tasks—from popout detection to pattern discrimination, from stereopsis to grating classification—but also in several characteristics of the learning process. For example, some of the perceptual learning effects investigated require only a few minutes of training, whereas others require hundreds or even thousands of trials. Similarly, in some experiments, learning manifests itself as a decrease in the error rate; in others, as a decrease in response time—and presumably therefore an increase in the speed of processing.

Many perceptual learning tasks involve abilities that would be considered as relatively basic. To discriminate between line orientations, for example, the visual system does not need much more than a set of orientation-selective feature detectors. Because these detectors are already found in area V1, an involvement of primary visual cortex in perceptual learning in such tasks may not be too surprising. Several of the tasks summarized in table 12.1, however, are clearly more demanding for the system. Pattern discrimination learning, for example, requires much more complex spatial discriminations.

For all these reasons, the perceptual phenomena summarized in table 12.1 have to be considered as representing a group of learning effects rather than a single type of learning. They may rely on quite different mechanisms and cell types in the visual system. With this in mind, it is even more astonishing that nearly all studies consistently found that learning

Table 12.1
Summary of results of various position transfer experiments

Learning paradigm	References	Smallest position shift tested	Transfer (F/P/N)	Notes
Stereopsis	Ramachandran 1976	2.5°	N/P	Some subjects no, others partial transfer.
Stereopsis	O'Toole and Kersten 1992	0.7°	N (P?)	Give no baseline; influence of selective spatial attention?
Popout detection	Ahissar and Hochstein 1996, 1997	0.7°	N/P	Transfer to homologous positions across the midline; correlation of positional specificity and task difficulty.
Vernier discrimination	Fahle 1994; Fahle, Edelman, and Poggio 1995	10°	N	Only with trained observers; unspecific learning with naive observers.
Vernier discrimination	Beard, Levi, and Reich 1995	2°	P	Some transfer along meridians; due to spatial attention?
Texture discrimination	Karni and Sagi 1991	3°	N	
Pattern discrimination	Nazir and O'Regan 1990; Dill and Fahle 1997	1°	N	
Line orientation discrimination	Shiu and Pashler 1992	11°	N	Cognitive influences.
Grating orientation discrimination	Schoups, Vogels, and Orban 1995	2.5°	N (P)	
Classification of Gabor patches	Rentschler, Jüttner, and Caelli 1994; Jüttner and Rentschler 1996	3°	P	Some transfer to homologous positions across the midline.
Motion discrimination	Ball and Sekuler 1987	2°	P	Some transfer even without stimulus overlap.
Spatial phase discrimination	Berardi and Fiorentini 1987	1°	N/P	Transfer to homologous positions across the midline.

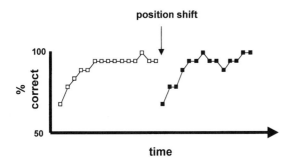

Figure 12.5
Stimulus specificity in grating discrimination learning. After a position shift (arrow), the percentage of correct responses falls back to the base level: a new learning process (filled squares) is started that apparently does not profit from initial training (open squares). Each point represents the percentage of correct responses in twenty consecutive trials. (Data from Berardi and Fiorentini 1987.)

does not—at least not completely—transfer to new locations in the visual field. Let us briefly consider three particularly clear examples.

12.3.2 Examples

Grating patterns are among the most frequently used stimuli in experiments on visual perceptual learning (see Fiorentini and Berardi, chapter 9, this volume). In one study (Berardi and Fiorentini 1987), subjects were trained to discriminate between complex grating patterns composed by superimposing two sinusoidal luminance profiles that differed with respect to the relative spatial phase of the two sinusoids. During the course of the training, observers' accuracy increased until only sporadic errors occurred. If the position of the stimuli relative to the fixation spot was now changed, performance immediately fell back to the base level (figure 12.5). This pattern of results is remarkably similar to the idealized curve in figure 12.4, top panel. Obviously, there is not even

partial transfer of learning across the visual field because performance after translation is not better than at the beginning of the training. The stimuli have to be relearned at the new location without any apparent benefit from the initial training.

Quite similar results—complete positional specificity of improvement—are found in several other paradigms, for example in vernier learning. As described in detail by Fahle (chapter 11, this volume), we can learn to detect tiny offsets of picture elements by extensive training over several hundred trials. This improvement is moderate, but significant, in the center of the visual field, but it is much larger for extrafoveal stimulation because the parafovea and periphery are less trained in everyday life. Fahle and coworkers (Fahle 1994; Fahle, Edelman, and Poggio 1995) trained subjects to improve vernier acuity at eight peripheral positions—one at a time over several days. At each location, subjects were trained for one hour to discriminate between vernier stimuli offset to the left versus to the right. In all sessions, a consistent pattern of results became apparent: the percentage of correct responses improved during training at one location by an average of about 7%, but decreased by the same amount immediately after the position of the stimuli was changed (figure 12.6). At each new location, subjects did not retain any improvement from other locations and had to be retrained from the start. Learning of vernier discrimination thus does not transfer to new locations but must occur at brain levels that retain at least some positional specificity.

Compared to vernier stimuli, random dot patterns such as the ones in figure 12.7 are relatively complex spatial arrangements. Humans are normally not very familiar with this kind of stimulus. When such patterns are presented only very briefly and at extrafoveal locations, most subjects are not able to tell more about the stimuli than that there was a cloud of

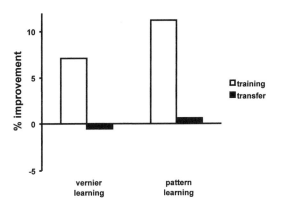

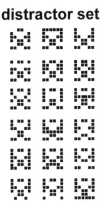

Figure 12.6
Positional specificity in vernier (*left*) and pattern discrimination (*right*) learning. White bars represent the improvement of performance due to perceptual learning. Black bars show the results directly after the position shift compared to base level.

Figure 12.7
Example of target pattern (*top*) and distractor set (*bottom*). Each pattern is bilaterally symmetric and consists of a 6 × 6 matrix of elements that are filled with a large black rectangle at 50% probability. One random pattern is defined as the target; eighteen distractors are created by changing a single element from black to white or vice versa.

dots. When one of these stimuli is presented to a defined position in the visual field and subjects have to decide whether a specific pattern—the target pattern—or one of several distractor patterns has appeared, their responses are highly erroneous at the beginning of the experiment. Subjects thus have difficulty discriminating novel dot patterns, but can learn to do so in training experiments.

In a typical experiment (Nazir and O'Regan 1990; Dill and Fahle 1997), performance improves within a few hundred trials, depending on the complexity of the stimuli and on other experimental conditions. When subjects eventually reach a criterion level of, say, 90% correct responses, training stops and they are tested at either the training or a transfer location. As shown in figure 12.6, performance at the transfer location falls off significantly compared to the training location, with accuracy at the new location no better than the base level at the beginning of the training. Pattern discrimination learning is thus completely specific to the location of training, as was

grating and vernier learning (see also section 12.5, where pattern discrimination learning is discussed in greater detail and these experiments related to how invariance of pattern recognition to retinal translations is achieved).

12.3.3 Exceptions

Task Difficulty
Although most studies found no transfer or only partial transfer to new locations, there are a few noteworthy exceptions. For example, Ahissar and Hochstein (1997) showed that task difficulty can be one factor influencing the degree to which learning is position specific. Simply stated, learning an easy

task transfers to new locations, whereas learning a more difficult task does not. Obviously, lower levels of processing get involved as soon as the task is too difficult to be solved completely by higher levels. It has been suggested (Ahissar and Hochstein 1997) that learning follows the visual processing hierarchy in a reverse direction: first, units on higher levels are selected that best solve the experimental task; then, if these units are not sufficient to achieve reliable performance, they recruit additional resources from lower levels. However, the trade-off for further improvement of performance from the participation of extra capacities is a lack of transfer to new locations.

Selective Spatial Attention

A second factor assumed to influence the degree of positional specificity is selective spatial attention: focusing attention on a particular location in the visual field can improve performance in visual tasks within a delimited window of attention while diminishing perceptual abilities in other areas of visual space. This well-established phenomenon, selective spatial attention, has been described in many classical studies. The ability to detect a stimulus increases significantly when the location of this stimulus is indicated beforehand by a position cue preceding the stimulus. On the other hand, in trials with an invalid position cue—one that misleads attention to a wrong location—subjects' ability to detect the stimulus is even lower than with no or neutral cues.

Interestingly, Moran and Desimone (1985)—and since then many others—found electrophysiological correlates for this behavioral phenomenon. Many cells in V4 and other visual areas alter their response behavior in a similar manner. If attention is directed to one visual field location, stimulation of other locations may be without effect, although the stimulus still lies in the classical receptive field of this cell.

Spatial attention can thus lead to positional specificity in both behavioral and physiological performance. Could it be that by training the visual system at just one location it is pushed to attend to this area, while ignoring the remaining parts of the visual field? If this is the case, positional specificity would have to be considered as an attentional artifact rather than as a characteristic of visual learning mechanisms.

O'Toole and Kersten (1992) investigated this possibility with regard to the positional specificity they found for learning stereoscopic depth perception. In their original experiments, they trained subjects at a single location and found reduced performance after transfer to another location. In a control experiment, however, they trained subjects with two patterns at two different locations. For example, pattern A was used only at position 1, whereas, within the same training session, pattern B was trained exclusively at position 2. Later, both patterns were recognized equally well at both locations. These additional results show that the acquired ability to discriminate depths can transfer as long as enough resources are allocated to both locations. Thus positional specificity in this class of experiments can, indeed, be attributed to selective spatial attention rather than to depth perception.

That vernier learning partially transfers along meridians of the visual field (Beard, Levi, and Reich (1995) indicates that the window of attention extends away from the fovea in a clublike fashion. Because, however, the extent of the attentional spotlight has not been assessed independently in this study, it is difficult to decide whether the partial transfer is the consequence of attentional mechanisms or of specializations of visual perception.

If attention plays a role in vernier learning at all, this role may be more general in the sense that observers learn how to attend to stimulation outside of the center of the fovea. Fahle and coworkers (Fahle

1994; Fahle, Edelman, and Poggio 1995), for example, reported that subjects who had never before taken part in psychophysical experiments involving extrafoveal stimulation showed some transfer of learning to other peripheral or parafoveal locations. This unspecific effect can most probably be attributed to learning how to divert attention away from the center of the visual field, where it is normally focused. Once subjects possess this know-how, further improvement of performance remains specific to the location of training.

For most of the perceptual learning paradigms, there are good arguments against an artifactual influence of selective attention. As mentioned above, some studies tested transfer over less than 1° displacement and found complete positional specificity. Experiments testing the minimal size of the window of spatial attention, on the other hand, have shown that observers cannot split attention between stimuli that lie within 1° of the visual field. Thus, at least in some cases, selective spatial attention can be excluded. Besides, there is no electrophysiological evidence to date that the modification of the receptive field by spatial attention is permanent. One might also expect that this tuning of high-level elements would deprive other spatial positions of processing resources, leading to performance levels even below the starting level after change of the location. There is no evidence, however, for an undershooting effect after spatial displacements: performance after position shift was never worse than at the beginning of training. Most studies seem to prove that learning at different locations is independent even in this respect.

Symmetrical Locations

Finally, a positional "anomaly" for symmetrical locations is worth noting. At least three studies (Berardi and Fiorentini 1987; Rentschner, Jüttler, and Caelli 1994; Ahissar and Hochstein 1996) found some transfer or even complete transfer of learning to homologous locations across the vertical midline of the visual field. This special role of symmetrical positions seems not to be attributable to callosal connections between the two hemispheres. Fiorentini et al. (1992) reported the case of a boy born without a corpus callosum who showed the same pattern of transfer as normal subjects: complete transfer to symmetrical locations, but no transfer to other places (cf., however, chapters 9, 10). Besides, a special role of positional symmetry relative to the fovea has also been found for the vertical dimension, that is, for symmetrical positions above and below the center of the fovea (Dill and Fahle 1999). Although the latter experiments did not involve learning, they suggest that the above findings are not the consequence of a special interhemispheric transfer.

12.4 What Positional Specificity Tells Us about the Locus of Plasticity—and What It Does Not

According to the rationale outlined in section 12.2, most authors have concluded that perceptual learning involves not only higher levels of the visual hierarchy, but also lower levels. Combining positional specificity with other results such as the orientation specificity and—in some cases—the monocularity of perceptual learning, some have argued that even the primary visual cortex, the very first visual area of the brain, may show some plasticity.

Although these interpretations may well be justified, when speculating on the locus of learning, one also has to be aware of several critical issues related to these tests for positional specificity. For example, a number of experiments tested transfer only very roughly, that is, stimuli were shifted between whole half-fields or quadrants of the visual field. Positional specificity at this rather coarse spatial grain may well result from higher levels. Despite an overall correlation between brain level and receptive field (RF) size, the variation of RF sizes within each visual area can be rather large. Because, even in area V4 or the posterior inferotemporal cortex, some cells have relatively small RFs of only a few degrees, some positional specificity may also stem from this level of processing.

But what about studies that tested transfer on a very fine spatial scale? As can be seen in table 12.1, many authors found no transfer or only moderate transfer to even very close locations. Learning orientation discrimination at a single location, for example, does not improve performance at a directly adjacent, but nonoverlapping, location (Schoups, Vogels, and Orban 1995). Similarly, Berardi and Fiorentini (1987) and Ahissar and Hochstein (1996, 1997) reported complete positional specificity to the location of training even when they tested transfer over 1° or less. Does not positional specificity on this fine resolution make an involvement of area V1 or other early stages of processing very likely?

Indeed, even though learning may be not just a high-level phenomenon, apparently position-invariant higher levels may produce a remarkable degree of positional specificity depending on the experimental conditions chosen. First, even those cells in area V4 and inferotemporal cortex that show the same stimulus preference over large parts of the visual field often display considerable variation of the overall response strength (figure 12.8). A neuron may respond more strongly when confronted with a triangle, say, than with a star, and this preference for triangles may be independent of the location. The contribution of this cell to the huge concerto of nervous responses in the brain may depend on visual

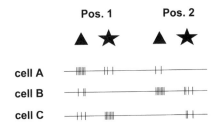

Figure 12.8
Schematic drawing of responses of three fictitious cells that respond both to a triangle and to a star pattern. Although cell responses are not position invariant, their selectivity is. Whereas selectivity, that is, the cell's preference for a triangle or a star, remains the same across different locations, the response strength differs between positions 1 (*left*) and 2 (*right*). The pattern of nervous responses from the whole set of cells, thus depends on visual field location.

field position. At some locations, its response may be so weak that other cells, which may respond to different features of the triangle, may vote down the first cell, with observers not recognizing the pattern where they would have, had its location not changed.

There is yet another possible explanation for positional specificity at more advanced stages of visual processing. Let us consider the pattern discrimination task discussed above (figure 12.9). The target pattern is recognized by a set of brain cells. Given that all distractors were very different from the target so that the cell sets recognizing target and distractors were largely disjunct, responses of a few cells, or even just one, would theoretically be sufficient to decide whether the target or a distractor was presented. On the other hand, when target and distractor stimuli are more similar to each other, the recognizing cell assemblies overlap. To specify whether the target has been seen, the system has to ensure that a larger number of target-detecting cells are responding. Although these cells may have rela-

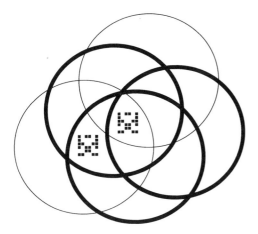

Figure 12.9
Similarity and invariance. Schematic drawing of the receptive fields of five cells around the presentation location of two patterns, showing how the output of "invariant" visual areas can depend on the position. Thick outline indicates cells that are responsive to a given stimulus pattern; thin outline, cells that are not. Depending on the similarity of target and distractor patterns, responses of either a few cells or the whole set of neurons are required for correct decisions.

tively large receptive fields, these fields are not necessarily identical. It is more likely that they overlap only partially. If target and distractor patterns are displaced to a new location, the probability that they will remain within the receptive field of all participating cells is relatively small. Because this probablility decreases with the number of cells actually required for recognition, the more similar (i.e., difficult) the discriminations, the smaller the maximum tolerated position transfer. Or, to phrase it slightly differently, in the completely disjunct case (OR relation), the target could be recognized within an area of visual space that corresponds to the envelope of the receptive fields of all cells specific for the target, whereas, in the more similar case (AND relation), the target could be recognized only within a rela-

tively small area that corresponds to the overlap of the minimum number of required cells. Positional specificity can thus be explained down to very fine resolution without requiring contributions from area V1.

Thus the available evidence on positional specificity by no means contradicts an involvement of lower levels of the visual hierarchy. Depending on the paradigm and experimental conditions, learning may be possible at different or even all stages of processing. Even the very first stages within the visual pathway may be able to learn. However, the final proof for perceptual learning by position-specific cells—for example, in area V1—has yet to be shown.

12.5 Perceptual Learning and Position Invariance

In section 12.4, we have seen how perceptual learning may lead to increased positional specificity. Here we will take a closer look at the possible relations of perceptual learning and position invariance. For that purpose, we will again refer to pattern discrimination learning. Having noted the central result of these experiments, that learning to discriminate random dot patterns is completely specific to the location of training, let us now go deeper into what actually happens in a subject's mind during such an experiment. This more introspective description may give us some understanding as to why perceptual learning is counterproductive for position invariance, and at the same time how it may be used by the brain to achieve translation-tolerant pattern recognition.

As already mentioned, subjects must decide whether a particular target pattern or one of a series of derived patterns (distractors) has been presented. At the beginning of a training session, the target is defined by presenting it ten times to the subjects. Later, the target is shown in half of the trials and a randomly selected distractor pattern in the other half. Each distractor differs from the target by only one element and its mirror-symmetric counterpart, which are changed from black to white or vice versa (see figure 12.7).

Because the presentation time (~150 msec) is too short for scrutinizing the patterns by directed eye movements, subjects at first do not see much more than an undefined cloud of dots. In most trials at the start of the training, observers can only guess, although, in some cases, they may recognize "something" in a particular pattern—much in the same way that we perceive, say, a face or an animal in the clouds. The recognized content may be an association with a familiar object, a simple shape, a characteristic elongated curve, or a particular configuration of dots. Many of these random images resemble human or animal faces, most probably due to their mirror symmetry. If the target looks like a strange monkey face, say, it will be very easy to distinguish it from a distractor whose appearance is not facelike because the "eyes" (two symmetric dots), present in the target, are now absent. In other cases, an isolated black dot surrounded by white fields may be very prominent in the target, so that it is rather easy to note when it is absent in a distractor.

This spontaneous recognition of familiar objects or simple shapes in an apparently novel pattern—let us call it "immediate input interpretation" (III)— helps subjects to identify at least some features, though not the whole stimulus domain, already during the ten presentation trials before the actual training. Quite often, therefore, initial performance is not at chance level, not even during the very first trials. III may allow reasonable, although not always perfect perceptual performance. To achieve a higher level of accuracy in our discrimination task, a learn-

ing process is necessary. During training, subjects refine their internal representation of the patterns step by step: they notice more and more discriminative features of a target (or of distractors), so that their performance improves until, after some time, they consistently give correct responses. Even if feedback is no longer given, accuracy stays at high levels as long as the position of presentation is kept constant.

As we have noted, when pattern location is changed, performance falls back, not to chance, but to the base level subjects reached at the beginning of the training. As at the beginning of the training, subjects after the position shift do not simply guess. Some information regarding the particular stimulus must have been transferred to the new location. That performance after transfer is remarkably similar to initial performance makes it very likely that III is position invariant. Any discrimination ability acquired during the course of training, on the other hand, is apparently specific to the location where it has been learned.

But why should the immediate input interpretation be position invariant, whereas perceptual learning is not? Introspection and common sense support the conclusion that III is position invariant. Because both the facelike appearance of a pattern and the existence of an isolated dot or another striking feature within it are conscious perceptions that can be communicated by subjects, it is reasonable to assume these high-level or even abstract characteristics of dot stimuli are detected independently of their location within the visual field. Subjects do not have to recognize that specific face or isolated dot again. They need only detect "a" face or "a" single dot.

That perceptual learning is position specific can be rationalized by the reverse hierarchy model (Ahissar and Hochstein 1997) mentioned above and explained in detail in chapter 14 of this volume. During the first trials of an experiment, the visual system learns only on higher levels that are invariant but restricted to relatively meaningful input—regular shapes, frequent and important objects, salient features. To refine performance and to make more difficult discriminations, the system has to learn more precisely, which involves information provided by lower levels.

Finally, discrimination learning may simply mean detecting and combining more and more features of a target. As we have seen in section 12.4, the need to consider responses from a large number of feature-detecting cells during the decision process can lead to increased positional specificity, even though individual feature detectors may well be relatively invariant to translation.

Although the question of how the position invariance of our immediate visual perception is achieved cannot be answered on the basis of these experiments, it is tempting to speculate that position-invariant recognition observed in an experiment is actually the result of perceptual learning at some time in the subjects' preexperimental lives. We have probably encountered geometrical structures such as triangles or more complex objects such as faces thousands or even hundreds of thousands of times during our lives. Because this massive and continued perceptual learning did not happen at just one location in the visual field, but most likely at many different locations, we recognize a triangle or a face wherever it is relative to the fovea. How this lifelong perceptual learning proceeds and how it eventually leads cells in the brain to give consistent responses independently of the visual field location remains to be investigated. Are several instances of perceptual learning later associated by some high-level mechanism? Or does training with variable position lead to translation-invariant memory? Clearly, much interesting experimental work remains to be done.

12.6 Conclusions

Positional specificity is an indication for—but no proof of—an involvement of area V1 or other low levels of visual processing in perceptual learning. Simple explanations for positional specificity based on cellular responses at these early stages of processing ignore the fact that vision and decision cannot be separated in learning processes and that a group of cells with largely position-invariant stimulus selectivity may well respond in a highly position-specific manner depending on how individual cell activities are joined to form the whole system's response. Perceptual learning may be a key mechanism in acquiring position-invariant visual recognition. Unfamiliar and complex patterns are not identfied as the same when they are presented to different locations unless they offer prominent features interpretable by high-level analyses. If these features are missing position invariant, recognition may only be achieved after repeated training at variable locations.

Acknowledgment

Marcus Dill was supported by Boehringer Ingelheim Fonds.

Higher-Level Psychophysics

The Role of Insight in Perceptual Learning: Evidence from Illusory Contour Perception

13

Nava Rubin, Ken Nakayama, and Robert Shapley

Abstract

The distinction between gradual and abrupt improvement in performance is commonly made in behavioral studies of learning. The learning of perceptual and motor skills is often characterized by gradual, incremental improvement and is found not to generalize over stimulus manipulations such as change in retinal size or location. In contrast, marked improvement in performance can occur suddenly—a phenomenon that has been termed "insight." Previously, insight has been studied in the context of problem solving and similar cognitive-level tasks. In this chapter, we use an illusory contours shape-discrimination task to present evidence that perceptual learning can exhibit characteristics of insight. Observers exhibited an abrupt, dramatic improvement in their performance, which resembled an incident of insight. At the same time, however, the improvement showed a degree of stimulus specificity that previously was thought to characterize incremental, gradual learning. This juxtaposition of abrupt and stimulus-specific improvement suggests that the dichotomy between the two forms of learning needs to be revised. This idea echoes Hebb (1949), who argued that the insight/incremental-learning dichotomy may be artificial and that the two forms of learning need to be addressed within a single theoretical framework. In terms of brain mechanisms, this means that all types of learning may involve interactions between low-level and high-level representations of the stimulus.

13.1 Introduction

Although recent studies of perceptual learning have taught us much about its behavioral and physiological aspects, most have focused on gradual and incremental improvement in performance. Much less is known about the mechanisms underlying another important form of plasticity—one that involves an abrupt improvement in performance known as "insight." An animal is said to show insight if a period of poor performance with no clear trend of improvement is followed by a sudden and marked increase in performance. Insight has been most extensively studied in the domain of problem solving, dating as far back as the seminal work of Wolfgang Köhler (1925) with chimpanzees and other animals, and continuing today (Kaplan and Simon 1990; Sternberg and Davidson 1995). But in fields such as visual psychophysics and electrophysiology, where perceptual learning has been extensively studied, the phenomenon of insight has been largely overlooked. One possible reason for this may be a tacit assumption that the neural changes that underlie insight are fundamentally different from the plasticity that gives rise to the more gradual forms of perceptual learning. It has been suggested that the incremental improvement observed in the acquisition of perceptual skills involves synaptic modifications in early cortical areas (see, for example, Karni and Sagi 1993; Poggio, Fahle, and Edelman 1992; Ahissar and Hochstein 1997; see also Fiorentini and Berardi, chapter 9, and Zenger and Sagi, chapter 10, this volume). The implication that perceptual learning may be understood as part of a continuum of activity-dependent plastic changes, like those which have been so useful in explaining neuronal development (Hubel, Wiesel, and LeVay 1977; Katz and Shatz 1996; Miller, Keller, and Stryker 1989), is obviously appealing. On the other hand, this point of view places the mechanisms underlying perceptual learning at a level quite separate from those that are traditionally associated with insight. The sudden improvements in performance observed in insight phenomena have been taken to indicate a cognitive event that occurs more centrally. Insight seems to be a process involving the whole animal, as in Köhler's apes (1925), who suddenly realize the potential relation of disparate elements in their visual field.

Nevertheless, the two forms of learning may be more related than is currently thought. Hebb (1949) suggested that the dichotomy between insight and rote learning may be artificial, and that the two forms of learning may share common mechanisms.[1] Hebb asked: "Is insight or hypothesis—or, in the broadest terms, intelligence—something distinct from the mechanism of association?" (p. 163). He observed that "learning is often discontinuous; error curves show sharp drops without warning, and the kind of error that is made on one day may be quite changed in the next" (p. 159). He concluded that "insight ... continually affects the learning of the adult animal" (p. 163), and that "it is not wholly separate from rote learning" (p. 164). Are Hebb's assertions valid for the case of perceptual learning? Is there evidence that insightlike phenomena are part of the process of learning to perform a perceptual task? In this chapter, we will argue that the answer to these questions is yes. Although we are used to think of insight in the context of high-level cognitive tasks (such as problem solving), abrupt improvements in performance, resembling an occurrence of insight, can be observed in visual perception, as well. A classic example is the perception of hard-to-segment pictures, such as the one shown in figure 13.1a, where a dramatic transition to the "correct" interpretation may occur spontaneously or as a result of a cognitive or visual hint. (After looking at figure

13.1a, readers may look at the original gray-scale image, in figure 13.1b, as a visual hint, and then go back to figure 13.1a to experience the changed perceptual organization.) Using a task that involves a similar (but much-simplified) transition in perceptual organization, we will show that, under appropriate experimental conditions, it is possible to cause the "sharp drops" in error curves mentioned by Hebb to occur at a predictable time. The ability to gain experimental control over *when* the unique event of insight occurs addresses a long-standing problem that researchers have faced, and suggests that perceptual learning may be a particularly suitable paradigm to study the role of insight in learning.

We will also address the relation between stimulus specificity and insight in perceptual learning. As discussed in chapters 9 and 10 of this volume, it is often found in studies of perceptual learning that the improvement in performance does not generalize across stimulus attributes such as retinal size and location, or shape (Ramachandran and Braddick 1973; Fiorentini and Berardi 1980; Karni and Sagi 1991; cf. chapters 9–12). Indeed, these findings have played a major role in driving theories that place the site of plasticity in perceptual learning at early cortical areas (e.g., area V1; Fiorentini and Berardi 1980; Karni and Sagi 1991). At first glance, we might expect improvements from insight not to be susceptible to such superficial changes of circumstances and thus to generalize to stimuli that differ only in low-level visual properties. But in our experiments, the insightlike abrupt learning does not generalize to a new retinal size. This finding echoes reports from the literature on problem solving, that subjects' ability to generalize an insightful solution, that is, to transfer the solution to a novel context, depends on the extent of surface-level similarity between problems (Gick and Holyoak 1980; see also Ippolito and Tweney 1995 on the specificity of expert insights).

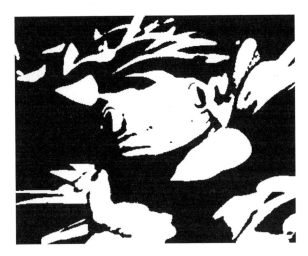

Figure 13.1a

Image obtained from gray-level original by blurring with a Gaussian filter, followed by two-toning (turning all the pixels above a threshold level to white, and those below, to black). In the resulting hard-to-segment image, the correct figural organization is not readily observed. Subjects may discover the embedded image spontaneously, or as a result of a verbal or visual hint. (The verbal hint is "ɐ ꓕɹoꓱ ɪu ɐ ꓕꟷᴧ doup"; the visual hint—the original image —is shown in figure 13.1b.) The transition from perceiving this image as a set of random ink blots to seeing the figure embedded in it occurs abruptly, as an all-or-none event, resembling an occurrence of "insight."

In this context, the stimulus specificity of abrupt learning calls for reevaluation of the way we think about insight and its role in perceptual learning, and about the source of stimulus specificity in learning phenomena in general.

13.2 Abrupt Learning Specific to Retinal Size

The task we used required subjects to discriminate between two possible shapes of an illusory surface that was globally defined by four inducers located at the corners of a "Kanizsa square" (Kanizsa 1979). Rotating the inducers about their centers made the illusory shapes appear "thin" or "fat" (see figure 13.2). Performance on this task is measured by the magnitude of rotation angle of the inducers needed to yield reliable discrimination between the two possible shapes. Previous studies using this task concluded that perception of the curved illusory contours (ICs) significantly increases the accuracy of discrimination, compared to how well the task can be done based on discriminating the orientation of the local inducers (Ringach and Shapley 1996; Rubin, Nakayama, and Shapley 1996). Our results offer independent support for this interpretation. The initial performance of subjects was quite poor, characteristic of judgments based on the orientation of the local inducers; the abrupt improvement in performance found subsequently was often reported to occur together with a change in perceptual organization, as subjects began to perceive the illusory contours.

To allow for substantial room for improvement, the parameters of the stimuli were chosen so as to make the task quite demanding. The side of the global (illusory) surfaces was 15 cm, which led to retinal sizes of 14.3° and 5.7° visual angle in the two viewing distances used (60 cm and 150 cm, respectively). The *support ratio*, defined as the ratio between the luminance-defined part of the illusory-surface edge and the total edge length, was 0.25 (except where noted, see below). The stimuli were presented briefly, followed by a blank screen and a mask (see figure 13.2). To establish that they understood the task, subjects were given a practice session before collection of the experimental data; in the practice blocks the illusory shapes were highly visible due to the larger inducers' size—the support ratio was 0.4 (the size of the global illusory surfaces was the same

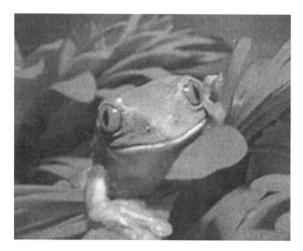

Figure 13.1b
Original gray-level image from which figure 13.1a was produced can be used as a "visual hint" to see the embedded figure.

as in the experimental blocks). The practice session consisted of four examples of long-duration stimuli, followed by 20 presentations of brief, masked stimuli. Subjects were required to give at least 17 out of 20 correct responses in their first or second practice block in order to participate in the experiment (3 out of subjects 33 were rejected from the experiment due to failure on this criterion). Once they passed this criterion, they were given the experimental blocks, where the IC stimuli were less salient, because of the smaller inducers' size. Subjects were given feedback in the form of a computer beep after correct responses throughout the practice and all experimental blocks.

Figure 13.3 shows the performance of an individual observer (A. H.) in seven consecutive blocks. The probability that the subject judged a given stimulus (i.e., a given value of inducers' rotation) as "thin" was computed for the twelve repetitions of that

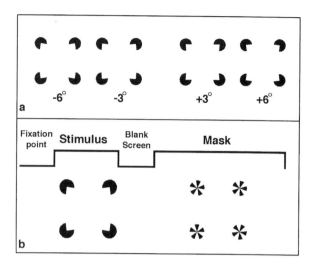

Figure 13.2
Shape discrimination task based on the perception of illusory contours. The inducers of a Kanizsa square were rotated about their centers by a variable degree, resulting in the perception of curved illusory surfaces of "fat" (*left*) or "thin" (*right*) shapes. Observers were required to choose between the two alternatives. (*a*) Direction and degree of inducer rotation determined the sign and amount of curvature of the illusory surfaces, respectively (our convention is to denote the direction of rotation that produced "fat" surfaces as negative). The range of curvatures used was varied from one experimental block to the other, thus allowing for control of the level of difficulty and the onset of the abrupt learning. (*b*) Each trial consisted of a brief stimulus presentation of either a "thin" or "fat" surface from the range of curvatures used in that block, followed by a blank screen and then a mask, which was designed to interfere with the perception of the inducers but not the global illusory surface. The stimulus was presented for 97 msec in the first experiment reported here, and for 97–194 msec in subsequent experiments (see text). The blank screen and the mask were presented for 69 msec and 250 msec, respectively.

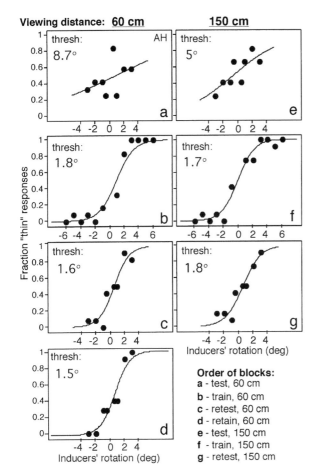

Figure 13.3
Performance of an individual subject (A. H.) in seven consecutive blocks of the "thin"/"fat" task. For each of the blocks, the fraction of times (out of 12 repetitions per stimulus value) that the subject judged the stimulus to be "thin" is plotted as a function of the inducers' rotation angle. A sigmoid curve, $[1 + \tanh(\beta(x - \alpha))]/2$, was fit to the data, with the slope (β) and bias (α) as free parameters. The threshold, defined as the inducers' rotation angle needed to reach 82% correct discrimination, was estimated from the fitted curve. For each block, the threshold is shown at the top left corner. The blocks shown in panels a–d were performed at a viewing distance of 60 cm. (*a*)

stimulus within each block. The psychometric functions depict performance in each block in terms of the probability of responding "thin" to a stimulus as a function of that stimulus's curvature. The data were fitted with a sigmoid function (see figure 13.3 caption) and thresholds were estimated from the fitted function. The first three experimental blocks were performed when the subject was seated at a viewing distance of 60 cm; each block took about 10 minutes; the whole session, including the practice and breaks, took about 45 minutes.

The first block ("test"; figure 13.3, panel a) consisted of stimuli where the inducers' rotation angles were small (0.5–3°). Performance was poor (threshold: 8.7°). In the next block ("train"; panel b), stimuli with larger inducer rotation angles (4–6°) were added to the stimulus set. In addition, large-curvature stimuli of longer exposure duration (139 msec + 56 msec blank screen) were inter-

"Test" block: when the range of rotation of the inducing elements was 0.5–3°, performance was poor. (*b*) "Train" block: when high-curvature stimuli (4–6°; as well as longer-duration stimuli; see text) were added to the set, the subject's performance improved markedly on the 2° and 3° stimuli, which were identical to those used in the "train" block. (*c*) "Retest" block: a repeat of the stimulus set used in the "test" block. After exposure to the "train" block, the subject was able to discriminate these stimuli reliably. (*d*) "Retain" block, run one week later: the subject still performed well on the low-curvature stimulus set, indicating that the learning was long-lasting. (*e*) The subject was moved to a viewing distance of 150 cm: performance in the "test" block, consisting of low-curvature stimuli, revealed that the learning exhibited in panels b–d was specific to the retinal size used. (*f, g*) Exposure to high-curvature stimuli again triggered marked improvement, and the subject's final performance in the "retest" block (panel g) was similar to that in the 60 cm viewing condition.

mixed. As is evident from panel b, the observer's performance improved dramatically: the threshold in this block was 1.8° (the data from longer exposure duration stimuli were not included for the calculation of the threshold). That the subject performed well on the higher-curvature stimuli is to be expected because they are inherently easier to discriminate. But note that performance improved markedly also on the low-curvature stimuli: A. H. correctly discriminated in this block between "thin" and "fat" figures with curvature values of 2° and 3° in 92% and 96% of the trials, respectively, compared to only 58% and 63% on identical stimuli in the previous block. This dramatic improvement was not due to a lack of cognitive understanding of the task in the first block—A. H. got 20 out of 20 trials correct in the practice block. Would good performance on low-curvature stimuli always require the presentation of high-curvature stimuli in the same block? This was tested in the third block ("retest"; panel c), which consisted of a stimulus set identical to that of the first block. The good performance was maintained (threshold: 1.6°), indicating that, compared to the poor performance exhibited in the "test" block, A. H. had undergone a rapid process of perceptual learning: he could now perform well on a set of stimuli that were too difficult for him before.

The remaining four experimental blocks were run a week later. The fourth block ("retain"; figure 13.3, panel d) was again a repeat of the low-curvature stimulus set. The good performance was maintained (threshold: 1.5°), indicating that the learning obtained a week before was long-lasting. Immediately following the "retain" block, the subject was moved to a new viewing distance of 150 cm, and here we found that the long-lasting perceptual learning described above was specific to the trained retinal size. Because the size of the stimuli on the screen was

unchanged, the greater viewing distance meant that the retinal size of the stimuli became smaller: the side of the illusory surfaces was now 5.7° visual angle (inducers' size: 1.4°), compared to 14.3° visual angle (inducers: 3.6°) at the 60 cm viewing distance. The first block at this new viewing distance ("test"; panel e) consisted of low-curvature stimuli, like those in the "test" and "retest" blocks at the 60 cm viewing distance. Performance fell markedly compared to before (threshold: 5°). Thus the learning observed in the 60 cm viewing distance did not generalize to the new retinal size. To ensure that good performance was in fact possible for this smaller retinal size, the subject was given a "train" block similar to that used at the 60 cm viewing distance, where high-curvature (4–6°) stimuli were mixed in with the low-curvature stimuli (panel f). This procedure again triggered a rapid improvement, leading to similar performance to that observed before (threshold: 1.7°). The final block at the 150 cm viewing distance was again a repeat of the low-curvature stimulus set ("retest"; panel g), but this time performance was good (threshold: 1.8°), indicating that the subject was able to learn the task at the new retinal size as well.

Figure 13.4 summarizes the results of six naive observers who were given the same sequence of blocks as A. H., in terms of threshold performance as a function of block type. All subjects showed sharp improvement in the transition from the "test" to the "train" blocks, and a lack of generalization of the learned performance to the new retinal size. As discussed earlier, the level of performance after the learning indicates that the subjects were basing their judgments on perceived illusory contours, whereas the poor level of performance in the "test" blocks is characteristic of a strategy based on making judgments based on the differences in the local inducers' orientation.

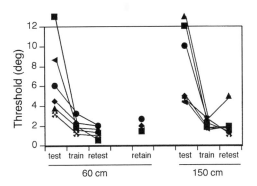

Figure 13.4
Results from six naive observers summarized in terms of threshold performance as a function of block type. The data for the first three experimental blocks were collected in one session, at a viewing distance of 60 cm. The initial performance ("test" block) varied greatly between observers, but all showed a marked improvement in the "train" block, and the good performance persisted in the "retest" block, which was a repeat of the stimulus set used in the first block. The data for the "retain" block, which was again run at 60 cm viewing distance, and for the three subsequent blocks, which were run at 150 viewing distance, were collected 1–7 days after the first session, to avoid fatigue of the naive subjects and to establish that the learning was long-lasting. (Results similar to those presented here were obtained from two experienced observers who performed all blocks on the same day.) The "retain" block was a repeat of the "retest" block stimulus set, and demonstrates that the learning is long-lasting; the poor performance in the "test" block at 150 cm demonstrates that the learning did not generalize to a new retinal size, but performance improved again after retraining.

13.3 The Time Course of Learning: A Trial-by-Trial Analysis of Performance

Thus far, we have seen that performance in the task can improve rapidly in the transition from the "test" to the "train" block. But in the data shown in figures 13.3 and 13.4, performance for each stimulus type is averaged across all twelve trials in the block. To

better examine the time course of the learning, we performed a trial-by-trial analysis of the performance of our subjects' group. Data points in figure 13.5 represent the percentage correct of discriminations for the pair of $+/-2°$ stimuli (upper panel) and the pair of $+/-3°$ stimuli (lower panel) as a function of time (i.e., the serial order of presentation of the stimulus in the block, or trial number). Each point in figure 13.5 represents the mean performance in that trial, averaged over all six subjects. For both the $+/-2°$ and the $+/-3°$ stimuli, the group performance shows an abrupt jump at the transition from the "test" to the "train" block (trials 13–24, shaded area), when the low-curvature stimuli were embedded in a set of high-curvature and long-exposure stimuli. The mean performance on the $+/-2°$ stimuli jumped from 58% in the "test" block to 84% in the "train" block (the numbers for the $+/-3°$ stimuli are 74% and 88%, respectively, a smaller but yet significant effect). In both cases, no improvement is observed within the "test" block: linear regression accounts for less than 3% of the variance in the data and the regression slopes are very shallow. The trial-by-trial analysis again shows that the good performance was maintained in the "retest" block (trials 25–36), and in the "retain" block (trials 37–48), which was run on the second session, one to seven days later. After the subjects were moved to the 150 cm viewing distance, a sharp drop in performance was observed on the first, "test" block (trials 49–60), followed by a rapid improvement on the "train" (trials 61–72) and "retest" (trials 73–84) blocks.

The time course of improvement manifested in figure 13.5 is different from what is usually reported in perceptual learning studies—a gradual, even if sometimes fast (Karni and Sagi 1993; Poggio, Fahle, and Edelman 1992; Fahle, Edelman, and Poggio 1995) increase in performance (Ramachandran and

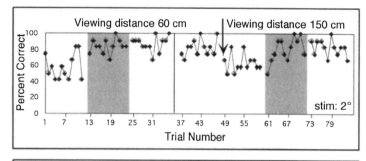

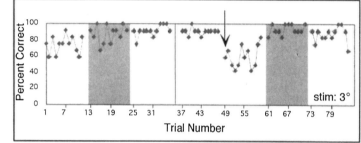

Figure 13.5

Trial-by-trial analysis of performance as a function of time. Percent correct discrimination for each successive pair of $+/-2°$ (*top*) and $+/-3°$ (*bottom*) curvature stimuli was separately tabulated, averaged over all six observers, and plotted as a function of time. Trials 1–12 were in the "test" block at the 60 cm viewing distance. Trials 13–24 (shaded zone) reflect the performance when identical stimuli were given in the "train" block, embedded in a set of higher-curvature and longer-duration stimuli. Trials 25–36 were in the "retest" block, which consisted of a stimulus set identical to that of the initial "test" block. The last four blocks, again of twelve trials each, were performed on a second session, between one and seven days later for different observers. The "retain" block (trials 37–48) was performed at the 60 cm viewing distance and the next three blocks were performed right after it, at the 150 cm viewing distance. Poor performance in the "test" block (trials 49–60) indicates that the learning did not transfer to the new viewing distance, although learning subsequently reoccurred in the "train" (trials 61–72) and "test" (trials 73–84) blocks for the new retinal size.

Braddick 1973; Ramachandran 1976; Fiorentini and Berardi 1980; Ball and Sekuler 1982; Karni and Sagi 1991; Ahissar and Hochstein 1993, 1997; cf. chapters 9, 11, 12). What is the relation between the abrupt, insightlike learning we observed and the more gradual form of learning reported in other studies? We shall return to the implications of this distinction in section 13.5.

Subjects' reaction times (RTs) also reflect a sudden, but stimulus-specific improvement. Figure 13.6

shows the trial-by-trial analysis of the RTs to the $+/-2°$ (top panel) and $+/-3°$ (bottom panel) stimuli. The pattern of performance parallels that found in the percentage correct data (figure 13.5), with a sharp drop in mean RTs at the transition between the "test" and "train" blocks at the 60 cm viewing distance, an increase in mean RTs as subjects were moved to the 150 cm viewing distance, and finally again a drop in mean RTs on the "train" block at the new viewing distance. In addition, a

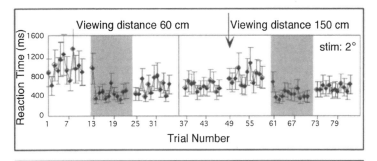

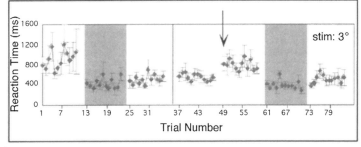

Figure 13.6
Trial-by-trial analysis of reaction times (RTs). Mean RTs for each successive pair of +/−2° (*top*) and +/−3° (*bottom*) curvature stimuli are plotted as a function of time (average of six observers). At the 60 cm viewing distance, trials 1−12 were in the "test" block; trials 13−24 (shaded zone), in the "train" block, where a marked drop in the RTs is observed; trials 25−36, in the "retest" block; and trials 37−48, in the "retain" block. At the 150 cm viewing distance, trials 49−60 were in the "test" block, where mean RTs increased and percentage correct performance fell off, as also observed in figure 13.5; trials 61−72, in the "train" block, where facilitation is observed again; and trials 73−84, in the "retest" block.

slight increase in mean RTs can be observed in the "retest" blocks (trials 25−36 and 73−84), indicating that observers were aware that these were more difficult than the preceding ones ("train"), although this increase in difficulty is not manifested in the percentage correct performance (figure 13.5). Note that the subjects were not told that their reaction times were being recorded; the only emphasis in the instructions was on the correctness of responses. In other words, the sharp drops in the mean values and variability of the RTs occurred even though the subjects were not instructed to respond as fast as possible, and suggest that a facilitation in performing the task took place.

The trial-by-trial analysis reveals a course of improvement that follows closely Hebb's behavioral criterion (1949, p. 160) for "insight": "There is a period first of fruitless effort in one direction, or perhaps a series of solutions. Then suddenly there is a complete change in the direction of effort, and a cleancut solution of the task." As mentioned earlier, the high thresholds in the "test" block are characteristic of performing the task based on the local inducers' orientation, whereas the good performance later indicates judgments based on illusory contour perception. This finding suggests that the improved performance was indeed associated with a changed strategy, or "direction of effort," as Hebb suggested.

The subjective reports of the observers are consistent with this idea. Several subjects reported that, in the first block, they did not see the global illusory shapes, and were basing their judgments on the local inducers; in the second block, they suddenly started seeing the global shapes (sometimes noting the well-known brightness effect associated with it; Kanizsa 1979; see also Petry and Meyer 1987). Thus both the subjective reports and the behavioral measures are consistent with a transition in subjects' strategy in performing the task, somehow triggered by the introduction of the "train" block. Interestingly, there was a notable difference between subjects who were practiced psychophysical observers (but were still naive about the purpose of our experiment), all of whom reported a transition in their strategy, compared with unpracticed subjects, who were much more likely to ascribe their improvement to their belief that the second block was "easier." That insightlike behavior can be triggered experimentally by appropriate "hints," even when subjects are unaware of the hints, has been known in the domain of problem solving for a long time (Mayer 1995).

Our results suggest that insightful learning may not be limited to domains such as problem solving, but rather may play a role in perception as well. This view is further supported by our findings about the role of external feedback in learning. During our pilot studies, we ran different subjects with and without feedback, and found that, on average, subjects who did not receive external feedback about their correctness did not show as robust learning as those who did. Again, this finding was particularly true of subjects who were not practiced psychophysical observers; in contrast, two practiced (but naive) subjects showed an abrupt and long-lasting improvement in the absence of any external feedback. On the other hand, recall that the insightlike

improvement in performance was specific to the trained retinal size, and retraining was necessary at the new retinal size. Thus there seems to be an interaction between the low-level (exposure to specific stimuli) and high-level (strategy, knowledge about the level of correctness) aspects of the abrupt learning; we shall return to this point in section 13.5 (cf. also chapters 11, 20).

13.4 Will Any "Easy" Stimulus Set Trigger Abrupt Learning?

We have seen that the abrupt learning did not generalize to a new retinal size, that is, the training procedure was effective only for the retinal size of the stimuli used in the "train" block. Next we examine further the extent to which the abrupt learning was sensitive to the specific attributes of the stimuli in the "train" block. First, we asked whether learning would take place when the large-curvature illusory surfaces had the same retinal size as before, but the inducing elements were of a different size. To test this, we ran a new group of ten subjects, which we designated "group B," on the first three experimental blocks of the "thin/fat" task (i.e., only the first session, at 60 cm viewing distance; the subjects received a practice block first, as before). The experiment performed by group B was identical to the first session in the experiment described before, except for the following change: the diameter of the inducers of the high-curvature stimuli (4–6°) was increased, leaving their centers at the same locations as before, so that the support ratio was 0.4. This change in diameter meant that the retinal size of the inducing elements was different from that used for the low-curvature stimuli, whereas the size of the *illusory* surfaces was the same for the two types of stimuli (see illustration in middle row of figure 13.7,

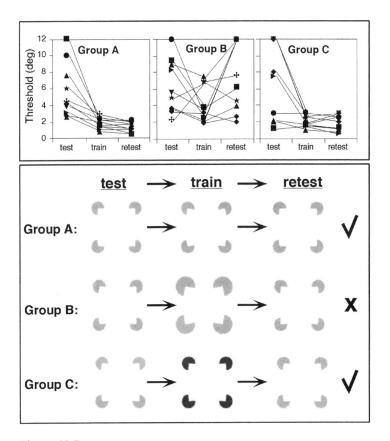

Figure 13.7
Specificity of the training stimuli. (*Bottom*) Schematic diagram of the different procedures used for the three experimental groups. Group A was given a "train" block with large-angle stimuli of the same inducer size as the small-angle ("test") stimuli (and those in the first three blocks in figures 13.3–13.6). Group B was given a "train" block where the high-curvature stimuli were of larger-size inducers than the "test" stimuli. Group C was given a "train" block that contained long-duration low-curvature stimuli, and no high-curvature stimuli (the longer-duration stimuli are illustrated here schematically by higher contrast). (*Top*) Subjects in group A (*left*) and group C (*right*) show a dramatic improvement in their performance, which is maintained after the training stimuli are again removed ("retest"). Subjects in group B (*middle*) show large individual differences; many do not improve during the "train" block at all, and those who do improve during the training block do not retain the good performance once the large-angle stimuli are taken away ("retest" block). The thresholds for the "train" block were estimated based on the data from the 1–3° short-duration stimuli only, for all three experimental groups.

bottom panel). Note that this manipulation makes discriminating the shapes of the high-curvature stimuli of the "train" block even easier than before. Would exposure to these stimuli lead to robust learning? The results are shown in figure 13.7 (middle panel on top) in terms of threshold performance as a function of block type. For comparison, we include the results of ten subjects who participated in the first session of the experiment described in section 13.2, where the "test" and "train" stimuli had the same support ratio (group A, left panel on top). It is evident that, whereas all the subjects in group A improved in the "train" block and retained their learning in the "retest" block, the subjects of group B showed large individual differences in their performance. Moreover, the performance of even those subjects who improved during the "train" block fell back to its initial ("test") level in the third, "retest" block. We conclude that the improvement in performance observed in group A, and the accompanying transition in the perceptual organization of the small-curvature ("test") stimuli into illusory surfaces, can only be triggered by large-curvature IC stimuli with similar size inducers (i.e., with the same support ratio). One reason for this result may be that illusory contours of different support ratios are generated or represented by different neural substrates, even though the illusory surfaces themselves look perceptually similar (e.g., different neurons respond to the local occlusion cues, or L-junctions, as the support ratio is changed, because those junctions fall on different retinal locations). Alternatively, the lack of learning observed in group B may be related to cognitive factors: the mixture of "very easy" and "very hard" stimuli that are easily discriminable (due to the different support ratios) in the same block may have led to a differential treatment of the two sets of stimuli by the subjects. Further experiments will be

needed in order to distinguish between these two possibilities (or to show the involvement of both).

The next question we asked was whether the "train" block had to contain high-curvature stimuli, or whether learning could be induced with other, "easy" stimuli. This question addresses a possible interpretation of the abrupt learning observed in section 12.2, which is that the introduction of the high-curvature stimuli allowed the subjects to establish two distinct categories, or templates, for the "thin" and "fat" surfaces. According to that interpretation, the minute differences in curvature given in the first ("test") block were not enough to establish two such distinct categories, and this led to the poor performance observed. Once subjects were able to form the categories, using the exaggerated examples given in the "train" block, they were able to classify the low-curvature stimuli correctly, too. This interpretation suggests the following prediction: significant improvement should not be observed when the "train" block is changed so that large-curvature stimuli are no longer given. This prediction, however, was not supported by the following experiment. A third group of subjects (group C) was given three consecutive experimental sessions, where the second ("train") session consisted of only low-curvature ($1-3°$) stimuli. To facilitate performance in this block, two sets of long-duration low-curvature stimuli were added to the stimulus set: 153 msec ($+69$ msec blank screen) and 194 msec ($+83$ msec blank screen); the rest of the $1-3°$ stimuli had exposure durations of 97 msec $+69$ msec blank screen, as in the "test" block). In other words, what made the additional stimuli in the "train" block easy this time was that they had, not higher curvature, but a much longer exposure duration. The results of group C are presented in figure 13.7 (right panel, top) in terms of threshold performance as a function of block type,

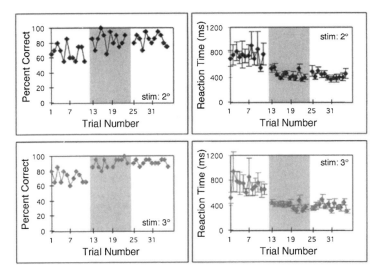

Figure 13.8
Trial-by-trial analysis of percentage correct (left-hand panels) and reaction time (right-hand panels) of group C, who received a "train" block that contained long-duration low-curvature stimuli, and no high-curvature stimuli (see figure 13.7, bottom panel, bottom row). Abrupt improvements, similar to those observed for group A (see figures 13.5 and 13.6), are seen at the transition (trial 13) from the "test" to the "train" block.

and show that long-exposure stimuli are sufficient to trigger learning. Figure 13.8 shows the trial-by-trial analysis of the percentage correct (panels on right) and reaction times (panels on left) performance, for the $+/-2°$ (top panels) and $+/-3°$ (bottom panels) short-duration stimuli. Abrupt improvements, similar to those observed before (see figures 13.5 and 13.6) are seen at the transition from the "test" to the "train" block. These results show that high-curvature stimuli are not necessary to trigger the learning. Therefore, the interpretation outlined above, which invoked the notion of a generation of two distinct categories for the learning to occur, must be rejected. Our results suggest instead that there may be several routes to facilitate learning (e.g., group A, group C), although not any set of "easy" stimuli is suitable (group B).

13.5 Discussion

Using a task of discriminating the shapes of global illusory surfaces, we were able to show that, under appropriate experimental conditions it is possible to induce a sudden and long-lasting improvement in performance. The overt measures of improvement—sharp drops in error rate and reaction times—were often accompanied by subjects' reports of a change in their strategy in performing the task, suggesting that the learning we observed was similar to the phenomenon of insight in humans and other animals (Köhler 1925; Sternberg and Davidson 1995). At the same time, however, the abrupt improvement in performance shared one of the main characteristics of perceptual learning: it was stimulus specific. The improvement did not generalize to a new retinal size, and retraining was necessary for the good performance to reoccur. The onset of the learning also showed great sensitivity to the spatiotemporal properties of the training stimuli, again demonstrating a strong perceptual component in the learning.

The paradigm presented here provides a unique situation in which these two properties of the improvement—abruptness and stimulus specificity—occur together. Usually, they tend to characterize quite different forms of learning. Stimulus specificity has been found mostly in cases where the learning was gradual and incremental—often requiring hundreds or even thousands of trials (Ramachandran and Braddick 1973; Ramachandran 1976; Fiorentini and Berardi 1980; Ball and Sekuler 1982; Karni and Sagi 1991; Ahissar and Hochstein 1993, 1997; Masson 1986; but see also Karni and Sagi 1993; Poggio, Fahle, and Edelman 1992). Insight, on the other hand, involves a sharp improvement by its very nature. Moreover, the name "insight" itself suggests that the subject has found some new "solution" to the problem at hand—a new understanding of how to perform the task or solve the problem. It implies that we should not expect the improved performance to be dependent on factors such as the context (e.g., in the case of problem solving) or the retinal size or location of the stimulus (in the case of a visual task). Research in problem solving, however, indicates the this expectation is not always met: in fact, subjects can show great susceptibility to the surface-level attributes of a problem they learned to solve, transferring the solution to another problem that shares these attributes, but failing to transfer it to a problem that has an identical deep structure but a different surface-level structure (Gick and Holyoak 1980). These findings echo those reported here, that an improvement which seems to involve an "insightful" solution can be stimulus specific.

The fact that abrupt (or insightful) and stimulus-specific improvements can happen within the same experimental paradigm suggests that there may be a connection between the mechanisms that underlie these two forms of learning, which were previously thought of as separate. One implication of this view is that perceptual learning should be thought of as *an active process*, where the subject's continual effort to process the incoming sensory information in the most efficient and meaningful way is crucial for the improvement to take place. According to this view, the fact that abrupt improvement can be induced experimentally should be viewed as a manifestation of the underlying active process of exploration on the part of the subject, a process that is taking place continuously. Indeed, studies by Shiu and Pashler (1992) and Ahissar and Hochstein (1993; see also chapter 14, this volume) provide further evidence for this idea. In their experiments, an identical set of visual stimuli could be presented in the context of two different tasks. They found that the extensive exposure that gave rise to the improvement in the "main" (trained) task affected performance in the other (untrained) task very little. One exception to this finding, however, may be when the task is "preattentive," in the sense of showing little or no performance loss as the attentional load is increased by enlarging the stimulus array (Treisman and Gelade 1980) or by introducing another, concurrent task (Braun and Sagi 1991). Ahissar and Hochstein (1993) found a significant amount of improvement in a popout task—a classical preattentive task—after subjects received extensive exposure to popout arrays in the context of a different task. Using a texture segregation task, Karni and Sagi (1993) distinguished two learning phases. The initial ("fast") phase, takes place over several hundreds of training trials (in their study this initial phase was associated with a drop in thresholds of more than a factor of two). Karni and Sagi (1993; see also Sagi and Tanne 1994) proposed that this phase involves top-down control and involves the establishments of connections that make the task automatic. The second, much slower phase of learning (which takes place over days and led to a further drop in thresholds of 30–40% in their study), is therefore hypothesized to be taking place in a passive, bottom-up way, requiring no active effort on the part of the observers.

The idea that incremental, stimulus-specific learning and abrupt, insightful improvements may be part of a common learning mechanism implies that it should be possible to show a continuous transition between these two forms of learning. There is evidence that such a continuum can indeed be observed. In the course of performing pilot experiments before those reported here, we ran a large group of subjects ($n = 34$) on variations of the paradigm described in this chapter. Our purpose was to characterize the distribution of performance across our subject population, in order to optimize stimulus conditions for abrupt learning. By changing the exposure duration of all stimuli, we varied the overall level of difficulty of the task while at the same time maintaining the "test-train-retest" structure reported here (low curvature in the "test" blocks; mixed high- and low curvature in the "train" blocks). We found that, for shorter exposure durations than those reported here (i.e., when the task was more difficult), subjects often did not show an abrupt improvement at the transition from the "test" to the "train" block, but instead showed a slower, more gradual improvement (and sometimes did not improve at all within the session). These results also shed light on the issue of why traces of abrupt or insightful improvements were not reported previously in perceptual learning studies. To allow for a substantial amount of improvement, researchers used parameter regimes that made their tasks extremely difficult, and thus also made gradual,

incremental improvements more likely than large, sudden ones. This observation was made already by Hebb (1949, p. 160), who noted that in order to induce insight, one needs "tasks ... of just the right degree of difficulty ... [the task] must neither be so easy so that the animal solves the problem at once, thus not allowing [experimenters] to analyze the solution; nor so hard that the animal fails to solve it except by rote learning in a long series of trials." Thus, while previous perceptual learning studies were not intended to optimize conditions for insightlike improvements to occur, it may well be the case that an appropriate change in the experimental procedure could promote such abrupt learning in other tasks as well (e.g., by using the method of constant stimuli to give a set of difficult stimuli followed by the same stimuli mixed in with easier ones, as we have done here). This in turn suggests that, by appropriate choice of the stimulus parameters and experimental procedure, perceptual learning may be used as a model for studying insight.

The resemblance between insight in problem solving and in perception has recently also been noted by researchers writing about the psychology of insight. Schooler, Fallshore, and Fiore (1995) found a strong correlation between insight in problem solving and the capability to find the shapes of objects in blurred pictures. Gruber (1995) specifically drew attention to similarities in the process of integration of fragmented images such as illusory contour stimuli and the integrative processes of insight in problem solving.

Another issue raised by the results presented in this chapter is the interpretation of stimulus specificity. The lack of generalization of perceptual learning to new stimulus parameters has been previously taken to imply that the learning occurred in early, retinotopically organized visual cortical areas, which are known to encode position, local orientation, and similar attributes at the level of individual cells (Ramachandran and Braddick 1973; Fiorentini and Berardi 1980; Karni and Sagi 1991; Poggio, Fahle, and Edelman 1992; Weiss, Edelman, and Fahle 1993; Fahle 1997; Ahissar and Hochstein 1997; see also chapters 9–11, this volume). Placing the site of plasticity at an early visual cortical site was consistent with two notable characteristics of the tasks and the learning course. First, the tasks were of a local nature, involving interactions between image points 1° apart or less (Ramachandran and Braddick 1973; Karni and Sagi 1991; Poggio, Fahle, and Edelman 1992; Fahle 1997; Ahissar and Hochstein 1997). Second, the improvement was incremental, often taking place over hundreds or even thousands of trials (Ramachandran and Braddick 1973; Fiorentini and Berardi 1980; Karni and Sagi 1991; Fahle 1997; Ahissar and Hochstein 1997). Even where fast learning phases were observed (Poggio, Fahle, and Edelman 1992; Karni and Sagi 1993), performance showed a steep, but gradual improvement, over several dozens of trials. In contrast, in the experiments reported here, there were large retinal distances between the inducers (more than 10° visual angle at the 60 cm viewing distance), which means that the relevant information was stored in widely separated neurons in early visual cortical areas. This in itself does not preclude models that assume that the visual *processing* required to perceive the illusory contours takes place in those early, small receptive field areas because information can propagate in a few iterations across several relays of lateral connections (Gilbert and Wiesel 1983; Gilbert et al. 1996; Lund 1988; Malach et al. 1993; for a model that makes use of such lateral connections to detect global shapes, see also Sha'shua and Ullman 1988). But here is where the abrupt nature of the learning we observed comes into play. For a model based on lateral connections to exhibit the kind of sharp im-

provement we observed, it would require the simultaneous modification of synaptic efficacies between multiple (neighboring) cells. The existence of neural mechanisms that could support such a "cooperative" form of synaptic plasticity is not presently known. Thus the abruptness of the learning, combined with the global nature of the task make it unlikely that a model based exclusively on quick synaptic modifications of local connectivity in early cortical areas, such as has been suggested previously for other tasks (Poggio, Fahle, and Edelman 1992), could work for the phenomenon presented here. The fact that the abrupt learning we observed was specific to retinal size indicates, however, that the site of plasticity cannot be limited to higher visual areas that encode shapes in a size-invariant way, either. It is therefore difficult to conceive of the learning as occurring at a single site. Instead, the improvement we observed is more consistent with changes in processes that involve interactions between multiple levels of representation of the stimuli, where activity in early visual areas is affected by stimulus-driven processing as well as top-down control (Edelman 1987; Grossberg 1987; Ullman 1995; Dayan et al. 1995; cf. chapters 18, 20).

To conclude, we have shown evidence that insightlike improvements in performance can take place in perceptual learning, and that the improvement may show stimulus specificity similar to that described before for more incremental, gradual learning. Our results suggest that the distinction between insightful and gradual, incremental learning may need to be revised. Rather than postulating two distinct mechanisms for the two forms of learning, our findings may be better understood within a single framework. This view was put forward already by Hebb (1949), who wrote that "insight ... continually affects the learning of the adult animal" (p. 163), and that "it is not wholly separate from rote learning" (p. 164). Hebb proposed a unitary mechanism, based on the associations of co-occurring internal states, within which to understand all learning phenomena. However, he emphasized that the sequence of internal states is not merely determined by external events, but is rather an active process in which the animal is attempting continually to discover structure and meaning in the incoming information. This is a very different view from the incremental and unsupervised form of learning with which Hebb is usually associated today (see, e.g., Rumelhart et al. 1986; Brown et al. 1990). Reading his seminal book fifty years later, it is striking to see how this neuroscientist was in fact acutely aware of the role of insight in learning—especially because he later came to be identified with the idea of "associative learning," which is today often equated with a passive, stimulus-driven and unsupervised form of synaptic plasticity. Our findings, as well as other evidence recently reported (Shiu and Pashler 1992; Ahissar and Hochstein 1993, 1997), vindicate Hebb's original ideas and call for a more integrative approach to studying the organization of learning.

Acknowledgments

We thank Merav Ahissar, Shaul Hochstein, Nancy Kanwisher, Michael Oren, Dario Ringach, Shimon Ullman, and Daphna Weinshall for helpful discussions. Special thanks to Anne Grossetete for experimental assistance and many insightful suggestions. Support from the McDonnell-Pew program in Cognitive Neuroscience and the Sloan Foundation, from the McKnight Foundation and Air Force Office of Scientific Research, and from the National Institutes of Health was received by Nava Rubin, Ken Nakayama, and Robert Shapley, respectively.

Note

1. *Rote learning* was the term used by Hebb to describe the gradual, incremental form of learning being studied in animals, primarily rats and pigeons, and modeled by the learning theorists of those days as a continuous process. The "mechanisms of association" Hebb mentions later refer to the central idea behind most theories of his time, that learning takes place as a result of the incremental strengthening of stimulus-response relations that gives rise to a desirable outcome (reward). Hebb himself, of course, is widely known for his contributions to learning theory; importantly for the present context, Hebb is probably best known today for his observation that learning via such a "mechanism of association" can occur in the absence of explicit supervision (reward or feedback), merely by the strengthening of pathways between co-occuring neural events.

14

The Role of Attention in Learning Simple Visual Tasks

Merav Ahissar and Shaul Hochstein

Abstract

Attention is essential for learning even simple perceptual tasks. Its role in learning far exceeds the simple gating mechanism often assumed in the context of "early-vision" tasks. Attention actively selects specific neural populations whose activity directly underlies task performance and where the modifications that account for task-dependent learning take place. The choice of a specific population is the neural implementation of a strategy. This chapter discusses the mechanisms dictating the attentional search for the appropriate neural population, in particular, the reverse hierarchy pathway of such a search. Once attention has been allocated, learning affects the entire population to which attention is paid. Thus attention is not only necessary for learning; it is also sufficient, in that stimulation at a particular site is not required. We propose that the role of attention in learning simple visual tasks is similar to its role in learning complex cognitive tasks.

14.1 Attention: A Brief Introduction

We and others have found that attention is a crucial factor in the ability to improve perceptual performance. In describing our experiments, we propose a theory for the specific mechanism by which attention affects perceptual learning. We present a view largely consistent with that presented by William James (1890) more than a hundred years ago: "Only those items which I notice shape my mind—without selective interest, experience is an utter chaos." Although we would temper this strong statement, dissociating attention from consciousness (perhaps "attempt to notice" would be more appropriate than "notice"), we believe that the long-term modifications underlying improvement in perceptual performance do indeed occur only for aspects we selectively attend.

Attention, as James (1890, 404) observes, "implies withdrawal from some things in order to deal effectively with others." The notion that attention is basically a selection mechanism still governs the field of psychology. What selective attention is, and whether it is limited to a single item, feature, or dimension at a time, are still open questions. Attempts to answer them are largely driven by different views of the fundamental bottleneck that underlies this selection (see review by Allport 1989).

Why is selection needed? Philosophers once bound attention and consciousness together and attributed the limit to our attention to the "unity of soul." The modern study of attention, largely pioneered by Broadbent, assumed a basic limit of our processing ability. To minimize unnecessary computation, relevant information is selected at early stages of processing (Broadbent 1956). "Late selection" was suggested by others (notably, Deutsch and Deutsch 1963), who assumed that the source of constraint is our inability to make simultaneous responses at the effector level. The need to make a single response imposes the need to select, although, according to this view, we should be able to process diverse sources of information simultaneously until we reach the stage of response planning. Less extreme views of late selection would place selection at the decision-making stage, regardless of whether an overt response is made or planned (Pashler 1998).

Proponents of early selection have drawn on findings that we can easily select on the basis of simple features but not on the basis of complex concepts. For example, Treisman and Gelade (1980) and Julesz (1981) showed that detecting (selecting) on the basis of a simple (primitive or early-encoded) feature (e.g., intensity, color, orientation) does not require attention, whereas searching (selecting) on the basis of a feature combination (conjunction) does. Treisman and Gelade found that, without sufficient attention, false conjunctions are perceived between basic features and elements. For example, when subjects are asked to report what they have seen at positions to which attention has not been focused in a brief display containing a green X and a red square, they are likely to report X, square, red, and green. But they will often confuse the conjunction between color and shape, reporting a red X and a green square. The finding of illusory conjunctions between basic features was the basis of Treisman's feature integration theory, which moved the dispute of early versus late selection toward understanding the mechanisms underlying selection. The theory characterized attention as the glue that binds basic features present at a single position (e.g., the orientation and the color of a light bar) to a unified percept.

What is the mechanism through which selection is implemented? One answer is facilitation—the attended information is processed faster. This idea was already suggested by James, and is largely accepted today (though still in dispute). Based on his personal observations, James (1890, 409) suggested that attention facilitates access to consciousness: "The smith may see the sparks fly before he sees the hammer smite the iron. There is thus a certain difficulty in perceiving the exact date of two impressions when

they do not interest our attention equally." Recently, Hikosaka, Miyauchi, and Shimojo (1993, 1996; but see Downing and Treisman 1997) have attributed a newly discovered motion illusion to the facilitatory effect of attention. In this illusion, a line, which is presented physically all at once, is perceived to be drawn from one side to the other, when attention has been captured by the first side due to a preceding visual cue.

The "early versus late" dispute that occupied attention research by cognitive psychologists also dominated the rare electrophysiological studies seeking the neural basis of attention. These studies measured the effect of the behavioral task performed by a monkey on the response characteristics of single neurons. Initial findings suggested that the responses of neurons in early visual (cortical) areas are determined by the retinal input (e.g., Wurtz, Goldberg, and Robinson 1982). Behavioral effects were only found at higher areas along both the dorsal (parietal lobe) and ventral (temporal lobe) processing streams. More recent studies (e.g., Motter 1993) indicate that when task performance requires selective spatial attention (such as when there are several elements in the display), responses are modified by attentional demands in the primary visual area (V1) as well as in higher areas (V2, V4).

Interestingly, these studies assume that attention follows the hierarchy revealed by bottom-up anatomical connections and neuronal response characteristics. That is, the earliest site of selection is the primary visual area, where basic features are represented. Thus, if attention operates at the level following feature representation, it operates just after area V1 (Julesz 1990). A late site of selection would be within inferotemporal areas (considering the ventral stream as an example), where objects may be represented (see Desimone and Ungerleider 1989 for review). In this chapter, we present an alternative hypothesis regarding the attentional hierarchy (see Ahissar and Hochstein 1997), namely, that attention proceeds along a reverse hierarchy, as revealed in feedback rather than in feedforward anatomical connections, a more natural flow for top-down effects that stem from extraretinal sources. Although this assumption seems obvious, its implications are broad. In terms of the neural basis of attention, "early attention" means selecting neural populations located at higher processing stages, and "late selection" means reaching "down" to early processing stages at low-level cortical areas. Our view of attention is presented in the context of perceptual learning, where this hypothesis accounts for seemingly conflicting and very variable sets of data.

Another aspect studied by electrophysiologists is the mechanism implementing attentional selection at the level of single neurons. Various changes in response characteristics were found as a function of behavioral state, providing "an existence proof" for attentional effects. In addition, the functional size of the receptive field was found to shrink around the attended stimulus, so that unattended stimuli within the receptive field induce substantially reduced responses (Moran and Desimone 1985). The extent of the modulation depends on the difficulty of the task. Responses of neurons are larger and more selective when the task is more difficult (Spitzer, Desimone, and Moran 1988). Niebur and Koch (1994) suggested a model for the neuronal implementation of selective visual attention based on temporal correlation among groups of neurons. Because psychophysical studies have not directly addressed the neuronal implementation of selective attention at the level of single neurons, we will focus on larger neuronal structures, at least at the level of neuronal assemblies (Churchland and Sejnowski 1988).

14.2 Learning a Simple Visual Task

14.2.1 Adults Improve Dramatically in Orientation Feature Detection

One of the best studied examples of effortless detection is feature search for a line segment whose orientation greatly differs from that of the surrounding distractor light bars, as illustrated in figure 14.1, panel A. The odd element "pops out" even without intended search suggesting a "preattentive" process. Furthermore, the response reaction time for this task is independent of the number of distractor elements, suggesting that search is parallel and not based on an attention-directed serial scan (Treisman and Gelade 1980; Julesz 1981; but see Joseph, Chun, and Nakayama 1997). Interestingly, Treisman (1996) now emphasizes the divided or spread attention rather than the preattentive nature of popout. The local characteristics of popout detection (Julesz 1986; Sagi and Julesz 1987; Nothdurft 1992) suggest that these tasks may be processed as early as areas V1–V2. This suggestion is supported by electrophysiological (Knierim and Van Essen 1992) and lesion (Merigan, Nealy, and Maunsell 1993) studies.

We used a backward-masked version of the simple popout stimulus to study perceptual learning. Our stimulus was an array of 7×7 light bars, which were identical except that on half the trials one bar was oddly oriented (deviating by $30°$; see figure 14.1, panel A). Because the stimulus was presented briefly and was followed shortly afterward by a masking stimulus, we could manipulate task difficulty by adjusting the stimulus onset asynchrony (SOA), thereby varying the time interval available for processing. We asked subjects to indicate the presence or absence of a target element by pressing a computer

A. stimuli for pop-out detection

with   **without**

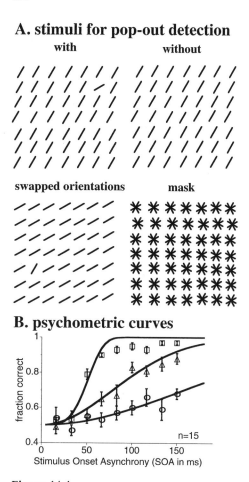

swapped orientations   **mask**

B. psychometric curves

Figure 14.1

(*A*) Schematic diagram of popout testing paradigm for orientation feature detection. Light bars in 7 × 7 array were presented briefly, either with (*upper left*) or without (*upper right*) an odd element, that is, a bar with a different orientation. A mask comprising bars of various orientations (*lower right*) was presented following each stimulus. We tested transfer of learning to new spatial conditions, such as detection with swapped target and distractor orientations (*lower left*). (*B*) Average performance improvement (all-positions paradigm) from the first and second thirds of the initial session (circles, triangles) to the posttraining final session (squares). Lines are Quick psychometric functions fit to data. Training induces a leftward shift and steepening

key ("1"/"0"). Plotting performance as a function of SOA, we obtained the psychometric function (see examples in panel B).

We found that subjects' performance in orientation detection improved dramatically following practice (Ahissar and Hochstein 1993, 1995). Although most subjects performed perfectly already on the first trials when given an unlimited amount of viewing time (> 200 msec), after training, they needed substantially less processing time (SOA) to achieve a threshold level of detection. For example, the psychometric curves of figure 14.1, panel B, are averages for 15 subjects for the first and second thirds of their first session (each session consisted of 1,400 trials), and for their final training session. With training, the psychometric curve gets steeper and is shifted leftward; that is, performance improves, with threshold (SOA for 82% correct) reduced by a factor of 3.

The finding of dramatic improvement over several thousand trials in adult subjects was especially impressive because this detection task seems almost automatic to begin with. Interestingly, other studies using simple tasks with backward-masking paradigms also found large improvement (Karni and Sagi 1991; Schoups and Orban 1996). It appears that tasks that pose temporal limitations on processing present a high prospect of dramatic and relatively fast improvement (days rather than months). Performance with similar tasks, which initially pose other types of constraints (e.g., lateral masking), may not be subject to such steep improvement (Wolford, Marchak, and Hughes 1988; Wolford and Kim 1992; see also Ahissar and Hochstein 1998a for review).

of the psychometric curve, substantially decreasing the threshold (stimulus onset synchrony, or SOA, for 82% correct). Threshold is the performance measure used in the following figures.

14.2.2 Can Learning Occur at an Early Cortical Site?

What type of neural plasticity underlies this dramatic behavioral improvement? During the 1960s, such an improvement would necessarily have been attributed to a high-level cortical area because low-level areas were assumed to lose their plasticity following a critical period of development. We now know that primary sensory areas may be modified in adults (e.g., Gilbert and Wiesel 1992). But which neural site and mechanism should serve as initial primary candidates for the modifications that underlie learning in the search for orientation features?

Our initial hypothesis followed a simple line of reasoning: (1) learning must occur at a site where the task is processed (or represented); (2) odd orientations are detected by processes at early cortical sites (as indicated by its being performed automatically and with parallel processing; see above); and (3) learning of orientation detection may therefore occur at an early cortical site. Our working hypothesis was that the site could be the earliest stage that explicitly codes for the task, that is, the earliest stage where neurons are selective for orientation (see for example, Karni and Sagi 1991). This hypothesis yielded several predictions, some of which turned out not to be true, as discussed in section 14.3.

14.3 Learning Can Occur at Multiple Cortical Levels

14.3.1 Learning Can Be Specific to the Trained Stimuli

To decipher the neural substrate underlying perceptual learning, we performed a series of learning studies using the feature search task (Ahissar and Hochstein 1993, 1995, 1996b, 1997). In these studies, we considered the stimulus characteristics for which we found learning specificity to indicate the cortical site of learning. This "psychoanatomy" mapping assumes that learning specificity reflects the response selectivities of the modified neurons. Two major conclusions emerged from these studies:

1. Learning can be very specific for basic visual dimensions, suggesting that learning can take place at very low-level cortical sites where neurons are selective for these basic visual dimensions.

2. The degree of specificity to the trained stimuli varies greatly across subjects and task conditions, suggesting that the learning site is not fixed.

The stimulation features that were tested for specificity include stimulus retinal position, stimulated eye, and stimulus size and orientation. In general, the scales of the specificities found were such that do not allow precise localization of a single underlying cortical area (see also chapters 8–13). After training with the target presented at a consistent retinal position, there was little improvement in performance with the target at other retinal positions (Ahissar and Hochstein 1995, 1996b; but see also qualified below). Substantial degradation in performance was found for a 0.7° shift in target (between training and testing sets) position within the array from near to farther away. Surprisingly, a shift twice as large, from one position right to one position left of fixation (or vice versa) did not hamper performance. The transfer across such distances, which are very large in terms of the size of receptive fields in area VI, suggests that, under these conditions, learning occurred, not in the primary visual area, but rather in areas that retain cruder retinal position selectivity. Although similar results were found for some other tasks (Berardi and Fiorentini 1987; cf. chapter 9; Karni and Sagi 1991;

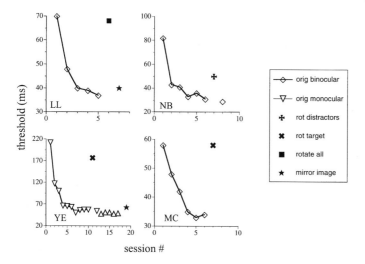

Figure 14.2
Orientation specificity to a variety of orientation manipulations in four subjects (L. L., N. B., Y. E., M. C.): rotating (rot) distractors (cross), rotating (rot) target only (X), and rotating all elements by 30° (square). All manipulations produce a substantial threshold increment, except left-right mirror reversal (star). Subject Y. E. was trained and tested monocularly (right eye: downward-pointing triangles; left eye: upward-pointing triangles), whereas other subjects were trained and tested binocularly. Subjects were presented a fixed 7 × 7 array, with target in any of central 5 × 5 position, except corners and fixation positions for subjects L. L. and M. C.; with target at one of two diagonal positions for subject N. B.; and with target as described in figure 14.6 for subject Y. E.

see chapter 10; Schoups, Vogels, and Orban 1995; see chapter 5), large degrees of spatial transfer (e.g., Treisman et al. 1992) and huge variability between different subjects (e.g., Fahle 1994; see chapter 11, Beard, Levi, and Rich 1995) were also observed using similar experimental procedures. Training with one eye and testing with the other, we did not find ocular specificity (figure 14.2; see Ahissar and Hochstein 1996), although some studies have (Karni and Sagi 1991; but see also Schoups and Orban 1996).

We observed specificity for a variety of orientation manipulations, including rotation of the target, the distractor elements, or both, or swapping their orientations (figures 14.2 and 14.3; see Ahissar and Hochstein 1993, 1996b). Orientation specificity was

also observed in all other reported studies that looked for it (Poggio, Fahle, and Edelman 1992; Fahle and Edelman 1993, Beard, Levi, and Reich 1995; Ramachandran and Braddick 1973; Shiu and Pashler 1992; Schoups, Vogels, and Orban 1995; Fiorentini and Berardi 1981; Treisman, Vieira, and Hayes 1992; Karni and Sagi 1991; Polat and Sagi 1994), although large between-subject variations for orientation specificity were also found, as illustrated in the distribution of orientation specificity across subjects plotted in figure 14.4 (see also Fahle and Edelman 1993). Size specificity was also observed (Ahissar and Hochstein 1993, 1996b; see also Fiorentini and Berardi 1981) together with a surprising asymmetry: no transfer occurred from big to small

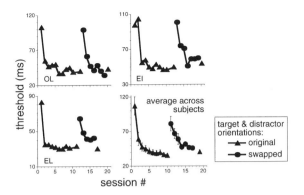

Figure 14.3
Learning and specificity for swapped orientations. The graphs show examples for three subjects (O. L., E. I., E. L.), and average for ten subjects (*lower right*) who trained with original orientations (triangles) and were subsequently tested and retrained with swapped target and distractor orientations (circles). Following several training sessions, subjects were retested with the originally trained orientations, to examine whether there was interference (final triangle). Note there is nearly no transfer to the swapped orientations condition (first circle), that is, learning had to begin again. Furthermore, learning for the swapped condition is somewhat slower than the original learning. On the other hand, after training with the swapped orientations, there was no interference when retesting with the original orientation condition—final triangle has just as low a threshold as asymptote before swapped orientation training—a finding contrary to the predictions of the hypothesis of modifications at the earliest site.

stimuli, but a large transfer was apparent from small to big (Ahissar and Hochstein 1996b).

In summary, among subjects trained with a consistent set of stimuli, learning is largely specific for position, orientation, and size (and sometimes for the eye trained), indicating a low-level cortical site for learning. However, the large variability of these specificities suggests that the site of learning may also be variable.

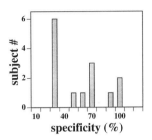

Figure 14.4
Distribution of percent specificity for 90° rotation across subjects. For each subject, the percent specificity is the increment in threshold induced by orientation manipulation relative to the total difference in threshold between first and asymptotic sessions. Note that the distribution is not normal. Data were collected from fourteen subjects trained with the task version illustrated in figure 14.6.

14.3.2 Learning Does Not Interfere with Seemingly Conflicting Stimuli

One training condition consistently yielded almost complete specificity to the trained orientations. In this condition, the target could be in any of 48 positions of a 7 × 7 array (all element positions excluding fixation). Despite the uncertainty of target position, training led to a dramatic improvement in performance, which was extremely specific to both target and distractor orientations. We asked whether the mechanisms underlying learning in this case involved neuronal changes within the earliest level that contained orientation-selective neurons (Ahissar et al. 1998). Such a mechanism would be simple, and would have the advantage of not needing a very sophisticated selective teaching mechanism (e.g., prior connections could be strengthened with training experience).

Our rationale was that several types of changes within the earliest level with orientation selective units could increase the salience of the odd element.

We rejected these changes one by one, as follows:

1. An increase in target detector sensitivity. If learning involved only this change, improvement would be selective only to the orientation of the target and would not depend on the orientation of the distractors. We found, however, that learning was specific for both orientations.

2. An increase in lateral inhibition among the distractor elements. The odd element would become more salient when background activity was reduced. If learning involved only such a change, then improvement would only be selective to the orientation of the consistently trained distractors and would not depend on target orientation because target detector activity would be constant and target salience would be just a by-product of interdistractor inhibition and its augmentation. We found, however, that though learning was specific to the orientation of the distractors, it was even more specific to that of the target.

3. An increase in lateral interactions between target and distractor elements, by increased facilitation from distractor detectors onto target detectors, by increased inhibition in the reverse direction, or, alternatively, by a combination of changes 1 and 2 above. If learning involved only these changes, the orientation of the trained target would have to be more salient than the orientation of the trained distractors. Thus, if we changed the array so that the orientations were swapped—the target assumed the previous distractor orientation and vice versa—initial performance should be even worse than in that of the naive state. Moreover, there should be no way that subjects could maximally enjoy training effects for practice both with one set of orientations and then with the swapped set of orientations. Improvement with one set of orientations should interfere and disrupt performance with the other because

these stimuli would induce conflicting directions of modifications (for a description of a specific model having this characteristic, see Peres and Hochstein 1994). We found, however, that none of these predictions proved true. Initial performance with swapped orientations (following original training) was not worse, and even somewhat better than naive performance. Optimal asymptotic performance was reached in both sets of orientations without interference, although learning of the swapped set was, for some subjects, slower than learning of the first set (as illustrated in figure 14.3).

These results refute the simplest, earliest-level hypothesis, indicating that the bulk of improvement in orientation detection does not stem from changes in lateral connections between simple orientation detectors. Changes underlying learning must occur at levels receiving their inputs from these earliest stages. Yet refuting a specific simple hypothesis does not indicate where learning does occur; indeed, it leaves many alternatives open. A more specific theory for choosing the site of modifications underlying behavioral improvement is discussed below.

14.3.3 Task Difficulty Determines Learning Specificity

While searching for the source of stimulus specificity and learning-site variability, we found that task difficulty plays a crucial determining role (Ahissar and Hochstein 1997). In a series of studies, we systematically manipulated the difficulty of the orientation detection task for different subject groups. Task difficulty was modified by training with different orientation gradients (target-distractor differences of 90°, 30°, and 16°), different target position conditions (target in 1 of 48 possible array positions; or in 1 of 2 easy horizontal positions or of 2 more difficult diagonal positions), and different processing times (SOAs). Consistently, in groups that trained with more difficult conditions, learning specificity for position and for orientation was larger than in groups training with easier conditions, as illustrated (for orientation) in figure 14.5, panel A. These results suggested that, for different groups trained with essentially the same task but with different degrees of difficulty, modifications underlying learning occur at different cortical sites.

Using a within-subject design, stimulus specificities at different processing durations (SOAs) were also compared (our training procedure employed blocks of different SOAs for each subject, as briefly described in the caption for panel A of figure 14.1; see Ahissar and Hochstein 1997 for further details). The dependence on SOA followed the same rule as the dependence on difficulty stemming from orientation gradient or target position. Increasingly difficult conditions (shorter SOAs) activated increasingly specific learning processes. Figure 14.5, panel B, demonstrates this dependence. The different degrees of stimulus specificities shown within each subject suggest that different learning sites, dictated by different degrees of task difficulty, may also characterize the learning process within a single individual.

As noted above, we attribute specificity to receptive field characteristics at the site of task performance and modification. Because receptive fields are more selective for basic stimulus dimensions at lower cortical levels, greater specificity is associated with lower-level task performance and learning. Thus the linkage between task difficulty and learning specificity indicates that easy learning takes place at high cortical levels (which generalize over basic stimulus dimensions), whereas difficult learning takes place at low cortical levels. Thus learning may take place at a variety of sites along the visual hierarchy, beginning at very high levels for easier task conditions, and

reaching down, for more difficult conditions, to levels which receive direct input from the lowest level that contains direct representation of the tested dimension.

14.4 The Role of Attention in Early Perceptual Learning

14.4.1 Selective Attention Is Necessary for Learning

Would learning of this simple detection task occur even without task-directed attention? To address this question, we designed a paradigm to ensure that subjects attended the stimuli, and became familiar with them, while performing a different task. We then asked whether implicit learning occurred, that is, whether practicing the different task with these stimuli improved their performance in orientation detection. To this aim, we modified the stimulus set so that in addition to odd-orientation detection, another task of similar difficulty could be trained and tested using the same set of stimuli (Ahissar and Hochstein 1993; see also Shiu and Pashler 1992; Treisman, Vieira, and Hayes 1992; Fahle 1997). The additional task required attention to another aspect of the same stimuli. Subjects were asked whether the entire array was vertically or horizontally aligned. Adding this task required modification of the original task, such that the array now consisted of either 5×6 or 6×5 elements, as well as being with or without an element of odd orientation (the four types of stimuli are illustrated in figure 14.6a). All four types of stimuli were equally likely. On the first two sessions, each subject was tested (and trained) with odd-element detection and array orientation, respectively. In the following sessions, half the subjects trained on one task and half trained on the other. When they reached a steady performance

A. learning curves & orientation specificity for 4 training conditions

B. orientation specificity

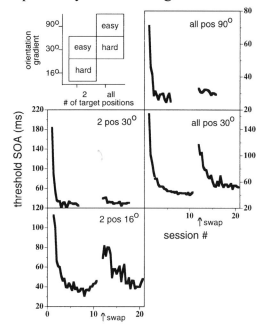

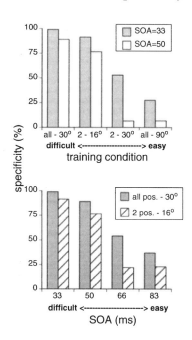

Figure 14.5

Linkage between task difficulty and learning specificity. (*A*) Comparison of learning specificity under four training paradigms. Target could appear at any array position (with equal probabilities) except fixation (all: right column) or at one of two positions (2 pos: left column). Target orientation deviated from that of distractors by 90°, 30°, or 16° (top, middle, bottom rows, respectively). Hard conditions are 2 pos 16° or all pos 30° and easy conditions are 2 pos 30° or all pos 90° (see inset at top left). Transfer to new orientations and positions was larger for easy than for hard task conditions. Average threshold is plotted as a function of thirds of session for each of the four subject groups. Note improvement, and transfer for easy conditions. (Bottom plot begins at the second third of the first session, because subjects barely noticed the target initially; threshold was 220 msec.) (*B*) Comparison of relative orientation specificity (performance decrement after orientation swapping as percentage of total gained improvement) for the four training conditions and different stimulus onset asynchronies (SOAs). Specificity for fixed SOA (*top*) decreases with decreased task difficulty; specificity for fixed paradigms and within subjects (*bottom*) decreases with increased SOA.

A
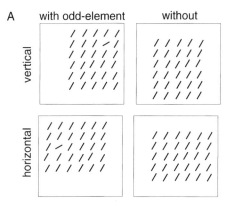

B
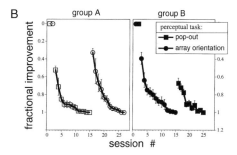

Figure 14.6a
Stimulus set of four stimulus types used to test cross-task learning transfer. Subjects trained on "local" odd-element orientation detection learned to differentiate between the left and right panels. Subjects trained on "global" array orientation detection learned to differentiate between upper and lower panels.

Figure 14.6b
Learning curves showing relative threshold change due to learning the "local" orientation detection task and to subsequent training on the "global" array orientation task (group A at left); and vice versa (group B at right). Note that learning in both cases is task specific, though there is some small degree of global to local task transfer.

level, all subjects were tested and trained with the complementary task.

We found that practicing orientation detection did not affect subjects' performance on the array alignment task. Practicing the array orientation task improved subjects' performance on the detection task, but only to a small extent. In both cases, further practice with the new task improved performance substantially. These effects are illustrated in figure 14.6b.

Our results indicate that attention is essential for learning even simple tasks. It is important to note that the role of attention in learning these two tasks was critical and robust. Whereas stimulus specificity characterized only some subjects under some conditions, task specificity characterized all trained subjects. The finding that learning odd-orientation detection can be specific to both basic stimulus spatial parameters and the attended task suggests that learning occurred at an early cortical stage and yet

was governed by attentional selection. Thus substantial top-down effects must influence low-level representations (Tsotsos 1990; Nakayama 1991; Motter 1993; Ahissar and Ahissar 1994; Rosenthal and Hochstein 1994; Ishay and Sagi 1995; Ullman 1995; Treisman 1996; see chapter 20).

The near absence of learning when subjects did not attend to the stimulus aspects that were relevant to task performance in simple feature detection tasks constitutes strong evidence against the possibility of learning irrelevant cues. Although one example cannot prove that such learning never occurs, we are not aware of any condition where learning unattended features has been unequivocally demonstrated. On the contrary, data that were previously interpreted as indicating learning without attention have recently been reinterpreted. For example, previous findings on learning rules without explicit instruction to attend to these rules were often interpreted as indicating unselective (automatic) learning of deep and global structures. However, it was recently shown that improvement may only be found when subjects can use what they are learning while they are learning it. Thus, before the training phase, subjects were told to attend the presented items, and after the training but before the test phase, they were told they were now to determine legality. Therefore, they could have used deep structure as a memory aid during the training phase, or they could have (intentionally) analyzed the memorized sequences to figure out their deep structure during the test phase. Indeed, if subjects are not instructed to judge legality, but implicit recollection is tested, for example, by asking about "pleasantness" of the stimuli, they do not recognize (i.e., consider as pleasant) novel items that follow the same deep structure as the test set. Thus there is no evidence for implicit learning of the rules when these are irrelevant (see Wright and Whittlesea 1998). Another phenomenon, priming for spelling homophone words presented to the unattended ear, was, on careful reexamination, also eliminated (Cowan and Wood 1997). These examples imply that while learning may not requires awareness, it requires selective attention. Indeed, Bar and Biederman (1999) have demonstrated subliminal priming for briefly presented object drawings. Their subjects were not able to consciously identify the objects, yet they actively attempted to identify them during both their first and second exposures. Thus, performance may improve without awareness of the learning process, but there is no evidence that it can occur without selective attention.

Taken together, these data seriously call into question whether any purely perceptual task of detection, discrimination, or identification can be learned without aspect-specific attention.

14.4.2 Selective Attention Is Sufficient for Learning

We have seen that attention is necessary for training, but is it sufficient? We have seen that stimulus pres-ence is not sufficient, but is it necessary? Suggesting the contrary may seem strange, having found that learning may be quite specific to the trained set of stimuli, that is, that no learning is found for stimuli that were not presented. Indeed, stimulus presentation is essential, but perhaps its importance does not stem from the need for bottom-up activation. Its importance may stem from the top-down search mechanism needing guidance. Sorting out these two alternatives is difficult. For example, we found, (as described above), that when subjects practice the detection of a target presented near fixation, they do not improve in detection of targets farther away from fixation. This position specificity may stem from the need for bottom-up activation to induce learning at this position. Alternatively, it may result from selective attention being allocated to this position, in which case, if we can induce subjects to pay "the right kind" of attention to a position where no target is presented, their detection at this position would improve. To test this, we had a group of subjects practice orientation detection with targets at one of two positions, two elements to the right or to the left of the fixation point (Ahissar and Hochstein 1996a, 2000). Because attending two separate positions with no "attentional link" between them was expected to be difficult, we reasoned that subjects might attend to a single "window of attention" extending from one target position to the other and including the area between them. We found that learning occurred for the entire area between and including the two target positions, but not for other areas of the array (as illustrated by the before and after "learning maps" of figure 14.7). Thus learning occurred where attention was allocated, regardless of whether a target was ever presented in these positions. Similar findings for interpolation of improvement in a vernier acuity task were reported by Beard et al. (1996).

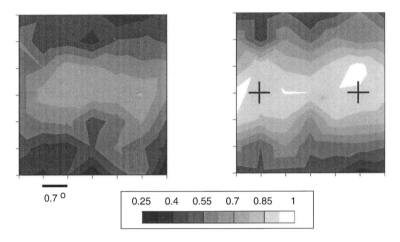

Figure 14.7
Detection maps before (*left*) and after (*right*) training with target at one of two nonadjacent horizontal positions (denoted by +). Improvement affected a single continuous area spanning intermediate positions. Brightness of map region indicates fraction of detection of targets at that position (see scale at bottom center) in pre- and postlearning sessions. The maps are measured by pre- and posttraining sessions with the target presented in any position in the 7 × 7 array.

These findings are consistent with the interpretation that the role of the stimulus in perceptual learning is mainly to guide the top-down search mechanism to select the appropriate population. A more specific hypothesis for this selection mechanism is presented below.

14.4.3 A Unified Hypothesis: The Reverse Hierarchy Theory

The well-studied anatomical and physiological hierarchy of cortical visual areas defines the sequence of stimulus processing (Van Essen et al. 1990). We propose that learning begins at high levels and proceeds downward in reverse direction along this hierarchy (see schematic illustration in figure 14.8). The reverse hierarchy theory rests on three basic concepts (Ahissar and Hochstein 1997):

1. *Multiple representations.* Multiple mechanisms exist within the visual hierarchical pathways for performing each perceptual task. Processing within a particular level of the hierarchy is chosen for determining the performance of the task. Perceptual learning is seen as a gradual refinement of the neuronal population selected as the best for implementing the task.

2. *Reverse hierarchy.* Selection of the neuronal population whose activity will determine task performance begins at the top of the visual hierarchy and proceeds downward. Selective attention chooses activity in higher-level populations (e.g., the inferotemporal cortical areas) as a default level. The advantage of these levels is that their representations are tuned to global entities in the external world, such as objects (rather than to local features, as in lower-level areas). Indeed, we see and attend to objects rather than features, unless otherwise specifi-

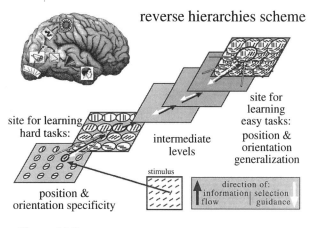

reverse hierarchies scheme

site for learning
hard tasks:

intermediate
levels

site for
learning
easy tasks:
position &
orientation
generalization

position &
orientation specificity

stimulus

direction of:
information | selection
flow | guidance

Figure 14.8
Schematic illustration of the reverse hierarchy theory. Circles denote neuron groups (e.g., cortical columns) and the
lines inside them their particular orientation preference.
Bold lines mark bottom-up stimulus-activated neuron
groups and paths interconnecting them. For example, target
element bar is shown to be initially encoded by orientation-
selective neurons at the lowest level. At subsequent levels,
there is substantial convergence across positions (second
level) and orientations (top level). Thus the orientation of
the original target signal is gradually undiscriminated, and
its salience diminished when neurons integrate over many
orientations (and convergence refines more abstract features). Spatial attention and learning are initially directed at
the highest, spatially generalizing levels. For easy conditions (e.g., large orientation gradient and long stimulus
onset asynchrony, or SOA) high levels suffice: even
diminished salience leaves some distinction between target
presence and absence. In this case, learning occurs at a high
level (e.g., by selecting among its inputs). If insufficient
signal remains at high levels, subjects may be stuck. Alternatively, if high-level mechanisms are pinpointed by easy
condition training, they may be used to direct attention
and learning to appropriate lower level mechanisms, within
the subdomain of their inputs. The learning cascade (figure
14.9) may reflect reverse order search along the hierarchy.
For these lower level mechanisms, learning will be restricted to trained orientations and positions, reflecting
increased spatial selectivity at this level. When a new
stimulus is presented (e.g. with swapped orientations),

cally instructed or required by the task at hand. Thus
neuronal populations in higher areas, which generalize over basic spatial stimulus dimensions, are used
(and dictate perception) in novel task conditions. In
tasks requiring some form of spatial resolution, such
as orientation detection, activity differences within
these higher-level populations are sufficient to make
easy discriminations. For resolving spatially difficult
task conditions, the search system needs to gain access to a better resolving representation. Thus successful performance under spatially difficult task
conditions requires selection of a neural population
in lower levels. The disadvantage of low-level learning is its specificity to the spatial attributes of the
trained stimulus.

3. *Search tree.* The selection mechanism seeks
better-resolving populations of neurons when these
are needed. Better-resolving populations are those
that yield a better signal-to-noise ratio with respect to
the presumed current task demands. Access to these
populations is achieved using a search tree. A downward search tree (Tsotsos 1990) is followed to the
subdomain of active input units, which provide a
better signal-to-noise ratio. Thus initial high-level
learning enables, but does not obviate, low-level
learning for hard cases.

common stimulus characteristics suffice for easy case (long
SOA) performance; high level mechanisms of the hierarchy, common for both orientation sets, result in large
transfer between orientations (figure 14.5—easy conditions). For difficult cases (small orientation gradient, short
SOA, or both), the lower-level mechanisms where learning
effects occur are spatially selective and inappropriate novel
stimuli. Reverse hierarchy paths from the common top-
level mechanism will have to be used again to redirect
learning to different low-level sites. This redirection may
account for short-SOA retarded learning when swapping
orientations (figure 14.3).

The reverse hierarchy theory maps behavioral patterns to a physiological framework and consequently provides a unified terminology. For example, specificity to basic spatial features was previously interpreted as stemming from learning at low cortical areas. However, some subjects show this specificity, whereas others, trained under the same conditions, do not. This variability, attributed to strategic differences, was not addressed by previous psychophysical studies. We now suggest that the broad range of specificities may be accounted for within a single set of rules, which dictate the pattern of choosing a site for learning rather than a specific site chosen for all subjects under given training conditions. Although the same rules apply to all subjects, the specific site chosen by the search mechanism depends on the saliency of the difference for each subject's visual system. Because, given different genetics and experience, the saliency of the same stimulus varies across subjects, attaining a specific level of saliency may lead to different choices of learning site in different subjects.

Interestingly, the reverse hierarchy theory unifies terminology of both stimulus-driven (e.g., physiological) processing and attention-driven (e.g., psychological) processing. Stimulus processing is bottom-up and its hierarchy follows a bottom-up sequence, as revealed in anatomical and physiological studies. In this respect, area V1 is "early" or low level. On the other hand, attention processing (which guides learning) follows a top-down sequence that begins at higher areas. From the attention perspective, area V1 is "later" or higher-level and is reached only when spatial resolution is needed. Thus an apparent paradox between interpretations is easily resolved. Treisman, Vieira, and Hayes (1992) found that learning an easy feature search transfers across positions, whereas learning a difficult conjunction search is largely position spe-

cific. Associating feature search with low-level areas and conjunction search with higher areas is at odds with physiological results indicating small receptive fields in lower-level areas and large receptive fields in higher areas. The reverse hierarchy theory claims, instead, that easy feature search is learned high along the bottom-up hierarchy, but "early" within the top-down hierarchy of attention. Difficult conjunction search requires more selective spatial attention choosing lower-level populations and consequently yielding position-specific learning.

14.5 Accounting for a Plethora of Behavioral Findings

14.5.1 Learning along a Continuum

A robust finding in both the laboratory and daily experience is the phenomenon of "learning along a continuum" described by Pavlov almost a hundred years ago (see Sutherland and Mackintosh 1971 for review). Pavlov used the conditioned reflex as a tool for studying the behavior of learning. He found that, when he induced conditioning with a single pure tone, the dog salivated also to the sound of neighboring tones, an effect he called "stimulus generalization." To obtain more specific conditioning, he had to train the dog to differentiate by repeatedly reinforcing (giving a reward for) one tone and not the other. But when these stimuli were very similar, the dog could not learn to differentiate between them even after training for a long time. Pavlov discovered that it was preferable to begin training with easy discriminations. He therefore first used stimuli that were very different from each other and then gradually diminished the difference between them. This type of experimental procedure is called "transfer along a continuum." One starts with an easy discrimination, and the easy learning transfers to somewhat more difficult discriminations, and so on. Since Pavlov's time, this procedure has been repeated often, notably, by Lawrence (1952) and Sutherland (et al. 1963), who found it has the air of a paradox: "Animals pre-trained with an easy discrimination perform more accurately on a difficult problem than animals trained from the outset on the same difficult problem" (Sutherland and Macintosh 1971). The surprising aspect is that, to achieve optimal performance with a difficult discrimination task, it would be best not to train with this difficult task for many trials, even if correct responses are rewarded. It would be best to first give easier, more informative trials.

Given our daily experience, "transfer along a continuum" is not intuitively surprising. That is, we all know that easy cases are a good introduction to hard ones. We come to appreciate the paradox when we try to account for this finding in terms of underlying mechanisms.

Learning is traditionally viewed as strengthening the connection between representation of the applied stimulus and that of the rewarded response. We would thus expect that the greatest stimulus-response strength would be achieved by repeated application of the desired stimulus-response association. Sutherland and Mackintosh (1971) tried to account for this seeming paradox by assuming intermediate stages between those activated by the stimulus and those underlying the choice of response. Differentiation is achieved by learning in stages that code the stimulus. The system needs to "figure out" which connections within these stimulus-coding stages should be strengthened. On the other hand, the repeated stimulus-response association strengthens only connections between the output of the stimulus-coding stages and those representing the specific re-

sponse. Thus, if the discrimination required at the onset of training is too difficult, the system will not figure out which changes should be made and differentiation will not be achieved. Still, the connections associating between the perceived stimulus and the reward will be strengthened. The reverse hierarchy theory is thus largely an extension of the learning theory proposed by Sutherland and Mackintosh, whereby "learning to attend" is described in a more concrete framework.

14.5.2 Learning Dynamics and Enabling: The "Eureka" Effect

The reverse hierarchy theory has two specific predictions with respect to learning dynamics:

1. Learning will proceed from easy to difficult cases even when these are presented in a mixed order. Analyzing the dynamics of learning by examining improvement within each SOA separately revealed a cascade of learning (figure 14.9, left): learning at each SOA was sigmoidal. The rising phase started earliest for easiest SOAs, and only after substantial improvement was obtained for these did improvement begin for harder, shorter SOAs. The slower improvement for short SOAs reached asymptote only after more than two sessions (figure 14.9, right).

The finding of a cascade of improvement is strong support for the assumption that learning of different degrees of difficulty occurs in separate neuronal populations. Consider the alternative, that learning affects different extents of a single network, depending on training condition. In this case, difficult tasks (for which we found stimulus specificity) would modify a subpopulation of that changed by easier tasks (for which there is more learning transfer to new conditions). In the context of our paradigm with interleaved blocks of easy and difficult trials, a

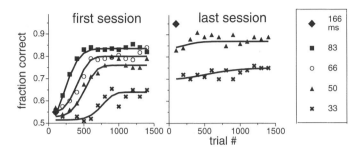

Figure 14.9
Dynamics of improvement for each stimulus onset asynchrony (SOA). Average fraction correct is plotted as a function of trial number for the group practicing with the target anywhere within the array and with target-distractor orientation gradient of 30°. Short blocks (20 trials) of different SOAs were presented in pseudorandom order so that, on average, various SOAs were presented within each 100-trial bin plotted here. During the first session (*left*), performance for each SOA remained at first near chance (50%), and improvement began only following some practice. The extent of this initial plateau was SOA dependent, being short (several dozen trials) for long SOAs and long for short SOAs (~400 trials for 50 msec SOA; >500 trials for 33 msec SOA). The slope of improvement was also SOA dependent, being steeper for longer SOAs. Toward the end of the first session, performance stabilized. Further improvement was gained on subsequent sessions, as seen by comparison to asymptotic performance in the last session (*right*).

natural outcome of the latter interpretation is that training easy conditions would induce immediate improvement for harder conditions. The temporal offset between improvement for different degrees of difficulty suggests that modifications occur at separate neuronal levels.

2. If training includes only difficult cases, even substantial practice may not yield improvement because the system will not have acquired a pointer to the appropriate lower-level site containing a detailed spatial representation. This phenomenon, as described above, had already been noted by Pavlov. We tested this in the context of orientation detection. A group of subjects was trained for a whole session with only 50 msec SOA (without feedback). This SOA was chosen because most subjects managed eventually to improve on 50 msec SOA trials substantially when they were intermixed with easier blocks of trials (figure 14.9). As predicted, when only

hard cases were trained, most subjects showed no improvement throughout the session (figure 14.10, left), even though they were shown a schematic illustration of the stimulus.

The more interesting prediction of the theory is that the system need only perceive one easy case to highlight the appropriate low-level region. Searching for a positive result, we tested another group of subjects with the difficult case following a long (30 sec) presentation of the whole array on the monitor screen, once with and once without an odd element. The results for this group were categorically different: most subjects showed dramatic improvement (figure 14.10, right). We called this large, single-presentation enabling of learning the "Eureka" effect (Ahissar and Hochstein 1997). Consistent results were also found in other paradigms involving subjective contours (Rubin, Nakayama, and Shapley 1997; see chapter 13) and texture discrimination (Papathomas et al. 1999).

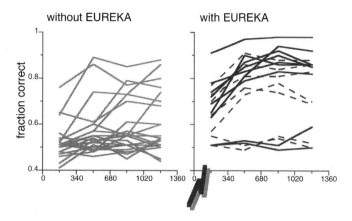

Figure 14.10
"Eureka" effect. Each curve plots performance of one subject. Subjects received verbal instructions and were shown pen and pencil drawings of the array with and without an odd element. (*Left*) When presented only with threshold-level trials of 50 msec stimulus onset asynchrony, most subjects failed to improve at all during their first session. Indeed, 16 out of 23 failed to reach 60% correct even in last quarter of first session (compare figure 14.9, left, triangles, where same 50 msec trials were interleaved with easier trials). (*Right*) Following an extended view of the stimulus, once with and once without the odd element, most subjects improved dramatically during the first session: 12 out of 16 exceeded 70% correct (dashed lines indicate subjects who were tested with swapped orientations relative to enabling stimulus, as in figure 14.1, panel A).

14.5.3   *The Drawbacks of Spoon-Feeding*

Intuitively, we think that spoon-feeding is not an effective training procedure if one wants to encourage creative, independent thinking. Perceptual training may follow the same rule. Spoon-feeding, in the context of the reverse hierarchy theory, is intensive training with explicit examples spanning a whole continuum of the easy to difficult range. Training may be effective because subjects can gradually learn to discriminate between similar examples (see above). Yet the cost may appear in subsequent training with a different, but similar set of examples. Initially, performance may gain from previous training. Higher-level nodes, used for the previous, similar set, may help to resolve the easy cases. But solving the more difficult cases, which require a more specifically tuned representation, may now be harder to achieve. The

extensively trained continuum has marked a path along the search tree leading to the populations best suited for the previously trained examples. Subsequent search may get trapped into following the marked path when seeking backward for appropriate nodes. Thus finding the best-suited population for resolving the novel examples may be harder and more laborious than initial learning. As in daily examples of problem solving, subjects will more likely choose the previously experienced solution than a potentially more appropriate novel one.

This seems to be the case in training orientation detection. Learning along the continuum is effective when training a whole range of SOAs. Later training, with swapped orientations, begins with somewhat better initial performance, but attains a similar asymptotic performance level and takes longer than training with the original set, as illustrated in figure

14.3. Interestingly, using a single Eureka presentation, thus bypassing some nodes (though not too many because that would result in a frustrating condition, with no learning at all), subsequent learning with different orientations is not slower than the original learning set (Ahissar and Hochstein 1997).

The reverse hierarchy thus defines guidelines for an optimal training procedure. Training should aim for conditions in which sufficient stimulation is provided to initiate and direct an appropriate attentional search. Yet it is better to avoid the full continuum so as not to overmark paths that need to be avoided in the future when conditions change.

14.6 Attentional Constraints

1. *We can learn only one thing at a time.* We have seen that learning needs attention. But perhaps this attention can be divided between several (two or more) tasks that subjects perform simultaneously. To test this, we trained a group of subjects under dual-task conditions (Ahissar and Hochstein 1998b; Ahissar, Laiwand, and Hochstein 2001). In each trial, given a single stimulus presentation, subjects were asked to perform two tasks. One task was detection of an oddly oriented element. The second task was identification of a letter (*T* or *L*) presented at the point of fixation. We expected that subjects performing the two tasks would gradually improve on both. Surprisingly, we found that even though we asked subjects to perform both tasks in each trial, improvement was almost always separate (19 out of 20 subjects). Consistently, subjects' performance first improved on the letter identification task at fixation, whereas their performance on the detection task was at chance level. Then there was a period lasting a few hundred to a few thousand trials during which performance with the central letter task was perfect, and yet no

improvement was apparent in performing the orientation detection task. Only later did improvement begin on the detection task (Ahissar, Laiwand, and Hochstein 2001). Task learning seems to require undivided attention. The order of learning for these tasks did not depend on the order of the response. Half of the subjects answered first "1"/"0" for odd-orientation presence/absence, and then "1"/"0" for *T/L*; and the other half answered in the reverse order. Nevertheless, the central letter task took priority in securing the undivided attention required for learning. Odd-orientation detection began to improve only after the central identification task was mastered.

2. *Performance always requires attention.* Subjects trained under dual-task conditions achieved successful dual-task performance. After several training sessions with each task separately, or with both concurrently, their performance of each task under the dual-task condition was almost as good as their performance of each task separately. We asked whether this gained success indeed reflected automatic performance unconstrained by the need for the limited attentional resources. We reasoned that if tasks were performed automatically and independently, making one task harder would degrade performance of this task, yet would not affect the other. Introducing novel stimuli largely reverses the effects of learning. We therefore expected that changing the stimuli for one task would degrade performance with this task. Thus changing the orientation of the array elements was expected to degrade performance in orientation detection, whereas changing the central letter was expected to degrade letter identification. Alternatively, processing for the two tasks might still require limited attentional resources even after training. In the latter case, we would expect cross-task interference.

We found an asymmetric pattern of interference. Changing all array elements by swapping the orientation of the target and distractor bars hampered orientation detection but had no effect on central letter identification. On the other hand, changing the central symbol from *T* or *L* to *Y* or ↑ hampered performance of both tasks (Ahissar, Laiwand, and Hochstein 2001). This pattern of interference suggests that, even when dual-task performance is almost as good as single-task performance, processing still requires (limited) attentional resources. In our case, the task that received priority, either by being performed first or by receiving more attentional resources, was central letter identification. The source of this preference may be that the letter was at fixation, whereas the orientation detection task required spreading out attention peripherally to a large portion of the array (Hochstein et al. 2000).

In summary, we have tried various methods of training a simple visual task. Although subjects' task performance substantially improved and they needed dramatically less processing time, their improved performance was not accompanied by acquired automaticity. Their performance became more efficient, but processing was still governed by the initial attentional limitations.

Acknowledgments

We thank Anne Treisman, Robert Shapley, Howard Hock, Ehud Zohary, and Ehud Ahissar for helpful discussions and comments. Work on this chapter was supported by grants from the Israel Science Foundation of the Israel Academy of Sciences and Humanities, the U.S.-Israel Binational Science Foundation (BSF), and the National Institute for Psychobiology in Israel.

High-Level Learning of Early Visual Tasks

Pawan Sinha and Tomaso Poggio

15

Abstract

Does learning shape perception? Recent experimental results have provided strong evidence demonstrating the experience-dependent malleability of perceptual processes. Several lines of reasoning suggest that the locus of learning in the reported instances is situated very early along the processing pathway. Whether high-level, object-specific learning can influence early perception is still a largely unresolved question. This chapter reviews recent models and experimental findings pertinent to this question in the context of a specific visual perceptual task—the recovery of three-dimensional structures from single two-dimensional line drawings. We discuss the limitations of shape recovery models devoid of high-level learning-based influences; we present experiments that explore whether high-level learning plays a role in three-dimensional form perception in humans; and we propose a computational model for incorporating high-level learning in early perception. The reviewed research points toward an impending unification of early perception and high-level (or "cognitive") visual learning. We conclude with a discussion of some of the basic open questions that need to be addressed to achieve this unification.

15.1 Introduction

The fundamental question of whether learning shapes perception has a rich history, going back more than two centuries to the early philosophical debates between empiricists such as John Locke (1632–1704) and George Berkeley (1685–1753), on the one hand, and idealists such as René Descartes (1596–1650) and Immanuel Kant (1724–1804), on the other. Over the past few decades, however, two lines of experimental evidence have convinced most cognitive scientists that learning does indeed shape perception.

The first of these lines clearly demonstrates the influence of early visual experience on the development of neural substrates that underlie perception. Hubel and Wiesel's pioneering studies (1970) showed that atypical early visual experience profoundly influenced the development of binocular cells and orientation tuning in the primary visual cortex (figure 15.1; cf. Introduction). They found, for instance, that a kitten forced to wear an eye patch while a few months old would subsequently exhibit severe deficits in stereoscopic depth perception. The inescapable conclusion was that unsupervised learning, mediated by early visual experience, was critically important for the normal development of perceptual processes. These findings have been confirmed and extended by several researchers over the past three decades (see Kaas 1994 for review).

The second line of evidence in support of the influence of learning on perception is amply represented in this volume (see especially chapters 9–14). Starting with Volkman's experiments (1858) on practice-dependent improvements in two-point thresholds, many behavioral studies have reported long-term effects of learning in simple perceptual tasks (see Ahissar and Hochstein 1998 for review). Figure 15.2 panel a, shows a perceptual learning curve from Fahle, Edelman, and Poggio's work (1995) on practice-dependent improvements in vernier acuity—a result representative of the findings of many other studies.

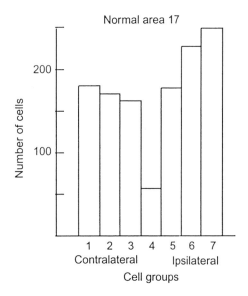

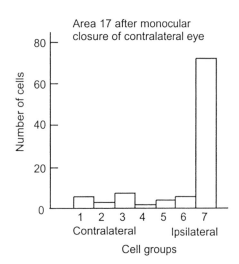

Figure 15.1
Distribution of cells in monkey striate cortex (area 17) from a normal animal (*top*) and from a monocularly deprived one (*bottom*). (Adapted from Hubel, Wiesel, and LeVay 1977.)

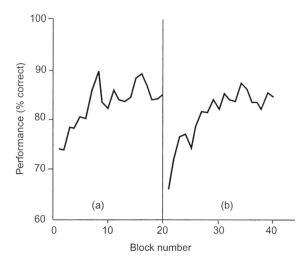

Figure 15.2
(*a*) Perceptual learning curve showing practice-dependent improvements on the vernier hyperacuity task. (From Fahle, Edelman, and Poggio 1995.) (*b*) Perceptual learning curve showing nontransference of learning to a differently oriented vernier task.

Although in the face of these two lines of evidence, the question of whether learning shapes perception can only be answered in the affirmative, there are still several fundamental issues that remain to be resolved. In this chapter, we shall focus on one of them.

15.2   An Open Issue in Perceptual Learning

The second part of Fahle, Edelman, and Poggio's perceptual learning curve (1995; see panel b of figure 15.2) shows the progress of learning when the vernier task is changed from a vertical to a horizontal stimulus. Clearly, this simple change in the stimulus requires a nearly complete relearning of the task. Such a result is typical; researchers have repeatedly found that the perceptual learning by subjects is strongly tied to some simple stimulus dimension. Thus, for example, learning often fails to generalize across stimulus orientation (Ramachandran and Braddick 1973; Berardi and Fiorentini 1987), retinal position (Nazir and O'Regan 1990; Dill and Fahle 1999; see chapter 12), retinal size (Ahissar and Hochstein 1993, 1995, 1996), and even across the two eyes (Karni and Sagi 1991, 1993; Polat and Sagi 1994; see chapter 10). It seems that improvements in subjects' performance cannot be attributed to the development of some abstract, stimulus-invariant, cognitive strategies. These results have led investigators to infer that the locus of visual learning is relatively early along the visual processing pathway, perhaps in cortical area V1. "Low-level" learning is thus believed to play an important role in shaping early perception. But is this the only avenue for changing early perception? Can learning at a later locus ("high-level" learning) also influence early perception? It is on this question that we shall focus.

Before proceeding, however, let us define our key terms. *High-level learning* refers to learning that is object or object class specific—that requires a prior recognition step to come to bear on a task; *early perception* refers to perception involving tasks supposedly performed by the early visual stages in a non-object-specific manner, such as three-dimensional shape recovery, edge detection, and image segmentation.

15.2.1   *Why This Question?*

The inherent incompatibility of our definitions of "high-level learning" (object specific) and "early perception" (*not* object specific) makes the issue of the possible influence of the first on the second a very intriguing one. The decision to focus on this issue is motivated by (1) its being a fundamental unresolved issue and (2) the possibility of revising our conceptualization of visual processing.

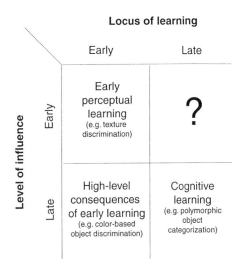

Figure 15.3
Of the four possible combinations of locus of learning and level of influence, three have been extensively studied. The fourth (*upper right*), which involves learned high-level influences on early perception, is still open to debate.

If, as in figure 15.3, we were to construct a 2 × 2 diagram of locus of learning versus level of influence (early perception or late perception), we find that of the four possible combinations, only one remains largely unresolved. Given the studies reviewed above, there is little doubt that low-level learning influences early perception, and therefore high-level perception as well. Also, there is no reason to doubt that high-level learning plays a role in high-level perception (e.g., learning about an object would influence how well it is subsequently recognized). However, the case for the fourth combination, high-level learning influencing early perception, is not quite so clear. Can cognitive knowledge actually influence the perception of basic visual attributes?

Conventionally, the visual system is believed to be organized hierarchically, with the computation of basic visual attributes such as depth, color, and mo-

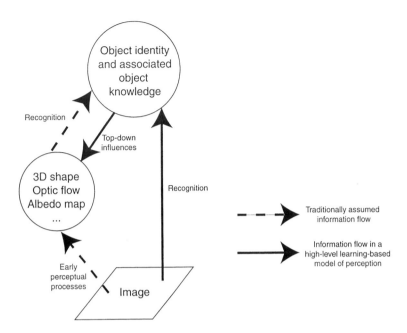

Figure 15.4
In conventional conceptualizations of visual processing, information is believed to flow primarily in the forward direction, from the image to the early visual areas and thence to the higher stations. That it may flow in the opposite direction represents a radical departure from the conventional scheme (cf. chapter 20, this volume). It is important to remember that the two schemes are not mutually exclusive. Both patterns of information flow may coexist.

tion being accomplished by early stages, and the results being sent on to the later stations concerned with visual cognition (figure 15.4). The possibility that learning at the later stages influences the computation of basic attributes can profoundly change this general hierarchical conceptualization. It may suggest that in addition to flowing from early perceptual stages to the later ones, visual information may also move in the reverse direction.

15.3   Previous Work

Here we review three important past attempts to determine whether early perception is shaped by high-level influences and then summarize the criti-

cisms that have been leveled against them. Our overall aim in this section is to suggest that, despite a rich history of research, the issue of high-level influences on early perception is still contentious and largely open.

15.3.1   High-Level Influences on Early Perception: The Case "For"

Prior Expectations
Several studies have shown a strong influence of prior expectations on the perceptual interpretation of ambiguous figures. Many of the stimuli used in these studies, such as the wife and mother-in-law picture in Boring 1930 (see figure 15.5, panel a) and the Dalmatian dog photograph reprinted in Gold-

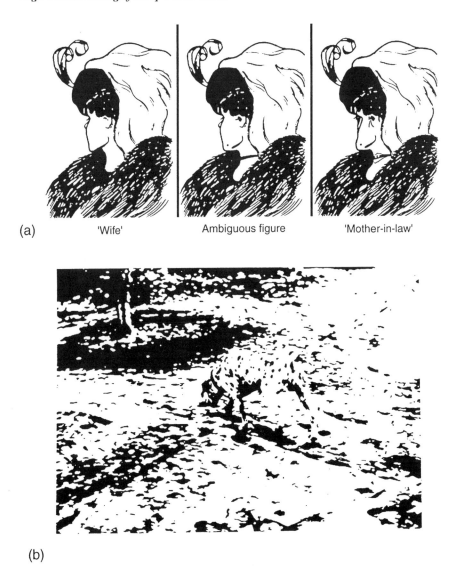

(a)   'Wife'   Ambiguous figure   'Mother-in-law'

(b)

Figure 15.5
Pictures that illustrate high-level influences on image interpretation. (*a*) "Wife" (*left*) becomes ambiguous figure (*middle*), which then becomes "mother-in-law" (*right*). (From Boring 1930.) (*b*) Dalmatian dog picture. (From Goldstein 1996.)

stein 1996 (see panel b) are now well known to any student of perceptual psychology. Typically, an ambiguous figure is interpreted differently depending on the prior biases inculcated in the observers. For instance, if observers look at the Boring picture after looking at a version disambiguated in favor of the wife, they are much more likely to perceive the picture as showing a young woman (wife) than an older one (mother-in-law). Naïve observers are equally likely to see either interpretation. Such results have been presented as evidence that high-level expectations can dramatically influence perception.

Personal Attitudes

Beginning with the influential work of Bruner (1951), several "new look" perceptionists suggested that personal attitudes and values can both render observers more attentive to certain aspects of a stimulus and actually distort their perception of the same. In one of the most famous experiments cited as evidence for this claim, Bruner and Goodman (1947) reported that the extent to which school children overestimated the size of a coin was a function not only of the coin's value, but also of the children's needs. Thus poor children overestimated the size of coins to a greater degree than rich children. Similar effects of attitudes on perception were reported by Bruner and Postman (1947). In their "perceptual defense" experiments, they found that observers' thresholds of perception were much higher for tachistoscopically presented socially taboo words than for other random words: "These phenomena suggest to the guileless investigator the image of the superego peering through a Judas eye, scanning incoming percepts in order to decide which shall be permitted into consciousness." A vast body of such experiments attempted to build a strong case for an intimate role of high-level attitudes in shaping basic perception.

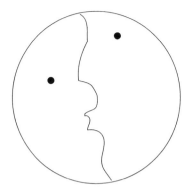

Figure 15.6
Ambiguous figure. (From Schafer and Murphy 1943.)

Reward and Punishment

Schafer and Murphy (1943) reported that the assignment of figure and ground in an ambiguous picture (figure 15.6) could be controlled by reinforcing one interpretation over the other through the use of monetary rewards. Although criticized on many grounds, this experiment prompted several other studies that sought to explore the influence of high-level rewards and punishments on early perception. Among these were Smith and Hochberg 1954, which employed electric shocks to influence figure-ground assignments, and Hochberg and Brook 1958, which showed that polygonal figures negatively reinforced with "chalk-on-blackboard screeches" were less well recognized than other figures.

Though a significant body of data was collected by the late 1950s, there were often disagreements between studies conducted by different laboratories. A case in point is Pustell 1957, which showed that shock associated figures were discerned more clearly than nonshocked figures—a finding contrary to those of Smith and Hochberg 1954 and Hochberg and Brook 1958. These differences notwithstanding, the overall implication in all these studies was that even relatively high-level reinforcement contingencies could modify subjects' perception.

15.3.2 High-Level Influences on Early Perception: The Case "Against"

Although the studies reviewed in section 15.3.1 appear to provide strong evidence in support of the idea that early perception may indeed be influenced by high-level cognitive processes, several researchers have challenged them on a variety of grounds. Three key criticisms are listed below.

1. The experimental data show changes in feature grouping rather than changes in the perception of attributes per se. Thus, for example, the change in an observer's percept from a meaningless collection of blobs to a meaningful scene in the well-known Dalmatian dog picture may involve, not a fundamental change in the basic perceived attributes such as edges and gray levels, but simply a cognitive regrouping of these attributes. For another example, the act of seeing faces in clouds may be based not so much on a change in the perception of basic visual attributes as on a cognitive restructuring of the available perceptual tokens.

2. It is not clear from the data whether responses are driven by a change in cognitive decision criteria or perception. Experiments most susceptible to this criticism purportedly demonstrate an influence of personal attitudes, values, and high-level reward-and-punishment contingencies on early perception, yet their results can as easily be accounted for by a deliberate change in response criteria as by any fundamental changes in perception per se.

3. Simple natural constraints can account for percepts. This criticism is motivated by whether it is at all necessary to invoke high-level influences to explain perception, or whether perception can be accounted for completely by simple bottom-up mechanisms that incorporate some general-purpose natural constraints. The usefulness and versatility of bottom-up mechanisms has been demonstrated in a few different domains, such as color perception (Land's Retinex model; Land and McCann 1971; Land 1983) and the perception of structure from motion (Ullman's use of the rigidity constraint; Ullman 1979). It is thus plausible that perception is simply a matter of identifying the right natural constraints and embedding them in perceptual mechanisms that can function in a bottom-up fashion without requiring high-level, object-specific knowledge. One of the most articulate proponents of this idea is Zenon Pylyshyn (1984, 1999), who has attempted to explain perceptual phenomena believed to be due to high-level influences more simply via appropriate bottom-up processes. He has championed the view that early perception is cognitively impenetrable, according to which it would be difficult, if not impossible, to demonstrate any high-level influences on early perception.

Thus it is fair to say that, despite a rich history of research, whether there exist high-level influences on early perception is still largely an open question. In the sections to follow, we describe some recent experimental and computational work that, by revisiting this question, provides stronger evidence that high-level learning does indeed influence early perception.

15.3.3 Does High-Level Learning Influence Early Perception? Recent Work

A few recent studies have provided evidence suggesting that high-level learning plays a role in different perceptual tasks. Notable among these are Peterson and Gibson 1993, 1994, which found that the first perceived figure-ground organization of briefly presented stimuli is strongly determined by the identity of the regions that make up the display. Moore and Cavanagh 1998 also found evidence that recognition of two-tone images is important for their interpretation as three-dimensional structures.

15.4 The Problem of Three-Dimensional Shape Recovery from Two-Dimensional Images

It is widely believed that one of the key objectives of early visual processing is to extract the three-dimensional structure of the visual world from the two-dimensional images impinging on the retinas (Clowes 1971; Waltz 1972; Horn 1975; Barrow and Tenenbaum 1981; Marr 1982; Yuille 1987). The visual system has to be able to perform this task even in the absence of binocular disparity, shading, texture, and motion parallax information, say, when looking at a single static two-dimensional line drawing (figure 15.7). What makes this perceptual task fascinating is the fact that it is highly unconstrained, that is, corresponding to any single 2-D image, there are infinitely many projectionally consistent 3-D structures (see figure 15.8). Yet, more often than not, the visual system can unambiguously zero in on the "correct" three-dimensional interpretation. Our choice of this particular task is motivated by three principal reasons:

1. Few other perceptual tasks are considered to be as central to the study of human vision as three-dimensional shape recovery.

2. Past work is overwhelmingly in favor of bottom-up, constraint-based explanations for how the visual system recovers three-dimensional shapes (Koffka 1935; Attneave and Frost 1969; Barrow and Tenenbaum 1981; Kanade 1981; Brady and Yuille 1983;

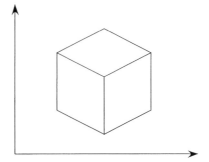

Figure 15.7
Planar line drawing. Despite the paucity of cues in such drawings, the visual system is often able to interpret them as three-dimensional structures. This remarkable ability has been the subject of much research, although significant gaps remain in our understanding of how this task is accomplished.

Marill 1992; Fischler and Leclerc 1992), widely believed to be an early visual task that provides inputs to the subsequent recognition processes.

3. Recent work examining high-level influences on the three-dimensional shape recovery task has involved a good mix of experimental investigations and computational modeling.

15.4.1 Capabilities of Bottom-Up Constraint-Based Models of Three-Dimensional Shape Recovery

Are high-level influences necessary for performing the task of three-dimensional shape recovery? According to most research thus far, the answer is no. As Pylyshyn (1999) argues, although such an early visual task may not be "cognitively impenetrable," general-purpose natural constraints should, by themselves, provide an adequate account of this perceptual ability.

In keeping with this hypothesis, nearly all proposals for three-dimensional shape recovery thus far have relied on the use of a few fixed, and perhaps

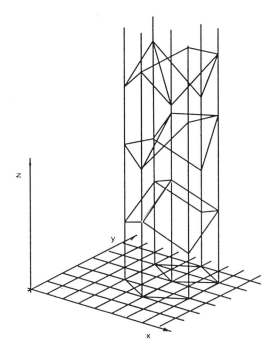

Figure 15.8
Underconstrainedness of three-dimensional shape recovery. Any planar line drawing is geometrically consistent with infinitely many 3-D structures, which makes the 3-D shape recovery task very challenging.

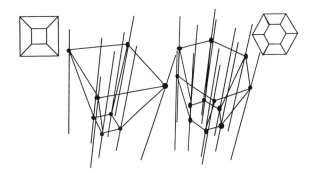

Figure 15.9
Two sample three-dimensional shape recovery results obtained by Sinha and Adelson's algorithm (1993).

innately specified, shape constraints (Koffka 1935; Attneave and Frost 1969; Barrow and Tenenbaum 1981; Kanade 1981; Brady and Yuille 1983; Marill 1992; Fischler and Leclerc 1992). The idea is to select the particular 3-D interpretation, from among the infinitely many, that best satisfies the chosen shape constraints. Typically, the constraints reflect the distinguishing characteristic of a perceptually favored 3-D interpretation: its low "complexity." Thus, for example, Sinha and Adelson (1993) and Sinha (1995) proposed that, to properly characterize the perceptually "correct" interpretations in the domain of polyhedrons, three types of measures are

required: angle variance, planarity of faces, and overcall compactness. They devised computer programs that incorporated these shape constraints (in essence, implementing a constrained optimization approach). Figure 15.9 shows two sample shape recovery results obtained using their program.

The Sinha and Adelson (1993) approach worked well on several input patterns, some of which are shown in figure 15.10. In each case, the approach recovered a three-dimensional shape that was consistent with the reported percepts of human subjects. Based on these successes, Sinha and Adelson concluded that the shape constraints they had identified had some perceptual relevance.

The critical next question was to assess the generality of these constraints. In other words, do these constraints provide a unified strategy for shape recovery across very different kinds of inputs? Further experiments by Sinha and Adelson (personal communication, 1993) suggested otherwise. Even though their procedure had worked well for several problem instances drawn from the class of polyhedra, it failed to generalize to inputs from more unconstrained domains, such as the class of natural objects.

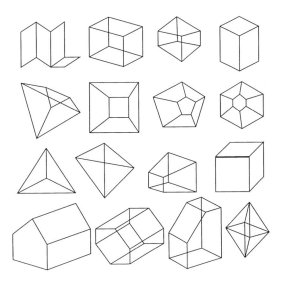

Figure 15.10
Sample test images for which Sinha and Adelson's algorithm (1993) produces perceptually correct three-dimensional shapes.

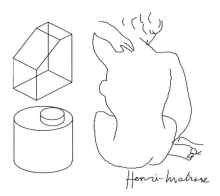

Figure 15.11
Two-dimensional images conveying a vivid sense of three-dimensionality. Computational schemes that employ a small set of prespecified shape biases have been able to mimic human 3-D shape perception with images of relatively regular geometric objects, such as the two shown on the left. They prove ineffective, however, in more general domains, which might contain images such as the Matisse line drawing shown on the right. (From Sinha and Poggio 1996.)

A simple line drawing from this class, which is uninterpretable by the procedure is shown in figure 15.11. Furthermore, there did not seem to be any obvious extensions of the procedure that would have enabled it to interpret these other inputs. This inability to generalize to inputs from different domains is not restricted to Sinha and Adelson's model. All other models of shape recovery proposed to date, without exception, share this shortcoming. Because the constraints employed by one model may bear little resemblance to those employed by another, it is not clear whether these constraint sets can ever be unified to have one procedure work across many different domains. As Hatfield and Epstein (1985) observed: "Our investigation leads us to believe that a global minimum principle, which acts as a cardinal principle of perception, will not be obtained." Even if we ignore the lack of a common set of constraints,

there remains a more fundamental shortcoming—the domains of applicability include only very geometric objects such as polyhedrons and cylinders. None of the models can interpret inputs drawn from the large class of natural objects.

Thus, at least in a few constrained domains, bottom-up strategies of employing a few fixed shape biases, such as those favoring symmetry and other structural regularities, have been shown to be effective for uniquely inverting the many-to-one three-dimensional to two-dimensional projection process. Efforts to design a general-purpose bias set applicable across different domains, however, have thus far been unsuccessful. This failure, though not conclusively proving that such a set does not exist, makes it unlikely. Given this limitation of general-purpose strategies, we need to consider the possibility of incorporating learned object-specific knowledge in the shape recovery task. In the next section we review experimental evidence that supports just such a possibility.

15.4.2 Experimental Evidence for a Role of High-Level Learning in Three-Dimensional Shape Perception

A learning-based approach can potentially provide a uniform mechanism to account for three-dimensional shape perception across diverse input domains, which might arise from a learned association between specific two-dimensional projections and the previously experienced correlated 3-D structures. This idea dates back at least three centuries to the early empiricists (Locke 1690/1939; de Condillac 1754; Hume 1738/1956; Helmholtz 1866/1911) and more recently to some seminal work by Wallach, O'Connell, and Neisser (1953). However, because their results can be accounted for by subjects' cognitive decisions having little to do with shape perception per se, studies demonstrating shape learning have been considered inconclusive. Two recent experiments present evidence that object-specific learning of 3-D shapes can actually modify observer's subsequent percepts. The first experiment (Sinha and Poggio 1996) shows postlearning changes in the perception of kinetic depth effect (KDE; Wallach and O'Connell 1953), whereas the second (Bülthoff, Sinha, and Bülthoff 1996; Bülthoff, Bülthoff, and Sinha 1998) demonstrates changes in stereoscopic depth perception.

Experiment 1
Sinha and Poggio (1996) developed an experimental paradigm to objectively verify the role of learning in shape perception by rendering the learning percep-

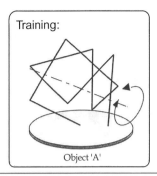

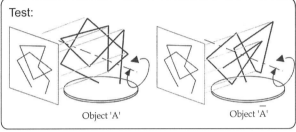

Figure 15.12
Sinha and Poggio's experimental paradigm. During the training phase (*top*), subjects saw a motion sequence of a rocking rigid three-dimensional object. In the subsequent test phase (*bottom*), after viewing either motion sequences of the training object or novel rigid objects, some of which had the same mean angle projection as the training object, subjects were asked to report whether the objects looked rigid or nonrigid. (From Sinha and Poggio 1996.)

tually manifest. They used this paradigm to show that the human visual system can learn an association between an arbitrary two-dimensional projection, which initially does not convey any impression of three-dimensionality, and a projectionally consistent but otherwise equally arbitrary three-dimensional structure.

Sinha and Poggio's experiment comprised a training and a test phase (figure 15.12). For use as stimuli, they generated random two-dimensional line drawings and assigned them arbitrary three-dimensional structures. During the training phase, to allow them to observe the correlation between the object's mean angle projection and its associated 3-D structure via the well-studied kinetic depth effect (KDE; Wallach and O'Connell 1953; Ullman 1979), subjects were shown one such object rocking through an angle of $\pm 20°$ about a frontoparallel horizontal axis passing through its centroid (the "training" object). The test phase commenced five seconds after the training session and was intended to assess subjects' shape learning. Subjects were shown either the training object rocking back and forth or another object having the same mean angle projection but a completely different 3-D structure (the "test" object). They were asked to indicate whether the objects shown looked rigid or nonrigid. Sinha and Poggio expected that if the subjects had indeed learned an association between the training object's mean angle projection and its 3-D structure, then, when presented with a test object having the same mean angle projection, they would perceptually impose on it the learned 3-D structure and the observed motion pattern would be mapped onto this learned structure. If the test object actually had a different 3-D structure, the sequence would appear to depict a nonrigid deformation. The experimenters expected that switching the roles of the training and test objects across different populations of subjects would lead to reversals in the patterns of results observed, and that subjects who had not undergone the training session would not perceive nonrigidity because of the well-known bias toward rigidity (Wallach and O'Connell 1953; Ullman 1979), possibly arising from visual experience over evolutionary timescales.

The subjects were placed in three nonoverlapping populations. Members of the first population individually underwent a training phase and then a test session, as described above. Each subject was tested with ten different objects, each object being used only once to prevent any given test session from serving as the training session for a later trial. To determine whether nonrigidity would be perceived even in the absence of any previous perceptual experience with a given object, members of the second (control) population did not undergo training sessions for any of the ten objects used. The procedure for the third population was identical in all respects to the procedure for the first except that the roles of the training and test objects were reversed. The experimenters expected to see a reversal of the pattern of results from population 1 to population 3 if the two-dimensional–three-dimensional association was truly a function of the visual experience during the training session.

Figure 15.13 shows the results from the three populations. The results are plotted as the percentage of trials (over all objects) during which subjects perceived nonrigidity in the object depicted in the motion sequence. Members of population 1 exhibit a clear effect of visual experience (panel a). While the training object appeared nonrigid for an average (across all four subjects) of 7.5% of the presentations, the test object (rotating about the same axis) appeared nonrigid in about 40% of the presentations. Members of population 2, on the other hand, perceived both the training and the test objects as being rigid in most of the presentations (panel b). Members belonging to population 3 exhibited a reverse pattern of results (panel c) relative to population 1.

The marked differences in the results of populations 1, 2, and 3 attest to the strong influence of visual experience on subsequent perception of three-dimensional form. One can conclude that it is possible for the human visual system to learn associations between arbitrary two-dimensional projections and 3-D structures, and that this learning subsequently

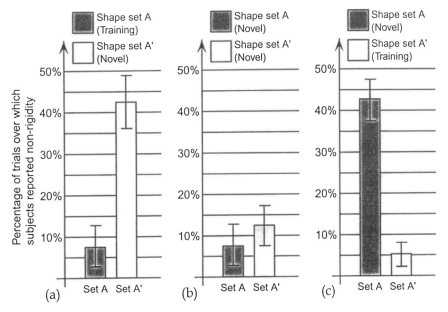

Figure 15.13
Results from three populations of subjects tested by Sinha and Poggio. Subjects were asked to indicate whether the objects shown in the motion sequences looked rigid or nonrigid. (*a*) Results from population 1 on training and test objects. (*b*) Results from population 2, who had not undergone any training sessions. (*c*) Results from population 3, for whom the training and test objects were switched relative to those for population 1. (From Sinha and Poggio 1996.)

influences 3-D form perception. At least for the kinds of objects considered in Sinha and Poggio's study, mutual temporal correlation seems more important for the formation of such associations than any intrinsic structural characteristics of the 2-D and 3-D shapes. Supporting this interpretation, subjects reported recognizing the test object as being the one they had seen during the training session.

To better characterize subjects' shape learning, the experimenters tested their performance under a few additional conditions. As figure 15.14, panel a, shows, the learning is long-lasting. Two subjects from population 1 who were trained for ten minutes on each of five objects (five training sessions of two-minute sequences evenly spaced over four hours on

each of the five objects) exhibited significant effects of learning upon being tested a day later. Their learning also seemed to be object specific in that the percept of nonrigidity declined with the addition of two-dimensional positional noise to the vertices of the original projection (panel b), although transformations that preserved the shape of the training projection, such as image scaling, did not have a large effect on subjects' responses (panel c).

Figure 15.15 shows two illusions devised by Sinha and Poggio related to the ideas presented above. Panel a shows a situation in which a completely rigid wire-frame object resembling a person, when rocked around the vertical axis (sequence shown in panel b), is perceived as a person walking (a nonrigid inter-

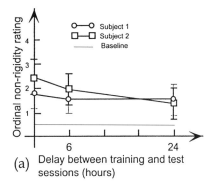

(a) Delay between training and test sessions (hours)

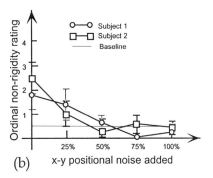

(b) x-y positional noise added

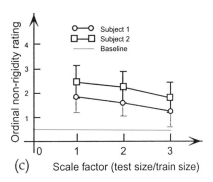

(c) Scale factor (test size/train size)

pretation). In this case, the association, learned in the course of our daily experience overrides the general bias towards a rigid interpretation. Panel c shows a noncuboidal object whose mean two-dimensional projection is the same as a cube's. A kinetic depth effect (KDE) sequence of this object rotating (panel d) looks highly nonrigid to most observers. Interestingly, if the vertices of this object are connected in a random fashion so it no longer looks like a cube (thus weakening the shape expectations), it begins to look like a rigid object.

The idea that three-dimensional shape perception might be mediated, at least in part, by object-specific learning has a direct corollary: 3-D shape perception may sometimes *follow* recognition rather than precede it (because the visual system has to be able to recognize the two-dimensional projection to access its associated 3-D structure). This idea, also suggested by Cavanagh (1991), runs contrary to the traditionally assumed hierarchy of visual processing, according to which recognition depends on the results of a bottom-up 3-D shape recovery process (Marr 1982).

These results have a strong bearing on the long-standing debate between empiricists and idealists on the issue of three-dimensional form perception. The latter have suggested that the human visual system might have some innately specified biases that allow even newborn infants to perceive simple two-dimensional pictures as 3-D forms. Sinha and Poggio's results suggest that these innate mechanisms might be complemented significantly by object-

Figure 15.14
Subjects were instructed to rate the perceived nonrigidity of training objects, which subtended, on average, a visual angle of 2.5°, on an ordinal scale, with "0" corresponding to a very rigid percept and "4" corresponding to a very nonrigid one. The gray horizontal line in all graphs is the baseline rating from a control group that did not undergo any training. (*a*) Persistence of shape learning over time. (*b*) Effect of adding two-dimensional positional noise to the mean projection of the test object. (*c*) Effect of changes in image scale on the percept of nonrigidity. (From Sinha and Poggio 1996.)

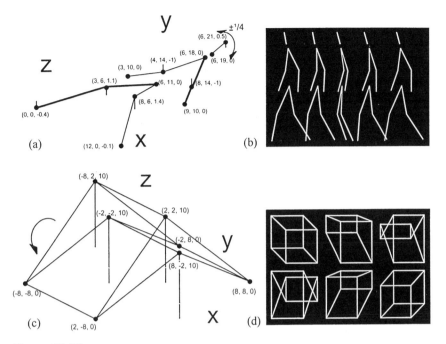

Figure 15.15

Two illusions devised by Sinha and Poggio to illustrate object-specific influences on the perception of kinetic depth effect (KDE) sequences. (*a*) This rigid structure, when rocked back and forth through an angle of 90° about the vertical axis, is perceived as a human walking (a nonrigid interpretation). (*b*) Frames from the motion sequence of structure in panel a. Mismatch between reality and perception is probably due to the recognition of the figure as a human, which leads the visual system to interpret the motion patterns in terms of how the human structure is expected to change, an expectation likely to have been learned through visual experience. The same vertex set, when not recognized as a human (say, when the vertices are connected up randomly) appears rigid upon rotation. (*c*) Object that projects to a cube (from a specific viewpoint) but has a very different three-dimensional structure. (*d*) Motion sequence of object in panel C, with cubelike projection, appears to depict a highly nonrigid object. When the vertices are connected randomly, the percept of rigidity is restored. Just as for the structure in panel a, the perceived nonrigidity here is likely to be due to the mismatch between the observer's expectations and the presented sequence. It is not clear whether the shape expectation for a cube (and other simple geometric objects) is learned during an observer's lifetime or is innate. (From Sinha and Poggio 1996.)

specific learning. Thus tasks conventionally assumed to be low level and hardwired might, at least in part, be learned through visual experience.

Experiment 2

Additional evidence showing high-level influences on early three-dimensional shape perception processes comes from Bülthoff, Sinha, and Bülthoff 1996 and Bülthoff, Bülthoff, and Sinha 1998 (see chapter 16). These studies differ from Sinha and Poggio's in two respects. First, they used dynamic nonrigid 3-D objects rather than rigid ones and second, they examined object-specific influences on stereoscopic depth perception rather than on KDE perception. Their basic finding was that subjects' high-level expectations about an object's 3-D structure could suppress the bottom-up depth information provided by binocular stereo.

The stimuli used by these three experimenters were variants of the biological motion displays popularized by Johansson (1973). Specifically, they were interested in the question of whether three-dimensional dynamic objects are represented using 3-D structural descriptions (Biederman 1987; Biederman and Gerhardstein 1993) or as two-dimensional motion traces. They started with the premise that if the internal representation for biological motion sequences is largely 2-D (Bülthoff and Edelman 1992), then scrambling the depth structure of such moving light sequences while leaving the 2-D traces unchanged should not adversely affect recognition performance. The three experimenters constructed a depth-scrambled human walker by adding uniform random noise to the depth positions of the points, while leaving their projections along the depth axis unchanged (figure 15.16). Subjects were shown stereoscopic motion sequences of this structure and asked to rate its structural goodness as a human figure on a scale from 1 (com-

pletely random) to 5 (completely human). Interspersed with these sequences, truly random and truly human (unscrambled) sequences were also presented to the subjects. As shown in figure 15.17, at a viewing position parallel to the depth axis depth-scrambled motion sequences were rated as high (4.54; standard error: 0.06) as unscrambled sequences (4.59; standard error: 0.07) by twenty-two subjects. The random sequences were rated much lower (2.45; standard error: 0.10). What caught the experimenters' attention was the seeming indifference on the part of the observers about whether they were viewing a depth-scrambled or a normal sequence: both such sequences were rated almost identically. There could be at least two explanations for this. Either the subjects were perceptually aware of the depth scrambling, but decided to base their ratings on 2-D "goodness," or they were perceptually unaware of the depth scrambling. This interesting open question led the three to design a second experiment to test for the existence of any recognition-dependent, top-down influences that might serve to suppress information about anomalous depth structure being provided by low-level binocular stereoscopic processes.

For use as stimuli, the Bülthoffs and Sinha created depth-scrambled biological motion sequences by adding six levels of arbitrary depth offsets to the trajectories of the body points, from 0% (no noise added) to 200% (a noise level of 100%). These offsets corresponded to a sequence of randomized depth positions of the individual points within the depth bounds of the original walker. The stimulus set also included x-y randomized versions of the depth-scrambled point walkers, which did not convey any impression of a human in motion. In each trial, after one walk cycle (about 1.5 sec), three points were highlighted by red outlines for 1 sec (about two-thirds of a complete walk cycle). Subjects had to

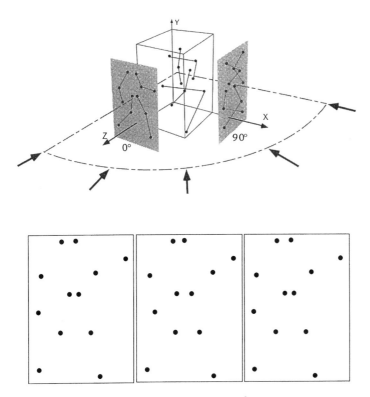

Figure 15.16
Depth-scrambling a three-dimensional motion sequence of a point walker (*top*) involves adding depth noise to the joint positions, while leaving their two-dimensional projections (in the *xy*-plane) largely unchanged. Stereograms of a single frame from a depth-distorted point walker sequence (*bottom*): left pair for cross-fusers and right pair for parallel fusers. (From Bülthoff, Bülthoff, and Sinha 1998.)

determine whether the three points lay in the same depth plane.

Figure 15.18 shows plots of false alarms (a response of "in same plane" when the points are in fact not in the same plane) for three conditions of stimulation (see figure caption) for the upright presentation as a function of depth noise level. The false alarm rate is highest for human sequences with points on the same limb. The three experimenters interpreted these results as pointing to the existence of a top-down influence capable of modulating the

information provided by the early processes of binocular stereoscopic depth perception. They hypothesized that recognition based on two-dimensional traces is accompanied by a strong top-down suppressive influence that renders observers less sensitive to anomalies in the depth structure of the presented stimulus. In keeping with its object-specific nature, this influence can be modulated by factors that change the recognizability of a stimulus. This hypothesis would explain why the false alarm rates for the human sequences are much higher than those for the

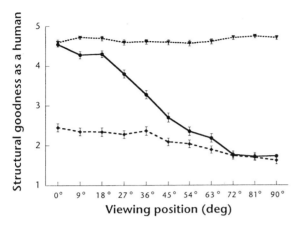

Figure 15.17
Results of goodness rating experiment averaged across twenty-two subjects. Subjects rated the presented sequences of a point walker on a scale from 1 (very random) to 5 (very human). At 0°, the walker is seen walking to the right with its depth axis parallel to the viewing axis; at 90°, the walker is seen walking toward the observer with its depth axis perpendicular to the viewing axis. Finely dashed curve = undistorted walker; solid curve = depth-distorted walker; coarsely dashed curve = walker distorted in x and z. (From Bülthoff, Bülthoff, and Sinha 1998.)

random ones. Also consistent with this hypothesis was the experimenters' finding that inverting the point walkers (an operation that reduces their recognizability while preserving all low-level cues) reduces the false alarm rate.

Summary

Experiments such as the two reviewed above have yielded data that strongly suggest the existence of learned object-specific influences on three-dimensional shape perception. As distinguished from studies reviewed in section 15.2, they render the high-level learning perceptually manifest; in other words, high-level learning changes observers' percepts per se, rather than merely changing their cog-

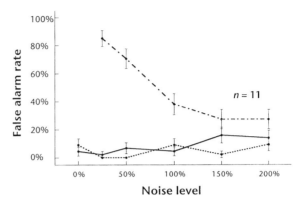

Figure 15.18
Depth discrimination for upright presentation. Dashed and dotted curve = human walker with the three marked points on the same limb; solid curve = human walker with the three marked points on different limbs; finely dashed curve = random sequence with three highlighted points. The false alarm rate is plotted against the maximum random depth distortion allowed in the sequence. (From Bülthoff, Bülthoff, and Sinha 1998.)

nitive decision criteria. It is also important to note that the perceptual processes undergoing change in these experiments (kinetic depth effect perception in experiment 1 and binocular stereoscopic depth perception in experiment 2) have traditionally been assigned to early vision, and therefore considered immune to top-down influences. Having reviewed evidence for the existence of learned high-level influences on early perception, we turn now to a recent attempt to computationally model these phenomena.

15.4.3 A Computational Model for Incorporating High-Level Learning in Early Perception

Let us first consider, in conceptual terms, what such a model must do. The model's overall task, to estimate perceptual attributes of an object in an image based on previously acquired knowledge about that object or its class, can be subdivided into four parts:

1. The model must recognize objects in images at the basic or subordinate level (Rosch et al. 1976).

2. The model must access previously learned knowledge (such as three-dimensional shape or location of depth discontinuities) associated with the recognized object; accordingly, it must be able to represent object- or class-specific knowledge or both.

3. If it lacks appropriate object-specific knowledge, the model must be able to generate it from class-specific knowledge.

4. Having generated perceptual attributes corresponding to the object in a top-down fashion, the model must combine it with information about the same attributes estimated by the bottom-up processes.

Some of these tasks clearly represent profound challenges in vision research. For example, we currently do not possess a general-purpose strategy for object recognition, nor do we know how top-down estimates are combined with bottom-up data under different circumstances. Clearly, a comprehensive model to perform all of these tasks is at present beyond our reach, although lesser models for restricted problem domains may be feasible. Jones et al. (1997) recently proposed a simple model that focused on items 2 and 3 from the list above.

Jones et al.'s Model for Incorporating Learned High-Level Influences in Early Perception

Jones et al.'s computational strategy (1997) for incorporating high-level influences in perception uses the concept of "flexible models" introduced by Vetter, Jones, and Poggio (Poggio and Vetter 1992;

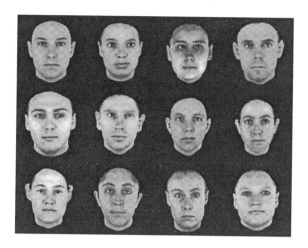

Figure 15.19
Twelve of the 100 prototype faces that were set in pixel-wise correspondence and then used for a flexible model of human faces. (From Jones et al. 1997.)

Jones and Poggio 1995; see also Beymer and Poggio 1996). Their flexible model is the affine closure of the linear space spanned by the shape and the texture vectors associated with a set of prototypical images (figure 15.19). First, pixel correspondences between a reference image and other prototype images are computed using an optical flow algorithm, and an image is represented as a "shape vector" and a "texture vector." The shape vector specifies how the two-dimensional shape of the example differs from a reference image and corresponds to the flow field between the two images (see figure 15.20). Likewise, the texture vector specifies how the image texture, that is, the pixel intensities (gray-level or color values) of the image, differs from the reference texture. The flexible model for an object class is thus a linear combination of the example shape and texture vectors. The matching of the model to a novel image consists of optimizing the linear coefficients of the shape and texture components.

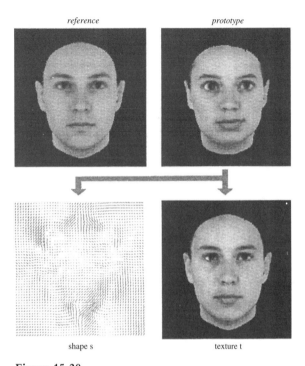

Figure 15.20
Image structure vectorized by shape and texture. Shape **s** (*bottom left*) consists of the displacements between each pixel in the reference image (*top left*) relative to its corresponding position in the prototype image (*top right*), whereas texture **t** (*bottom right*) is the texture of the prototype image warped to the shape of the standard reference image. The shape **s** field warps the reference image (*top left*) into the prototype image (*top right*). (From Jones et al. 1997.)

Once estimated, the parameters of the flexible model can be used for effectively learning a simple visual task, such as three-dimensional shape recovery for face images, in the following way. Assume that a good 3-D shape estimate is available for each of the prototypical gray-level images (obtained initially in a bottom-up fashion perhaps via haptic inputs or binocular stereo). Then, given the image of a novel face, the Jones et al. strategy (1997) is to estimate the parameters of the best-fitting gray-level flexible model and to plug the same parameter values into a second flexible model built from the prototypical 3-D shape estimates. This strategy can be regarded as learning the mapping between a gray-level face image and its 3-D shape from a set of examples. To demonstrate their ideas, Jones et al. (1997) implemented a slightly different version of the shape recovery task. Instead of explicit shape estimation (depth recovery for each point on the object), they focused on the task of implicit shape recovery in the form of novel view estimation. The view estimation problem is an implicit shape recovery task because even though it is tied to the 3-D shape of an object, it does not require an explicit computation of the 3-D structure. This problem arises in recognition tasks in which an object, for which only one example image is available, has to be recognized from a novel view. Poggio and Vetter (1992) had also considered this problem for linear object classes and concluded that an object belongs to a linear class if its 3-D structure can be exactly described as a linear combination of the 3-D structure of a small number of prototypes. A new, "virtual" view of an object that belongs to a linear class can be generated exactly from a single example view, represented as a two-dimensional shape vector, provided appropriate prototypical views of other objects in the same class are available (under orthographic projection). In this way, new views of a specific face with a different pose can be estimated and synthesized from a single view (the procedure is exact for linear classes; empirically, faces seem to be close to a linear class, so that the procedure above provides a good approximation for pose and expression). Again, this procedure can be formulated in terms of the learning metaphor in which a learning box is trained with input-output pairs of prototypical views representing each prototype in the initial and in the desired pose.

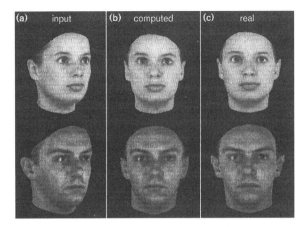

Figure 15.21
Results of using the Jones et al. algorithm to generate novel views of three-dimensional objects such as human heads. (*a*) Input images; (*b*) computed frontal views; (*c*) real frontal views, included in order to allow an assessment of the fidelity of the computed results. (From Jones et al. 1997.)

Then, for a new input image, the system synthesizes a virtual view in the desired pose (figure 15.21).

The model is not limited to the task of implicit three-dimensional shape recovery. Explicit estimation of 3-D structure from a single image would proceed in a very similar way, provided the image and the 3-D structure of a sufficient number of prototypical objects of the same class were available (Poggio and Vetter 1992; Vetter and Poggio 1996). In Jones et al.'s learning box metaphor (1997), the system, trained with pairs of prototype images as inputs (represented as two-dimensional shape vectors) and with their 3-D shape as output, would effectively compute shape for novel images of the same class (compare with the somewhat different approach of Redlich et al. 1996).

In discussing the generality of their model, Jones et al. (1997) suggested that a similar approach might

be extended to other supposedly early perceptual tasks such as edge detection, color constancy, and motion analysis, where the desired information about edge locations, color, or motion would need to be provided in a learning-from-examples scheme based on the use of a class-specific flexible model. To substantiate their claim of generality, Jones et al. considered the problem of edge detection at length. We briefly summarize their approach and results on this task next.

Jones et al. (1997) started with the premise that an edge map corresponding to a gray-level image should ideally capture all the "relevant" edges of the object, in a way similar to an artist's line drawing. As many years of work on edge detection have shown (for review, see Marr and Hildreth 1980; Haralick 1980; Canny 1986), the problem is difficult, in part because physical edges—meant as discontinuities in three-dimensional structure and albedo that convey information about the object's shape and identity—do not always generate intensity edges in the image. Conversely, intensity edges are often due to shading, therefore depend on illumination and do not reflect invariant properties of the object. Several years ago the Turing Institute circulated a photograph of a face and asked fellow scientists to mark "edges" in the image. Some of the edges found by the subjects of these informal experiments corresponded, not to any change in intensity in the picture, but rather to locations where the subjects knew that the 3-D shape had a discontinuity, for example, the chin boundary. The traditional approach to edge detection—to use a general-purpose edge detector such as a directional derivative followed by a nonlinear operation—is bound to fail in the task of producing a good line drawing, even if coupled with algorithms that attempt to fill edge gaps, using general principles such as good continuation, and colinearity (Shashua and Ullman 1988). A quite different approach, and the one adopted by Jones et al., is to exploit specific knowledge about faces in order to compute the line drawing. This approach runs contrary to the traditional wisdom in computer vision, because it assumes that object recognition is used for edge detection—almost a complete subversion of the usual paradigm. A possible implementation of this approach is based on a learning metaphor. Consider a set of prototypical (gray-level) face images and the corresponding line drawings, drawn by an artist. The task is to learn from these examples the mapping that associates to a gray-level image of a face its "ideal" line drawing. Computationally, this task is analogous to the problem of view prediction described above.

Jones et al. (1997) implemented an even simpler version of the scheme. They assumed that the ideal line drawing corresponding to the average prototype is available from an artist, as shown in figure 15.22. Matching the flexible model obtained from the prototypes (some of which are shown in figure 15.19) to a novel gray-level image provided a shape vector that was a linear combination of the prototypes and that effectively prescribed how to warp the average shape of the gray-level prototype in order to match the shape of the novel gray-level image. Because

the line drawings were supported on a subset of the pixels of the corresponding gray-level images, the line drawings associated with novel images could be straightforwardly obtained by warping the line drawing associated with the reference prototype using the estimated shape vector (see figure 15.20). Figure 15.23 shows a few examples of novel images (not contained in the set of Jones et al. prototypical examples) and the line drawing estimated from each of them by Jones et al.'s "ideal edge detector." To

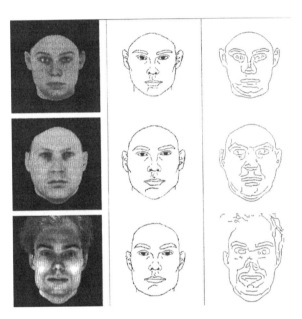

Figure 15.23
Examples of ideal edges found by the Jones et al. algorithm. The left column shows the input novel images. The middle column shows the line drawings estimated automatically by the algorithm, which matches the flexible models to the novel images and then appropriately modifies the ideal edges of the reference image. For comparison, the right column shows the edges found by a bottom-up edge detector (Canny 1986). Note that the ideal edges emphasize the perceptually significant features of the face much better than the Canny edges. (From Jones et al. 1997.)

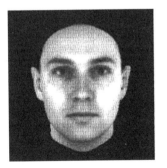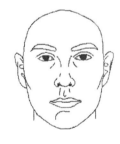

Figure 15.22
Reference face (*left*) and corresponding line drawing (*right*) created by an artist. (From Jones et al. 1997.)

contrast this approach to a low-level gradient-based approach, figure 15.23 also shows the edges found for each face image by a Canny (1986) edge detector. Figure 15.24 shows the ideal edge estimated for a partially occluded input image. As is evident from the examples, Jones et al.'s algorithm can detect and complete edges that do not correspond to any intensity gradients in the image. The power of the algorithm derives from the high-level knowledge about faces learned from the set of prototypical images.

Thus the scheme proposed by Jones et al. (1997) is an example of a class of algorithms that can be used to learn visual tasks in a top-down way, specific to object classes. From the point of view of a neuroscientist, these demonstrations are nothing more than plausibility proofs that a simple learning process can successfully incorporate object-specific knowledge and thereby learn to perform seemingly "low-level" visual tasks in a top-down manner (Cavanagh

1991; Mumford 1992; Ullman 1995). We conjecture that visual perception in humans may rely on similar processes to a greater extent than commonly assumed. Of course, biological vision may use bottom-up verification routines to validate the top-down "hallucination." A similar verification approach (top-down and bottom-up) could also be effectively used in machine vision implementations such as the one described here.

Logically, our conjecture consists of two somewhat independent parts. First, at least in some cases, our visual system may solve low-level vision problems by exploiting prior information specific to the task and to the type of visual input. And second, visual systems may learn algorithms specific to a class of objects by associating in each "prototypical" example an "ideal" output to the input view—the main thesis of this chapter. The "ideal" outputs may be available through other sensory modalities, sequences of images in time, or even explicit instruc-

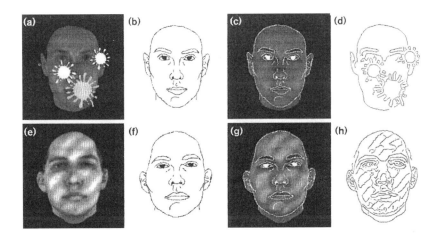

Figure 15.24
Examples of ideal edges found for degraded inputs. (*a, e*) Of the two input face images, the first (*a*) is partially occluded, whereas the second (*e*) has spurious edges such as those caused by patterned shadows. (*b, f*) Edges found by the Jones et al. algorithm for inputs in panels a and e. (*c, g*) Ideal edges superimposed on the gray-level images. (*d, h*) Edges estimated by a bottom-up operator. (From Jones et al. 1997.)

tion. The notion of what constitutes an "ideal" output corresponding to a certain class of inputs may change and evolve over time as the learning process encounters new examples. The second part of our conjecture predicts that human subjects should be able to learn to associate arbitrary outputs to input images and to generalize from these learned associations, a prediction confirmed by recent psychophysical evidence, as we saw in section 15.2. The strong form of this second part is that the learning follows the linear combination algorithm Jones et al. used in their plausibility demonstration; the weak form, which we favor, leaves open the specific learning scheme. Further work may enable us to verify whether the strong or weak form is to be preferred and if the weak, to determine which learning scheme is used by the visual system.

15.5   Summary and Conclusions

We began this chapter by asking whether learning shapes perception. Experimental results over the past four decades have provided strong evidence demonstrating the experience-dependent malleability of perceptual processes (Hubel and Wiesel 1970; Kass 1994). Several lines of reasoning suggest that the locus of learning in the reported instances is situated very early in the processing pathway (Karni and Sagi 1991; Ahissar and Hochstein 1998).

Answering the question of whether high-level, object-specific learning can influence early perception is important for understanding the overall organization of information flow in the brain. Early experimental data supporting the position that it does (Schafer and Murphy 1943; Bruner and Postman 1947; Bruner and Goodman 1947; Hochberg and Brooks 1958) have been criticized on the grounds that such data reflect changes in cognitive

decisions rather than modifications of perception per se (Gibson 1969). Several authors (e.g., Fodor and Pylyshyn 1981; Pylyshyn 1999) have argued for the cognitive impenetrability of early perception. Early perception, in their view, is governed by general natural constraints and is immune to learned object-specific knowledge.

We examined this question in the context of a specific visual perceptual task—the recovery of three-dimensional structures from single two-dimensional line drawings, long considered one of the key early vision tasks and widely believed to be performed by relying on the use of general natural constraints. We started by describing a constraint-based shape recovery system and its limitations as a comprehensive model of the corresponding perceptual process. Tests of the implemented system suggest that, though it mimics human perception in specific domains, it does not possess the ability to generalize to other, more naturalistic, domains. All constraint-based shape recovery schemes proposed thus far, without exception, share this limitation. Although such a limitation certainly does not prove that the constraint-based account is untenable, it does point to the need for exploring an alternative high-level learning-based account for the task.

We next described recently reported experiments to determine whether the three-dimensional percept corresponding to a given two-dimensional image can be accounted for in terms of the observers' prior visual experiences. The results suggest that this may indeed be the case. Observers can learn to associate a projectionally consistent but otherwise arbitrary 3-D structure with a randomly generated 2-D line drawing, with two significant perceptual consequences: misperception of KDE sequences (rigid rotating objects appear highly nonrigid) and misperception of stereoscopic depth. The learning is long-lasting and specific to particular line drawings. These results provide compelling evidence in support of a role of high-level object specific learning on 3-D shape perception.

As a follow-up to these experimental results, we discussed a simple computational model for how object-specific learning may be brought to bear on the performance of supposedly early perceptual tasks. Given the identity of an object in an image, or perhaps just its class membership, the model attempts to facilitate the computation of basic attributes such as three-dimensional shape and contour structure, and to bring previously learned knowledge about the object class to bear on this task. The model relies on a prior stage of recognizing the object in an image but is agnostic about precisely how this may be done. It then represents the image as a combination of training instances. The parameters of the combi-

nation are finally used to compute the desired attributes such as shape corresponding to the input. It is interesting to note that the information flow being proposed here (image → recognition → perceptual attributes) is quite the reverse of what has conventionally been assumed (image → perceptual attributes → recognition).

15.6 Open Questions

Recent experimental results have made significant headway in resolving the question of whether high-level learning can influence early perception. Interesting computational models have also been proposed to account for these experimental findings. These efforts are bringing us closer to a unification of cognition and perception. Such a unification—

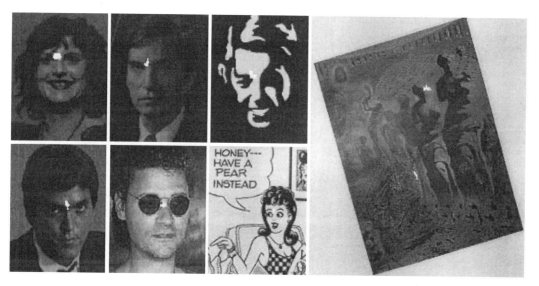

Figure 15.25
Preliminary object recognition results with "minimalist" representations, quasi invariants constructed from pairwise ordinal brightness relationships over different regions of the images. In the examples shown here, the task is to detect human faces irrespective of the illumination conditions, identity, and complexion. Detections are marked by white spots in the center of the head.

critical if we hope to achieve a comprehensive understanding of how information flows and is processed across the different stages in the brain—is nevertheless still quite out of reach. Several open questions remain. We end this chapter by considering two that we believe are the most important.

15.6.1 *What Are the Neural Mechanisms by Which High-Level Learning Influences Early Perception?*

Clearly, corticocortical feedback projections are obvious candidates for such mechanisms (Mumford 1992; Ullman 1995), although there is only a small body of experimental data implicating the projections in this role. Hupé et al. (1998) have found area V5 lesions to reduce responses in areas V1 and V2, presumably due to disruption of cortical feedback. Roelfsema, Lamme, and Spekreijse (1998) have found heightened edge responses to the attended stimuli, perhaps due to high-level modulatory influences. Zipser, Lamme, and Schiller (1996) have reported contextual modulation of responses of area V1 cells, although it is not clear whether the modulation is due to lateral connections in area V1 itself or top-down influences from extrastriate areas, and if the latter, which extrastriate areas and whether the influence is object specific.

Demonstrating, as the aforementioned studies do, that the feedback connections have some modulatory influences is only part of the story. What is important, and thus far unknown, is whether these modulatory influences are high-level and object-specific influences. After all, object-specific influences need not necessarily modify the activity of early areas. They could be combined with bottom-up information and thus incorporated in perception by areas even further along the processing pathway. Thus still another fundamental open question is, do high-level influences actually modify the activity of early areas or do they merely modify the conscious percept that may have a later genesis?

15.6.2 *How Can the Visual System Recognize Objects in Images without Relying on Sophisticated Perceptual Constructs?*

In a high-level, learning-based scheme of visual processing, the first step is recognition. Without this bootstrapping step, relevant object- and class-specific knowledge cannot be brought to bear on a perceptual task. The challenge of devising a recognition scheme here is made more difficult by the requirement that the strategy not rely on any sophisticated perceptual constructs such as three-dimensional shape estimates of objects in the image (because that is what the high-level, learning-based scheme is supposed to yield as its output). We have an ongoing effort to explore "minimalist" object representation schemes constructed from elementary image measurements (Sinha 1994, 1995; Thorek and Sinha 2001). Although still in an early stage of development, the results thus far have been very encouraging (figure 15.25). Other fascinating open issues that deserve close research attention in future models of top-down processing include methods for initial acquisition of high-level knowledge from bottom-up measurements and schemes for combining bottom-up data with top-down expectations.

The prospect of tying together early perception and high-level learning is an extremely exciting one. It represents a qualitative change in how we view the brain's processing hierarchy and promises to help unify the efforts in perception and cognition, leading to faster progress on both fronts.

Learning to Recognize Objects

Guy Wallis and Heinrich Bülthoff

16

Abstract

This chapter reviews a large body of literature describing how experience affects recognition. Results both from neurophysiology and psychophysics provide clear evidence for the development of recognition over time. In particular, we explain how perceptual learning in recognition can be directly linked to learning in feature-tuned inferotemporal lobe neurons. We argue that all of the available evidence points to the representation of objects as groups of associated, two-dimensional views. Further, we argue that the natural environment is so structured that potentially very different images appearing in close temporal succession are likely to be views of the same object, and that this temporal structure allows the visual system to associate diverse views into coherent representations of individual objects.

As an introduction to the subject we review the case of S.B., a patient whose insusceptibility to visual illusions and failed perception of depth all point to the fact that much of our ability to interpret the form of objects and scenes is learned. We go on to describe how, by using novel stimuli, it has been possible for researchers to complement patient studies with controlled studies of normal populations, providing us with a more precise description of how object representation and recognition develops.

The results described in this chapter strongly support the empiricist view that object recognition and categorization is largely an ongoing process, affected by experience of our environment. Taken as a whole, the results serve to underpin the main tenet of this book, namely, that perception is mediated via a dynamic learning system, the modification of which continues throughout our lives.

16.1 Introduction

In the process of everyday life we are continually analyzing and interpreting our visual environment.

We effortlessly convert the flat retinal images supplied by our eyes, into a rich three-dimensional world, filled with licorice and ladybugs, shipyards and woods. The apparent speed and ease with which we do this is deceptive. The images cast on our retinas by objects change drastically as a function of viewpoint, lighting, size, or location. Consider, for example, the scene depicted in figure 16.1, in which the same office chair appears several times. We seem to find it trivial to distinguish cast shadows or wall paintings from the genuine article, and it seems self-evident that the chair on the desk is small enough to hold in the hand, whereas the chair in the adjacent office is large enough to sit on. We happily conclude this from various cues in the image, even though the images formed on our retinas by the two chairs are actually identical. This chapter describes theories of how humans solve the recognition problem, and particularly, how our perception of objects changes with experience. The question of how we recognize objects is an active area of research, and part of this chapter is dedicated to a summary of the proposals that have been made. This is followed by a review of the evidence for perceptual learning in object recognition, ranging from the level of single neurons to that of human behavior. The chapter concludes by considering how we might learn to associate very dissimilar views of an object, describing how temporal as well as spatial correlations present in our environment can be used to make the necessary associations.

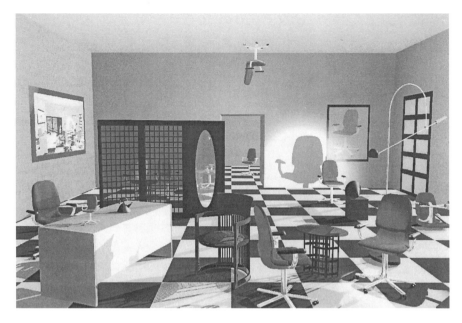

Figure 16.1
Complex scene comprising many chairs seen with different sizes, viewpoints, lighting conditions, and so on, demonstrating the range of problems faced in recognizing and categorizing objects.

16.2   Interpreting Our Visual World

16.2.1   Philosophical Beginnings

The question of how we construct an internal representation of our visual world has provided fruitful labor for philosophers, psychologists, and engineers for many years. The first recorded ruminations on the topic appear in the writings of the ancient Greeks. Plato was particularly interested in how we recognize and categorize objects. He came to wonder what it was about a cat, for example, that let it be classified as a cat and yet remain distinct from all other cats. He proposed an innate fund of perfect, universal forms, to which all seen objects are likened. Plato's

ideas find parallels in current theories of prototypes (Rosch 1973; Posner and Keele 1968; Edelman 1995), but the proposal that such categories are innate gifts has been replaced by the belief that much about visual perception is learned, and is therefore shaped by our environment. This belief was first voiced in the early seventeenth century in the writings of René Descartes, and within fifty years it became the guiding principle of a new philosophical movement called "empiricism."

The founding father of empiricism was John Locke. Locke rejected all theories of innate knowledge, and although he was prepared to accept a certain amount of prenatal knowledge, he attributed it mainly to sensory experience within the womb. This rather extreme stance ultimately led to a damning rebuke. Idealist philosophers such as Kant argued that perception requires a framework, an assumed space and time, and a concept of categories to be able to begin to represent the real world. This argument was later championed by the Gestalt movement, which strongly influenced thinking in the first half of the twentieth century. Gestalt psychologists such as Köhler and Koffka took the view that human perception is littered with assumptions that are used to transform the retinal image into an object. They both believed the principles of organization that they proposed to be fundamental, like laws of physics, enforcing unavoidable and universal constraints on perception.

Köhler (1947, 277) condemned the empiricist view, stating:

Now, when the concept of organization was first introduced, we were at every step hampered by empiricist explanations.... It has been shown, I hope, that [Gestalt laws] do not allow of explanations in terms of learning, and that therefore, organization must be accepted as a primary phase of experience. At present we may go further and claim that, on the contrary, any effects which learning has on subsequent experience are likely to be after-effects of previous organization.

Nowadays, many of the Gestaltist laws seem rather vague and anecdotal, but their work did succeed in highlighting a large number of instances in which humans infer form and shape on the basis of a few built-in assumptions. Perhaps their only disservice to science was their success, which stifled progress on perceptual learning throughout the early part of the twentieth century. It was not until the 1960s and 1970s that interest in the seminal work of late-nineteenth-century empiricist writers such as Helmholtz and James enjoyed a resurgence of interest. One of the tasks for current researchers is to provide evidence for how much of visual perception is altered by experience and how much is innate.

16.2.2 The Case of S.B.

Having reviewed the idealist versus empiricist debate, let us consider some of the evidence for the two philosophies. The earliest arguments in favor of perceptual learning stem from the work of the early empiricists. Of course, being philosophers rather than scientists in the modern sense, they relied more on reasoning than on experimentation. Their preferred approach was to present readers with a mental conundrum followed by an elegant explanation that furthered their cause. Nevertheless, through such mind games, they made at least some seemingly testable predictions. One favorite concerned a man born blind, who is suddenly able to see. They speculated on how his tactile experience of the world would transfer to his interpretation of a visual world.

Commenting on a draft of Locke's *Essay on Human Understanding* in early 1693, Molyneux (Locke 1708, 37−38) concluded with "a jocose problem: Suppose a man born blind ... and taught by his touch to distinguish between a cube and a sphere. Suppose then ... the blind man made to see; query whether by his sight ... he could now distinguish and tell which the globe and which the cube." Both Locke and Molyneux thought not.

Did anyone ever "live out" Molyneux's gedanken-experiment? Several hundred years ago a man born blind was almost certain to remain so, and in more modern times operable cases are usually dealt with soon after birth. It turns out, however, that there are a very few cases of people recovering their sight after years of blindness. Gregory and Wallace (1963) review several such cases making reference to the discussions of the empiricist philosophers, describing in detail experiments conducted with S.B., a man who lost his sight at the age of ten months and then had it restored some fifty-two years later. Finally, after two hundred years of waiting, it seemed that S.B. could provide scientists with the opportunity to supplant the empiricists' reasoning with facts.

The first remarkable thing about S.B. was that some tactile information clearly transfered almost instantaneously to his seeing world. In other words, things that S.B. had felt with his hands could often be readily perceived with his eyes. He could, for example, read the time on a clock face across a room. He could also read printed capital letters, although lowercase letters meant nothing to him because he had not been taught to read them as a blind schoolboy. Clearly, this type of transferral is at odds with the predictions of Locke and Molyneux. Far from being an exception, there is now good evidence that the transferral from touch to visual perception is quite normal. This has led theorists to propose a much closer link between the two sense modalities than the early empiricists would have expected. With this notable exception, many of their predictions did stand the test of time. For example, Locke (1721, 107) proposed that depth cues such as shading and perspective are only useful after experience of their meaning: "When we set before our Eyes a round Globe ... 'tis certain, that the Idea thereby imprinted in our Mind is of a flat Circle variously shadow'd.... But we having by Use been accustomed to perceive, what kind of appearance convex Bodies are wont to make in us ... the Judgement presently ... alters the Appearances into their Causes ... and frames to it self the perception of a convex Figure...."

Gregory and Wallace (1963) tested S.B. on various illusions and found him abnormally insusceptible to those shown in figure 16.2, revealing an unusual insensitivity to depth cues. Indeed, S.B. described looking from an upstairs window and feeling that he could step to the ground several floors below without harm. This misapprehension of depth accords both with Locke's words above and with those of

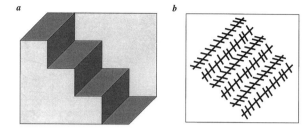

Figure 16.2
Examples of optical illusions to which S.B., blind for more than fifty years and now able to see, was exposed during testing. (*a*) Staircase illusion, in which S.B. failed to infer depth from the oblique lines, hence avoiding the usually bistable percept. (*b*) Zöllner illusion, in which S.B. described seeing straight, parallel lines rather than the collection of bowed black lines described by normal observers.

George Berkeley whose Euphranor argues (Berkeley 1732, 164–165): "Now, I find by Experience that when an Object is removed still farther and farther off ... its visible Appearance still grows lesser and fainter.... That is to say—we perceive Distance, not immediately, but by mediation of a Sign, which hath no Likeness to it, or necessary Connexion with it, but only suggests it from Experience as Words do Things." Not surprisingly, Berkley (1713, 413) concludes a similar conversation in *Three Dialogues Between Hylas and Philonous* thus: "Now, is it not plain, that if we suppose a Man born blind was on a sudden made to see.... He would not ... have any Notion of Distance annexed to the things he saw ..."

Gregory and Wallace's findings support the idea that a great deal of S.B.'s tactile experience of essentially two-dimensional views (of letters and clock faces) carried over to the visual world, but that his perception of depth and the use of cues to three-dimensional form were missing, which is to some extent surprising because S.B. probably went blind at the age of ten months. Although there is no record of his visual development before this time, had it been normal, developmental studies have shown that by this age he would have gained some ability to process depth information, including the rigidity assumption (Gibson, Owsley, and Johnston 1978), and the use of stereoscopic disparity (Held 1999). None of this early experience seems to have been retained, however; instead, S.B.'s experience with his tactile world appears to have formed the basis for what he later saw. Indeed, there is some evidence that, shortly after the operation that restored his sight, his previous tactile experiences caused curious misperceptions of objects. For example, he initially saw buses as having spoked wheels, as they had had at the turn of the century when he last had cause to touch them as an inquisitive boy. He only correctly perceived the modern solid wheels months after his operation. On the other hand, he had no difficulty in correctly perceiving the shape of a quarter moon, which as a blind man he had imagined would be sliced like quarter of a cake!

Over the next few months, S.B.'s conception of things around him continued to improve. Gregory and Wallace (1963, 35) noted that since leaving the hospital, S.B. had become fascinated by the varying appearance of objects: "Quite recently he had been struck by how objects changed their shape when he walked round them. He would look at a lamp post, walk around it, stand studying it from a different aspect, and wonder why it looked different and yet the same." It is clearly tempting to read a great deal into S.B.'s words, but as Gregory and Wallace point out, this temptation is dangerous because we cannot see directly into the mind of a blind man. A blind man's vocabulary derives from that of the sighted, and one should therefore exercise caution in interpreting his descriptions of visual experience. Indeed, a recent brain imaging study by Sadato et al. (1996) has demonstrated that the visual cortex of blind people becomes recruited for tasks such as Braille reading in

a manner quite unlike that in normal subjects. This was confirmed by Cohen et al. (1997), who used magnetic stimulation to disrupt processing in particular brain areas to show that blind people require visual cortex to interpret Braille, once again, unlike normal subjects. Bearing this in mind, we should shy away from extrapolating too much from S.B.'s experiences. Nevertheless, the case does raise some intriguing questions about the influence of experience in interpreting our visual environment.

16.2.3 Pragmatism in Perception

For many years, researchers (e.g., Gregory 1972; Fahle, Edelman, and Poggio 1995) have been aware of perceptual differences arising directly from people's experience, even as adults. One example receiving renewed attention concerns an illusion described by Pollock and Chapais (1952). This illusion causes subjects to overestimate the length of vertical lines relative to horizontal ones, which Baddeley (1997) explains in terms of the level of image correlation occurring at different orientations within natural scenes. Evidence supporting this hypothesis comes from the reliable difference in the magnitude of the horizontal-vertical line length illusion between country folk from the Norfolk Fens and townsfolk in the City of Glasgow (Ross 1990), environments containing very different amounts of image correlation at different orientations (figure 16.3). This work requires further corroboration, but if correct, it provides remarkable evidence that the characteristics of our everyday visual environment directly affect basic perceptual judgements such as line length.

Despite the considerable evidence supporting perceptual learning, there are many counterexamples in the literature. For example, an earlier study by Ross and Woodhouse (1979) on the same population of city and country dwellers found no influence of en-

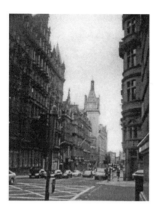
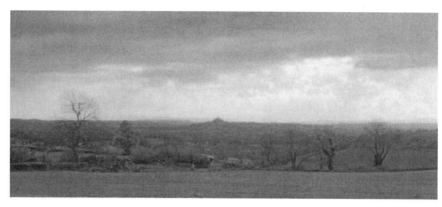

Figure 16.3
Images of Glasgow (*left*) and the Somerset Levels (*right*). Like the Norfolk Fens, the Somerset Levels were large, flat flood-lands that have been drained for farming. Glasgow, in contrast, is a large industrial city littered with tall, closely packed buildings. Daily exposure to vertical structures typical of cities may be responsible for the reduced size of the classical horizontal line length illusion in city dwellers compared with country folk, as reported by Ross (1990). Such results provide evidence that our visual diet affects fundamental perceptual judgements. (Pictures © 1997 Martin Smith, and © 1998 Pete Harlow, reproduced with permission.)

vironment for sensitivity to differences in line orientation. Also, in the field of depth perception, it has been shown that we perceive depth from cast shadows on an built-in assumption that the light source is situated above and to the left of the viewed object (Ramachandran 1988). Preliminary evidence that this assumption is innate was provided by Hershberger (1970), who showed that without prior experience of shadows, chicks perceive depth from cast shadows.

Apart from innate assumptions for interpreting our environment, some psychologists have also claimed that certain cues or sensory modalities are immutable in the presence of conflicting evidence, forming the framework within which other cues are adapted. For example, Harris (1963) showed that the relearning of hand-eye coordination when wearing eyeglasses with displacing prisms is purely motor based, rather than vision based. Spelke (1990), too, suggests that

some systems do not adapt, arguing, for example, that the impression of distance derived from apparent object motion during head movements (motion parallax) is not adaptable, and that it forms an anchor for adapting other sources of information such as stereoscopic vision. On the other hand, recent work has revealed a great deal of evidence that all cues to depth can be overridden in the presence of strongly competing cues (Landy et al. 1995), and that the cues interact in a nonlinear manner (Bradshaw and Rogers 1996). Indeed Wallis and Bülthoff (1998) have shown that in the presence of additional depth cues, stereoscopic information recalibrates perceived depth from motion, directly countering the argument made by Spelke.

The point in raising these examples is to make it clear that neither the idealist nor empiricist view is exclusively correct. It is important to bear in mind that the force that has shaped us, evolution, is both eclectic and pragmatic. If some advantage is to be had from hardwiring certain assumptions, while leaving others to be discovered, then there is nothing to say that evolution has not devised such a compromise. It is also possible that some of the basic assumptions shared with animals as distant from us as chickens, are useful leftovers from before the rapid expansion of the neocortex. As Ramachandran (1985) puts it, we should not be surprised to find that evolution has supplied us with a "bag of tricks" for interpreting the world. Ultimately, what is interesting for those investigating perceptual learning is how many of these tricks are inherited assumptions and how many are extrapolated from our environment. For that reason, recent perceptual models have focused on the use of Bayesian mechanics, in which assumptions can be formally incorporated as statistical priors (Bülthoff and Yuille 1996).

In the rest of this chapter we shall concentrate on the mechanisms underlying the representation and recognition of objects, attempting to get to the core of why, as S.B. put it, an object can "look different and yet be the same." In particular, we shall explain why we believe that the theories of the early empiricists have relevance to the problem by detailing the role of experience both in representing and recognizing objects.

16.3 Object Recognition Paradigms

16.3.1 Extracting Three-Dimensional Information

One of the most influential writers in the field of object recognition was David Marr (1982), who believed that recognition of an object requires the matching of elemental parts of that object to the parts of three-dimensional models which we have memorized. The correct apprehension of those

3-D features was, for Marr, achieved in three consecutive stages: first, the primal sketch, a wholly two-dimensional representation which contains information about lines and edges visible in the scene; second, a $2\frac{1}{2}$-D sketch derived from these edges and depth information, describing closed surfaces in space; and finally, a full, three-dimensional representation of our environment built from the identified surfaces.

The third stage, Marr argued, provided all of the information required to recognize objects. Recognition itself involved taking the shapes drawn from the environment and matching them to stored three-dimensional models. These models were themselves built up of constituent parts, or building blocks, which defined an object's shape at various levels of abstraction and detail. Within such a scheme, the form of a standing human, say, could be said to fill the volume of an upright cylinder, as could a tree or a high-rise, but not a car or a bed, whose major axis is horizontal. Beyond this we recognize the six major bodily divisions of the head, trunk, and four limbs, which afford discrimination from most nonanimal object categories. This recursive analysis then proceeds to the level required to solve a particular discrimination task or make a specific categorization judgment.

Although strongly associated with this type of hierarchical approach, Marr was neither the only nor the first person to propose using it in categorization and recognition. Indeed, the idea underpins a whole series of theories (Guzman 1971; Marr and Nishihara 1978; Brooks 1981; Tversky and Hemenway 1984) that can be traced back to early attempts to build artificially intelligent systems in the 1970s. Irrespective of the detailed implementation, the approaches are united in the assumption that we use 3-D information from our environment to extract 3-D parts, and that objects are represented as configurations of

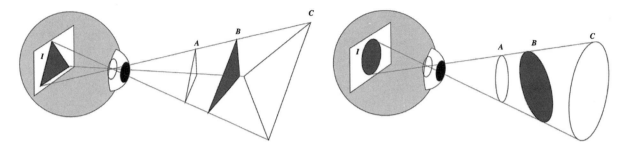

Figure 16.4
When we view a surface at some random orientation in space, it often results in a characteristic two-dimensional pattern on our retina from which we can infer its true shape. Although triangles remain triangles and ellipses remain ellipses irrespective of viewpoint, we must decide which of the many possible shapes is responsible for the image seen. In the above examples, the image *I* is due to object *B*, but it could equally well have been due to object *A* or object *C*.

these parts. One can think of it as a "LEGO representation." The only major difference in each case is the precise shape and range of LEGO bricks used. Examples include: polyhedrons (Waltz 1975), spheres (Badler and Bajcsy 1978), cylinders (Nevatia and Binford 1977; Marr and Nishihara 1978), and "superquadrics" (Pentland 1986).

16.3.2   Projective Invariants

A quite different approach to identifying objects is the use of projective invariance. Projective invariance refers to the fact that projection of a three-dimensional shape onto a flat surface (like our retina) produces certain characteristic patterns irrespective of the angle at which that 3-D feature is being viewed. For example, because a triangle remains a triangle from all but the most contrived viewing directions, if we detect any surface with three sides, we can label it as a triangle (figure 16.4; cf. chapter 15). We can then use the presence of the triangle as the basis for working out what the object is that includes this feature. Other useful invariances are that parallel lines suggest parallel lines in the object

and that ellipses are views of ellipses of equal or smaller aspect ratio.

There are several different levels of tolerance to projective distortion that the human visual system might exhibit. At one extreme, there is full projective invariance (Duda and Hart 1973; Cutting 1986; Weiss 1988), which assumes that full three-dimensional information can be recovered from the two-dimensional image on our retina, although projective transforms can leave objects unrecognizable —suggesting that humans cannot achieve this. Alternatively, humans might simply ignore the effect linear perspective has on the appearance of objects, namely the narrowing of straight lines with distance (Hoffman 1966; Lamdan, Schwartz, and Wolfson 1988; Koenderink and van Doorn 1991). Unfortunately, this type of "affine" approximation cannot distinguish simple shapes such as rectangles because they are all affine transforms of each other.

The third and most promising type of invariance to be investigated is perspective invariance (Mundy and Zisserman 1992; Pizlo 1994). Perspective invariance relies upon the types of predictable mappings of triangles, circles, and the like mentioned above, and authors have argued that such invariances can form a basis for recognition. There is a problem, however. Because infinitely many triangles oriented in three-dimensional space map to any one triangle on our retina, and infinitely many ellipses map to a single ellipse, some heuristic has to be used to decide which one of the family of possibilities to select (see figure 16.4). Possible constraints include assuming that the true shape corresponds to the form in which the ratio of an object's area to its perimeter is maximized (Brady and Yuille 1984), or that the true form has bilateral symmetry (Vetter and Poggio 1994). By applying these constraints, variability in appearance due to viewing angle can be eliminated in many cases.

16.3.3 Geon Structural Description

One development of the part-based, Marrian approach to recognition is the "geon structural description" due to Biederman (1987), who, once again, suggests that objects are represented by explicit relationships of a small set of LEGO-like blocks, which he calls "geons" (figure 16.5, panel a). For example, a house might be represented as the base of a pyramid on top of a cube, and a U.S. mailbox as a cube on top of a narrow cylinder. In this manner a few (thirty-six in Biederman's opinion) volumetric primitives can be used to describe any object.

Despite the similarity to Marrian ideas, geon theory also owes something to the idea of perspective invariants. Biederman's approach specifically excludes any textural or similar depth cues, concentrating instead on the mapping of two-dimensional space relations to inferences about three-dimensional shape. Biederman cites Lowe's list of nonaccidental 2-D properties (Lowe 1984), in his discussion of

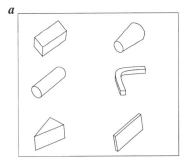

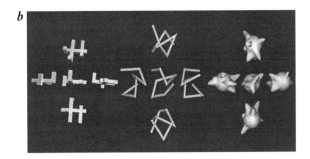

Figure 16.5
(a) Examples of geons, volumetric shape primitives for categorizing and recognizing natural shapes, adapted from Biederman (1987), who describes how a set of thirty-six geons can exhaustively describe all everyday objects. (b) Examples of three data sets used by Bülthoff and Edelman (1992) and Tarr and Pinker (1989) to investigate within category view generalization in novel objects. *From left to right*: aerials, paper clips, and amebas.

how 2-D cues such as colinearity, skew symmetry, and coincident line termination can be used to infer 3-D shape.

16.3.4 Active Shape Matching

Another alternative to have received consideration—especially from researchers hoping to build working recognition systems—is template matching. The precise details of how to implement such a system vary considerably, but in practice all matching approaches are one of two conceptually important types. The first uses stored models containing explicit three-dimensional shape information, and therefore assumes that it is possible to extract the location of three (or more) anchor points in 3-D space, which are matched to those in the stored models. Matching the anchor points requires a 3-D rotation and scaling of the stored model until the anchor points are most closely aligned. Recognition then proceeds by measuring the amount of overlap in the two views (e.g., Ullman 1979).

The second approach relies on representations based upon groups of two-dimensional views. For example, in elastic pattern matching a nonlinear image transformation is made to the incoming image of the object being viewed. A measure of how well the model matches the stimulus is derived by attributing a cost to how far points in one image have to be moved to find a similar-looking feature in the other. Features which have been tried include: Gabor-like patches or "jets" (Buhmann, Lades, and von der Malsburg 1990), specific features such as end-stopped lines or junctions (Hinton, Williams, and Revow 1992), and edge-based facial features such as ovals for eyes and a triangle for a nose (Yuille 1991).

16.3.5 Recognition Based on Two-Dimensional Image Features

Although the recognition of familiar, everyday objects proceeds almost effortlessly, some views are generally easier to recognize than others, both in terms of reaction times and accuracy. Such views are referred to as "canonical" in the recognition literature (Palmer, Rosch, and Chase 1981). Many researchers have since studied view specificity using novel objects trained in particular views (see figure 16.5, panel b).

Results consistently point to a decrease in recognition performance as a function of the viewpoint's disparity from a previously learned view (Shepard and Cooper 1982; Rock and DiVita 1987; Bülthoff and Edelman 1992; Tarr and Pinker 1989; Jolicoeur 1990). Similar drops in recognition performance with viewing angle have also been reported for unfamiliar faces (Troje and Bülthoff 1996).

These results have led to a new alternative for how objects are represented and recognized, namely, the feature-based, multiple-view approach (Bülthoff and Edelman 1992). Although it bears some relation to earlier two-dimensional matching theories and similarly benefits from the result of Ullman and Basri (1991) that any 2-D projection of a three-dimensional object can be written as a *linear* combination of 2-D views, the multiple-view model differs from that of the classical 2-D models in two important respects. First, the views are not deformed to match each incoming image, and second, the views are represented, not as single templates, but as a collection of small picture elements, each tolerant to small view changes. In the feature-based scheme, individual neurons are selective to features that occur frequently in the environment. Although these features may be selective for identifiable things such as noses or eyes, most will be responsive to more abstract combinations of edges and surface textures. An ensemble of many hundreds of cells would then be required to act in unison to uniquely identify any one object. The emergent properties of robustness to small variations in the input image (from changes in view, size, or location) and to cell damage, have long been realized by the neural network community (Hinton, McClelland, and Rumelhart 1986).

Unlike other two-dimensional representation schemes, the feature-based, multiple-view approach represents a significant departure from object-based models because it requires neither the extraction of depth information nor the exhaustive matching of three-dimensional models. It is also consistent with a great deal of neurophysiological evidence, as we shall describe in section 16.4. (For a more detailed discussion of the pros and cons of this and the other representation schemes, see Wallis and Bülthoff 1999; Pizlo 1994; Tarr and Bülthoff 1995; Biederman and Gerhardstein 1993.)

16.4 Learning from Examples

16.4.1 Neurophysiology

From lesion studies and cellular recording it has been proposed that a series of cortical regions starting in area V1 and running ventrally through the occipital into the temporal lobe (V1-V2-V4-intraparietal areas) solves the problem of what we are looking at. In contrast, a second stream leading dorsally and into the parietal lobe (V1-V2-V3-intraparietal areas) has been implicated in the role of deciding *where* that object is (Farah 1990; Ungerleider and Mishkin 1982; Goodale and Milner 1992; Young 1992; see figure 16.6).

Cells in the latter part of the ventral stream, in the inferotemporal (IT) areas, are of particular relevance to object recognition because of their tolerance to changes in the precise appearance of their preferred stimuli. Transformations tolerated by IT cells include changes in an object's position, viewing angle, or size, as well as in its overall image contrast or spatial frequency content (Rolls 1992; Desimone 1991; Tanaka et al. 1991; see chapter 4)—indeed, they include all of the types of transformation invariance required for view-invariant object recognition. These neurons are also of interest in that they provide a source of evidence of learning in the recognition system. Evidence for experience-dependent

learning in inferotemporal cortex has now been reported by many researchers (Rolls et al. 1989; Miyashita 1993; Logothetis and Pauls 1995; Kobatake, Tanaka, and Wang 1998; see chapter 6). The link from view-based recognition to representations in inferotemporal cortex was strengthened through recording work by Logothetis and colleagues (Logothetis and Pauls 1995; Logothetis, Pauls, and Poggio 1995), in which monkeys were trained to recognize particular aspects of the paper clip stimuli originally used by Bülthoff and Edelman (1992) (see figure 16.5, panel b). After training, many neurons were shown to have learned representations of particular paper clips, including some selective to specific views. In addition to longer-term changes to cell selectivity, there is also good evidence of almost instantaneous learning in IT cells. Tovee, Rolls, and Ramachandran (1996), for example, presented images of strongly lit, two-tone (black-and-white) faces, referred to as "Mooney faces" in the literature (figure 16.7, panel a). Some IT neurons that did not respond to any of the Mooney faces did so if once exposed to the standard gray-level version of the face (see panel b), which accords with findings in humans, who often struggle to interpret Mooney face images the first time, but then have no difficulty in seeing them as faces a second time, even weeks later (Ramachandran 1994).

16.4.2 Psychophysics

There is considerable psychophysical evidence that our perception of objects is affected by experience. Even a few days or hours of training can affect the speed and accuracy with which we recognize objects. Bülthoff and Edelman (1992), for example, were able to show that if subjects learn to recognize two views of a novel object, recognition performance is better for new orientations located between the two train-

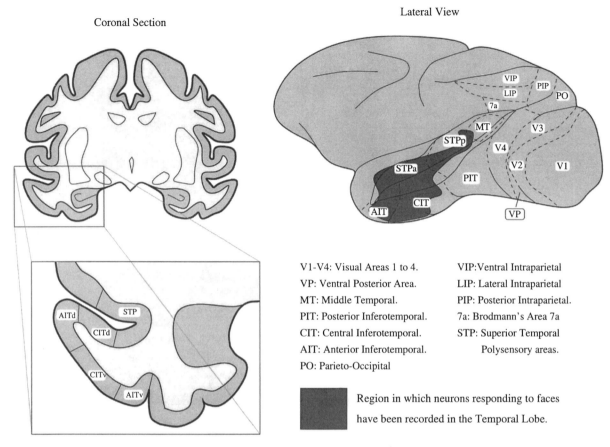

Coronal Section

Lateral View

V1-V4: Visual Areas 1 to 4.
VP: Ventral Posterior Area.
MT: Middle Temporal.
PIT: Posterior Inferotemporal.
CIT: Central Inferotemporal.
AIT: Anterior Inferotemporal.
PO: Parieto-Occipital

VIP:Ventral Intraparietal
LIP: Lateral Intraparietal
PIP: Posterior Intraparietal.
7a: Brodmann's Area 7a
STP: Superior Temporal
       Polysensory areas.

Region in which neurons responding to faces
have been recorded in the Temporal Lobe.

Figure 16.6
Lateral view (*upper right*) and coronal section (*upper left*) of the primate cortex, showing some of the significant visual processing areas. The expanded coronal section (*lower left*) portrays some of the important subdivisions of the temporal lobe. (Adapted from Rolls 1992; Perrett et al. 1992.)

ing views (INTER) than outside them (EXTRA), which in turn is better than for orientations away from the axis linking the trained views (ORTHO; see figure 16.8). A first step to explaining these results, within a feature-based representation scheme, is to understand why recognition performance drops with distance from a learned view. We can start by first imagining what happens when leaning a single view.

When a view of a novel object is presented, many feature-selective neurons respond, and the associated pattern of responses they produce comes to represent the presence of that object. Now identification of a novel view of the object will clearly be easiest for views nearest to the one trained because these views are most likely to contain one or more of the features supporting the representation of the learned view.

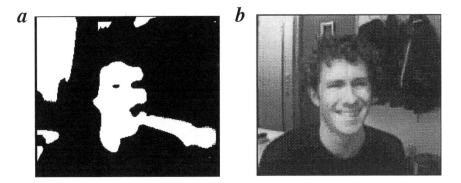

Figure 16.7
(*a*) Example of a Mooney face, similar to those used by Tovee, Rolls, and Ramachandran (1996). Subjects or face-selective neurons exposed to such a two-tone image often fail to see a face. (*b*) On seeing the veridical image, both neurons and subjects can now identify the face and will continue to do so in the future, providing evidence for rapid and lasting learning.

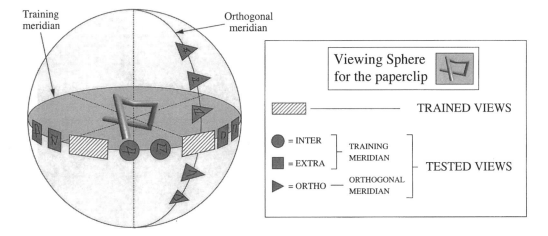

Figure 16.8
If two views of a novel object are learned, recognition is better for new viewing angles located between the two training views (INTER) than outside them (EXTRA), itself better than for orientations away from the axis linking the trained views (ORTHO).

Using a similar line of argument, if two views of the object have been learned, and both are identified as being the same object, then the presence of any of the features seen in either learned view will tend to evoke recognition of that same object. This second step is important because the INTER and EXTRA results follow as a natural consequence, because any view falling within the range of the two trained views is more likely to have features in common with either or both of the trained views than a view of the object from outside that range, INTER views are more likely to be easily recognized than EXTRA views.

The ORTHO effect stems from the type of training used. The training views used were not stationary but rather rocked back and forth through a few degrees, which had the effect that only cells tolerant to changes in the object's appearance along the training meridian (see figure 16.8) were strongly activated during learning, and hence only they strongly supported recognition of the object. Because views of the object lying along the training meridian (i.e., INTER and EXTRA views) are much more likely to contain the features for which these cells are selective than views lying on an orthogonal meridian (ORTHO views), INTER and EXTRA views are more readily recognized.

Edelman and Bülthoff (1992) investigated the effects of extensive training to see whether it could override view specificity. After training large numbers of views, they were able to change the shape of the recognition curves. Not only did reaction times decrease and accuracy increase, but view-specific effects, such as canonicality, gradually disappeared. This issue has been raised again recently in several studies investigating how continued exposure to an object class may affect the manner in which the objects within the class are represented. Schyns, Goldstone, and Tribaut 1998 and Schyns 1998 argue

that sufficient exposure to a particular stimulus type causes the representation of these stimuli to alter and be enhanced. This finding in turn relates to the those of researchers studying learning in IT neurons (Miyashita 1988; Logothetis and Pauls 1995; Kobatake, Tanaka, and Wang 1998; see chapters 4, 6), whose work showed that extensive experience of a class of images or objects causes a rise in the amount of cells selective for those stimuli. By devoting more neural hardware to the representation of the features present in an object class, one would presumably be better able to discriminate subtleties in their form, as suggested by the Schyns studies.

Gauthier and Tarr (1998) also make this point. Their study revealed that experience of an originally novel object class heightens the subjects' awareness of small changes to objects within the same class, and they argue that our highly sophisticated ability to recognise faces is simply due to a natural concentration of neural resources from our lengthy exposure to the particular object class we call "faces" (see chapter 17). Some researchers, drawing on studies of the neurological disorder prosopagnosia, would counter that face recognition is special. Prosopagnosia is characterized by normal ability to recognize common objects coupled with extreme difficulty in recognizing people's faces (De Renzi 1997). That the locus of the brain damage in prosopagnosia patients was a part of the temporal lobe homologous to that of cells selective for faces in monkeys (Rolls 1992; Desimone 1991) made a strong case for the suggestion that prosopagnosia was caused by damage to these cells (Farah 1990). Although psychological studies (Tanaka and Farah 1993; Fiser, Biederman, and Cooper 1996) have revealed a dissociation between face and object recognition in the past, the latest picture from the neurophysiological evidence is not as clear as some theorists had first hoped. Direct attempts to find the illusive area responsible for face recognition in monkeys has been controversial and until now unfruitful (Perrett et al. 1992; Cowey 1992), which in turns lends greater weight to Gauthier and Tarr's proposal (1998) that prosopagnosia may reveal a general deficit in the area dedicated to fine-level discriminations of highly trained objects, rather than to a specialist face area per se.

Apart from questions of recognition speed and accuracy, there is also the question of familiarity, which by definition is experienced based. Nevertheless, one interesting prediction to come out of the feature-based approach to recognition is that a face made up of previously experienced features, though itself novel to the observer, should appear familiar. This hypothesis has been tested by Solso and McCarthy (1981), whose subjects were presented with photo-fit pictures of people and then tested on a familiarity task. The test set of faces contained either familiar faces, wholly novel faces, or novel faces containing combinations of features present in the familiar ones. The most intriguing result was that subjects chose the composite faces as more familiar than both the unfamiliar and the familiar faces. This result not only provides further support for the distributed-feature-based approach; it also demonstrates that perceived familiarity need not correlate with true familiarity.

16.4.3 Temporal Continuity as a Cue to Invariance Learning

Although a broadly tuned feature-based system of the type advocated in this chapter would be sufficient to perform recognition over small transformations (Poggio and Edelman 1990), associating images over larger shape transformations would require either separate prenormalization for size and translation of the image or separate feature detectors, which would

then be fed into a final decision unit. As it turns out, the use of prenormalization is contrary to the evidence we have from the responses of real neurons implicated in object recognition. Invariance seems to be established over a series of processing stages, starting from neurons with restricted receptive fields and culminating in the types of cell responses found in inferotemporal cortex mentioned earlier. With this in mind, it remains to be explained how one might learn to associate very different views of an object.

One possible solution to this problem is that in the real world, we tend to see discrete sequences of images of an object, images that often undergo transformations. Regularity in time may act as an important cue for predicting the identity of an object as it undergoes transformations, due to a change of position relative to the object. This change in viewing position may be simply due to our approaching the object, watching it move, rotating it in our hand, and so on. If the time domain is truly influential in setting up representations of objects, then there should presumably be some evidence for this in the learning of inferotemporal neurons. In effect, one should expect to see quite different views of an object being associated to the same neuron in preference to other very similar images, simply on the basis of the sequence in which they are presented. This last section discusses evidence that temporal relations in the appearance of object views do indeed affect learning.

The temporal association hypothesis has been discussed in the past, and has been successfully used in various neural network models of recognition (Edelman and Weinshall 1991; Földiák 1991; Wallis and Rolls 1997). In particular, Wallis and Baddeley (1997) demonstrated how the temporal statistics of the real world can be optimally used to establish transform-invariant representations of objects. The hypothesis has also found direct experimental sup-

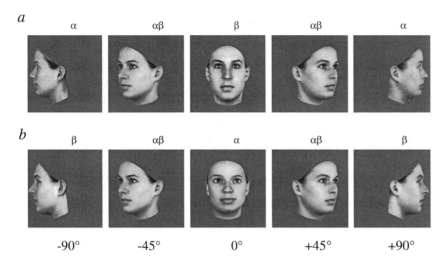

Figure 16.9
Example of a pair of faces used in Wallis and Bülthoff (2001). Each association sequence consisted of the two faces (α and β) in profile and frontal view, and a morphed face ($\alpha\beta$) shown at $\pm 45°$. Subjects saw both sequences (*a*) and (*b*) during training.

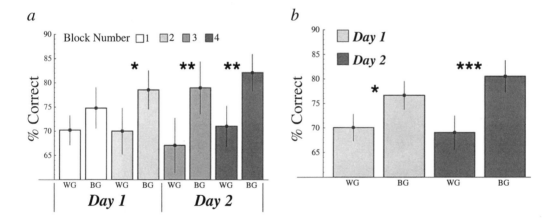

Figure 16.10
Results from Wallis and Bülthoff (2001). Subjects were asked to discriminate faces previously seen in morphed sequences. (*a*) Discrimination performance across training blocks, measured as percentage correct in the mismatch trials, showing for comparison within-group (WG) and between-groups (BG) scores. (*b*) Same results broken down across the two training days. * = $p < 0.1$, ** = $p < 0.01$, *** = $p < 0.001$.

port from neurophysiological recordings (Stryker 1991; Miyashita 1993). Miyashita (1988), for example, was able to show that repeating a temporal sequence of randomly selected fractal images establishes cells in inferotemporal cortex that respond to one stimulus in the series very strongly, but also to those patterns appearing in close succession. He was also able to show that the efficacy of a stimulus declined purely as a function of temporal disparity between stimuli.

Until recently, there was little or no psychophysical evidence to support the theoretical and neurophysiological findings. However, in 1996 Sinha and Poggio (see chapter 15) used temporal sequences to establish the perception of the form of ambiguous wire-frame objects, and Wallis and Bülthoff (2001) considered the effect of temporal sequences for natural objects such as faces. Wallis and Bülthoff (2001) hypothesized that exposing observers to sequences of different faces would cause them to confuse the identity of faces seen together in a sequence, which should then become apparent by the increased number of discrimination errors for faces that were seen in sequences, as opposed to faces that were not. Figure 16.9 puts this hypothesis in a more graphical light by displaying two possible sequences, each containing two different people's faces. The temporal association hypothesis predicts a higher confusion rate for pairs of faces associated in this way than for pairs of faces coming from two different sequences. During the experiment, subjects were exposed to thirty-six such pairings of heads and then tested on their ability to discriminate them. The results of their experiment are displayed in figure 16.10. "WG" indicates that the tested faces were from within a group, that is, appeared in a training sequence together; "BG," that the faces tested were once again familiar but came from separate groups, thus had not been seen in the same training sequence. The results

clearly demonstrate that discrimination performance was indeed worse for faces associated in sequences. The difference between the WG and BG condition is also seen to increase with each session of training.

Also looking at the influence of temporal order on the representation of objects, Stone (1998) used amoeba-like shapes, similar to those in Edelman and Bülthoff (1992), rather than wire-frame or familiar facial objects. During a learning phase, subjects had to discriminate four objects from numerous distractors. In this first phase, all stimuli rotated in one particular direction. During testing, certain of the trained objects were rotated in the opposite direction, which caused a falloff in discrimination performance, and an increase in reaction times. In fact, although similar to the results described above, the Stone (1998) results suggest something new, that temporal information forms part of the representation of the object.

A time-based association mechanism that correctly associated arbitrary views of objects without an explicit external training signal could overcome many of the weaknesses of using supervised training schemes or of associating views simply on the basis of physical appearance. For this reason, the three experiments described above may well represent a significant new step in establishing the two-dimensional multiple-view approach to object recognition.

Learning New Faces

Vicki Bruce and Mike Burton

17

Abstract

As children, we become particularly sensitive to the configuration of upright faces and to variations that discriminate faces within our own race, although we have difficulty recognizing faces when they are presented upside down or show variations with which we are unfamiliar. Throughout our lives we continue to learn to recognize each specific new face we encounter. During learning the visual representation shifts away from external face features and toward internal ones, particularly the eyes, and allows us to recognize a familiar (learned) face across a range of viewpoints, lighting, and expressions. After reviewing what is known about how we learn faces—both generally and specifically—this chapter outlines a theory that links the learning of new faces to the mechanisms responsible for repetition priming of familiar items.

17.1 Introduction

The human brain is a perceptual learning machine par excellence. Different demands are made of this machine at different times in its life. Developing infants quickly learn to differentiate and to individually recognize the important object categories in their world. At about the time children become familiar with most of the basic object categories they will ever encounter, they meet the new visual perceptual challenge of learning to read.

The further task of distinguishing between objects of the same overall type is one that will continue to tax the perceptual learning system throughout adulthood: almost every chosen profession, trade, or hobby requires its practitioners to acquire new per-

ceptual categories based on subtle differences between items, unnoticed by the untutored eye. Moreover, all of us, whether we also become accomplished radiographers, bird-watchers, or car buffs, will continue throughout our lifetimes to meet new people in the flesh, in films, or on TV. Through these encounters, each of us will continue to learn new members of the most important social category of all—the human face.

Familiar face recognition represents a considerable challenge for the human recognition system because known faces must be recognised across a variety of transformations. Like other objects, faces must be recognized across different viewing angles and in different lighting conditions. Unlike most other objects, however, faces also deform nonrigidly during expression and speech; slower, age-related changes in weight, wrinkles, hairstyle, and color, and sometimes rapid changes in hairstyle, also pose major challenges to the recognition system.

Early consideration of the processes of face recognition produced some apparently extraordinary demonstrations of "one-trial" face learning in experiments reported in the late 1960s and 1970s. A number of researchers (e.g., Shepard 1967; Standing 1973) showed that recognition memory for once-viewed pictures was extremely accurate and that this accuracy was maintained when pictures were drawn from homogeneous meaningful sets of items such as faces or pictures of houses. Memory for faces, however, generally exceeded that for other comparable groups of items. For example, Yin (1969) asked subjects to study for three seconds each image from a series of forty pictures drawn from two different groups (e.g., faces and houses). An immediate forced-choice recognition test followed in which subjects were asked to choose the studied item from each of twelve pairs of pictures of each type of object. The faces were all clean-shaven, adult males chosen to "be similar with respect to general age, expression and lack of outstanding distinguishing features ..." (p. 142). The houses were less uniform, to Yin's eye, than the faces. Nonetheless, recognition memory for upright faces was 93% correct, compared with 81% for pictures of houses.

Similar high rates of recognition memory have been found using "old-new" rather than forced-choice recognition memory tests, where decisions must be made to each individual face in a series of previously studied and new, distractor items. For example, Bruce (1982, experiment 1) presented a series of 24 unfamiliar male faces for study, for 8 seconds each, and later asked participants to decide whether each of a series of 48 male faces was old or new. When the "old" faces were shown in identical pictures to those studied, recognition rates of 90% were recorded, with a false positive rate of 12%. Importantly, however, in this study recognition rates for faces shown with changed viewpoint or expression were considerably less accurate. Thus what the early recognition memory experiments usually demonstrated was very good memory for specific pictures of faces, rather than any rapid learning of representations useful for generalising to novel views.

Indeed, in a meta-analysis of 128 eyewitness and facial identification studies, Shapiro and Penrod (1986) found that one important metafactor affecting recognition memory for previously unfamiliar faces is the extent to which the test conditions re-create the study conditions—in terms of facial image characteristics and associated context. Initially highly picture-specific performance with unfamiliar faces somehow transforms into the kind of visual memory that allows us to recognize highly familiar faces in difficult and novel circumstances.

This chapter will review what is known about the learning process which is relevant to the nature and acquisition of representations of familiar faces, and will not consider other important and interesting questions about memory for pictures, memory for relatively unfamiliar faces (as in eyewitnessing), or computer models of human face recognition, except where these topics illuminate the main thrust of the chapter. We start by considering the developmental learning process by which children gradually improve in face recognition abilities until they reach adult levels of expertise. The expertise acquired seems to include a particular sensitivity to the configural or relational properties of face patterns in general, plus a knowledge of the discriminating dimensions of the specific types of faces encountered during development. Despite this expertise, however, adults must learn each individual face they encounter. Briefly exposed, thus poorly learned faces are extremely difficult to recognize; the process of learning an individual face seems to shift its representation from one of extreme image specificity to a consolidated representation of a familiar face that can allow recognition across a range of natural transformations. This process of learning new faces will form the major focus of this chapter.

17.2   Comparisons between Face and Object Recognition

Before considering the detail of how we learn faces, it is interesting to inquire whether there is any difference between learning to recognize faces and learning to recognize other categories of objects. To what extent do the principles of learning faces illuminate (or become illuminated by) those applying to other categories? (For a fuller comparison of face and object recognition, see Bruce and Humphreys 1994.)

17.2.1 Multiple Levels of Categorization

Faces, like other objects, can be categorized at a number of different levels. First there is the "basic-level" categorization (Rosch et al. 1976; Biederman 1987): this pattern is a face, as opposed to some other kind of thing, such as a dog or a car. The system responsible for object recognition may deliver this categorization of a face as a face—or it may be part of a specific hardwired face detection module, which may be crucially important for infant-mother interactions and for social interactions in adults (see, for example, Goren, Sarty, and Wu 1975; Johnson et al. 1991).

Another level of categorization is of the face as a kind of face—for example, as a male face, as a Japanese face, or even as a nice-looking face. This requires that we derive meaning from the visual characteristics of the face alone (what Bruce and Young 1986 termed *visually derived semantics*), whether familiar or unfamiliar. This process is somewhat like recognizing what breed of dog or what make of car is present. Finally, we are able to determine, for familiar faces, to whom the face belongs. This process is more like recognizing an individual dog or our own car. It is this final level of face identification that is the most visually demanding because differences between individual faces can be extremely modest and can defy description.

17.2.2 Other Uses of Information from Faces

Besides serving as unfamiliar objects to be categorized in particular ways or as familiar objects to be successfully identified, all faces serve a variety of other functions that involve other mappings between visual form and meaning. We recognize emotions from facial expressions and can also make phonemic decisions based on perceived mouth shapes. We make use of head and eye gaze direction to understand where others are directing their attention. These social messages are derived from mapping between different nonrigid (expressive, speaking) movements and rigid (head direction) variations and other meaning categories. Such variations in the facial conformation are likely to make the task of face categorization and particularly face identification difficult because the range of rigid and nonrigid transformations of the face provides essential input to other social processes. Owing to the subtleties of the social demands of face processing, the representational requirements of recognition are likely to be different for faces compared with most other objects, although other varieties of *expert* identification, categorization, or both may well resemble face processing.

17.2.3 Expertise with Faces

Born with the ability to track facelike patterns with their eyes and head immediately after birth (Goren, Sarty, and Wu 1975; Johnson et al. 1991), babies very rapidly learn at least some faces: within the first few days of life, they will look more at the face of their mother than at another woman of similar appearance in conditions where olfactory cues are masked (Bushnell, Sai, and Mullin 1989). Despite these early proficiencies, however, face processing in early childhood is considerably less accurate than in adulthood. Chung and Thomson (1995) review the development of face recognition skills through childhood, and a recent study of our own (Bruce et al. 2000) shows how a range of face-processing skills, including the ability to process expression, facial

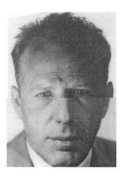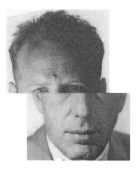

Figure 17.1
Composite faces of the type developed by Young, Hellawell, and Hay (1987), here formed from the top half of Bruce Willis's face and the bottom half of Humphrey Bogart's. It is much easier to recognize these individuals in the offset (*right*) than in the aligned (*left*) composite.

speech, and gaze, develop alongside face recognition skills from three through to ten years of age.

One hallmark of adult face recognition performance was first explored in pioneering work by Robert Yin (1969), who found that inverted faces were recognized much more poorly than upright faces; indeed, the effect of inversion was greater for faces than for other categories of objects. The basis of the inversion effect has been explored in detail in recent years; one hypothesis is that inversion disrupts the processing of configural information on which our expertise with upright faces depends.

In an interesting study of the effects of inversion on configural processing, Young, Hellawell, and Hay (1987) produced composite faces (figure 17.1) from the top half of one famous face and the bottom half of another. When the two halves were aligned, it was much more difficult to identify to whom the half faces belonged than when the two halves were offset. The alignment created a "new" face, which seemed to interfere with the perception of its parts. When the composites were inverted, however, this

effect disappeared, and the separate halves of the aligned composite faces became relatively easier to identify. That inverted faces are not subject to as much configural processing as upright faces is normally disadvantageous to recognizing inverted faces. This more piecemeal processing, however, allows the identities of the separate halves of the inverted composite faces to be retrieved equally well for aligned and nonaligned faces.

Valentine (1988) provided a detailed review of studies of the inversion effect, arguing that there was no unequivocal support for the notion that inverted faces were processed by *qualitatively* different processes from upright ones. Since 1988, however, a number of studies (Bartlett and Searcy 1993; Tanaka and Farah 1993; Rhodes, Brake, and Atkinson 1993; Leder and Bruce 1998) have provided more convincing evidence for the quite specific disruption of configural processing of inverted faces. We will consider some of these studies in more detail later in this chapter.

Whether or not inverted faces are processed in a qualitatively different way from upright ones, it is clear that the processing of upright faces involves an enhanced sensitivity to face configuration. It has been argued that this configural processing results from expertise acquired during a lifetime of processing faces. In this view, young children process faces in more "piecemeal" fashion than adults do; it is the development of configural processing skills that underlies the older child's enhanced recognition abilities. The evidence for this is equivocal, however. Although several studies have shown that young children are less disrupted by the inversion of faces than are older children and adults, Carey and Diamond (1994) showed that six- to seven-year-olds, ten- to eleven-year-olds, and adults showed the same "face composite" effect reported by Young, Hellawell, and Hay (1987). At all ages tested, the halves of aligned composites were more difficult to identify than those of nonaligned composites when displays were upright, but there was no difference between aligned and nonaligned versions when displays were inverted. Thus, to the extent that "configural" processing is tapped by the composite effect, it seems well established in early childhood. Nonetheless, in these same experiments, Carey and Diamond found an age-orientation interaction—with adults showing stronger overall decrements from the inversion of faces than children.

Carey and Diamond (1994) explain their apparently paradoxical findings by distinguishing between the access of parts of faces and the recognition of faces on the basis of relational features. They argue that young children, like adults, clearly find it difficult to access parts of faces from within whole ones (aligned composites); hence the composite effect is evident at all age groups. Nonetheless, experience with faces through childhood enhances the sensitivity to configural relationships in the representations used to identify faces: adults are much more disadvantaged when faces are inverted, and their configural relationships thus become more difficult to code. To use a simple analogy, the young child may have a very unsophisticated representation of familiar faces, for example, that one face has big eyes and another has small ones, but the processing of the whole configuration of an aligned composite could still interfere with the process of separately accessing the eyes to determine their size. The adult may have a much more elaborated representation of the relative shapes and separation of the eyes and their relationship with other facial features. Alignment of composites will make such descriptions equally hard to recover, but inversion will additionally disrupt the derivation of these kinds of relationships.

In this view, learned experience with faces creates expertise at encoding the spatial relationships that distinguish between different members of the class "face." Diamond and Carey (1986) distinguished between first-order spatial relationships, which define a basic-level category such as face (eyes above nose above mouth), and second-order spatial relationships, which differentiate members of this class. They reasoned that if expertise in distinguishing faces resulted from increasing sensitivity to these configural relationships, then perhaps experts in domains involving other classes of objects having the same first-order representation would also show heightened sensitivity to spatial relationships. If so, such experts should show inversion effects like those found with faces. Diamond and Carey (1986) tested this hypothesis with dog experts (judges of specific breeds of dog) and showed that such individuals suffered as much in terms of decreased recognition rates from inverting pictures of dogs as pictures of faces. Nonexperts showed greater effects of inverting pictures of faces than dogs. Although there are some problems with the results of this study (the dog experts were not actually superior to the nonexperts on upright pictures of dogs, which Diamond and Carey attributed to the experts' being much older than the control subjects), they nonetheless support the general theory that expertise creates sensitivity to discrimination of second-order spatial relationships.

17.2.4 Cross-Race Effect

Although adults are expert with faces of the type they have learned through exposure, they are much worse at recognizing faces of unfamiliar types than younger people are. Europeans find Japanese faces difficult to recognize, and vice versa (see Brigham 1986 for a brief review). Such effects cannot be explained in terms of inherent difficulties of one kind of face or another, or we would not observe cross-over interactions of this kind. The best-supported explanation is that experience with faces of our own race allows us to learn just the features that are discriminating within that race. In this view, increased contact with members of another race should reduce or even eliminate the cross-race effect. Some evidence supports this "contact" hypothesis, though the data are rarely unambiguous. For example, Chiroro and Valentine (1995) found that black African students who had a great deal of exposure to white faces recognized white faces as well as black ones, but the results obtained in the other half of the design with white observers were not so clear-cut.

Thus evidence from the development of face recognition and sensitivity to inversion combines with that from the cross-race effect to provide a reasonably consistent picture. Our facility at recognizing upright faces arises as a result of years of exposure to faces during childhood, exposure that enables us to discriminate types of faces from their subtle configural variations on the basic face pattern.

The recognition skills we have considered here apply to faces in general, not just to familiar ones. But what happens when a face becomes familiar? How do we learn new faces? To answer these questions, we need to understand the nature of the visual representations used when faces are unfamiliar, and how these change as a face is learned.

17.3   What Is the Difference between Unfamiliar and Familiar Faces?

Although visual memory for initially unfamiliar faces appears to be dominated by details of the particular picture or image of the face encountered, our representations for familiar faces appear to be more abstract.

17.3.1   Unfamiliar Face Representations Are Image Specific

A good illustration of the difference between representations for familiar faces and those for unfamiliar ones comes from an ongoing project of our own on the identification of people shown from closed-circuit television (CCTV) images (see Bruce 1998 for an overview). In some of our studies, observers are asked to choose the person from a photo array who matches the person shown on video, and in others asked to verify whether a video image matches a photographic still for identity. Observers make substantial numbers of errors identifying images of unfamiliar faces, even when the quality of the video image is high, whereas they are highly accurate in identifying and verifying images of familiar faces shown on video, their rates being at or near ceiling, even when video image quality is poor (Bruce et al. 1999; Burton et al. 1999; Bruce, Henderson et al. 2001).

In a recent study (Bruce, Henderson, et al. 2001), Zoe Henderson showed observers still images or short clips of a person walking into the University of Glasgow Psychology Department, where a CCTV system records a short clip of each entrant, of an image quality typical of commercial systems. They were given a still photograph of either the same person, or a different person, chosen to bear some resemblance to the target person in the video clip and asked to decide whether the two matched or not. A group of sixty observers who were chosen to be familiar with the people shown in the video images averaged 94% correct in this task, whereas observers unfamiliar with any of the faces seen in video or still images averaged only 73% correct. Note that there is no memory component at all in this task—observers must simply compare the visual image of one face against another, and have unlimited time to make their decision. Performance when faces are unfamiliar shows that the visual images of the two faces alone cannot be used to make an accurate comparison of the face features. Images of an already familiar face, however, can be independently identified even from the poor-quality video images, and these preexisting visual categories, and the nonvisual (identity) information that they access, can effectively mediate the comparison of the two images.

In another of our experiments, observers were shown target images of unfamiliar faces extracted from high-quality video and asked which of an array of ten male faces of similar overall appearance matched the identity of the image at the top. Although observers knew that the target was present on every trial, they made about 20% false matches in this task (Bruce et al. 1999), even when the target image was chosen to match the full-face viewpoint and neutral expression of the array faces as closely as possible.

Such studies suggest that our visual representations of unfamiliar faces are highly image specific (see also Hill and Bruce 1996; Kemp, Towell, and Pike 1997). Even when no memory load is involved, two different images of the same person can easily be confused with images of two different but similar-looking people. Yet we do not appear regularly to make such confusions between people we know well, although certain kinds of errors and difficulties in everyday person recognition are reasonably frequent (Young, Hay, and Ellis 1985). Clearly, there must be some shift in the representational process as we learn faces.

17.3.2 *Unfamiliar Face Representations Do Not Allow for Generalization*

Recognition of unfamiliar faces is considerably disrupted by changed image conditions, such as a change in viewpoint or lighting. Indeed, this disruption occurs even in tasks with no memory component at all, where the task is simply to compare two faces and determine whether they are the same person. For example, Hill and Bruce (1996) found matching accuracy was reduced when two images of the same person were shown in different viewpoints or with different lighting directions. Bruce et al. (1999) found that matching video images to full-face photo arrays was more difficult when the head pose of the video target was changed from full face to 30°. Thus the image specificity of face matching does not appear to be a function of memory, but of the way we perceive unfamiliar faces.

Familiar faces are not immune to all such effects, however. Johnston, Hill and Carman (1992) found that recognition of friends' faces was disrupted if these were shown with a highly unusual lighting direction (lit from below). Moreover, familiar face recognition, like unfamiliar face processing, is dramatically disrupted by inversion of the image in the picture plane (see Valentine 1988 for a review) and by reversal of polarity when images are shown in photographic negative (see, for example, Galper 1970; Phillips 1972). Bruce and Langton (1994) showed that where observers were forewarned of the list of celebrities whose faces might appear, identification of famous faces dropped from 95% in upright, positive images to 55% upright negative and 70% inverted positive. The two transformations combined virtually abolished recognition altogether, with recognition dropping to a mere 25% correct. It seems, then, that expertise with faces in general and familiarity with individual faces lead to representations that can tolerate transformations *within* the range usually experienced (e.g., of angle and of lighting) but *not outside* it (see Bruce 1994 for further discussion).

17.3.3 Internal versus External Features

Using recognition memory and matching tasks, Ellis, Shepherd, and Davies (1979) and Young et al. (1985) showed that representations of unfamiliar faces are dominated by the external features of hairstyle and face shape. This is consistent with similarity sorting studies reported by Shepherd, Davies, and Ellis (1981), where the three main dimensions extracted from multidimensional scaling of similarity judgments corresponded to hairstyle, face shape, and age. In contrast, however, the recognition and matching studies reported by Ellis, Shepherd, and Davies (1979) and Young et al. (1985) found that representations for familiar faces are weighted more toward internal features. Ellis, Shepherd, and Davis found that the external feature advantage in unfamiliar faces competely switched to an internal feature advantage in familiar ones, whereas Young et al. found that external and internal features were rather more equally weighted in familiar faces, but still showed the shift from external feature dominance in unfamiliar faces.

The shift in feature salience is consistent with the idea introduced earlier that unfamiliar face representations are based primarily on image properties of the specific pictures in which they are encountered (termed *pictorial codes* by Bruce and Young 1986). Although the hairstyle and external features represent a relatively large proportion of the total image encountered, hairstyles and face shapes change quite substantially over time, as people restyle their hair, change weight, or age—much more so than do internal features, whose characteristics change relatively slowly with age. In contrast, internal features are mobile and communicative and their momentary postures must be attended to in interpersonal communication. Perhaps these are the reasons why representations for learned (familiar) faces become shifted to capture this area of the face more strongly.

Importantly, Young et al. (1985) found that the shift toward internal feature processing occurred only when the identities of familiar faces had to be matched across different pictures. When familiar faces were used in a picture-matching task, the relative ease of internal and external feature matching was the same as shown with unfamiliar faces. Thus it is in the more abstract "structural" codes, which allow the recognition of familiar faces across changes of viewpoint, that internal features acquire their salience.

17.3.4 Dynamic Properties

There also seem to be differences in the ways that dynamic properties of unfamiliar and familiar faces are used for recognition. In a study since replicated in our own laboratory (Lander, Christie, and Bruce 1999), Knight and Johnston (1997) showed that negative images of famous faces were better recognized when an animated sequence was shown than when a single static image was shown. Such a result might arise simply because an animated sequence conveys more information than a static image does in the different viewpoints and expressions shown. In her doctoral research at the University of Stirling, Karen Lander has shown convincingly that this cannot be the only explanation. Using faces made hard to recognize through thresholding (figure 17.2) rather than negation, she has found that the beneficial effects of motion depend critically on motion characteristics rather than on the number of frames shown. Thus animated image sequences are best recognized when the face is shown at its original frame rate, as opposed to more quickly, more slowly, or in reverse or disrupted sequence (Lander, Christie and Bruce 1999; Lander and Bruce 2000).

Findings from unfamiliar face recognition are slightly different. Christie and Bruce (1998) found

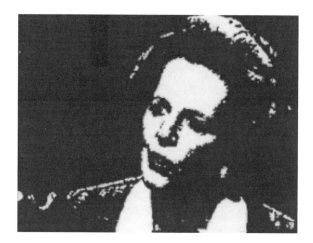

Figure 17.2
Thresholded image of the type used by Lander, Christie, and Bruce (1999). When images are reduced to one bit per pixel (black on white), they are more difficult to recognize, but become easier if shown in an animated sequence.

that studying unfamiliar faces in short animated sequences conferred no recognition memory advantage over studying them in fixed frame after fixed frame of these same sequences. In contrast, Pike et al. (1997) did find such an advantage, though subsequent work (personal communication) suggests that only rigid motion provides this advantage. The beneficial effects of movement in Pike et al. 1997 may have arisen because the lighting conditions for recognizing novel faces at test differed from those encountered at study. In this situation, formation of a three-dimensional description of the face may be of greatest use for subsequent recognition. Importantly, the recognition memory advantage for familiar faces that seems to arise from seeing nonrigid as well as rigid motion patterns does not extend to relatively unfamiliar faces (cf. chapter 15). This finding suggests that as part of, or in parallel with, structural representations of the *form* of familiar faces, exposure

to familiar faces leads us to learn a representation of how they *move*.

17.4 Representational Candidates for Face Recognition

Here we consider different possible types of representation for the internal description of faces and, in particular, how representations may become consolidated as a face is learned.

17.4.1 *Representational Options*

What are the representational "primitives" used by the visual system to describe and recognize faces? Does our internal representation of a face consist of a list of types of features and their relationships, of three-dimensional surfaces and their arrangement, or of some less abstract representation of patterns present within images of faces? Although the sensitivity of unfamiliar face recognition to image properties suggests that these properties must be represented in relatively unanalyzed image-based form, is this also true of familiar faces? First, let us consider the options.

Basic-level object recognition may be based in part on volumetric or other primitives derived from an edge-based "sketch" of the significant intensity changes present in an image (Biederman 1987; but see chapters 6, 16 for alternate accounts). Although such a representational scheme might suffice to categorise a face from a nonface, it seems highly unlikely that it can be used for more specific representational purposes. If something like a primal sketch of the major face features formed the basis of a set of measurements used to recognize faces, it is difficult to understand why unelaborated line drawings of famous faces are so difficult to recognize (Davies, Ellis, and Shepherd 1978; Bruce et al. 1992). Good representations for identity seem to require that the overall pattern of light and dark be preserved: negative images of faces are difficult to recognize because they invert the usual pattern of light and dark.

Bruce and Langton (1994) and Kemp et al. (1996) report studies exploring in greater detail why negative images are hard to recognize. Bruce and Langton (1994) showed that the recognition of nonpigmented, three-dimensional surface images of faces derived from scanning the shapes of faces with a laser range finder was affected rather little by negation. They used this result to suggest that the inversion of brightness of pigmented regions of the face (e.g., light skin to dark skin) was responsible for the effects of negation, rather than the reversal of shading patterns that were preserved in 3-D surface images. Kemp et al. (1996) showed that the alteration of hue of pigmented regions did not affect recognition of familiar faces, and suggested that the negation effect arose at least in part from how negation affected shape-from-shading processes.

Nevertheless, because even highly familiar faces are extremely difficult to recognize from three-dimensional shape alone, representations for face recognition seem unlikely to be based wholly or even largely on 3-D shape descriptions derived from shading patterns (Bruce, Healey, et al. 1991). Findings such as these have encouraged our group (e.g., Hancock, Burton, and Bruce 1996; Hancock, Bruce, and Burton 1998) to explore low-level image-based coding schemes such as principal components analysis (PCA) of image pixels (e.g., Kirby and Sirovich 1990; Turk and Pentland 1991) and graph-matching of Gabor wavelet patterns (e.g., Wurtz, Vorbruggen, and von der Malsburg 1990) as possible analogies for how the human visual system describes faces for recognition. In PCA, the intercorrelations between the variations in image intensity between each pixel are computed and used to derive underlying dimen-

sions (principal components) that can describe a set of faces economically. The different components extracted can be depicted graphically as "eigenfaces"; individual faces can then be described and reconstructed from the sum of a set of eigenfaces suitably weighted. Thus far, we have found that the PCA coding scheme certainly seems to capture, at least in part, how humans encode faces, though the wavelet-based graph-matching model may be a better model of how we recognize faces across pictorial transformations (Hancock, Bruce, and Burton 1998).

In sum, poor recognition of line drawings and the effects of photographic negation support the idea that patterns of light and dark are critical for representing faces. Shading patterns may lead to the derivation of an explicit three-dimensional description of the facial surface, which is clearly important for some tasks (for example, we cannot stroke someone's face unless we understand the 3-D layout of its surface). However if 3-D shape were computed explicitly as part of the representation for recognition, it is difficult to understand why we are so poor at recognizing faces from new viewpoints. We suggest instead that 3-D shape is coded only implicitly via the direct analysis of two-dimensional intensity patterns that mediate our recognition of identity.

17.4.2 Features versus Configuration: Holistic Representations

One of the attractions of low-level image-coding approaches such as those mentioned in the last section is that these analytic techniques extract global dimensions rather than local features for describing faces. A frequent finding in recent studies of face processing has been that the configuration of face features is at least as important as the local features themselves. In section 17.2.3, we described Young, Hellawell, and Hay's investigations (1987) of the face

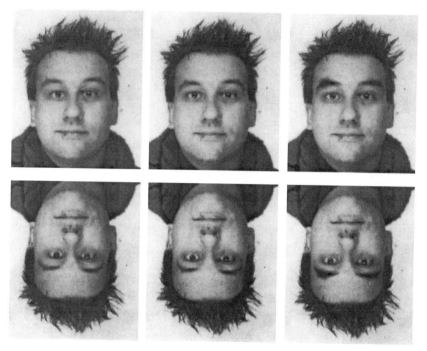

Figure 17.3

Images illustrating the work of Leder and Bruce (1998). The central image is distorted by changing the configuration (*left*) or local feature (*right*). Both changes are equally salient in upright faces, but only the local feature change remains more distinctive than the original when the image is inverted.

composite effect, where new face identities emerged from the juxtaposition of the top half of one face with the bottom half of another, provided these were closely aligned. Of the many similar demonstrations of the importance of configural information for face processing (e.g., Tanaka and Farah 1993; Rhodes, Brake, and Atkinson 1993; Bartlett and Searcy 1993; Searcy and Bartlett 1996), Leder and Bruce 1998 is notable for the realism of its configural and feature manipulations. Original faces with hairstyle concealed were rendered more distinctive either by making a change to a local feature (e.g., making the eyebrows more bushy) or by altering the relationship between features (e.g., by moving the eyes closer together; see figure 17.3). When such faces were shown upright, then both types of faces were rated as more distinctive and found to be more memorable than the originals. When shown upside down, however, only the distinctive local versions maintained their advantage over the original versions. The distinctiveness of those with configural alterations completely disappeared. Experiments such as these raise the thorny issue of what exactly is meant by "configural" processing of a face. Do we mean the coding of the spatial relationship between face features—or is a face processed as an undifferentiated "whole" pattern, within which there is no discrete analysis of features such as eyes, nose, and mouth at all? Although many researchers are unclear about this issue, others have expressed distinct positions: Diamond and Carey (1986) clearly point to the importance of the spatial relationships between different face features, and Tanaka and Farah (1993) suggest that faces might be processed as nondecomposed wholes.

The PCA (or eigenface) approach to automatic recognition is attractive in this context because of the global nature of the individual components (i.e. "representational primitives") it uses. The issue of part-based versus holistic face processing arises in part from an intuition that faces are made up of component parts, and that these different parts can be arranged in different configurations. Because recognition appears to be influenced both by the parts and by their configuration, it becomes hard to define either independently. Using PCA as a representational primitive has the advantage that faces are built of sets of features (or dimensions or primitives) but each of these covers the entire face. Thus the intuition that there are two aspects of faces, the primitives and their configuration, may have to be replaced with a representational scheme combining the two. PCA is not the only scheme available in this regard. Other systems, such as Gabor-filter-based matching systems also rely on primitives that cover a very large part of the face, rather than just common-usage features such as mouths or eyes. Technical solutions to engineering problems of pattern recognition may shed light on the nature of the primitives in face recognition; psychological research is under way to establish whether these representations may be useful in understanding human recognition.

17.4.3   *Prototype Face Representations?*

Thus far, we have considered what might form the basis of our representational primitives for face recognition, but not how picture- or image-specific representations first become more abstracted in the process of learning individual faces. Starting with a representation that captures image-based properties of the regions and interrelationships seen in one or a very few images of an unfamiliar face, we somehow gain, over the course of many encounters with that face, perceptual learning of a consolidated visual memory that now emphasizes internal over external features, and allows a degree of generalization to novel images of that face in a way not possible for the unfamiliar.

One possibility is that the different image-based encounters with the face literally become averaged in some process of overlaying or merging of successive images of the face to form a prototype representation. Another is that each exemplar is stored independently and that generalization emerges from the increasing opportunities for overlap between any new instance and one of the collection stored. Baron (1981) provides a clear early computer model of how both averaging and retention of distinct exemplars could coexist. According to his model, as each instance of a known face is encountered, its similarity to already stored representations of that face is compared, with the fate of the new instance dependent on its degree of resemblance to what is already stored. If its overlap with a stored exemplar is very high, then the new instance is simply discarded, whereas, if its resemblance is very low, then the new instance is stored as a novel exemplar of that person. If similarity is intermediate between these two extremes, then the new exemplar is averaged with the record already stored. In this way, for example, faces might acquire a set of consolidated or abstracted representations at each of a distinct number of canonical viewpoints.

Evidence consistent with this kind of storage process has been obtained in experiments on the storage of face "prototypes" from variant facial exemplars.

Bruce et al. (1991) gave observers a series of faces to rate for apparent age. The series contained several different variants of each of a number of distinct individual faces, where variations were created by displacing the internal features of the face upward or downward by regular amounts around a starting or "prototype" arrangement of the features. We found that, in a later unexpected recognition memory test, observers found these "prototype" faces highly familiar, even if they had never been seen in the study series. Such findings were reminiscent of those by Posner and Keele (1968) using varying dot patterns from which the protypical pattern arrangement was apparently learned.

One way of explaining these data is to suggest that successive instances of a face become superimposed as a face is learned, so that the "average" of the encountered traces seems more familiar than any individual trace. Importantly, Bruce (1994) and Cabeza et al. (1999) reported limits to this superimposition effect. When face variations were based on *angular* changes in head pose, there was little evidence for a prototype effect unless angular variations were very small indeed, whereas variations in *feature placement* (internal configuration) led to prototype effects, even when the feature variations shown were very large (Cabeza et al. 1998).

Thus our suggestion is that, as an initially unfamiliar face is learned, different instances of the same face become superimposed to provide a structural code (or, most likely, a set of such codes spanning different viewpoints), which represents the central tendencies in all the variations of the face encountered.

Finally, we should note that within the large literature on prototype or "typicality" effects in perceptual and conceptual learning there has been a fairly lively debate between "prototype" theories and "exemplar" theories, with the weight of evidence tending to favor the exemplar account (see Medin

1989 for an overview). On the other hand, although it is easy to think about the separation of exemplars within the learning of a concept such as "bird" (where each exemplar might be one type of bird—sparrow, robin, ostrich, etc.), it is not so easy within the domain of perceptual learning of categories such as "John's face." Even though our laboratory experiments may separate John's face into a number of discrete training or test exemplars (photographs or pictures), in everyday life, a new face will be encountered in the continuous transformations of expression, gesture, and speech. In such a context, a process of averaging and abstraction—at least within small variations of the same viewpoint—would seem more likely on logical grounds. Finally, we note that neither of these broad approaches seems well suited to capture the dynamic properties of faces that also seem to be represented as a result of learning (see section 17.3.4).

17.4.4 Categorical Effects

Another shift occurs as a face is learned through the process of abstraction outlined above. The function of such learning seems to be to make differences between different instances of the same face less easy to see because they are united by the common representational entity that allows each of them to be recognized. In contrast, differences between one face and other similar looking people become easier to see, and when faces are familiar they appear to be largely immune from the kinds of confusion we find in matching images of unfamiliar faces.

This function of categorical perception is a familiar one when applied to certain kinds of perceptual categories, such as colors (Bornstein and Korda 1984), phonemes (Liberman et al. 1957), and even facial expressions (Etcoff and Magee 1992; Young et al. 1996). In all these domains, it has been shown that it is harder to discriminate between two different exemplars that fall within the same perceptual category (e.g., two different shades of red or two different happy expressions) than between two exemplars of equivalent physical dissimilarity that straddle a category boundary (e.g., a red with an orange or a happy face with a sad one).

Interestingly, these same kinds of effects have also been demonstrated in familiar face recognition. Beale and Keil (1995) presented observers with images that were morphed in graded steps between two familiar faces such as Bill Clinton's and John F. Kennedy's. At one end of the continuum lay morphs (e.g., 90% Clinton and 10% Kennedy or 80% Clinton and 20% Kennedy) that were readily categorized as one or the other person (e.g., Clinton). Near the middle of the continuum were morphs that were much more difficult to categorize (e.g., 50% Clinton and 50% Kennedy). They found that discrimination between two different Clinton-Kennedy morphs straddling the boundary between their identities was much better than discrimination between two morphs both judged to belong to the same identity, although importantly, such categorical effects were not found for pairs of faces unfamiliar to participants (but see Levin and Beale 2000).

Stevenage (1998) was able to chart the process of learning familiar but difficult face categories using photographs of the faces of identical twins. As observers became able to discriminate one twin from another, their similarity ratings came to exhibit categorical effects. After training with numerous images of each twin's face, they judged different exemplars of the same twin to be more similar in appearance, and different exemplars of different twins to be more dissimilar in appearance, than they had before training.

Such categorical effects are pervasive, although their explanation is also controversial. It is unclear how much categorical perception arises from perceptual learning, and how much from verbal labeling as a result of such learning.

17.4.5 What Changes as Faces Become Familiar?

The preceding sections have suggested that representations for familiar faces are based upon the superposition of image-based descriptions in a way that selectively enhances their internal facial features. Can we experimentally chart the process of acquiring new representations of previously unfamiliar faces and see the changes in visual representation emerge in more detail? This interesting idea was tested in an unpublished experiment by Hadyn Ellis and colleagues, who showed observers a set of video sequences of a to-be-learned set of faces every day for several days. They found that performance on a face-matching task shifted from external feature dominance toward internal feature dominance over the course of this training. These preliminary findings have been replicated in recent studies within our own group.

Adriana Angeli (see Angeli, Bruce, and Ellis 1999) attempted a similar study at the University of Stirling: on each of nine successive days, observers were introduced to short video clips of thirty individuals accompanied by some descriptive information about who the people were. Each day included a face familiarity decision test where observers had to discriminate thirty familiar from thirty unfamiliar faces using whole faces, internal features, or external features (ten familiar and ten unfamiliar items in each condition each day). The results from this study were very promising, with a switchover from external feature dominance to internal feature dominance over the course of the experiment, as shown in the summary of data in table 17.1.

A further promising study has just been completed by Chris O'Donnell, a doctoral candidate at the

Table 17.1
Mean discrimination of familiar from unfamiliar faces and latency of familiarity decisions as new faces were learned (Angeli, Bruce, and Ellis 1999)

	Accuracy (d′)	Correct Reaction Time (msec)
Mean Days 1–3		
Internal	1.26	2,285
External	1.48	1,970
Whole	3.19	1,736
Mean Days 4–6		
Internal	3.22	1,443
External	2.40	1,350
Whole	4.87	1,124
Mean Days 7–9		
Internal	4.30	1,099
External	3.60	1,198
Whole	5.93	945

University of Stirling. He asked observers to learn a small number of individuals who were shown repeatedly on video until all could be identified correctly by name. Observers then moved to a face-matching task where they were asked to decide as quickly but accurately as possible whether pairs of faces were identical or different. When faces were unfamiliar, only changes to the hair were well detected, whereas changes to all other features including the eyes were not. On the other hand, performance on pairs differing in the region of the eyes alone was selectively enhanced for faces that had been familiarized compared with novel (unfamiliarized) faces, consistent with a shift to internal feature processing (O'Donnell and Bruce 2001). This research suggests that it is the eyes specifically, rather than internal features more generally, that are learned as faces become familiar.

The above studies suggest that we can chart a shift from external to internal feature processing during familiarization, and that the eyes in particular benefit from at least the early stages of familiarization.

17.5 Modeling the Learning of New Faces

Most computational models of face recognition are based on recognition of individual pictures of faces. For example, the Face Recognition Technology (FERET) test (Phillips 1998) has been used to compare a number of engineering tools for face recognition on their performance at recognizing large numbers of individual face images. Recently, there has been increased interest in the coding of image sequences of individual faces (e.g., Graham and Allinson 1998; Psarrou, Gong, and Buxton 1995), showing how, for example, viewpoint invariance can result from such coding sequences. Thus far at least, this work has made little contact with psychological models of face recognition, though we have just embarked on a new research project aiming to redress this. To examine possible models for the learning of new faces, we turn first to repetition priming and then to models of cognitive processes in face recognition.

17.5.1 *Repetition Priming of Face Recognition*

Within the psychological literature, the phenomenon of repetition priming, which appears to arise from the updating of representations of familiar faces, may hold the key to how we learn new ones. Repetition priming, the gain in recognition accuracy or speed from earlier exposure to an item, has been demonstrated in recognition of words, objects, and faces (see, for example, Bruce et al. 2000). It is of interest because it is domain specific—faces prime faces but names do not—thus must arise within the system representing the visual appearances of faces.

Moreover, repetition priming seems to require item identities be retrieved: sex decisions do not prime sex decisions, for example (Ellis, Young, and Flude 1990).

Repetition priming of faces is sensitive to variations in facial appearance that seem to reflect representations used for recognition. Priming is reduced when face viewpoint, expression, or both are varied (Ellis et al. 1987), reduced when gray-level "format" is altered (Bruce et al. 1994), but not affected by a change in image from color to gray scale or vice versa (Bruce, Terry, and Smith 1998). Repetition priming can be shown from faces viewed entirely incidentally, for example, on subject recruitment posters (Bruce, Carson, et al. 1998).

In their interactive activation and competition (IAC) model of the stages of person identification, Burton, Bruce, and Johnston (1990) suggested that repetition priming arises from the strengthening of connections between units involved in identifying a face. Following earlier functional models (and particularly Bruce and Young 1986), they proposed pools of face recognition units (FRUs) corresponding to the stored visual representations of faces. These units are connected via processing links to a pool of units called "person identity nodes" (PINs), which code individuals rather than faces and can receive information from other recognition domains (e.g., names or voices). These PINs are themselves connected via a further stage of links to personal information for each of the persons to be identified. Burton, Bruce, and Johnston proposed a simple Hebbian link update mechanism, one that has the effect of strengthening the links used. In this way, if a face has been seen recently (and the link between a particular FRU and the corresponding PIN therefore strengthened), processing will proceed faster on the second presentation of the same face. (For details of

the architecture and simulations, see Burton, Bruce, and Johnston 1990.)

This simple idea that repetition priming involves strengthening the links (or pathways) used within a model has been extended to more recent versions of the Burton, Bruce, and Johnston (IAC) model of the cognitive aspects of face recognition. Burton, Bruce, and Hancock (1999) describe how the IAC model can be interfaced with an image-processing "front end," based on PCA of facial images. Face images are represented by the values of a few of their components (eigenfaces), represented as input units and linked to the face recognition units described above. Because the Hebbian link update mechanism is used throughout this version of the IAC model, repetitions of exactly the same image give maximum priming: all links strengthened during the first presentation are subsequently used during the second presentation. Because there is considerable overlap between the principal component (PC) representations of the two images, presentation of two different images of the same person produces some priming; because the overlap is not total, however, priming is reduced.

This model seems to provide a natural account of the processes involved in repetition priming. Burton, Bruce, and Hancock (1999) go on to show that a model incorporating both image processing and cognitive stages of face recognition offers a much larger predictive range than models limited to the "perceptual" or "cognitive" domains alone.

17.5.2   Burton's Model of Learning New Faces (IACL)

Although our discussion of repetition priming in section 17.5.1 may seem a digression from the main focus of this chapter, one of the few computational models of face learning available relies on the idea that exactly the same processes are involved in new face learning and in priming.

Burton (1994) proposes that priming observed in behavioural experiments is simply the residue of a mechanism whose chief purpose is to learn faces in the first place. Of the criteria a model of face learning should satisfy, Burton emphasizes three: such learning should be modeled as automatic, gradual, and cumulative. By "automatic," Burton means that learning should be unsupervised: the same procedures that allow us to recognize a known face should also allow us to recognize a face as unfamiliar, and to begin to learn it (cf. chapters 18.4, 20 for types of learning models). The argument is that there is no humunculus in our brains who knows the right answer and can alert us to faces that are or are not genuinely new; instead, the process appears to be automatic. Second, the model should allow for gradual learning. We mentioned above that there are grades of familiarity; intuitively, we appear to know some people's faces better than others. And third, face learning in the model should be cumulative; we seem to learn new faces with no consequent effects on representations of known faces. The IACL model (IAC with Learning) is intended as a model of adult face learning, *not* developmental face learning. This final criterion is particularly important in comparisons with some connectionist models of learning. Indeed, many connectionist models capture the transition from no knowledge whatever to total knowledge, for example, by presenting the to-be-learned corpus blocked many times (e.g., Farah, O'Reilly, and Vecera 1993). The IACL model is an attempt to capture a more realistic process in which new faces are learned throughout adulthood.

In the IACL model, the pools of FRUs and PINs are large enough to allow space for many more representations than are used at any one time, whereas, in models using both localist and distributed representations, such space is achieved by having redundancy in the number of units available. In the IACL model, these unused representational patterns are connected with very small randomly varying connections to the units coding input dimensions (see section 17.5.3). When an input pattern is known, it will traverse strong, well-used links and cause excitation of units corresponding to a known person. When, however, the pattern is not known, no particular such unit will become active. Instead, a random "spare" unit will become selected as the most highly active unit. Simple Hebbian update on all links in the model will ensure that this new unit will come to specialize on the new pattern. After several presentations, the links connecting the input pattern and the new person will become as strong as the links connecting previously known faces.

The procedure of recruiting new units automatically is, on the surface, cognitively rather odd. However, it is mathematically exactly the same procedure as recruiting a new pattern in a distributed representation. It also has the advantage that it meets all three criteria set out for it: it is automatic, gradual, and cumulative. (For full simulations see Burton 1994; for a detailed discussion of the computational efficiency of the procedure, as compared to distributed systems, see Burton 1998.)

We have not yet applied the theoretical model of learning based on hypothetical face patterns to the realistic face images that form the input to the most recent version of the IAC model (Burton, Bruce, and Hancock 1999). That version takes PCA-coded faces as its input, based on individual static views of faces. A further challenge will be to consider how image sequences with their variation over time can be coded and learned in models of this type. At this much later stage, we will be able to see whether this kind of model reproduces the same effects of familiarization we find in human learning of new faces.

For now, we present one additional thought about the kind of learning algorithm that may be appropriate to model learning new faces.

17.5.3 Need Learning Be Unsupervised?

Burton's learning algorithm (1994) involves the gradual association of conjunctions of face features with face recognition units by the simple, unsupervised mechanism of Hebbian update, which is comparable to the gradual emergence of a representation for a familiar face from repeated encounters with its visual image. In the simulations of IACL to date, the input "feature" units for learned and new faces remain constant in repeated encounters. An obvious need is to extend IACL to a situation that convincingly models the process of learning representations across variations of the input pattern as viewpoints, expressions, and lightings change. Given our observations of unfamiliar face matching—where frequent confusions are made between different individuals when the task is to match one view of an unfamiliar face with another—how can such a learning system possibly cope with such variation? Importantly, the system described by Burton is doing a harder job than it strictly needs to. When we encounter new faces in the real world, there is plenty of scope for supervised learning. To mention just three important factors:

1. As a face changes in its appearance—through viewpoint and expression—the temporal sequence provides constraints so that each image viewpoint is only a slight modification on the one before. It is extremely important that current computational work on coding temporal sequences be brought to bear on psychological models of learning new faces, and our own future work will do this.

2. As a face is presented in all its variations, other aspects of the learning context remain constant. For example, we know that this continues to be Fred because the remainder of Fred remains in the same place even as his face pattern varies before us. Fred has a body and Fred has a voice.

3. When a face is presented to us, we rarely see it without some accompanying information about who the person is (their character in a film; the fact that they live in your street when met at home, and so forth). In the terms of the IACL model, activity will be being stimulated and changed in the semantic information units and their connections back via the PINs to the developing face recognition units. Thus the process of acquiring new face representations will have top-down support from a range of other sources of information. In our own future program of research, we will investigate whether such nonvisual constraints affect the way that visual representations are learned.

We have argued that image-based representations of each new face encountered become consolidated through a process of abstraction. This process can be implemented within our IACL framework, though we have yet to extend this to varying exemplars and have yet to explore the IACL mechanism using real images of faces, as in Burton et al. 1999. We expect that familiarization with new faces, once implemented, will lead to the emerging properties of generalization, categorical effects, and shifts from external to internal feature processing. However, the representation of dynamic properties from moving faces will require a different or additional means of image coding from that implemented to date.

Acknowledgments

Our research is currently supported by grants from the U.K. Economic and Social Research Council, and the Engineering and Physical Sciences Research Council.

Modeling

Models of Perceptual Learning

Shimon Edelman and Nathan Intrator

18

Abstract

This chapter addresses learning on a general computational level, reviewing a series of broadly relevant theoretical notions to identify the dimensions along which varieties of learning can be classified. In particular, we discuss (1) the goals of learning, (2) the mechanisms that can support learning, (3) the cues that a learning system can rely on to improve its performance, and (4) the paradigms or metaphors used to describe learning computationally. Our hope is that this review of the computational underpinnings of learning will make the relationships among existing models, including those mentioned elsewhere in the book, more readily apparent.

18.1 Introduction

A generation ago, mathematical psychology, then the premier discipline in charge of modeling behavior, appeared to be in poor shape. One prominent mathematical psychologist, William Estes (1957, 609), described the situation: "Look at our present theories ... or at the probabilistic models that are multiplying like overexcited paramecia. Although already too complicated for the average psychologist to handle, these theories are not yet adequate to account for the behavior of a rodent on a runway." During the following decades, when mainstream psychology underwent a major paradigm shift, the modeling of perceptual learning fared better than what one might have expected from the view expressed by Estes. A new theoretical outlook, which encouraged thinking now termed *representational* or *computational*, took over

the field, and the models became, if anything, more complex than those of 1957.

Encouragingly, the models are now also more successful in explaining behavior (rather than merely predicting the probability of a certain response to a given stimulus), while giving no undue troubles to the psychologists (for an interesting historical perspective on these issues, see Hintzman 1994). Insofar as there is progress, it seems to stem mainly from (1) the improvement in the experimental techniques that subserve data collection in behavioral and physiological psychology, and (2) the revision of the theoretical basis on which models are built. The "rodent on a runway" example mentioned above serves well to illustrate both these points. On the theoretical or conceptual side, the current explanation takes the route presaged by Tolman (1948) and based on the concept of cognitive maps (O'Keefe and Nadel 1978). On the experimental side, the existence of cognitive maps in the rat brain could not have been demonstrated without modern multiple-electrode recording methods and the information-processing tools that accompany them.[1]

In this chapter, we shall concentrate on approaches to the modeling of perceptual learning, rather than on its phenomenology or on specific models—the standard fare of the reviews one finds in the literature (Gibson 1969; LaBerge 1976; Walk 1978; Barto 1989; Gallistel 1990; Gluck and Granger 1993; Berry 1994; Gilbert 1994; Sagi and Tanne 1994; Ahissar and Hochstein 1998). In perceptual learning, of course, periodic reviews are as important as in any other discipline blessed with a steady stream of empirical findings. Such reviews stress the relative merits of learning mechanisms, often at the expense of computational theory itself (Marr and Poggio 1977). This preoccupation with mechanisms reflects the classical methodological stance, codified by Popper (1992), according to which empirical studies should begin with a discussion of the models to be tested and should end by refuting some of the models.

It is indeed easier to refute a specific model, mechanism, or wiring diagram than to gain support for a general theory. Nevertheless, a field of study stands to gain more from the latter endeavor: by providing an explanation for the observed phenomena, a good theory can subsume an entire range of models of the underlying mechanisms within the same formal framework (Deutsch 1997). Following this line of reasoning, to understand perceptual learning, we must, first and foremost, address basic questions such as "What does it mean, from a general information-processing standpoint, for a system to learn something?" Note that the answer "To learn a perceptual task means to acquire an adequate low-dimensional internal representation of the stimulus set" would be proper in this case (even if it eventually proved to be factually wrong) because it is coached in general information-processing computational terms (see Marr and Poggio 1977). By comparison, the answer "Learning something means growing extra dendrites" would constitute a category mistake—as would the seemingly more abstract answer "Learning is the recruitment of extra memory," unless the need for this memory is explained in functional terms that are algorithm and implementation neutral.

18.2   Goals of Learning

The main distinction at the task level that conceptually precedes any discussion of learning mecha-

nisms is between merely exercising memory, on the one hand, and using experience with familiar stimuli or problems to process or solve new ones, on the other.

18.2.1   Memorization

Early quantitative studies of the acquisition of declarative information used lists of items to be memorized as stimuli. For example, the subjects could be asked to memorize lists of nonsense syllables, whose recall was subsequently tested by the experimenter. In this setting, popularized by Ebbinghaus (1885), rehearsal of the stimulus is certainly a sensible strategy, repetition being the mother of learning (see chapter 17 for repetition learning of faces). Likewise, in learning that can be described as procedural (i.e., learning to perform a perceptual discrimination or a motor task), repetition was found early on to bring about an improvement of performance (see discussion of Volkman's 1858 study of cutaneous spatial acuity in Gibson 1969).

In the century and more since the pioneering work of Volkman and Ebbinghaus, repetition was shown to lead to improved performance in virtually every perceptual and motor domain tested; at the same time, the scope of memorization as a paradigm for learning was shown to be limited. Specifically, it became clear that performance gain from repetition is transferred only partially to novel situations (Gibson 1941; Ellis 1965). The extent and the nature of the transfer depends on the relationship between the sets of perceptual stimuli (or the repertoire of movements in motor learning) and between the tasks defined over these stimuli in the original and novel situations (Osgood 1949). To cite some relatively recent examples, limited transfer was reported by Fiorentini and Berardi (1981), who found that practicing discrimination between spatial contrast gratings at one orientation does not improve the performance at an orthogonal orientation (see Fiorentini and Berardi, chapter 9, this volume). An analogous situation prevails in motor learning; for example, an acquired ability to perform precise elbow flexions was found to transfer only partially from one set of joint angles to another (Gottlieb et al. 1988).

The distinction between memorization and transfer is of crucial importance to any theory of learning. A theory that fails to make this distinction succumbs to the same confusion that surrounds the much-publicized inability of an early neural network model of learning, the perceptron (Minsky and Papert 1969), to solve the "exclusive OR" (XOR) problem (figure 18.1). This problem is special: every nearest neighbor of each input belongs to the opposite class, thus no cluster structure (i.e., no similarity structure, where nearby points belong to the same class) exists.

The prospects of perceptrons (and of any models of perceptual learning that share their limitations) would be indeed bleak if real-life scenarios tended to resemble the XOR setup, in which generalization is ill defined (Bishop 1995). As we shall argue next, however, learning scenarios that focus on memorization—testing subjects (1) in a fixed task and (2) with the same stimuli encountered during the learning phase—cover only a part of the great variety of everyday situations in which learning is known to occur.

18.2.2   Generalization

The behavioral importance of transfer of learning, or generalization, to novel conditions (as contrasted with memorization) has been pointed out and discussed by philosophers, psychologists, and neurobiologists. In philosophy, the "naturalistic" approach to epistemology (Kornblith 1985) involves the concept of natural kinds—categories of objects that share sufficiently many features to support associative

recall, inference (prediction) of unobserved properties, and valid generalization from one stimulus to another (Quine 1969; Dretske 1995).

In psychology, empirical data gathered in the 1940s and 1950s prompted Guttman (1963) to view stimulus generalization as a central theoretical challenge. Shepard (1987) responded to the challenge by proposing a "universal law" to describe the quantitative relationship between the likelihood of two stimuli receiving the same response and their perceived similarity. More precisely, Shepard showed, on the basis of data from a wide range of perceptual experiments, that stimuli in each experiment could be arranged in a low-dimensional metric feature space so that the probability of generalization between any two stimuli was monotonic in their proximity (i.e., similarity). Shepard's treatment of this issue included a derivation of the monotonic dependence law from some basic assumptions on the probability measure used to quantify generalization.

In theoretical neurobiology, generalization underlies the "fundamental hypothesis" of Marr's theory of the cerebral neocortex (1970, 150–151): "Where instances of a particular collection of intrinsic properties (i.e., properties already diagnosed from sensory information) tend to be grouped such that if some are present, most are, then other useful properties are likely to exist which generalize over such instances. Further, properties often are grouped in this way." Although this hypothesis seems at present every bit as convincing as it must have appeared to Marr, it remains, unfortunately, empirically unsubstantiated; its vindication or refutation is likely to bear on statistical theories of brain function, such as those of Uttley (1959) and Marr (1970), and the neural network theories of their recent successors (more on this below).

The foundational status of generalization in visual perception and cognition can be easily illustrated

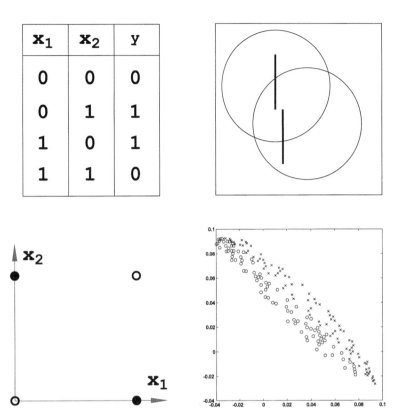

Figure 18.1
(*Upper left*) Truth table definition of a two-variable exclusive OR (XOR) problem. (*Lower left*) Note how the points belonging to the two classes are interspersed among each other. The common characteristic of this kind of problem, which impedes generalization, is that the probability of two neighboring points belonging to the same class is at chance. (*Upper right*) Outlines of size and position of two Gaussian receptive fields (RFs; see Poggio, Edelman, and Fahle 1992) in vernier discrimination problem. (*Lower right*) Representations of 200 vernier stimuli in the space of the outputs of these same two RFs. The simulation that produced this plot used a 100×100 image, and two Gaussian filters with $\sigma = 30$, positioned at $(70, 30)$ and $(30, 70)$. The two symbols, $\circ$ and $\times$, correspond to the two senses of vernier displacement, making this a class-conditional probability density plot of a sort. The vernier displacement in this experiment ranged from 5 to 15 pixels. The crucial characteristic here are the clusters of points belonging to the same class, which are simply connected and unimodal (human observers find learning more difficult when the class-conditional distributions are disjunctive or multimodal; Flannagan et al., 1986). It seems safe to conjecture that in general the class-conditional densities arising from perceptual tasks can be relatively easily made to look like this, facilitating decision making (unlike the case of the XOR example). In this chapter, we argue that learning can be construed as the formation of a representation space in which the problem at hand is well-behaved in this sense.

in intuitive terms, on an everyday task. Consider, for example, learning to recognize a face from several snapshots. The observer's ability to recognize the face in this case most probably extends to new images (obtained, say, under various combinations of viewpoint and illumination). Moreover, the observer is also expected to be able to solve a range of perceptual problems involving that face (e.g., to estimate its direction of gaze, to categorize its various expressions, etc.). These latter abilities effectively require that learning be transferred from one set of stimuli (i.e., images of the many faces previously processed by the subject) to another (i.e., images of the new face). Thus any theory of perceptual learning must include a component that would account for generalization across stimuli and across tasks, over and above rote memory (figure 18.2). The central role of generalization in learning underscores the importance of experiments such as those of Fiorentini and Berardi (1981), which define the limits of generalization in the human perceptual system, and thereby make a crucial contribution to the discovery of the principles and the mechanisms that support it.

18.3   Mechanisms of Learning

The characteristics of learning discussed thus far have to do with the nature of the task, where the main distinction is between memorization and generalization. We now consider the mechanisms employed by models of learning to explain the improvement of the performance with practice. At the highest level of abstraction, a common (though not entirely warranted) distinction is between symbolic mechanisms and neuromorphic ones. Whereas in symbolic learning the building blocks of models are propositions and rules (Carbonell, Michalski, and Mitchell

1983), the components of neural models of learning are activation states of simple computing elements and their interconnection patterns (Selfridge 1959; Hinton 1989; Rumelhart and Todd 1993).

It is now widely acknowledged that the principles of operation of neural learning models apply also to more traditional computational paradigms and data structures (Omohundro 1987). Even more importantly, neural networks turn out to be amenable to mathematical analysis that invokes well-established statistical tools dealing with inference and decision making (Bishop 1995). For example, Widrow's "Adaline" (adaptive linear element) networks (1985) can be identified with linear discriminant functions, and multilayer perceptrons with multivariate multiple nonlinear regression. (For further parallels between the neural network terminology and that of statistics, see Sarle 1994.)

Inferential statistics thus constitutes a useful foundation for the understanding of the computational capabilities of neural networks. If this foundation is to be useful in the development of specific models of learning in the nervous system, statistical samples of stimuli must be shown to contain information necessary for learning. Having been downplayed for decades by Chomsky and his school, the notion that statistical inference can support learning even in markedly "symbolic" domains such as language acquisition is now making a comeback. This process is aided by the growing evidence that humans (both adults and infants) are sensitive to statistical cues present in linguistic stimuli. For example, from such cues, subjects can implicitly extract information about boundaries between the underlying morphological units (Saffran, Aslin, and Newport 1996), word meaning (Markson and Bloom 1997), and even grammarlike rules (Berns, Cohen, and Mintun 1997). Consequently, models built around symbolic

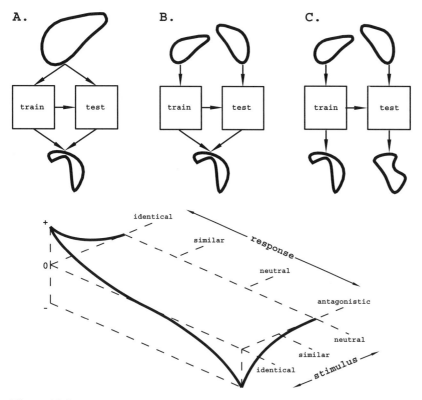

Figure 18.2
(*Top*) Schematic diagrams of three varieties of data- and task-related situations in learning. (*A*) When inputs and required outputs are the same in both training and testing phases, learning amounts to memorizing the input-output association, such as that of a name with a face. The arrow leading from the train to the test box represents the parameters acquired by the adaptive mechanism during the learning process. (*B*) If new data are to be mapped into the same output space, the system must generalize the previously learned association, such as by naming a familiar face seen under novel conditions (e.g., peculiar illumination). (*C*) If both the input and the output spaces change between training and testing, the problem turns into that of transfer of learning to a new task, such as matching two views of an unfamiliar face on the basis of prior experience with other face stimuli. (*Bottom*) Schematic diagram of the dependence of transfer on the relationship between the characteristics of two tasks. (Adapted from Osgood 1949.) The degree of transfer grows with the similarity between the stimuli in the two tasks, and, for highly similar stimuli, is reduced if the required responses are different.

abstraction (rule inference) must now routinely compete with models that posit similarity-based processing (Berry 1994; Goldstone and Barsalou 1998).[2]

In visual perception, three-dimensional object recognition is one domain where the hegemony of symbol manipulation models is increasingly challenged by statistical or connectionist learning approaches. Visual recognition gives rise to a variety of learning-related tasks like those encountered in face processing (mentioned briefly above). For many object classes, the main challenge inherent in learning recognition—achieving invariance over transformations or deformations of the stimulus—disappears if the objects are represented structurally (Biederman 1987). This observation leads to the assumption that learning to recognize an object entails the identification of its parts and the determination of their spatial relationships. Under this assumption, the possession of a library of generic parts that can be assembled in various ways would also endow the system with the ability to represent and process novel objects—the ultimate kind of generalization.

Recently, a different approach to invariance and to the ability to process novel shapes has been proposed and implemented in a series of models (Poggio and Edelman 1990; Edelman and Duvdevani-Bar 1997; Riesenhuber and Poggio 1998; Edelman 1998a; Edelman and Intrator 2000). The computational underpinnings of this alternative approach are discussed elsewhere (see section 18.5.2; see also Sinha and Poggio, chapter 15, and Wallis and Bülthoff, chapter 16, both this volume). For now, we shall take the encroachment of alternative learning models into territory hitherto reserved for structural methods as license to focus our review on neural, rather than symbolic, computation.

18.4 Cues for Learning

A central question to be addressed in the modeling of a perceptual learning task is that of supervision: what are the sources and what is the form of the information that guides the learning process? The usual distinction found in the literature is between supervised models, which require each training stimulus to be accompanied by the desired output, and unsupervised ones, which are able to extract some statistical information from the data, without guidance.

Classifying an experimental setup on the basis of supervision available to the learning model is not always as straightforward as it may seem, however. Even when the learning process is fully and explicitly controlled by the experimenter, subjects have access to, and are likely to make use of, information that transcends the experimental design. For example, when subjects are required to learn the names of some unfamiliar faces, their ensuing confusion rates will be higher among some faces than among others.

The reasons for the advantage of some stimuli over others are simple, and have nothing to do with the labels (i.e., names) provided explicitly by the experimenter. Rather, they stem from the choice of faces selected for the experiment, and from the computational makeup of the subjects' visual systems. The necessary commitment on the part of any system to the use of some features at the expense of others gives rise to representational idiosyncrasies, which in turn cause some faces to be mapped into more crowded regions of the internal "face space" (Valentine 1991; Edelman 1998b) than others, and thus to be more easily confused. Analogous phenomena are observed in situations that require subjects to generalize, say, from one view to another, a generalization easier to learn for typical than for atypical faces (Nosofsky 1988; Newell, Chiroro, and Valentine 1999), typicality being defined as proximity to the center of the cluster corresponding to the set of stimuli in the face space.

18.4.1   Unsupervised Learning

Because the human visual system spontaneously perceives some things as more similar to each other than others, it is able to group stimuli by similarity intrinsic to a given test set and influenced by the context, but it does not require that class membership be dictated or revealed by an external supervisor. The information-processing task in this case is known as "unsupervised clustering" (Duda and Hart 1973); it constitutes one of the most challenging problems in computational learning.

Both "hard" and "soft" or fuzzy versions exist for many clustering algorithms. In hard clustering, each point can only belong to one cluster, whereas fuzzy algorithms allow a graded membership index. The latter approach is probably better suited to the modeling of perceptual categorization decisions: the boundary between classes in forced-choice tasks is never clear-cut. The dependence of the probability of membership in a given category on the location of the stimulus that falls "in between" clusters is typically sigmoidal. The slope of the sigmoid in the transition zone may be quite steep both in discrimination and in identification tasks, a phenomenon known as "categorical perception" (Harnad 1987).

In general, clustering algorithms decide whether or not to attribute points from a given data set $\{x_i\}$— in the present context, descriptions of stimuli in some feature space—to the same category on the basis of interpoint distances.[3] A typical algorithm employs standard combinatorial optimization techniques to minimize some function of V_w/V_b, where $V_w =$ $\sum_k E[x_k - \bar{x}_k]^2$ is the total within-cluster variance ($x_k \in C_k$, the latter being the kth cluster), and V_b is the between-clusters variance for the given data set $\{x_i\}$.

In some situations, prior knowledge about the nature of the problem provides hints that make unsupervised clustering easier. Consider, for example, the problem of learning to recognize several faces from their snapshots. The formation of the initial representation here is equivalent to clustering the snapshots (in whatever feature space the system uses as its front end). This clustering will be facilitated if the snapshots appear in a natural order, corresponding to the succession of views seen by the subjects, as the head to which the face belongs revolves in front of them. Such facilitation can be supported by a Hebbian learning mechanism, whereby association between successive views is made stronger in proportion to their temporal proximity (Hinton 1989; Stone 1996).

18.4.2   Supervised Learning

Whereas unsupervised learning algorithms have only the feature space distances between the stimuli to go by, the training data for supervised learning algorithms comprise a set of input-output pairs: $T = \{(x_i, y_i)\}$. The model in this case is required to learn a mapping $f : \mathcal{X} \to \mathcal{Y}$ such that $\forall i$, $y_i = f(x_i)$.

For the purpose of memorization, the functional requirement imposed on the learning algorithm in the fully supervised case is fulfilled either by a lookup table or by an associative network (Willshaw et al. 1969; see also Marr 1971 on simple memory). If generalization is required (i.e., if the model needs to estimate $\hat{y} = f(x)$ for some $x \notin \{x_i\}$), the problem becomes that of interpolation (or extrapolation, depending on the location of the new x relative to $\{x_i\}$) of the function f.

An efficient distributed implementation of function interpolation exists in the form of regularization networks (Poggio and Girosi 1990; Girosi, Jones, and Poggio 1995), of which radial basis function (RBF) networks constitute a special case, having a certain biological appeal (Poggio 1990). The simplest Gaussian RBF model approximates the input–output mapping f as a superposition of basis function values:

$$y = f(x) = \sum_i c_i e^{-\|x - x_i\|^2 / \sigma_i^2},$$

although extensions to vector-valued output, other basis functions, and other input space metrics also exist.

18.4.3 Self-Supervised Learning

An interesting variation on supervised learning is achieved by setting the output of a learning system to be identical to its input, while forcing the input-output mapping to pass via an intermediate representation stage. Such self-supervised learning can be implemented conveniently by a three-layer perceptron in which the number of units in the middle ("hidden") layer is smaller than in the input or output (Cottrell, Munro, and Zipser 1987). When this "bottleneck" network is trained successfully on a set of data, the activities of its hidden units form a lower-dimensional representation of the data. In traditional theories of perception, this coding or feature extraction operation is held to be a central characteristic of learning (LaBerge 1976).

Intuitively, having access to the right features is expected to greatly facilitate the performance of the system (Gibson 1969). More formally, the effectiveness (indeed, the very feasibility) of learning from examples depends critically on the availability of a low-dimensional description of the problem. Such a description facilitates learning because it avoids the curse of dimensionality—the exponential dependence of the number of examples needed for valid generalization on the number of dimensions of the representation space (Bellman 1961; Stone 1982; Huber 1985).

18.5 Paradigms of Learning

Psychologists had been aware of the central role of feature discovery in learning for a long time before any systematic attempts to cast this idea into computational terms were made.[4] To cite a prominent example, Eleanor Gibson (1969) concluded in her review of perceptual learning that the skilled perceiver is able to gain extra information from the stimulus by detecting features and "higher-order structure" to which the naive viewer is not sensitive. In this section, we shall offer a straightforward computational formulation of this insight with regard to the formation of new representations. We shall consider two distinct kinds of representations, the first suitable for regression problems (having continuous variables), and the second for classification problems (having mostly discrete variables; see figure 18.3). Finally, we shall examine a common framework that subsumes both kinds of tasks.

18.5.1 Learning as Forming New Representations

The power of forming new representations or, more specifically, of adjusting the representation to the problem at hand stems largely from the singular computational advantage conferred by the possibility of a linear solution. In regression tasks, such a solution is possible when a high linear correlation exists between the variables; in classification tasks, when the classes are linearly separable. Thus a representation is good if it allows a linear solution.

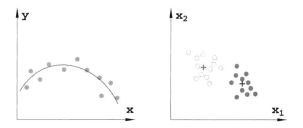

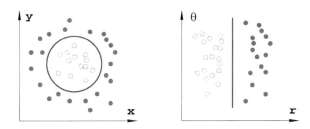

Figure 18.3
(*Left*) Regression problem. When expressed in terms of probabilities, the performance goal of the learning system in this case can be stated as the estimation of the posterior probability $p(y \mid x)$. (*Right*) Classification problem. Here the performance goal can be formulated as the estimation of $P(C_k \mid \mathbf{x})$, where C_k signifies membership in class k, and $\mathbf{x} = (x_1, x_2)^T$. In either case, the posterior probabilities can be learned directly (as in some neural network models), or computed from class-conditional probabilities estimated during a prior learning stage using the Bayes theorem: $P(C_k \mid \mathbf{x}) = p(\mathbf{x} \mid C_k) P(C_k)/p(\mathbf{x})$. (See Bishop 1995 for an accessible exposition of these approaches.)

Figure 18.4
Nonlinear (*left*) is translated to linear (*right*) discrimination problem via a coordinate transformation. The mapping $(x_1, x_2) \leftrightarrow (r, \theta)$ is itself nonlinear ($x_1 = r \cos \theta$; $x_2 = r \sin \theta$).

Consider the example illustrated in figure 18.4, where the task is to discriminate between the interior and the exterior of a circle. Solving this problem using a linear mechanism (left panel) is difficult because of the need to create many instances of such a mechanism to approximate the curved decision boundary. Thus a system that tries to solve this problem in the original representation space will use more resources and is likely to take longer than a system confronted with the same problem stated in polar coordinates (right panel), which can be solved using a linear mechanism. This distinction has implementational parallels: the representation on the left is suitable for interpolation by "bump" functions (e.g., radial basis functions), whereas the representation on the right is suitable for "ridge" functions, such as those implemented by the inner-product unit in a perceptron (or the hidden units in a multilayer perceptron, or MLP).

If a linear solution is ruled out in the original space, and if the system is biased toward using linear mechanisms, it may attempt to learn a new, better representation, that is, to remap the data into another representation space, in which linear regression or separability is possible. It should be quite obvious that a universal mechanism capable of such a remapping would go a long way toward solving just about any problem posed to it (because of the relative ease of solving the linear version of the problem in the new representation space). Some recently developed linearization methods do claim such universal applicability. For example, the support vector machines for classification and regression remap the original problem into an extremely high-dimensional space, where it becomes linear; the curse of dimensionality is avoided by making the solution dependent on a small number of examples ("support vectors") that lie close to the regression surface or to the class boundary (Vapnik 1995).[5] If the human visual system uses anything like the support vector algorithm, it should learn faster when given the more informative (and more difficult) examples first. We could not find evidence to this effect in the perceptual learning literature: human vision seems to be rather more limited than a support vector machine in this respect.

Interestingly, the attempts on the part of a learning system to improve its performance under the limitations imposed by its architecture are precisely what may pass as the manifestation of the process of learning to an external observer. For example, a system constrained to use RBFs may start by "tiling" the inside and the outside of the circle in figure 18.4, using up many basis function units. It may then shift to the more economical representation in which the inside and thus the outside of the circle are represented by a single basis—an event that would look like the kind of feature discovery mentioned by Gibson. In other words, learning can be defined computationally as the art of creating the most suitable representation of the data, given the constraints of the model at hand.[6]

18.5.2 Learning Visual Manifold Geometry: Regression

For a resource-constrained system, attempting to solve the learning problem in the original feature space may prove too complicated, as illustrated by the application of RBFs to the circle example. At the same time, attempting to remap the original problem into a new representation space where it would become linear may be equally hard, rendering the problem intractable. Fortunately, it appears that many perceptual problems possess an inherent structure that makes them amenable to learning methods that rely neither on the exhaustive tiling of a high-dimensional space (intractable because of the curse of dimensionality) nor on a sophisticated remapping (possibly beyond the visual system's capabilities). The structure in question is that of a smooth low-dimensional manifold, which arises for two reasons: (1) problem spaces in a typical perceptual task are parameterized by only a few variables (Edelman and Intrator 1997), and (2) the "front end" of a typical visual system—its

measurement space—largely preserves the local geometry of the distal problem space (Edelman 1999).[7]

The first reason can be illustrated by a series of examples taken from all areas of perception. Consider, for example, the vernier discrimination task in which the observer is to judge the sense of the relative displacement of two abutting line segments (see figure 18.1, right). The solution in this case is parameterized by a single variable, which controls the displacement of the segments perpendicular to their extent. Stepping this variable by small increments through a range of values between, say, $-15''$ and $+15''$ would cause the measurement space representation of the resulting stimulus to ascribe a one-dimensional manifold.[8] All that a visual system would have to do to learn vernier discrimination would be to interpolate this manifold from a set of examples (i.e., input-output pairs), as described in section 18.4.2.

As another illustration, we may consider the problem of learning to recognize an object from examples (i.e., a few of its stored views, each view being construed as a snapshot of the multidimensional measurement space). For a rigid object allowed two rotational degrees of freedom, corresponding to the two axes of rotation in depth, the manifold spanned in the measurement space will be two-dimensional, and will be amenable to learning from examples, as shown in Poggio and Edelman 1990. An entire range of other learning tasks having to do with object recognition can be solved on the basis of related principles, as shown in Edelman 1999 and Duvdevani-Bar et al. 1998.

In psychology, the well-behavedness of the internal representation space of various visual qualities has been noted repeatedly, beginning with the shift toward representational theories of vision in the 1960s. The concept of an internally represented stimulus space was mentioned by Guttman (1963, 144), who pointed out in a discussion of generalization in animal learning that the pigeon "knows the spectrum, in an important sense of the word 'know'"—it exhibits the kind of orderly generalization between colors that psychologists routinely observe, and must, therefore, possess an internal "color space." More than two decades later, Shepard (1987) formulated his law of generalization in terms of proximities in an internal psychological space, observing that structure inherent in various distal "quality spaces" (Clark 1993), such as the color continuum discussed by Guttman, is faithfully represented internally.

It is interesting to compare the observations concerning the low dimensionality and the smoothness of the internally represented quality spaces to similar observations made by statisticians and neural network researchers. In nonparametric statistics, for example, the surprisingly good performance of nearest-neighbor methods, which rely on raw feature space distances, has been explained intuitively: the relevant points in these spaces—that is, the examples—tend to be confined to smooth low-dimensional subspaces (Friedman 1994). In neural network research, an analogous observation can be found in Bregler and Omohundro 1995.

Realizing that the problems at hand typically possess such a convenient structure is, however, only the first step toward their solution. Lowering the dimensionality of the space in which the stimuli are originally encoded is a nontrivial operation; as we pointed out above, in human visual perception the original dimensionality of any stimulus is, nominally, on the order of 10^6, which is the number of fibers in each optic nerve. The illustration (figure 18.3, left) of the manifold embedded in two-dimensional space, is thus highly simplified. Many of the computational approaches devised for the extraction of low-dimensional manifolds do not scale well with

the dimensionality of the embedding space. This includes the self-organizing map algorithm (Kohonen 1982), and the different varieties of autoencoders or bottleneck networks (Cottrell, Munro, and Zipser 1987; Leen and Kambhatla 1994).

The performance of such unsupervised or self-supervised manifold-extracting algorithms can be improved if additional knowledge is brought to bear on the problem. Typically, this is done by making the learning mechanism observe certain invariances known to apply to the problem (Földiák 1991; Wiskott 1998). A particularly simple way to do that is to provide the label of the category to which each stimulus belongs.[9] To see how this information helps the algorithm isolate the relevant manifold, note that directions orthogonal to it can be effectively specified by forcing stimuli that differ along those directions to be mapped to the same category (Intrator and Edelman 1997).

18.5.3   Learning Visual Category Structure: Classification

From the perspective of the task, the main difference between regression and classification is that in regression the location of the point within the low-dimensional structure matters, whereas in classification it does not. For example, the location of the point representing a face in a face space (the manifold corresponding to the different possible views of the same face) would encode its orientation, which is a piece of information that should not be discarded. In comparison, in the vernier task, where the problem is that of classification, only the membership in one of the two clusters in the representation space matters to the system.

Despite this difference, the basic considerations identified before in the discussion of regression apply also to classification. In particular, the curse of dimensionality still has to be taken into account. Huber (1985) illustrates this point quantitatively, by showing how difficult it is to find a three-dimensional Gaussian bump (which could, in terms of figure 18.3, right, correspond to one of the class-conditional clusters), when it is embedded in a ten-dimensional space. Although neurally inspired models of learning that are tailored specifically for categorization and mixture estimation do exist (Carpenter and Grossberg 1990; Carpenter et al. 1992; Williamson 1997), they are not expected to deal better with realistically high-dimensional cases than the knowledge-based models mentioned earlier (which were designed for manifold extraction, yet should be equally capable of clustering).

18.5.4 *Learning Joint Input-Output Probability Density*

When learning is treated as a problem in statistical inference, the observations we made in section 18.5.3 can be rephrased using the concept of the underlying generator of the data—the entity that causes whatever regularities are present in the data set. In visual perception, this entity is the distal stimulus, which gives rise to the observed values of features through a complex process (reflection and scatter of light, propagation in the medium, refraction by the optics of the eye, phototransduction, etc.). In regression-like tasks, the distal stimulus space is continuous by nature, for example, the continuum of views of an object that undergoes rotation in front of the observer (in figure 18.3, left, it is the smooth curve underlying the sausagelike cloud of points). In classification, the distal stimulus space is discrete, for example, the set of categories to which the viewed object may belong (in figure 18.3, right, this space

consists of the centroids of the two clusters of data points).

Thus both regression and classification can be subsumed under a common framework, which calls for estimating the joint probability density of all the variables included in the data set. It is well known that this information reveals everything there is to know about stochastic data, such as the measurements performed by a perceptual system on the world. Although the underlying generator of the data (thus the quantities needed for regression or classification) can then be estimated optimally from the density function, the first step in this process—the inference of an unconstrained density function from data—is prone to the curse of dimensionality, as shown in the seminal work of Stone (1980, 1982).

In view of this problem, researchers typically take two approaches, which are not mutually exclusive. The first is to make some assumptions about the density function. For example, they may assume that the density function is smooth, then estimate it using splines (Wahba 1979) or radial basis functions (Poggio and Girosi 1990). They may instead assume something about the structure of the density. For example, it may be postulated to belong to an additive model, making it expressible as a sum of functions of some low-dimensional projections of the data (Stone 1985, 1986). Or they may assume that the density is factorial, namely, a product of marginal densities of one variable (Dayan, Hinton, and Neal 1995). The latter two methods, though they do not lower the dimensionality of the density function, make the estimation process more efficient and less prone to the curse of dimensionality.

The second general approach, which bypasses the problem of density estimation, is based on the observation that, for many practical problems, only a certain function of the density is required. The hope is that such a function can be easily computed directly from the data, without having to make the full density estimation, which happens, for example, when the desired function is defined over a low-dimensional manifold embedded in the original space or, more generally, when the desired function has a simpler structure compared to the full density. In such cases, the learning system may attempt to extract the low-dimensional representation of the problem from the data, using an unsupervised approach such as principal component analysis and its generalizations, or using a supervised approach tailored to the desired target function, as in many feedforward network models.

In all these cases, a model would do well by applying the methods listed in sections 18.5.2 and 18.5.3, which dealt with learning manifold extraction (regression) and clustering (classification). On the other hand, those methods cannot be practically subsumed under the aegis of density estimation unless the estimation algorithm (1) aims for learning a certain target function of the density, which is usually problem specific, and (2) relies on some prior assumptions about the properties of the desired representation, such as low dimensionality and smoothness (Intrator 1993).

18.6 Discussion

The theoretical stance adopted thus far equates learning with the acquisition of efficient representations, a computational procedure that can be regarded as a kind of statistical inference. Although we may seem to have strayed far from the gritty details that must be dealt with by any model aiming to simulate human learning behavior, we believe that a good model starts at the top, with a clear notion of what is being modeled and why.

18.6.1 On the Levels of Explaining Learning

The overarching concern in the modeling of a perceptual phenomenon is getting the performance right. Beyond that, however, there is a considerable variation in what is deemed acceptable: whereas some comprehensive models treat both the computational (theoretical) and the implementational aspects of the problem, others tend to concentrate on the issues of implementation and mechanism. Models built around neural networks most likely belong to the second group, going straight from the phenomenology to a hypothesis about the underlying mechanism, perhaps also attempting to emulate along the way the real biological neural network.

We illustrate this observation with a striking example of perceptual learning, found in the task of detecting a small low-contrast Gabor patch projected onto a certain retinotopically defined location. The detection threshold in this task depends on whether the target patch is flanked at a distance by patches of similar orientation and spatial frequency (Polat and Sagi 1993). The effect of the flanking patches is amenable to learning: the spatial range of the effect (i.e., the maximum effective distance between the target and the flanking patches) grows with practice (see Zenger and Sagi, chapter 10, this volume). Significantly, learning is only possible if the original, untrained range is extended gradually by exposing the subject to configurations of progressively larger and larger extent (Polat and Sagi 1994).

A phenomenon such as this seems to positively demand an explanation at the mechanism level, invoking receptive fields of retinotopic "units," linked laterally and exerting facilitatory influence on each other. Polat and Sagi (1994) offered just such an explanation for their psychophysical findings. As we claimed in section 18.1, however, because they concentrate on the wiring details at the expense of leaving the computational goal of the system out of the picture, models formulated primarily in the language of units and connections achieve less than what a model can and should achieve. To support this argument, let us reconsider the "lateral learning" scenario, keeping in mind the taxonomy of learning paradigms discussed earlier.

Assume for the moment that the goal of the system is to detect the faintest possible line element (a real-life counterpart to a Gabor patch) in a given retinal location. Merely lowering the decision threshold for that location will likely just increase the false-alarm rate there; additional information must be brought to bear on the decision if it is to be reliable. The presence of other line elements in the vicinity would count as the necessary additional support if they are compatible with the original hypothesis (i.e., if their orientation is consistent with that of the element whose fate they are about to seal). Thus the task at hand can be reformulated as that of (literal) interpolation between the flanking lines, or of extrapolation if the continuation of an "end-stopped" segment is sought.

This formulation makes it possible to uniformly treat a range of perceptual learning tasks. Indeed, on an abstract level, learning to detect a Gabor patch flanked by similar patterns is now seen to be the same as learning to recognize an object "sandwiched" between two familiar views from a novel viewpoint. The analogy drawn between these two tasks hinges on a parallel between the view space of the object, on the one hand, and the "space" space—that is, the retinal location space—of the Gabor patch, on the other. Once this analogy is accepted, cross-fertilization may occur in both directions. Whereas models of object recognition may benefit from postulating a mechanism that carries out interpolation by growing lateral links between neighboring units in a view representation space, models of line detec-

tion may benefit from exploring the possibilities originally developed in the context of object recognition (e.g., interpolation with feedforward basis functions).

An edifying perspective on the issue of levels of modeling is provided by recalling some of the "old-fashioned" models of brain function (and learning) produced by neurobiologists. Two such models that were prominent in their own time, one dealing with "universals" or the problem of invariance (Pitts and McCulloch 1947/1965) and the other with probabilistic generalization (Marr 1970), actually did link theory and mechanism. Marr's model of the neocortex (1970), for example, spans the entire possible range of levels. It starts with a general, yet succinctly phrased hypothesis concerning the probabilistic structure of the world (the "fundamental hypothesis," mentioned in section 18.2.2), and ends with a detailed explanation of the possible ways in which neuroanatomy and neurophysiology of the cortex may be tuned to put the observed probabilities to work. This style of modeling, which integrates different levels of explanation, requires a combination of encyclopedic knowledge with considerable ingenuity on the part of the modeler. Unfortunately, it is now quite rare, having been replaced by a methodology that allows the levels—computational, algorithmic, and implementational—to be kept separate.

18.6.2 Prognosis

In visual perception, learning is a pervasive phenomenon, which, when properly studied, offers the researcher a unique searchlight on the inner workings of the system. Although it would be rash to predict what this searchlight might reveal, there are four strategies we would like to see adopted in modeling perceptual learning:

1. *Integrate past achievements.* Attempts to develop mathematical models of learning date back more than half a century. Much of the work carried out before mid-1960s has now been branded "behaviorist" and effectively buried in the libraries. Reexamining that work may lead to interesting insights into the nature of the present-day models (see Hintzman 1994).

2. *Look at learning differently.* A diametrically opposite trend is that of complete rejection of both the old and the contemporary models of learning in favor of esoteric theories that involve concepts such as catastrophes, self-organized criticality, or phase transitions in dynamical systems. Although the trend is in response to legitimate challenges, such as the need to explain abrupt learning and related phenomena (see Rubin, Nakayama, and Shapley, chapter 13, this volume), we believe that perceptual learning research will be best served by the widest variety of different approaches, from the very traditional to the very novel.

3. *Explain as much as possible.* The "dynamical" models attempt to explain the behavior of the perceptual system by appealing to an isomorphism between its physics (i.e., the differential equations that describe it) and the physics of other systems exhibiting a similar behavior. In that, they resemble the behaviorist models, which skirt the issues of representation, and deal with disembodied equations aimed at mimicking the phenomenology of the target system. Nor are they alone in this regard. Purely representational models also end up dealing only with the phenomenology; a good example is Shepard's law of generalization (1987; mentioned in section 18.2.2), which makes no claims as to the reality of the "psychological similarity space" it postulates. In contrast to all these, explanations offered by the more daring connectionist models (which bite the bullet and hope for the best) include parallels both on the level of behavior, and on the level of architecture.

4. *Go after the big question.* To understand the brain, we need a really comprehensive explanation, one that starts from a concrete premise, yet spans all the levels of the "hierarchy" of computation, representation, algorithm, and implementation—a postulate about what the brain actually does. Several such postulates are available, for example, Marr's probabilistic inference (1970), Barlow's redundancy reduction (1990), and Poggio's function approximation (1990). A more intense competition in this arena is likely to lead to some exciting developments in the modeling of learning.

The ability to learn, at all levels and under all circumstances, is the most striking attribute of human cognition. What would it take to really understand it? Just as Gounod's Faust asked Mephistopheles for youth—the treasure that contains all others—so we wish for a model of the brain that would make the modeling of perceptual learning superfluous.

Notes

1. Cognitive maps in the rat brain are thought to reside in the hippocampus, a cortical structure implicated in perceptual (spatial) and other kinds of learning. Information about the spatial location of the animal turns out to be represented in the firing patterns of hippocampal "place" cells, whose ensemble activity constitutes an internal cognitive map of the rat's environment (Wilson and McNaughton 1993). Another class of cells in the hippocampus are the "head direction" cells, which serve as an internal compass to orient the cognitive map. The functional properties of place and head direction cells emerge from a complex and as yet poorly understood interaction between internally generated, self-motion cues (e.g., vestibular information) and external sensory input (e.g., visual landmarks; Knierim, Kudrimoti, and McNaughton 1995).

2. At a certain level of abstraction, the distinction between symbolic and "connectionist" computational paradigms ceases to make sense, as attested by the possibility of implementing rules and variables in neural networks (see, for example, Ajjanagadde and Shastri 1991).

3. The distance $d(x_i, x_j)$ between two points in the feature space can be assumed to vary monotonically with the inverse of the perceived dissimilarity between the corresponding stimuli. For a discussion of this issue, and of the choice of metric to be used in the computation of distance, see Shepard 1987.

4. Indeed, one of the most influential figures in the field, James J. Gibson, consistently resisted any attempts to invoke computation as an explanatory tool in perceptual psychology.

5. Conceptually, the reliance on a small number of support vectors that exemplify the distinction that the system must learn is close to Winston's use of "near miss" examples (1975) in his system that learned concepts from symbolic descriptions.

6. This formulation mixes two "levels of understanding"— the abstract and the implementational—that would have been kept separate according to the methodology propounded by Marr and Poggio (1977).

7. *Measurement space* can be defined through the vector of measurements performed by the visual system on the world and is well exemplified by the million-dimensional space of all possible activities of the retinal ganglion cells, whose axons constitute the optic nerve.

8. In figure 18.1, right panel, both the displacement of the vernier and its location in the visual field were varied, which is why the clouds of points belonging to each of the two classes are not exactly one-dimensional manifolds.

9. This labeling technique can be compared to the "stimulus predifferentiation" method, shown in the past to boost the generalization rate in learning (Ellis 1965, 58).

Learning to Find Independent Components in Natural Scenes

19

Anthony J. Bell and Terrence J. Sejnowski

Abstract

The brain may operate in an arbitrarily complex way, while its self-organizational, or learning, processes, to the extent that they can be distinguished from normal operation, may be quite simple. Therefore one research program is to define learning rules using candidate abstract principles, and apply these algorithms to natural data to see if they produce processing systems similar to those found in neurons exposed to the same data.

In this chapter, we apply information-theoretic learning to noiseless sigmoidal neurons exposed to natural images. The neurons learn localized oriented receptive fields qualitatively similar to simple cells in area V1 of visual cortex. The algorithm maximizes the information contained about the input while choosing a coordinate system that makes each element of the resulting code as independent as possible. To a first approximation, the recoding of visual input in early perceptual processing may follow simple information-theoretic principles.

Both the classic experiments of Hubel and Wiesel (1968) on neurons in visual cortex and several decades of theorizing about feature detection in vision (Marr and Hildreth 1980) have left open the question most succinctly phrased by Barlow and Tolhurst (1992) "Why do we have edge detectors?" Barlow (1989) has suggested that the line and edge selectivities of neurons found in primary visual cortex of cats and monkeys should emerge from an unsupervised learning algorithm that attempts to find a factorial code of independent visual features. Along similar lines, Field (1994) has argued that a sparse, distributed representation of natural scenes should be goal of early visual representations.

These hypotheses can now be tested with unsupervised learning algorithms whose goal is to either find maximally independent linear filters (Bell and Sejnowski 1995a, 1997) or to maximize sparseness (Olshausen and Field 1997), applied to an ensemble of natural scenes. Both of these approaches produce sets of visual filters that are localized and oriented, including some filters whose associated basis functions are Gabor-like. These results are quite different from the filters produced by other decorrelating filters produced by principal components analysis (PCA) and zero-phase components analysis (ZCA). The set of filters produced by independent component analysis (ICA) has more sparsely distributed (kurtotic) outputs on natural scenes (Bell and Sejnowski 1997). They also resemble the receptive fields of simple cells in visual cortex, which suggests that these neurons form a natural, information-theoretic coordinate system for natural images.

Most studies that have examined the statistics of natural images for the purpose of reducing redundancy, and thereby making a more efficient code, have used only the second-order statistics required for *decorrelating* the outputs of a set of feature detectors. Although Hebbian feature-learning algorithms for decorrelation have been proposed (Linsker 1992; Miller 1988; Oja 1989; Sanger 1989; Földiák 1990; Atick and Redlich 1993), in the absence of particular external constraints the solutions to the decorrelation problem are nonunique. One popular decorrelating solution is principal components analysis (PCA), but the principal components of natural scenes amount to a global spatial frequency analysis (Hancock, Baddeley and Smith 1992). Thus, second-order statistics alone do not suffice to predict the formation of localized edge detectors.

Additional constraints are required. Field (1987, 1994) has argued for the importance of sparse, or "minimum entropy," coding (Barlow 1994), in which each feature detector is activated as rarely as possible. This has led to feature-learning algorithms with a "projection pursuit" flavor (Huber 1985, Intrator 1992, Baddeley 1996, Olshausen and Field 1997).

An alternative constraint is to start with an information-theoretic criterion that maximizes the joint entropy of a nonlinearly transformed output feature vector. This is the approach taken by "independent components analysis" (Comon 1994) which can achieve the blind separation of mixed sources (Jutten and Hérault 1991; Bell and Sejnowski 1995a, 1996). Finding independent components is equivalent to Barlow's redundancy reduction problem; therefore if Barlow's reasoning is correct, the independent components should produce filters which are localized and oriented, and in fact it does. In addition, when applied to natural images, the outputs of the resulting filters are more sparsely distributed than those of other decorrelating filters, thus supporting some of the arguments of Field (1994) and helping to explain the results of Olshausen and Field (1997) from an information-theoretic point of view.

We will return to the issues of sparseness, noise and higher-order statistics. First, we describe more concretely the filter-learning problem.

19.1 "Causes" in Natural Images

A perceptual system is exposed to a series of small image patches, drawn from one or more larger images. Imagine that each image patch, represented by the vector $\mathbf{x}$, has been formed by the linear combination of N basis functions. The basis functions form the columns of a fixed matrix, $\mathbf{A}$. The weighting of this linear combination (which varies with each image) is given by a vector, $\mathbf{s}$. Each component of this vector has its own associated basis function, and represents an underlying "cause" of the image. The *linear image synthesis* model is therefore given by:

$$\mathbf{x} = \mathbf{As} \tag{19.1}$$

which is the matrix version of the set of equations

$$x_i = \sum_{j=1}^{N} a_{ij} s_j \tag{19.2}$$

where each x_i represents a pixel in an image, and contains contributions from each one of a set of N image "sources," s_j, linearly weighted by a coefficient, a_{ij}.

The goal of a perceptual system, in this simplified framework, is to linearly transform the images, $\mathbf{x}$, with a matrix of filters, $\mathbf{W}$, so that the resulting vector:

$$\mathbf{u} = \mathbf{Wx} \tag{19.3}$$

recovers the underlying causes, $\mathbf{s}$, possibly in a different order, and rescaled. Representing, by $\mathbf{P}$, an arbitrary permutation matrix (all zero except for a single "one" in each row and each column), and, by $\mathbf{S}$, an arbitrary scaling matrix (nonzero entries only on the diagonal), such a system has converged when:

$$\mathbf{u} = \mathbf{WAs} = \mathbf{PSs} \tag{19.4}$$

The scaling and permuting of the causes are arbitrary, unknowable factors, so consider the causes to be defined such that $\mathbf{PS} = \mathbf{I}$ (the identity matrix).

Then the basis functions (columns of $\mathbf{A}$) and the filters that recover the causes (rows of $\mathbf{W}$) have the simple relation: $\mathbf{W} = \mathbf{A}^{-1}$.

All that remains in defining an algorithm to learn $\mathbf{W}$ (and thus also $\mathbf{A}$) is to decide what constitutes a "cause." We concentrate here on algorithms producing causes that are decorrelated, and those attempting to produce causes that are statistically independent.

19.2   Decorrelation and Independence

The matrix, $\mathbf{W}$, is a *decorrelating* matrix when the covariance matrix of the output vector, $\mathbf{u}$, satisfies:

$$\langle \mathbf{u}\mathbf{u}^T \rangle = \text{diagonal matrix} \qquad (19.5)$$

In general, there will be many $\mathbf{W}$ matrices which decorrelate. For example, when $\langle \mathbf{u}\mathbf{u}^T \rangle = \mathbf{I}$, then:

$$\mathbf{W}^T \mathbf{W} = \langle \mathbf{x}\mathbf{x}^T \rangle^{-1} \qquad (19.6)$$

which clearly leaves freedom in the choice of $\mathbf{W}$. There are, however, several special solutions to Eq. (19.6).

Principal components analysis (PCA) is the orthogonal solution to Eq. (19.5). The principal components come from the eigenvectors of the covariance matrix. The filters are orthogonal. When the image statistics are stationary (Field 1994), the PCA filters are *global* Fourier filters, ordered according to the amplitude spectrum of the image. Example PCA filters are shown in figure 19.1a.

If $\mathbf{W}$ is forced to be symmetrical, so that $\mathbf{W}_Z^T = \mathbf{W}_Z$, then the resulting decorrelating filters are zero-phase (ZCA). ZCA is in several ways the polar opposite of PCA. It produces *local* (center-surround type) whitening filters, which are ordered according to the phase spectrum of the image. That is, each filter whitens a given pixel in the image, preserving

the spatial arrangement of the image and flattening its frequency (amplitude) spectrum (Goodall 1960; Atick and Redlich 1993). Example ZCA filters and basis functions are shown in figure 19.1b.

Another way to constrain the solution is to attempt to produce outputs that are not just decorrelated but statistically independent (Jutten and Hérault 1991; Comon 1994). The values of the u_i are independent when their probability distribution, $f_{\mathbf{u}}$, factorizes: $f_{\mathbf{u}}(\mathbf{u}) = \prod_i f_{u_i}(u_i)$. There are many ICA algorithms, based on different approaches (Cardoso and Laheld 1996; Karhunen et al. 1996; Amari, Cichoki, and Yang 1996; Cichocki, Unbehauen, and Rummert 1994; Pham, Garrat, and Jutten 1992; Bell and Sejnowski 1995a).

ICA produces decorrelating filters that are sensitive to both phase (locality) and frequency information, just as in transforms involving oriented Gabor functions (Daugman 1985) or wavelets. These filters are thus semilocal, depicted in figure 19.2 as partway along the path from the local (ZCA) to the global (PCA) solutions in the space of decorrelating solutions. Example ICA filters are shown in figure 19.1d and their corresponding basis functions are shown in figure 19.1e.

It is important to recognize two differences between finding an ICA solution, $\mathbf{W}_I$, and other decorrelation methods: (1) there may be no ICA solution, and (2) a given ICA algorithm may not find the solution even if it exists, because there are approximations involved. In these senses, ICA is different from PCA and ZCA, and cannot be calculated analytically, for example, from second-order statistics (the covariance matrix), except in the Gaussian case (when second-order statistics completely characterize the signal distribution).

The approach developed in Bell and Sejnowski 1995a was to maximize by stochastic gradient ascent the joint entropy, $H[g(\mathbf{u})]$, of the linear transform

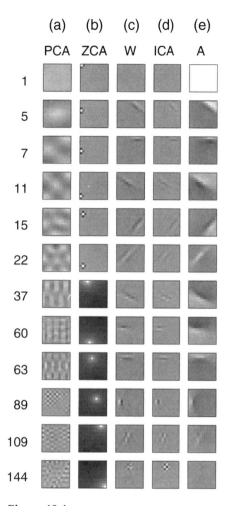

squashed by a sigmoidal function, g. When the nonlinear function is the same (up to scaling and shifting) as the cumulative density functions (CDFs) of the underlying independent components, it can be shown (Nadal and Parga 1995) that such a nonlinear "infomax" procedure also minimizes the mutual information between the u_i, exactly what is required for ICA.

However, in most cases we must pick a nonlinearity, g, without any detailed knowledge of the probability density functions (PDFs) of the underlying independent components. The resulting mismatch between the gradient of the nonlinearity used and the underlying PDFs may cause the infomax solution to deviate from an ICA solution. In cases where the PDFs are super-Gaussian (meaning they are peakier and longer-tailed than a Gaussian, having kurtosis greater than 0), we have repeatedly observed, using the logistic or hyperbolic tangent nonlinearities, that maximization of $H[g(\mathbf{u})]$ still leads to ICA solutions, when they exist, as with our experiments on speech signal separation (Bell and Sejnowski 1995a). An extended version of this algorithm can be used when there are mixed sub-Gaussian and

Figure 19.1
Selected decorrelating filters and their basis functions extracted from the natural scene data. Each type of decorrelating filter yielded 144 12×12 filters, of which we only display a subset here. Each column contains filters or basis functions of a particular type, and each of the rows has a number relating to which row of the filter or basis function matrix is displayed. (*a*) Principal components analysis (PCA, or $\mathbf{W}_P$): The 1st, 5th, 7th, etc. principal components, showing increasing spatial frequency. There is no need to show basis functions and filters separately here, since for PCA they are the same thing. (*b*) Zero-phase components analysis (ZCA, or $\mathbf{W}_Z$): The first six entries in this column show the one-pixel-wide center-surround filter which whitens while preserving the phase spectrum. All are identical, but shifted. The lower six entries (37, 60 ... 144) show the basis functions instead, which are the columns of the inverse of the $\mathbf{W}_Z$ matrix. (*c*) The weights, $\mathbf{W}$, learned by the independent component analysis network trained on $\mathbf{W}_Z$-whitened data, showing (in descending order) the DC filter, localized oriented filters, and localized checkerboard filters. (*d*) The corresponding ICA filters, in the matrix $\mathbf{W}_I$, look like whitened versions of the $\mathbf{W}$-filters. (*e*) The corresponding basis functions, columns of $\mathbf{W}_I^{-1}$ (or $\mathbf{A}$). These are the patterns that optimally stimulate their corresponding ICA filters, while not stimulating any other ICA filter, so that $\mathbf{W}_I \mathbf{A} = \mathbf{I}$.

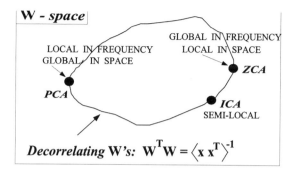

Figure 19.2
Schematic depiction of weight space. A subspace of all matrices, **W**, here represented by the loop (of course it is a much higher-dimensional closed subspace), has the property of decorrelating the input vectors, **x**. On this manifold, several special linear transformations can be distinguished: principal components analysis (PCA), global in space and local in frequency; zero-phase components analysis (ZCA), local in space and global in frequency; and independent components analysis (ICA), a privileged decorrelating matrix which, if it exists, decorrelates higher as well as second-order moments. ICA filters are localized, but not down to the single-pixel level, as ZCA filters are.

super-Gauassian sources (Lee, Girolami and Sejnowski 1999).

The filters and basis functions resulting from training on natural scenes are displayed in figures 19.1 and 19.4. Figure 19.1 displays example filters and basis functions of each type. The PCA filters (figure 19.1, panel a) are spatially global and ordered in frequency. The ZCA filters and basis functions are spatially local and ordered in phase. The ICA filters, whether trained on the ZCA-whitened images (figure 19.1, panel c) or the original images (figure 19.3, panel d) are semilocal filters, most with a specific orientation preference. The basis functions (figure 19.1, panel e), calculated from the ICA filters (figure 19.1, panel d), are not local and look like the edges that might occur in image patches of this size. Basis

functions in figure 19.1, panel d, are the same as the corresponding filters because the matrix **W** is orthogonal, as is the case for the PCA filters, $\mathbf{W}_P$. This is the ICA-matrix for ZCA-whitened images.

Figure 19.4 shows, with lower resolution, all 144 filters in the matrix **W**. The general result is that ICA filters are localized and mostly oriented. There is one DC filter and fewer than ten unoriented checkerboard filters.

Figure 19.5 shows the result of analyzing the distributions (image histograms) produced by each of the three filter types. As emphasized by Ruderman (1994) and Field (1994), the general form of these histograms is double-exponential ($e^{-|u_i|}$), or "sparse," meaning peaky with a long tail, when compared to a Gaussian. This shows up clearly in figure 19.4, where the log histograms are seen to be roughly linear across twelve orders of magnitude. The histogram for the ICA filters, however, departs from linearity, having a longer tail than the ZCA and PCA histograms. This spreading of the tail signals the greater sparseness of the outputs of the ICA filters, and this is reflected in the kurtosis measure of 10.04 for ICA, compared to 3.74 for PCA, and 4.5 for ZCA.

Univariate statistics can only capture part of the story, so in figure 19.5, panels a, c and e, are displayed, in contour plots, the average of the bivariate log histograms given by all *pairs* of filters, for ICA, ZCA and PCA respectively. In contrast with these joint probability distributions, figure 19.6, panels b, d and f, show the corresponding distribution if the outputs of the filters were independent (i.e., the outer product of the marginal, or univariate, distributions in figure 19.4). Only the ICA joint histogram captures well the diamond-shape characteristic of the product of the sparse univariate distributions, thus satisfying, to a greater extent, the independence criterion: $f_{u_1 u_2}(u_1, u_2) = f_{u_1}(u_1) f_{u_2}(u_2)$.

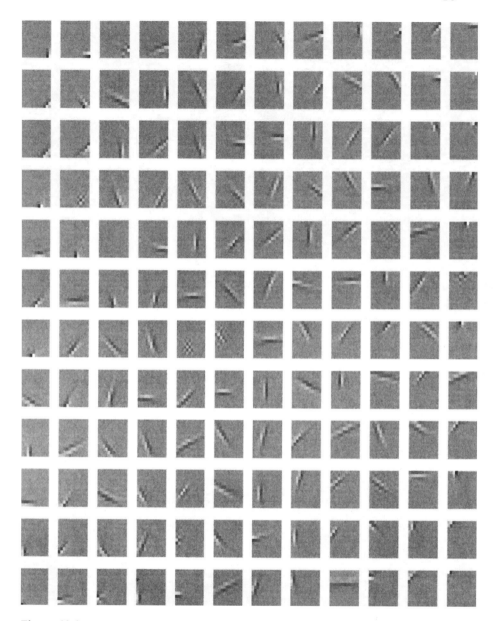

Figure 19.3
Matrix of 144 filters obtained by training on natural images whitened by zero-phase components analysis. Each filter is a row of the matrix **W**. The independent components analysis basis functions on ZCA-whitened data are visually the same as the ICA filters. On nonwhitened data, the filters look like high-pass versions of the filters shown here, and the basis functions look like low-pass versions of them.

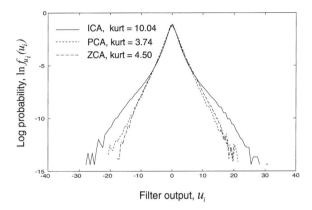

Figure 19.4
Log distributions of univariate statistics of the outputs of independent, zero-phase and principal components analysis (ICA, ZCA, and PCA) filters, averaged over all filters of each type. All three are approximately double-exponential distributions, but the more kurtotic ICA distribution is slightly peakier and has a longer tail, showing that it is *sparser* than the others. This distribution (and the two dimensional ones in figure 19.5), although averaged over the outputs of all filters, are extremely similar to the distributions output by individual filters (respectively, pairs of filters). The only exception is the DC filter (top left in 19.3) which has a more Gaussian distribution.

In summary, the filters found by the infomax ICA algorithm with a logistic nonlinearity are localized, oriented, and produce outputs distributions of very high kurtosis.

19.3 Comparisons with Other Approaches

A substantial literature exists on the self-organization of visual receptive fields through factors such as learning. Many contributions have emphasized the roles of decorrelation and PCA (Oja 1989; Sanger 1989; Miller 1988; Hancock, Baddeley, and Smith 1992; Földiák 1990). Often this has been accompanied by information-theoretic arguments. The first

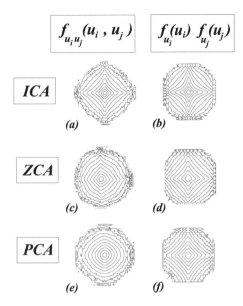

Figure 19.5
Contour plots of log distributions of pairwise statistics of the outputs of independent, zero-phase, and principal components analysis (ICA, ZCA, and PCA) filters. (*a*, *c*, *e*) Joint log distributions averaged over all pairs of output filters of each type, and all images. (*b*, *d*, *f*) Product of marginal (univariate) distributions. The ICA solution best satisfies the independence criterion that the joint distribution has the same form as the product of the marginal distributions.

work along these lines was by Linsker (1988), who first proposed the "infomax" principle that underlies our own work. Linsker's approach, and that of Atick and Redlich (1990), Bialek, Ruderman, and Zee (1991), and van Hateren (1992) uses the second-order (covariance matrix) approximation of the required information-theoretic quantities, and generally assumes Gaussian signal and Gaussian noise, in which case the second-order information is complete. The explicit noise model and the restriction to second-order statistics mark the two differences between these approaches and our approach to infomax.

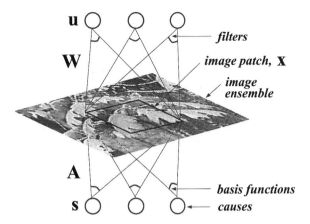

Figure 19.6
The blind linear image synthesis model (Olshausen and
Field 1997). Here each patch, **x**, of an image is viewed as a
linear combination of several (here three) underlying basis
functions, given by the matrix **A**, each associated with an
element of an underlying vector of "causes," **s**. Causes are
viewed here as statistically independent "image sources."
The causes are recovered (in a vector **u**) by a matrix of
filters, **W**, which attempt to invert the unknown mixing of
unknown basis functions constituting image formation.

The assumption of a noise model has been generally thought to be a necessary ingredient. In the case
where the decorrelating filters are of the local ZCA
type, the noise model is required (Atick and Redlich
1990) to avoid center-surround receptive fields with
peaks a single pixel wide, as in figure 19.3, panel b
(see also Atick and Redlich 1993). In the case of the
PCA-style global filters, noise is automatically associated with the filters with high spatial frequency
selectivity whose eigenvectors have small eigenvalues.

In both cases, it is questionable whether such
assumptions about noise are useful. In the case of
PCA, there is no a priori reason to associate signal
with low spatial frequency and noise with high spatial
frequency or, indeed, to associate signal with high
amplitude components and noise with low ampli-

tude. On the contrary, sharp edges, presumably of
high interest, contain many high-frequency, low-
amplitude components. In the case of local ZCA-
type filters, some form of spatial integration is
assumed necessary to average out photon shot noise.
Yet we know photoreceptors and the brains associated with them can operate in the single-photon
detection regime. Therefore shot noise is, in at least
some cases, not considered by neural systems to be
something noisy to be ignored, and such systems
appear to operate at the limit of the spatial acuity
allowed by their lattices of receptors.

In a general information-theoretic framework,
there is nothing to distinguish signal and noise a
priori, and we therefore question the use of the
concept of noise in these models. Of course there are
signals of lesser or greater relevance to an organism,
but there is no signature in their spatial or temporal
structure that distinguishes them as important or not.
It is more likely that signal and noise are subjective
concepts having to do with the prior expectations of
the organism (or neural subsystem). In the case of the
simple linear mappings we are considering, there is
no internal state (other than the filters themselves)
to store such prior expectations, and therefore we
consider "noiseless infomax" to be the appropriate
framework for making the first level of predictions
based on information-theoretic reasoning.

The second difference in earlier infomax models,
the restriction to second-order statistics, has been
questioned by Field (1987, 1994) and Olshausen and
Field (1997). This has coincided with a general rise
in awareness that simple Hebbian-style algorithms
without special constraints are unable to produce
local oriented receptive fields like those found in
area V1 of visual cortex, but rather produce solutions
of the PCA or ZCA type, depending on the constraint put on the decorrelating filter matrix, **W**.

The technical reason for this failure is that second-order statistics correspond to the amplitude spectrum of a signal (because the Fourier transform of the autocorrelation function of an image is its power spectrum, the square of the amplitude spectrum.) The remaining information, higher-order statistics, corresponds to the phase spectrum. The phase spectrum is what we consider to be the informative part of a signal, since if we remove phase information from an image, it looks like noise, while if we remove amplitude information (for example, with zero-phase whitening, using a ZCA transform), the image is still recognizable. Edges and what we consider "features" in images are "suspicious coincidences" in the phase spectrum: Fourier analysis of an edge consists of many sine waves of different frequencies, all aligned in phase where the edge occurred.

As in our conclusions about "noise," we feel that a more general information-theoretic approach is required, an approach taking account of statistics of all orders. Such an approach is sensitive to the phase spectra of the images, and thus to their characteristic local structure. These conclusions are borne out by the results of ICA, which demonstrate the emergence of local oriented receptive fields, which second-order statistics alone fail to predict.

Several other approaches have arisen to deal with the unsatisfactory results of simple Hebbian and anti-Hebbian schemes. Field (1987, 1994) emphasized, using some of Barlow's arguments (1989), that the goal of an image transformation should be to convert "higher-order redundancy" into "first order-redundancy." These arguments led Olshausen and Field (1997) to attempt to learn receptive fields by maximizing sparseness. In terms of our figure 19.6, they attempted to find receptive fields (which they identified with basis functions—the columns of our $\mathbf{A}$ matrix) that have underlying causes, $\mathbf{u}$ (or $\mathbf{s}$), and are as sparsely distributed as possible. The sparseness constraint is imposed by a nonlinear function that pushes the activity of the components of $\mathbf{u}$ toward zero.

Thus the similarity of the results produced by Olshausen and Field's network and ours may be explained by the fact that both produce what are perhaps the sparsest possible u_i distributions, though by different means. In emphasizing sparseness directly, rather than an information theoretic criterion, Olshausen and Field do not force their "causes" to have low mutual information, or even to be decorrelated. Thus their basis function matrices, unlike ours, are singular, and noninvertible, making it difficult for them to say what the filters are that correspond to their basis functions. Recently, Lewicki and Olshausen (1999), working with overcomplete representations, have overcome these problems.

Our approach, on the other hand, emphasizes independence over sparseness. Examining figures 19.4 and 19.5, we see that our filter outputs are also very sparse. This is because infomax with a sigmoid nonlinearity can be viewed as an ICA algorithm with an assumption that the independent components have super-Gaussian PDFs. It is worth mentioning that an ICA algorithm without this assumption will find a few sub-Gaussian (low-kurtosis) independent components, though most will be super-Gaussian (Lee, Girolami, and Sejnowski 1999).

Sparseness, as captured by the kurtosis, is one projection index often mentioned in projection pursuit methods (Huber 1985), which look in multivariate data for directions with "interesting" distributions. Intrator (1992; see chapter 18), who pioneered the application of projection pursuit reasoning to feature extraction problems, used an index emphasizing *multimodal* projections, and connected it with the BCM (Bienenstock, Cooper, and Munro 1982) learning rule. Following up, Law and Cooper

(1994) and Shouval (1995) used the BCM rule to self-organize oriented and somewhat localized receptive fields on an ensemble of natural images.

The BCM rule is a nonlinear Hebbian/anti-Hebbian mechanism. The nonlinearity undoubtedly contributes higher-order statistical information, but it is less clear than in Olshausen's network or our own how the nonlinearity contributes to the solution.

Another principle, predictability minimization, has also been brought to bear on the problem by Schmidhuber, Eldracher, and Foltin (1996). This approach attempts to ensure independence of one output from the others by moving its receptive field away from what is predictable (using a nonlinear "lateral" network) from the outputs of the others. Finally, Harpur and Prager (1996) have formalized an inhibitory feedback network that also learns nonorthogonal oriented receptive fields.

19.4   Biological Significance

The simplest properties of classical V1 simple cell receptive fields (Hubel and Wiesel 1968) are that they are *local* and *oriented*. These are properties of the filters in figure 19.4, while failing to emerge (without external constraints) in many previous self-organizing network models (Linsker 1988; Miller 1988; Atick and Redlich 1993; Troyer et al. 1999). However, the transformation from retina to V1, from analog photoreceptor signals to spike-coding pyramidal cells, is clearly much more complex than the $\mathbf{W}_I$ matrix, with which we have been working.

Nonetheless, evidence supports a feedforward origin for the oriented properties of simple cells in the cat (Ferster et al. 1996). Also the ZCA filters approximate the static response properties of ganglion cells in the retina and relay cells in the lateral geniculate nucleus, which, to a first approximation, prewhiten inputs reaching the cortex.

If we were to accept $\mathbf{W}_I$ as a primitive model of the retinocortical transformation, then several objections might arise. One might object to the representation learned by the algorithm: the filters in figure 19.3 are predominantly of high spatial frequency, even though spatial frequencies have been found to spread over several octaves in cortex (Hubel and Wiesel 1974). The reason there are so many high spatial frequency filters is because they are smaller, therefore more are required to "tile" the 12×12 pixel array of the filter. However, active control of fovea-based eye movements and the topographic nature of V1 spatial maps means that visual cortex samples images in a very different way from our random, spatially unordered sampling of 12×12 pixel patches. Changing our model to make it more realistic in these two respects could produce different results.

Another important issue with regard to redundancy reduction is the significant redundancy across the encodings of neighboring image patches. The spatial decorrelation of natural images in a wavelet representation leads to suppressive interactions between filters in neighboring patches (Schwartz and Simoncelli 1999), similar to what has been reported in the primary visual cortex (Das and Gilbert 1999).

The approach taken here can also be extended to redundancy that occurs in sequences of images (van Hateren and Ruderman 1998). Here the inputs are three-dimensional spatiotemporal patterns and the filters have the properties of directionally selective simple cells found in the primary visual cortex.

The properties of neurons in the visual cortex depend on experience as well as genetically determined mechanisms, so it is natural to ask whether there are biological ways that an ICA algorithm could be implemented. Although the learning rule we used is nonlocal, it involves a feedback of information from, or within, the output layer. There are many ways that such a biophysical self-organizational processes could be accomplished using local spatial media where the feedforward and the feedback of information are tightly functionally coupled (Bell 1992; Eagleman et al. 2001).

Regardless of whether any biological system implements an unsupervised learning rule such as ICA, the results allow us to interpret the response properties of simple cells in visual cortex as a form of redundancy reduction, as Barlow conjectured. Care must be taken, however, in drawing strong conclusions about visual cortical encodings, from models consisting of only a single static linear transformation.

19.5   Conclusion

What coding principles predict the formation of localized, oriented receptive fields? Barlow's answer was that edges are suspicious coincidences in an image. Based on the principles of information theory (Cover and Thomas 1991), Barlow proposed that our visual cortical feature detectors might be the end result of a redundancy reduction process (Barlow 1989; Atick 1992), in which the activation of each feature detector is as *statistically independent* from the others as possible.

We approached this problem through unsupervised learning in a single layer of linear filters based on an ensemble of natural images. The localized edge detectors that were produced have phase sensitivity as a result of the sensitivity of ICA to higher-order statistics.

Edges (or rather, areas of local contrast) are the first level of structure in images, being detectable by linear filters alone. The analogous cells in area V1, called "simple cells," are the last in the visual system to fit a "cardinal cell" model (von der Malsburg 1999)—that is, there is one cell for each location and

type of object (i.e., orientation). Complex cells in area V1, which are somewhat location invariant, and neurons further up the visual processing pathways, which have many invariant properties, present a huge challenge to unsupervised learning models. Can their properties be predicted (or retrodicted) and their coding properties thus explained?

We believe the answer to this question is yes, and that it will involve the formulation of algorithms related to ICA, in which group-theoretic symmetries in probability distributions are identified with the subspaces in which they are embedded. Von der Malsburg has argued convincingly for many years that invariant coding and "feature binding" are the same problem, so we expect such learning algorithms will help bridge, in an information-theoretic way, the difficult gap between sensory and perceptual learning.

This will also greatly increase the computational power of abstract unsupervised learning techniques.

20

Top-Down Information and Models of Perceptual Learning

Michael H. Herzog and Manfred Fahle

Abstract

Current neural network models, mostly concerned with bottom-up processes, such as finding optimal parameters for a given set of data (which correspond to the stimuli of experiments), do not incorporate top-down information, such as preselecting features or internal knowledge. New experimental results, however, show that attention and other higher cortical processes play an important role in perceptual learning issues. After briefly reviewing current (mathematical) learning models, we present these new results and sketch out a framework of perceptual learning that takes top-down influences into account.

20.1 Introduction

One predominant feature of perceptual learning is its specifity for certain stimulus dimensions such as orientation, spatial frequency, direction of motion, retinal position, and the eye of presentation (e.g., Fiorentini and Berardi 1980; Karni and Sagi 1991; Shiu and Pashler 1992; Fahle, Edelman, and Poggio 1995; Schoups, Vogels, and Orban 1995; Ahissar and Hochstein 1997; Crist et al. 1997; Rivest, Boutet, and Intriligator 1997; but see also Liu 1999; Liu and Weinshall 2000; chapters 9–12). Models of perceptual learning have been mainly concerned with describing these specificities and mainly focused on the isolated set of data (figure 20.1). Both supervised and unsupervised learning schemes show good agreement with the data (see Moses, Schechtman, and Ullman 1990; Poggio, Fahle, and Edelman 1992; Sundareswaran and Vaina 1994). Bootstrapping models (a mixture of supervised and unsupervised learning) using stimuli that the system can classify internally have also been suggested (see Weiss, Edelman, and Fahle 1993; Fahle and Edelman 1993). Simulations with so-called radial basis function (RBF) networks have replicated the effect of orientation specificity for vernier stimuli (Poggio, Fahle, and Edelman 1992), offering a possible explanation for the process underlying perceptual learning: the stimuli were used to synthesize highly specific centers used as the bases for interpolation (see Sinha and Poggio, chapter 15, this volume). Because finding these centers is task specific, no transfer of improvement occurs even between similar tasks. In this chapter, we show that in addition to these purely feedforward mechanisms top-down aspects such as attention are also important for perceptual learning.

Because we will often refer to experiments using a vernier discrimination task, let us briefly describe this paradigm (for a more detailed description, see chapter 11, this volume). A vernier consists of two almost aligned straight bars of the same orientation that are slightly displaced relative to each other by an offset that might be much smaller than the smallest diameter of a retinal photoreceptor. Despite the small size of this spatial offset, most observers are able to discriminate its direction. More importantly, most subjects improve this ability with practice. The phenomenon of spatial resolution below the diameter of a retinal photoreceptor is called "hyperacuity." It is also possible to define hyperacuity tasks with three-dot verniers (figure 20.2, panel a). It is believed that changes on the very early stages of visual processing

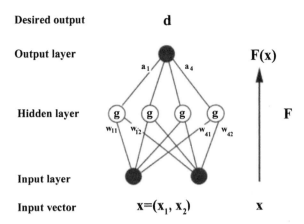

Figure 20.1
Three-layer neural network with a single output unit, the most common architecture for supervised learning. Here the output for a particular input vector $x = (x_1, x_2)$ is $F(x) = \sum_{i=1}^{4} a_i g(x * w_i) = \sum_{i=1}^{4} a_i g(\sum_{j=1}^{2} x_j w_{ij})$, where a_i represents the "synaptic" weights between the hidden units and the output layer unit, and w_{ij} represents the weights between the two input units and the four hidden layer units. Not all "synaptic" weights are indicated.

in the cortex are involved in the learning process because improvement through learning is specific both for the orientation and the eye used during training (e.g., chapter 11, this volume; Gilbert 1994; but see also Mollon and Danilova 1996). Neurons that are monocularly driven and orientation selective are mostly found in the primary visual cortex, area V1 (Hubel and Wiesel 1959), which proves to be more plastic even in adult animals than previously thought (see Eysel, chapter 3, this volume; Gilbert 1994).

20.2   Learning Models

In mathematical terms, learning is viewed as classifying a given set of stimuli $X = \{x^1, \ldots, x^s\}$ con-

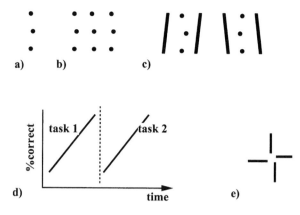

Figure 20.2
(*a*) Three-dot vernier, whose middle point is shifted slightly to the left or right of the imaginary line through the outer points. (*b*) Nine-dot stimulus, for which 84 three-dot spatial tasks can be defined, including diagonals, "triangles," and the like. Additional tasks can be defined with more or less than three points; the possible number of tasks grows exponentially with the number of (homogeneous) features of the stimuli (dots). (*c*) Features correlated to the target dots. If the middle dot is offset to the right, the bars are always rotated clockwise; if the middle dot is offset to the left, the bars are always oriented counterclockwise. (*d*) Schematic graph of performance for sequential training of two possible tasks, with percentages of correct responses plotted against time (or block numbers). (*e*) Vernier discrimination might use the two vertical segments on task 1 and the two horizontal segments on task 2. Throughout the whole experiment, vertical and horizontal verniers are presented simultaneously. Only attention to the particular task is different. If observers attend to task 1 first, an improvement of performance is found that does not transfer to task 2. Thus passive viewing does not yield learning (cf. chapter 11.13).

taining *s* samples. Models for which classification of stimuli is a necessary component are called "supervised"; those for which it is not, "unsupervised." The dependency on feedback is one of the major features used to characterize learning models.

For the sake of simplicity, we focus mainly on feedforward networks, where information propagates in only one direction and neurons belonging to the same layer are not connected with each other. Models where all neurons are interconnected encounter problems that do not arise in feedforward networks. Recurrent models, for example, have to reach a "convergent" state to classify a given stimulus. In Hopfield networks, this state is reached when the reciprocal weights of two neurons are identical, whereas, in cortical networks, the reciprocal connections between two neurons, if they exist at all, will rarely by of equal strength. It should also be mentioned that, in the brain, neither the assumptions of feedforward networks of full connectivity nor of lack of connectivity inside a layer are met. For example, in the primary visual cortex most, but not all, connections of a neuron terminate on other primary visual cortex neurons (Peters, Payne, and Rudd 1994). The relevance for modeling of the experimental results presented here is largely independent of the connectivity of the architecture.

A feedforward neural network (figure 20.1) usually consists of a number of layers, each composed of a defined number of units. Mathematically, such networks can be described as a function $F : \mathbb{R}^n \to \mathbb{R}^m$, where *n* is the number of input units. Their activation is the input vector $x = (x_1, \ldots, x_n)$ and *m* is the number of output units. The output of any particular unit *i* is calculated as the dot product $y * w_i$, where

$$y * w_i = \sum_{j=1}^{r} y_j w_{ij}, \qquad (20.1)$$

with the weight vector $w_i = (w_{i1}, \ldots, w_{ir})$ of unit *i* and the activation vector $y = (y_1, \ldots, y_r)$ of the preceding layer (containing *r* units). The scalar $y * w_i$ is fed into an activation function *g*. Popular activation functions are sigmoid functions such as the common $\sigma_\beta(x) = \dfrac{1}{1 + e^{-2\beta x}}$.

20.2.1 Supervised Learning with a Teacher

Supervised learning means adjusting the "synaptic" weights to obtain the desired output d^k for every given x^k of a set of training data $X = \{x^1, \ldots, x^s\}$. The goal is to minimize the norm $\|d^k - F(x^k)\|$ for all pairs of data values and desired outputs (x^k, d^k). The adjustment can be achieved with a learning rule written as

$$w_{ij}^{t+1} = w_{ij}^t + \alpha L(G^t, x^k, (d^k - F(x^k))), \qquad (20.2)$$

where G^t is the set of all weights of the neural network at time *t*. The vectors x^k and G^t completely determine the state of the net at time *t*. The teacher term $(d^k - F(x^k))$ indicates the error the network produced at time *t* after the presentation of the vector x^k. This procedure is called "data labeling" because the teacher is attaching a label d^k to each data point x^k. In the case of no error, $L(G^t, x^k, 0) = 0$; thus no modifications occur. The learning rate α determines the speed of the learning process, and the function *L* specifies the different on-line techniques such as backpropagation. In supervised learning with a teacher, two components are necessary: (1) a desired output has to be given for every stimulus presentation; and (2) the difference between the actual and the desired output has to be evaluated. It is important to note that not every feedback signal can serve as a teacher signal (see, for example, the experiment providing block feedback in section

20.3.2). Supervised models with a teacher do not allow learning *without* a data labeling mechanism.

20.2.2 Unsupervised Learning

In unsupervised learning models, only the data $X = \{x^1, \ldots, x^s\}$ are given; the model learns by extracting "features" just from the data. Well-known examples are competitive or Hebbian learning rules. Most of these models describe learning as a system of exposure-dependent rules adjusting the strengths of connections (weights) between their elements strictly according to the stimulus. These procedures are totally independent of any top-down effects. As in supervised learning models, the input vector propagates through the network, and the output of a particular unit is determined in the same way. However, no teacher term $(d^k - F(x^k))$ is present in the learning rule, which may be written as

$$w_{ij}^{t+1} = w_{ij}^t + \alpha L(G^t, x^k). \qquad (20.3)$$

To give an example: during the experiments, owing to noise (e.g., eye tremor), the repeated presentation of stimuli may form two classes of inputs for the two fixed vernier offsets (and not only two vectors). A winner-take-all mechanism might find the appropriate weights to separate these classes. Purely exposure-dependent unsupervised learning rules clearly allow learning without feedback; they predict that learning will be independent of the particular feedback condition.

20.2.3 Other Models

Many of the models for which feedback is a necessary component belong to the class of reinforcement learning architectures, and most of them encounter serious problems in describing perceptual learning.

Indeed, none of these models was ever proposed for this purpose; thus we do not discuss them here. Moreover, most of the problems of supervised learning models, as discussed below, apply to these architectures as well.

20.2.4 Summary

In all models described above, learning exclusively focuses on the set of data. Neither preprocessing, such as a selection of interesting coordinates of the input vectors, nor any other top-down information is incorporated. All modifications made with respect to the stimuli presented are implicit. For example, the probability distribution of the stimuli is implicitly built into the synaptic weights but is neither estimated explicitly nor stored in an independent memory that may control the learning process. The same holds true for the rate of feedback signals. A bias of feedback signals favoring one decision class over another is not explicitly represented, thus cannot influence the learning process directly. The learning rate α in equations 20.2 and 20.3 above is a scalar, whereas, in most models, α has to approach zero to ensure convergence. If α does not decrease, the output of the network may differ widely when the same stimulus is presented at different times. Most learning rules thus use α^t with $\alpha^t \to 0$, which is to say that, with time, the system loses its plasticity. Moreover, the amount of modification achieved by a single presentation of an input vector may be quite limited.

20.3   Experimental Results

Which features are important for modeling perceptual learning? Three features are of paramount importance: (1) selection processes, such as attention; (2) external information, such as the processing of feedback; and (3) internal criteria and information. We present new experimental findings on all three.

20.3.1 Selection Processes

Most neural networks treat the stimulus as a whole, incorporating neither a task-guided selection of features of the stimuli nor any other top-down information. In contrast, general (external) knowledge about particular features may play an important role for perceptual learning. What happens, for example, if two (or more) tasks can be defined for a set of stimuli (see figure 20.2)? Are all tasks learned or only the instructed ones? If only the instructed tasks, a selection of particular features of the set of stimuli has to occur, which can be considered to involve attention. The typical experiment to test whether attention is involved in a learning task is to present a set of stimuli for which at least two tasks can be defined (see figure 20.2). Observers train on the first task in the first sessions and on the second in succeeding sessions; the amount of improvement transferred from the first to the second task is determined. Note that the set of stimuli is always the same; only the tasks differ.

Shiu and Pashler (1992) presented lines differing in both orientation and luminance. Training on the luminance discrimination task did not improve performance on the orientation discrimination task afterward. This result proves that learning does not transfer between two "visual dimensions." A similar finding was made by Boutet, Intriligator, and Rivest (1995) on a color versus motion task. Investigating the transfer from a globally to a locally defined texture discrimination task and vice versa, Ahissar and Hochstein (1993) found no transfer from the global to the local task, and only a small partial transfer vice versa, indicating that attention was involved in spatial discrimination tasks. Similar results were obtained by

Meinhardt and Grabbe (in press) for spatial frequency discrimination. When Herzog and Fahle (1994) presented a vertical and a horizontal (line) vernier simultaneously, they found only partial transfer between the stimuli presented at different orientations (chapters 11–13). This result shows that attention can actively select between the learning even of very similar tasks and between neighboring stimuli. In a neurophysiological study, Ahissar et al. (1992) found that monkeys trained on an auditory task learned only the behaviorally relevant features. Taken together, these results suggest that selection processes based on general knowledge about the set of stimuli as a whole (e.g., What are the relevant features?) play an important role in perceptual learning.

Why Is the Brain Not Learning All Possible Tasks?

A stimulus configuration does not determine the task: many tasks can be defined for almost all sets of stimuli, and sheer complexity, makes it impossible to learn all tasks. In figure 20.2, panel b, 84 different three-dot tasks might be defined. In principle, the number of tasks grows exponentially with the number of features in the stimulus: to every subset of features (i.e., the dots in panel b), a task can be defined. Because no knowledge about the relevant stimulus features can be incorporated and because a given task can be performed with almost infinitely many sets of stimuli, this problem is a major challenge for unsupervised learning models. Consider the three-dot vernier discrimination task in figure 20.2, panel a. The same task can be performed with the stimuli displayed in panel b, which have six additional neighboring dots; although the task remains the same, the set of input vectors has changed dramatically.

Where the stimuli are correlated, the problem might be even harder. Additional features correlated with the target stimuli might be used to solve the task—especially if these features have a larger d', that is, if they are "more easily" discriminated than the "original" features. Figure 20.2, panel c, illustrates such correlated features. The two targets to be discriminated from each other consist of a dot vernier, with the middle dot offset to the left or right. If the middle dot is offset to the right, the bars are always rotated clockwise and if the middle dot is offset to the left the bars are always rotated counterclockwise. If the vernier discrimination task is "more difficult" than the orientation discrimination task defined by the correlated bars, the latter task might be "learned" instead of the vernier discrimination task. In supervised learning models, weights may be changed according to the correlated features because feedback is also correlated to them. After decorrelating the tasks, a deterioration of performance will result.

Thus the set of stimuli does not determine the task, nor vice versa. Because not all tasks can be learned, it is important to incorporate knowledge about the features relevant for the task. Attention-like mechanisms might contribute to the solution of the problem of selecting features, which becomes more prominent if different tasks have to be learned in succession (see also section 20.3.3).

20.3.2 External Information

Role of External Feedback
One of the main characteristics used to classify neural networks is their dependency on external feedback, which can be viewed as additional external information (about "correct" classifications) for *each particular* stimulus. Because, as noted above, supervised neural networks with a teacher have to rely on external feedback to label the data, they propose that perceptual learning without external feedback is impossible, whereas (pure) unsupervised learning models propose quite the contrary, and are indifferent to whether or not feedback is provided.

How do humans use external feedback? A pioneering study on the dependency of feedback for perceptual learning was conducted by Shiu and Pashler (1992) using an orientation discrimination paradigm. Here we discuss data from a more recent, larger study (Herzog and Fahle 1997) that used a vernier discrimination task to investigate perceptual learning. Vernier stimuli were presented under different but comparable feedback conditions:

1. *Correlated trial-by-trial feedback.* An incorrect response was followed immediately by an acoustical error signal, whereas no tone occurred after a correct response.

2. *No feedback.*

3. *Block feedback.* At the end of each block of eighty stimuli, a score of correct responses was displayed; during a block, no error signals were provided.

4. *Uncorrelated trial-by-trial feedback.* All responses were labeled as incorrect with a probability of 0.5.

Correlated trial-by-trial or block feedback (condition 1 or 3) improved the speed of learning as well as overall performance, whereas uncorrelated trial-by-trial or no feedback (condition 2 or 4) slowed down or even abolished improvement of performance (see also Ball and Sekuler 1987; Shiu and Pashler 1992; chapters 11, 12). With the setup described above, we did not find a significant improvement of performance if no feedback was provided, although some subjects improved their performance under this condition, and in similar experiments, observers improved significantly even in the absence of error feedback (e.g., McKee and Westheimer 1978; for long-term learning, see Shiu and Pashler 1992; chapters 11, 12). Thus learning without external feedback is possible; whereas the improvement of performance is slower without than with feedback, the positive effect of feedback is neither very specific nor accurate: reduced feedback in the block feedback condition does not change the results dramatically. On the other hand, manipulated feedback abolishes learning. Because unsupervised learning models incorporate no feedback-dependent computations, they cannot explain this graded dependency on external feedback. And because external feedback is not used to label the data and to compute a teacher signal, supervised learning models with an external teacher cannot be used to explain the effects of feedback on perceptual learning either.

Why Is External Feedback Not Used to Label the Data?

The average number of connections of a neuron in the monkey neocortex is about $4 * 10^3$ to 10^4 synapses (Beaulieu et al. 1992), creating networks with an incredibly large number of weights to be adjusted. As an example, imagine that an output neuron is coding for a particular task in a three-layer feedforward network and a supervised learning algorithm tries to backpropagate the error. This output neuron is connected to $4 * 10^3$ neurons in the hidden layer and each of the $4 * 10^3$ neurons has $4 * 10^3$ connections to the input layer. In total, at least $1.6 * 10^7$ weights are involved in this network to improve only one particular task. But the situation in the brain is even more complex. Not all connections projecting to a neuron in the cortex originate exclusively from areas "below," nor are all related to the particular task. Connections originate from noncortical structures, from neurons in the same area, and from other areas. Less than 10% of the inputs to neurons in area V1 originate from the lateral geniculate nucleus (Peters, Payne, and Rudd 1994). An error backpropagation procedure might change some of these weights, at the same time erasing weights adjusted for different tasks. Because so many synapses need to be modified (a quantitative problem) and because a mechanism is needed to prevent adjusting the "wrong" ones (a qualitative problem), the ap-

propriate connections for the task must be found before adjusting the appropriate sizes of the weights, which may in part explain why the experimental results do not supply any positive evidence for the existence of a supervised procedure with a teacher in perceptual learning.

Learning with Insight

If after a period of nonimprovement with stimuli very difficult to discriminate (small d'), stimuli with a large d' are briefly presented, an immediate and strong improvement may follow, the "Eureka" effect (Ahissar and Hochstein 1995; Rubin, Nakayama, and Shapley 1997; Rubin, Nakayama, and Shapley, chapter 13, this volume; Meinhardt 2001). Because, however, the amount of modification after each stimulus is determined by the learning rate and thus may be quite limited, many learning models cannot reflect this behavior by incorporating the additional crucial information. Moreover, in supervised models, correctly classified stimuli that result from a large d', corresponding to a zero error $d - F(x) = 0$ (see equation 20.2), do not yield any modification. Therefore, information already "known" by the system does not contribute to the learning process.

20.3.3 Internal Criteria and Information

The last two subsections described the influence of external top-down information on perceptual learning. Here we present results of experiments showing that the brain builds up and uses internal criteria and information to *actively* control the learning process.

In experiments providing biased feedback, Herzog and Fahle (1999) found their subjects used internal criteria about the correctness of responses. They provided manipulated feedback on a binary choice task using vernier stimuli with different offset sizes, where one of the stimuli was labeled as belonging to

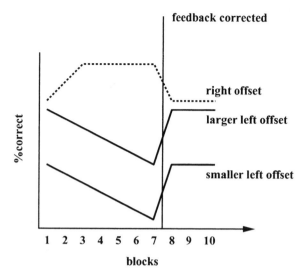

Figure 20.3
Three verniers were presented, two offset to the left and one offset to the right. The vernier offset to the right and the vernier with the larger offset to the left had the same offset size and received correct feedback, whereas the vernier with the smaller offset to the left received reverse feedback: a correct response was labeled as incorrect and an incorrect response as correct. After the seventh block (vertical dividing line), correct feedback was provided for all stimuli. Subjects were not informed about the display conditions in general nor about the correction of feedback after the seventh block. A significant deterioration of performance occurs for *both* verniers offset to the left. The correction of feedback leads to an immediate and strong rebound of performance. In the first seven blocks results for the vernier offset to the right are always superior than for the verniers offset to the left. After correction of feedback a deterioration of performance occurs for this stimulus. If feedback would have been used to classify the data, performance for the vernier with larger offset to the left should be constant or improved: this stimulus was correctly labeled. Only performance for the vernier with smaller offset to the left should deteriorate because of the reverse feedback indicating offset to the right. This proves again that external feedback is not used as a labeling signal. Subjects only changed their decision criteria—voting more often for the stimulus offset to the right. The fast rebound in block

the other, incorrect class (for details see figure 20.3). This stimulus was always followed by a reverse feedback, that is, an error feedback followed correct responses, and vice versa. Observers changed their decision criterion according to the manipulated feedback, that is, they partly reversed their responses to this stimulus, which resulted in a deterioration of performance because feedback and physical offset size did not tally. But they were not really learning (i.e., a permanent change of performance probably due to synaptic weights) since reestablishing correct feedback almost instantaneously reversed the effects of biased feedback (figure 20.3).

In experiments investigating the influence of the statistics of stimulus source, no learning occurred when verniers offset to the left and right had sufficiently different probabilities (Herzog, Broos, and Fahle 1999). We suggest that subjects assumed that the stimuli were uniformly distributed, that is, presented with equal probabilities. Because deviations from this assumption resulted in a suppression of the learning processes, we conclude that a priori assumptions about the external characteristics of the set of stimuli can play an important role in perceptual learning.

Why Are Internal Criteria and Internal Knowledge Important?

If some neurons code for a specific task, subsequent cortical areas of the brain (such as motor effectors) must locate these neurons and know the way they code. This problem challenges mainly unsupervised learning rules and indicates that learning has to occur in a rather integral way. Which neuron classifies for

---

7 indicates the involvement of *internal* criteria: reversing the decision behavior is much faster than its slow adjustment was with biased feedback in the first seven blocks (schematic results of five observers).

which class of stimuli in unsupervised learning models depends on the (unknown) initial weights and the (unknown) order of presentations. How can subsequent neurons know which preceding neurons code for which class? The same problem applies to supervised learning of the hidden units. Because the coding of these neurons cannot be determined without knowledge about the initial weights and the order of stimulus presentations (none of the $r!$ possible permutations of the hidden layer units alters the output), the coding of these units cannot be used explicitly. It follows that, to ensure that succeeding neurons receive the "correct" input, the coding of neurons may not be arbitrary.

To avoid these problems, we suggest that internal criteria, depending on a self-monitored decision behavior, *actively* control the learning process. For example, any unexpected bias of the decision rate might result in a suppression of synaptic modifications. There is another reason for active control of the learning process. In most neural network models, an additional mechanism is required to control the learning process to ensure convergence and to prevent overlearning—achieved by a controlled decrease of the learning rate α^t. However, with decreasing α^t, the system loses its plasticity—the well-known plasticity-stability dilemma (see Hertz, Krogh, and Palmer 1991, p. 228; Carpenter and Grossberg 1987). This problem arises in many models because the control of the time course is not locked to the "success" of the learning process. Active control of the learning process, control that depends on internal estimations extracted from the learning process, may solve the problem of keeping the system plastic when required. Yet another problem arises when the supervised learning process is captured in local minima, as is sometimes the case. To escape from these minima is impossible because no explicit

monitoring of performance is incorporated. The system does not "know" about being "trapped." It is hard to see how previous adjustments can be erased and how the learning process can start again from a "tabula rasa" or an earlier "branch point." We observed that, under manipulated feedback conditions, such as uncorrelated feedback, learning courses exhibit a deeply cleft behavior, with many ups and downs (Herzog and Fahle 1997). This result is also hard to explain for unsupervised learning models because a rapid decay of performance after a strong improvement is counterintuitive. If performance has improved once, the weights should be kept relatively constant. Taken together, these experimental results suggest that the learning process might become more flexible with active control of the learning rate. In section 20.4, we suggest a framework that uses both external and internal feedback to control the learning processes via the learning rate. Our experiments show that information from external sources and from the monitoring of the internal decision and learning process is evaluated in perceptual learning. This information is used for *active* control of the learning process to ensure that "correct" classifications are learned and that the system is kept plastic as long as necessary.

20.4 Summary

In discussing selection processes, external information, and internal criteria and information—all important top-down information-processing features of perceptual learning—we noted that models mainly focusing on the raw data cannot explain the experimental results we have presented. Unsupervised learning rules or parts of interpolation schemes such as RBF networks may still be useful tools to describe perceptual learning. However, we believe that simply extending the existing models with some additional "independent" structures will not improve them: top-down information must be incorporated in an *integral* way.

It should be noted that the components of neural network models were criticized (Shepherd 1990; Gardner 1993). One problem here is that many aspects of neurons, like their compartment structure or (nonlinear) intersynaptic computations, are over-simplified or not modeled at all. The importance of these aspects for a biologically realistic description of neural processing cannot be judged yet. Moreover, most neurons are either excitatory or inhibitory, but not both, implying that they cannot change their synaptic weights from positive to negative values and vice versa (Dale's law; Shepherd 1990; Kandel and Schwartz 1991).

In summary, a serious problem in modeling perceptual learning consists in how remote information related to the task and stored in higher cortical areas can control learning in the very early processing stages. Only these early levels contain neurons with small receptive fields that might provide the information necessary to process the selected task (see section 20.1; and chapter 11, this volume). Unsupervised learning rules use purely local information, but cannot integrate top-down knowledge about the required task. Supervised models, on the other hand, can incorporate general knowledge but cannot realize the local changes necessary for perceptual learning while obeying biological constraints.

20.5   Toward a Framework Incorporating Top-Down Information

It follows from the discussion above that a model of perceptual learning has to use feedback connections, possibly of a cholinergic nature (see chapter 2.1.7).

Neurons in higher cortical areas have to send task-related information to the appropriate lower level areas to overcome the various selection problems. Because many tasks have to be performed using the same neurons, we suggest that information is gated in a task-dependent way through a processing stage. In sketching out our framework for perceptual learning, we propose that models may be divided into three parts: the first to consist of conventional feedforward propagation of the stimulus; the second to evaluate any available feedback; and the third to control the propagation of information, using recurrent operations to change the gating properties of processing units. Because of the huge number of synaptic connections, neurons, and modules, selection processes must be involved that modify just a few of the many combinations of the processing units, depending on the chosen task (figure 20.4). In our framework, internal and (if provided) external feedback evaluates the "success" of this choice and controls the temporal application of the update (i.e., learning) mechanism. Depending on the result, the next element in the selection process is chosen according to feedback evaluation, a priori knowledge, and other top-down influences (figure 20.4).

Incorporating selection mechanisms can solve the problem of choosing relevant features. If no exact information about the "best" choice exists, different choices may be evaluated successively. In this scenario, it does not matter whether different tasks are learned simultaneously or in succession, thus bypassing the plasticity-stability dilemma. The selection mechanisms can also solve the problem of choosing which of the many weights must be modified. In this framework, feedback is not used to calculate a teacher term that depends on the known classification of stimuli. Internal and external feedback evaluates performance, thus *actively* controlling the learning process via the learning rate. Learning

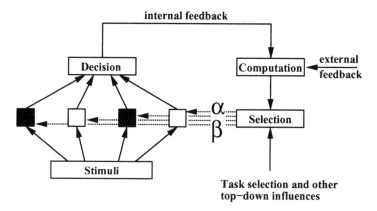

Figure 20.4

Major components of a recurrent model involving top-down influences and a feedback-controlled learning rate α. A stimulus is presented and, depending on a selection mechanism, its representation is gated through one (or more) processing layers to a decision stage. The selection mechanism chooses particular processing units and modifies their properties to achieve a "correct" classification of the stimulus. Processing units may be single neurons, groups of neurons, whole modules, or just axons of neurons. Based on the gating, a decision is made about the stimulus resulting in a motor response (not shown in this figure); this decision creates an internal feedback term, which depends on the discriminability, i.e., determined by both the physical properties of stimuli and the properties of gating. The value of the feedback term is evaluated, together with external feedback (if provided), and fed into the selection mechanism, which is also controlled by top-down mechanisms such as attention. Each time a particular task is carried out, a corresponding selection action is chosen. The goal of learning is to find "good" actions to discriminate between the features that are "important" for the task. However, it is not necessary to design a special detector for this task as long as the features are discriminated separately. In the framework depicted here, two mechanisms are involved: a selection mechanism, β, to control which of the units are chosen (in this figure the black squares) and an update mechanism, α, to control the processing changes of the units chosen by β. Both mechanisms interact with each other. The control of α depends heavily on internal and external feedback. For example, β selects a group of neurons and a Hebb-rule is applied to change the synaptic weights of these neurons. Feedback controls the speed of the update process by controlling the learning rate α. Modifications in the top-down parts are also allowed. The major difference from the neural network models reviewed in this chapter is that feedback *actively* controls the learning process in a closed loop with an (implicit) feedback memory. Additional top-down aspects are easily incorporated.

without external feedback is possible because internal feedback is employed, although learning without external feedback is slower because the update process cannot be accelerated. Learning by insight may help make good choices: easily discriminated stimuli "suggest" which modules are "important" for the particular task, thus facilitating the learning process. If, in comparison, there are disturbances in the processing of stimuli (such as those mediated by feedback)

and internal criteria (such as a priori assumptions about the statistics of stimuli), learning via the mechanism α is suppressed. Learning by insight and external feedback may be related. Stimuli that are more easily discriminated can guide learning of stimuli that are harder to discriminate by providing *internal* feedback about correctness of responses (see above). Thus providing "easy" and "hard" stimuli might be interchangeable with providing only "hard" stimuli and external feedback. (Here it should be noted that the amount of learning depends on the individual baselines of subjects. Faster improvement is found for subjects training with a vernier with a larger offset compared to observers training with a smaller offset size—even the starting performance levels of the subjects, measured in percentages of correct responses, are virtually identical; see also Fahle and Henke-Fahle 1996.)

In our framework, components are *integrally* interconnected. Models may take into account the functional differences between excitatory and inhibitory systems, as is known from several anatomical and electrophysiological investigations (e.g., Shepherd 1990; Kandel and Schwartz 1991). The feedforward pathway may be modeled as the excitatory part, with feedback loops assumed to exert recurrent inhibition on the feedforward excitation. (For a concrete example of modeling learning in a vernier discrimination task, see Herzog and Fahle (1998). Although many other models are conceivable; see, for example, Williamson 1999).

An important feature of our framework is the volatility of the proposed gating operations, which are enabled only when the corresponding task is performed. Thus no *long-lasting* neurophysiological modifications, such as a permanent change of tuning curves of neurons, are expected. This feature agrees well with recent psychophysical and neurophysiological findings. Schoups (chapter 5, this volume) did not find any changes in the responses of area V1 neurons after learning a perceptual orientation discrimination task. Fahle (chapter 11, this volume) showed that no transfer of learning occurs between discrimination tasks employing verniers with a difference of orientation as small as 10°, a surprising result because the half-width of receptive fields of V1 neurons is believed to be 30° (Movshon and Blakemore 1973) and thus an interaction between

the different vernier tasks is believed to occur. Fahle (1997) also found no transfer between discrimination tasks employing verniers, chevrons, and lines with different orientations, all three stimuli believed to be processed by orientation sensitive cells in V1. A *long-lasting* modification of receptive fields according to one of these tasks should modify performance on the other tasks. However, this proposition could not be confirmed. We suggest that receptive fields are modified via gating but only as long as the task is performed to avoid any interference with other tasks.

20.6   Conclusions

In the last ten years, many pioneering studies have discovered mechanisms of perceptual learning; many models have reproduced the results of these studies, largely by focusing on the stimuli themselves. More recent experimental results suggest, however, that the stimuli are only one part of the story. Other aspects, as yet not included in models, are important as well. In this chapter, we showed that the role of feedback for the learning process was misunderstood, and the role of selection and control processes underestimated.

It seems that the learning of even *simple* stimuli, such as those used in most experiments on perceptual learning, cannot be tackled by *simple* models. Rather, perceptual learning requires highly sophisticated architectures. The experimental results suggest that most learning phenomena cannot be tracked down, and that a single, comprehensive model of perceptual learning thus cannot be fully specified. We may never find the basic elements of learning that might be used as an "alphabet" for learning more complex tasks because these elements work together. On the other hand, because top-down influences and other important aspects play an important role in perceptual learning, they might be studied with the simple stimuli of perceptual learning, and perceptual learning might itself become an important tool to investigate the entire universe of learning phenomena.

Acknowledgments

Michael Herzog and Manfred Fahle were supported by the SFB 517 "Neurocognition" of the German Research Council (Deutsche Forschungsgemeinschaft). Manfred Fahle was supported in addition by the von Humboldt Society (Max Planck Prize). We are grateful to Sven Heinrich for his valuable comments on the manuscript.

Glossary

AMPA Alpha-amino-3-hydroxy-5-methyl-4-isox-azolo-propionic acid. **Glutamate** agonist for a glutamate receptor that gates fast channels permeable for sodium and potassium.

anterograde A movement or influence acting from the neuronal cell body toward the axonal target (opposite of **retrograde**).

area 17 Cytoarchitectonic cortical area located at the occipital pole of the brain (**primary visual cortex; V1**), terminology of the anatomist Brodmann (1909), who divided the human cortex into consecutively numbered **cytoarchitectonic areas**.

BDNF Brain-derived neurotrophic factor. Trophic factor similar to **NGF** that acts during development (and after lesions of the brain) to stabilize and maintain neuronal connections.

binocular deprivation Deprivation of sight in both eyes (in experiments, achieved by suturing the lids of both eyes shut).

CaMKII Calcium calmodulin kinase II. Important intracellular enzyme, involved in the intracellular signaling cascade of **LTP**.

cerebellum Prominent hindbrain structure concerned with motor coordination, posture, and balance. Composed of a three-layered cortex and deep nuclei; attached to the brain stem by three sets of cerebellar peduncles.

cerebral cortex Superficial **gray matter** of the cerebral hemispheres.

classification Task of attaching a category label to each point in a data set.

clustering Task of grouping the points in a data set on the basis of their mutual proximity. The computation of proximities requires that the data space be endowed with a metric.

colinear Arrangement of line segments along a straight line that is parallel to their orientation (opposite of parallel).

collateral Axon arbor branching from the main axon.

computational model Said of a perceptual task, a model that aims at explaining (1) the representations involved in fulfilling the task, and (2) the nature and the reasons behind their transformations.

corpus callosum Large midline fiber bundle that connects the cortices of the two cerebral hemispheres.

cortex **Gray matter** of the cerebral hemispheres and **cerebellum**, where most of the neurons in the brain are located.

course of dimensionality In learning, the exponential dependence on dimensionality of the number of examples required to cover the representation space for the purpose of robust model estimation. Because of this dependence, learning from examples in high-dimensional spaces requires additional assumptions about the structure of the feature space.

cytoarchitectonic areas   Distinct regions of the neocortical mantle identified by differences in cell size, packing density, and laminar arrangement.

dark-rearing   Raising of animals in complete darkness (in a dark room).

distal   Farther away from a point of reference (opposite of **proximal**).

EPSP   Excitatory postsynaptic potential. Depolarizing event at the postsynaptic membrane of a synapse caused by the action of a transmitter substance at ligand-gated (fast) or metabotropic receptor–coupled (slow) channels that are permeable for sodium and potassium. Increases the probability of reaching the **firing threshold**.

firing threshold   Membrane potential level (normally in the range of −50 to −60 mV) that has to be reached to elicit a regenerative sodium action potential.

GABA   Gamma-aminobutyric acid. Most important inhibitory transmitter substance in the brain.

GABA$_A$ Receptor for **GABA** coupled to a ligand-gated channel permeable for chloride. Action: fast inhibition due to hyperpolarization (to about −70 mV) and shunting.

GABA$_B$ Metabotropic receptor for **GABA** that activates a G-protein-coupled channel permeable for potassium. Action: slow inhibition due to hyperpolarization (up to about −90 mV) and inhibitory postsynaptic potential (**IPSP**).

Gabor patch   Circular striped pattern (alternating dark gray/light gray) that is generated by modulating a sine or cosine wave grating with a two-dimensional Gaussian envelope. Gabor patches selectively excite cells tuned to a specific orientation, spatial frequency, and spatial location.

GAD   Glutamate decarboxylase. Enzyme for the production of **GABA** from **glutamate**.

generalization   The ability of a learning system to classify novel patterns (e.g., to respond adequately to a novel stimulus), to which it has not been previously exposed.

generator   Entity or process underlying stochastic data that is responsible for the regularities existing in a data set. Typically, the underlying regularities are obscured by measurement imperfections, extraneous factors, and noise, and must be uncovered, for example, through learning.

glutamate   Most important excitatory transmitter substance in the brain. Acts on **NMDA** and non-NMDA (**AMPA**, kainate) as well as metabotropic glutamate receptors.

gray matter   General term for regions of the central nervous system rich in neuronal cell bodies and neuropil, characteristically gray in outward appearance; includes the cerebral and cerebellar cortices, the nuclei of the brain, and the central portion of the spinal cord. See also **white matter**.

Hebbian learning rule   Postulated by Donald O. Hebb in 1949, this rules states that a synapse is strengthened when its pre- and postsynaptic elements are synchronously activated. Theoretical background of long-term potentiation (**LTP**).

hippocampus   Cortical structure in the medial portion of the temporal lobe; in humans, associated with short-term declarative memory, among many other functions.

hyperexcitability   Activity state above normal. Can be due to reduced firing threshold, depolarization of a cell, or increased transmitter levels.

immunohistochemistry Method of labeling specific cells by means of an antigen-antibody reaction or an irreversible receptor agonist.

intracortical Within the cortex.

in vitro Literally, "in glass." Outside the living body. Brain tissue studied in vitro is cut in about 400 μm slices that are put into oxygen/carbogen bubbled bath of artificial cerebrospinal fluid (aCSF). Cells can be recorded extra- or intracellularly or by patch clamp methods in a stable situation under microscopic control.

in vivo Literally, "in living." Within the living body. In vivo is the only way to study nerve cells under natural conditions with original sensory input or intact motor output and in the intact system environment.

IPSP Inhibitory postsynaptic potential. Hyperpolarizing event at the postsynaptic membrane of a synapse. Involved ion channels are permeable for chloride or potassium. Reduces the probability of reaching the **firing threshold**.

LTD Long-term depression. Weakening of synapses induced by low-frequency stimulation (causing a situation not in accord with the **Hebbian learning rule**). Correlated with a low intracellular calcium level. In neurophysiology, persistent weakening of synapses based on past patterns of activity.

LTP Long-term potentiation. Long-lasting (hours to days) strengthening of synapses induced by high-frequency stimulation (causing a situation in accord with the **Hebbian learning rule**). Correlated with an increased intracellular calcium level. The effect is mediated by postsynaptic mechanisms (e.g., phosphorylation of membrane receptors) as well as presynaptic mechanisms (e.g., increased transmitter release). LTP is specific: only the suprathreshold synapse that is stimulated with high frequency is potentiated. LTP is associative: weak synapses when activated synchronously with stronger inputs to the same cell can be strengthened as well.

magnification factor Factor describing the relation between a peripheral sensory surface and the size of its central representation. The magnification factor is as a rule directly related to the receptor density in the periphery: the fovea of the retina, the frequencies related to speech in the cochlea, and the lips and fingertips of the skin have the largest cortical magnification factor.

manifold Smooth "surface" embedded in a higher-dimensional space, such as a curve drawn on a sheet of paper and the sheet of paper itself, embedded in the three-dimensional space.

MAP-2 Microtubuli-associated protein 2. Associated with axonal transport.

measurement space If the output of each unit in a sensory pathway is thought of as a dimension along which the signal can vary, the entire ensemble of units (e.g., the ganglion cells in the retina) is seen to span a measurement (representation) space whose nominal dimensionality is equal to the number of units.

MLP Multilayer perceptron. Layered neural network architecture in which the response of each unit is determined by computing the inner product between its inputs and a vector of weights, and by passing the result through a nonlinearity. MLPs are usually trained (i.e., the weights are adjusted) by backpropagation of errors.

monocular deprivation Deprivation of sight in one eye. See also **binocular deprivation**.

MRI Magnetic resonance imaging. Brain imaging technique based on the detection of changes in an artificially created magnetic field.

neocortex Six-layered cortex that covers the bulk of the cerebral hemispheres.

neuronal plasticity Property of the nervous system that makes it modifiable in response to use and disuse, damage, and disease. The natural events of development are often also associated with the term *plasticity*. Adult central nervous system plasticity is often related to mechanisms active as well in developmental plasticity.

neuropil Dense tangle of axonal and dendritic branches, and the synapses between them, that lies between neuronal cell bodies in the **gray matter** of the brain and spinal cord.

NGF Nerve growth factor. First obtained from salivary glands of male mice by Rita Levi-Montalcini (Nobel prize 1985). Regulates axonal outgrowth and maintains the survival of cells when taken up from the target cells and retrogradely transported to the soma. The trkA receptor is the specific receptor for NGF.

NMDA *N*-methyl-D-aspartate. Artificial **glutamate** agonist of one type of glutamate receptors. The NMDA receptor–gated channel is permeable for sodium, potassium, and calcium. NMDA is blocked at resting potential by magnesium (magnesium block) and can only be activated after the magnesium block has been released by depolarization. NMDA channels are associated with **LTP**.

NT-3 Neurotrophin 3. Another member of the family of neurotrophins and nerve growth factors that includes **NGF** and **BDNF**.

ocular dominance columns Segregated termination patterns of thalamic inputs representing the two eyes in primary visual cortex of some mammalian species.

primary visual cortex Cortical area in the occipital lobe of the brain (Brodmann's **area 17**), first cortical stage of visual scene analysis.

proximal Closer to a point of reference (opposite of **distal**).

RBFs Radial basis functions. Method for function approximation and classification in which the target function is represented as a superposition of values of basis functions, which in turn depend only on the distances between the input and their respective centers. Also, a two-layer neural network architecture implementing this approximation method.

receptive field Region of the body surface where stimulation causes a sensory nerve cell (or axon) to respond. In the visual system, region in visual space where presentation of a stimulus causes a neuron to respond.

regression Task of determining the mean of a distribution of points in a data set along some of the dimensions, conditional on their location along the remaining dimensions.

retinotopy Property of central parts of the visual system. The retina is mapped in these structures (lateral geniculate nucleus, superior colliculus, primary and higher visual cortices) in a topographic way, where neighboring regions of the retina are represented in neighboring regions in the central visual pathways. The maps are nonlinear with an overproportional representation of the central retina (**magnification factor**).

retrograde A movement or influence acting from the axonal target toward the neuronal cell body (opposite of **anterograde**).

scotoma Blind area in the visual field. The blind spot of the retina is due to the optic nerve head (region free of receptors) in the eye and thus a "physiological scotoma." Pathological scotomas can be due to retinal as well as central damage all along the visual pathway.

smooth mappings Mappings under which a small change in the input results in a small change in the output.

squint See **strabismus**.

statistical inference Acquisition of information concerning the probability distribution of the data (e.g., the examples in a learning scenario), which can then be used in decision making (e.g., as in a Bayesian framework).

strabismus Misalignment of the two eyes such that normal binocular vision is compromised.

striate cortex Primary visual cortex. Located in the occipital pole of the brain, the first cortical area that receives subcortical input from the retina via the lateral geniculate nucleus of the thalamus.

support vectors Data points lying close to the would-be decision boundary in the task of learning a discrimination curve. These points have a much greater influence on the boundary location (discriminant curve) than others, and can be used to speed up learning and make it more efficient.

synapsin Substance associated with synapse formation in development and plasticity.

tangential connections Fiber pathways in the cerebral cortex that extend in a direction parallel to the cortical surface (also termed *horizontal* or *intralaminar*), in contrast to vertical connections that run perpendicular to the cortical surface, from layer to layer.

threshold Stimulus intensity at which an observer detects a stimulus (or is able to discriminate it from another stimulus) with a defined accuracy level, most commonly 75%.

tracer In neurobiology, substance used to trace (label or visualize) nerve cell connections.

transfer Process of learning to perform one task and then using the acquired knowledge to perform a different task. See also **generalization**.

2-AFC Two-alternative forced-choice. Common experimental design in psychophysical experiments. Presented with a target during one of two subsequent stimulus presentation intervals, observers have to indicate whether the first or the second interval contained the target. This design eliminates subjective bias observes may have with detecting the presence of a target in a single stimulus interval (yes/no response).

vertical meridian Vertical midline of the visual field.

Weber law When the task is to discriminate two stimuli of intensity I and $I + \Delta I$, the discrimination **threshold** ΔI is proportional to the pedestal I. This law is usually violated when stimulus intensities are low (close to the detection threshold).

white matter General term for large axon tracts in the brain and spinal cord, which characteristically have a whitish cast when viewed in freshly cut cross section. See also **gray matter**.

References

Abbott, L. F., Rolls, E. T., and Tovee, M. J. (1996). Representational capacity of face coding in monkeys. *Cereb. Cortex* 6: 498–505.

Abeles, M. (1991). *Corticonics: Neural Circuits in the Cerebral Cortex*. Cambridge.

Adcock, N. V., and Mangan, G. L. (1970). Attention and perceptual learning. *J. Gen. Psychol.* 83: 247–254.

Adini, Y., Sagi, D., and Tsodyks, M. (1997). Excitatory-inhibitory network in the visual cortex: Psychophysical evidence. *Proc. Natl. Acad. Sci. U S A* 94: 10426–10431.

Aertsen, A. M., Gerstein, G. L., Habib, M. K., and Palm, G. (1989). Dynamics of neuronal firing correlation: Modulation of "effective connectivity." *J. Neurophysiol.* 61: 900–917.

Aglioti, S., DeSouza, J. F. X., and Goodale, M. A. (1995). Size-contrast illusions deceive the eye but not the hand. *Curr. Biol.* 5: 679–685.

Aglioti, S., Smania, N., Atzei, A., and Berlucchi, G. (1997). Spatio-temporal properties of the pattern of evoked phantom sensations in a left index amputee patient. *Behav. Neurosci.* 111: 867–872.

Ahissar, E., Abeles, M., Ahissar, M., Haidarliu, S., and Vaadia, E. (1998). Hebbian-like functional plasticity in the auditory cortex of the behaving monkey. *Neuropharmacol.* 37: 633–655.

Ahissar, E., and Ahissar, M. (1994). Plasticity in auditory cortical circuits. *Curr. Opin. Neurobiol.* 4: 580–587.

Ahissar, E., Vaadia, E., Ahissar, M., Bergman, H., Arieli, A., and Abeles, M. (1992). Dependence of cortical plasticity on correlated activity of single neurons and on behavioral context. *Science* 257: 1412–1415.

Ahissar, M., and Hochstein, S. (1993). Attentional control of early perceptual learning. *Proc. Natl. Acad. Sci. U S A* 90: 5718–5722.

Ahissar, M., and Hochstein, S. (1995). How early is early vision? Evidence from perceptual learning. In T. V. Papathomas, C. Chubb, A. Gore, and E. Kowler, eds., *Early Vision and Beyond*. Cambridge, MA: MIT Press.

Ahissar, M., and Hochstein, S. (1995). Time course of perceptual learning probes underlying mechanisms. *Perception* 24: 22a.

Ahissar, M., and Hochstein, S. (1996a). Perceptual learning transfer over space and orientation. *Invest. Ophthalmol. Vis. Sci.* 37: 3182.

Ahissar, M., and Hochstein, S. (1996b). Learning pop-out detection: Specificities to stimulus characteristics. *Vision Res.* 36: 3487–3500.

Ahissar, M., and Hochstein, S. (1997). Task difficulty and the specificity of perceptual learning. *Nature* 387: 401–406.

Ahissar, M., and Hochstein, S. (1998). Perceptual learning. In V. Walsh and J. Kulikowski, eds., *Perceptual Constancies*, 455–498. Cambridge: Cambridge University Press.

Ahissar, M., and Hochstein, S. (2000). The spread of attention and learning in feature search: Effects of target distribution and task difficulty. *Vision Res.* 40: 1349–1364.

Ahissar, M., Laiwand, R., and Hochstein, S. (2001). Attentional demands following perceptual skill training. *Psychol. Sci.* 12: 57–63.

Ahissar, M., Laiwand, R., Kozminsky, G., and Hochstein, S. (1998). Learning pop-out detection: Building representations for conflicting target-distractor relationships. *Vision Res.* 38: 3095–3107.

Ajjanagadde, V., and Shastri, L. (1991). Rules and variables in neural nets. *Neural Comput.* 3: 121–134.

Albrecht, D. G., Farrar, S. B., and Hamilton, D. B. (1984). Spatial contrast adaptation characteristics of neurones recorded in the cat's visual cortex. *J. Physiol. (Lond.)* 347: 713–739.

Albus, K., and Wolf, W. (1984). Early post-natal development of neuronal function in the kitten's visual cortex: A laminar analysis. *J. Physiol.* 348: 153–185.

Allman, J., Miezin, F., and McGuinness, E. L. (1985). Stimulus specific responses from beyond the classical receptive field: Neurophysiological mechanisms for local-global comparisons in visual neurons. *Annu. Rev. Neurosci.* 8: 407–430.

Alloway, K. D., and Aaron, G. B. (1996). Adaptive changes in the somatotopic properties of individual thalamic neurons immediately following microlesions in connected regions of the nucleus cuneatus. *Synapse* 22: 1–14.

Allport, D. A. (1989). Visual attention. In M. I. Posner, ed., *Foundations of Cognitive Science*, 631–682. Cambridge MA: MIT Press.

Amari, S., Cichocki, A., and Yang, H. H. (1996). A new learning algorithm for blind signal separation. In *Advances in Neural Information Processing Systems*, vol. 8. Cambridge, MA: MIT Press.

Angeli, A., Bruce, V., and Ellis, H. D. (1999). Getting familiar with faces. *Perception* 28, Suppl. 115.

Anton, B. S, Player, N. I., and Bennett, T. L. (1981). Transfer of perceptual learning: Role of tactual-kinesthetic feedback reexamined. *Percept. Mot. Skills* 52: 195–202.

Arckens, L., Schweigart, G., Qu, Y., Wouters, G., Pow, D. V., Vandesande, F., Eysel, U. T., and Orban, G. A. (2000). Cooperative changes in GABA, glutamate and activity levels: The missing link in cortical plasticity. *Eur. J. Neurosci.* 12: 4222–4232.

Artola, A., and Singer, W. (1987). Long-term potentiation and NMDA receptors in rat visual cortex. *Nature* 330: 649–652.

Ashbridge, E., Perrett, D. I., Oram, M. W., and Jellema, T. (2000). Effect of image rotation or size change on object recognition: Responses of single units in the macaque monkey temporal cortex. *Cogn. Neuropsychol.* 17: 13–34.

Atick, J. J. (1992). Could information theory provide an ecological theory of sensory processing? *Network* 3: 213–251.

Atick, J. J., and Redlich, A. N. (1990). Towards a theory of early visual processing. *Neural Comput.* 2: 308–320.

Atick, J. J., and Redlich, A. N. (1993). Convergent algorithm for sensory receptive field development. *Neural Comput.* 5: 45–60.

Attneave, F., and Frost, R. (1969). The determination of perceived tridimensional orientation by minimum criteria. *Percept. Psychophys.* 6: 391–396.

Axelrod, S. (1959). *Effects of Early Blindness: Performance of Blind and Sighted Children on Tactile and Auditory Tasks.* New York: American Foundation for the Blind.

Baddeley, R. (1996). Searching for filters with "interesting" output distributions: An uninteresting direction to explore? *Network* 7: 409–21.

Baddeley, R. (1997). The correlational structure of natural images and the calibration of spatial representations. *Cogn. Sci.* 21(3): 351–372.

Badler, N., and Bajcsy, R. (1978). Three-dimensional representations for computer graphics and computer vision. *Comput. Graph.* 12: 153–160.

Bakin, J. S., and Weinberger, N. M. (1990). Classical conditioning induces CS-specific receptive field plasticity in the auditory cortex of the guinea pig. *Brain Res.* 536: 271–286.

Bakin, J. S., and Weinberger, N. M. (1996). Induction of a physiological memory in the cerebral cortex by stimulation of the nucleus basalis. *Proc. Natl. Acad. Sci. U S A* 93: 11219–11224.

Baldassi, S., and Burr, D. C. (2000). Feature-based integration of orientation signals in visual search. *Vision Res.* 40: 1293–1300.

Baldi, P., and Heiligenberg, W. (1988). How sensory maps could enhance resolution through ordered arrangements of broadly tuned receivers. *Biol. Cybern.* 59: 313–318.

Ball, K., and Sekuler, R. (1982). A specific and enduring improvement in visual motion discrimination. *Science* 218: 687–698.

Ball, K., and Sekuler, R. (1987). Direction-specific improvement in motion discrimination. *Vision Res.* 27: 953–965.

Baltes, P. B., and Lindenberger, U. (1997). Emergence of a powerful connection between sensory and cognitive functions across the adult life span: a new window to the study of cognitive aging? *Psychol. Aging* 12: 12–21.

Bar, M., and Biederman, I. (1999). Localizing the cortical region mediating visual awareness of object identity. *Proc. Natl. Acad. Sci. U S A* 96: 1790–1793.

Bara-Jimenez, W., Catalan, M. J., Hallett, M., and Gerloff, C. (1998). Abnormal somatosensory homunculus in dystonia of the hand. *Ann. Neurol.* 44: 828–83.

Barbas, H. (1992). Architecture and cortical connections of the prefrontal cortex in the rhesus monkey. In *Advances in Neurology*, vol. 57, ed. P. Chauvel et al., 91–115. New York: Raven Press.

Barlow, H. B. (1950). The receptive fields of ganglion cells in the frog retina. In *Proceedings of the Eighteenth International Physiological Congress*, 88–89. Copenhagen: Bianco Lunos Bogtrykkeri.

Barlow, H. B. (1972). Single units and sensation: A neuron doctrine for perceptual psychology? *Perception* 1: 371–394.

Barlow, H. B. (1985). The twelfth Bartlett Memorial Lecture: The role of single neurons in the psychology of perception. *Q. J. Exp. Psychol.* A37: 121–145.

Barlow, H. B. (1989). Unsupervised learning. *Neural Comput.* 1: 295–311.

Barlow, H. B. (1990a). A theory about the functional role and synaptic mechanisms of visual after-effects. In *Vision: Coding and Efficiency*, ed. C. Blakemore, 363–375. Cambridge: Cambridge University Press.

Barlow, H. B. (1990b). Conditions for versatile learning, Helmholtz's unconscious inference, and the task of perception. *Vision Res.* 30: 1561–1571.

Barlow, H. B. (1994). What is the computational goal of the neocortex? In C. Koch and J. L. Davis eds., *Large-Scale Neuronal Theories of the Brain*. Cambridge, MA: MIT Press.

Barlow, H. B. (1995). The neuron doctrine in perception. In M. Gazzaniga, ed., *The Cognitive Neurosciences*, 415–435. Cambridge, MA: MIT Press.

Barlow, H. B., and Tolhurst, D. J. (1992). Why do you have edge detectors? *Opt. Soc. Am. Tech. Digest* 23: 172.

Baron, R. J. (1981). Mechanisms of human facial recognition. *Int. J. Man-Mach. Stud.* 15: 137–178.

Barrow, H. G., and Tenenbaum, J. M. (1981). Interpreting line-drawings as three-dimensional surfaces. *Artif. Intell.* 17(1–3): 75–116.

Bartlett, J. C., and Searcy, J. (1993). Inversion and configuration of faces. *Cogn. Psychol.* 25: 281–316.

Barto, A. (1989). From chemotaxis to cooperativity: Abstract exercises in neuronal learning strategies. In R. Durbin, C. Miall, and G. Mitchison, eds., *The Computing Neuron*, 73–98. New York: Addison Wesley.

Baskerville, K. A., Schweitzer, J. B., and Herron, P. (1997). Effects of cholinergic depletion on experience-dependent plasticity in the cortex of the rat. *Neurosci.* 80: 1159–1169.

Baudry, M. (1998). Synaptic plasticity and learning and memory: Fifteen years of progress. *Neurobiol. Learn. Mem.* 70: 113–118.

Baylis, G. C., Rolls, E. T., and Leonard, C. M. (1985). Selectivity between faces in the responses of a population of neurons in the cortex in the superior temporal sulcus of the monkey. *Brain Res.* 342: 91–102.

Baylis, G. C., Rolls, E. T., and Leonard, C. M. (1987). Functional subdivisions of the temporal lobe neocortex. *J. Neurosci.* 7: 330–342.

Beale, J. M., and Keil, F. C. (1995). Categorical effects in the perception of faces. *Cognition* 57: 217–239.

Beard, B. L., Klein, S. A., Ahumada, Jr. A. J., and Slotnick, S. D. (1996). Training on a vernier acuity task does transfer to untrained retinal locations. *Invest. Ophthalmol. Vis. Sci.* 37: S696, 3180.

Beard, B. L., Levi, D. M., and Reich, L. N. (1995). Perceptual learning in parafoveal learning. *Vision Res.* 35: 1679–1690.

Beaulieu, C., Kisvarday, Z., Somogyi, P., Cynader, M., and Cowey, A. (1992). Quantitative distribution of GABA-immunopositive and -immunonegative neurons and synapses in the monkey striate cortex (area 17). *Cereb. Cortex* 2: 295–309.

Bedford, F. L. (1993). Perceptual and cognitive spatial learning. *J. Exp. Psychol. Hum. Percept. Perform.* 19: 517–530.

Bedford, F. L. (1995). Constraints on perceptual learning: Objects and dimensions. *Cognition* 54: 253–297.

Bedford, F. L. (1997). Are long-term changes to perception explained by Pavlovian associations or perceptual learning theory? *Cognition* 64: 223–230.

Bell, A. J. (1992). Self-organisation in real neurons: Anti-Hebb in "channel space"? In J. Moody et al., eds., *Advances in Neural Information Processing Systems*, vol. 4, pp. 59–66. San Francisco: Morgan-Kaufmann.

Bell, A. J., and Sejnowski, T. J. (1995a). An information maximization approach to blind separation and blind deconvolution. *Neural Comput.* 7: 1129–1159.

Bell, A. J., and Sejnowski, T. J. (1995b). Fast blind separation based on information theory. In *Proceedings of the International Symposium on Nonlinear Theory and Applications*, Las Vegas, December 1995.

Bell, A. J., and Sejnowski, T. J. (1996). Learning the higher-order structure of a natural sound. *Network* 7: 2.

Bell, A. J., and Sejnowski, T. J. (1997). The "independent component" of natural scenes are edge filters. *Vision Res.* 37: 3327–3338.

Bellman, R. E. (1961). *Adaptive Control Processes*. Princeton, NJ: Princeton University Press.

Benardete, E. A., and Kaplan, E. (1999). The dynamics of primate M retinal ganglion cells. *Vis. Neurosci.* 16: 355–368.

Bende, M., and Nordin, S. (1997). Perceptual learning in olfaction: Professional wine tasters versus controls. *Physiol. Behav.* 62: 1065–1070.

Benedetti, F. (1991). Perceptual learning following a long-lasting tactile reversal. *J. Exp. Psychol. Hum. Percept. Perform.* 17: 267–277.

Bennett, C. H., and Mackintosh, N. J. (1999). Comparison and contrast as a mechanism of perceptual learning? *Q. J. Exp. Psychol. B.* 52: 253–272.

Bennett, P. J., and Banks, M. S. (1987). Sensitivity loss in odd-symmetric mechanisms underlies phase anomalies in peripheral vision. *Nature* 326: 873–876.

Bennett, T. L., and Anton, B. S. (1972). Critical periods for early experience in transfer of perceptual learning. *Percept. Mot. Skills* 35: 743–746.

Bennett, T. L., Levitt, L., and Anton, B. S. (1972). Effect of exposure to a single stimulus on transfer of perceptual learning. *Percept. Mot. Skills* 34: 559–562.

Benson, P. J., and Perrett, D. I. (1991a). Synthesising continuous-tone caricatures. *Image Vis. Comput.* 9: 123–129.

Benson, P. J., and Perrett, D. I. (1991b). Perception and recognition of photographic quality facial caricatures: Implications for the recognition of natural images. *Eur. J. Cogn. Psychol.* 3: 105–135.

Berardi, N., and Fiorentini, A. (1987). Interhemispheric transfer of visual information in humans: Spatial characteristics. *J. Physiol. (Lond.)* 384: 633–647.

Berardi, N., and Fiorentini, A. (1991). Visual field asymmetry in pattern discrimination: A sign of asymmetry in cortical visual field representation? *Vision Res.* 31: 1831–1836.

Berardi, N., and Fiorentini, A. (1997). Interhemispheric transfer of spatial and temporal frequency information. In: *Cerebral Asymmetries in Sensory and Perceptual Processing*, ed. S. Christman. Amsterdam: Elsevier.

Berkeley, G. (1713). *Three Dialogues Between Hylas and Philonous*. London: Innys. Reproduced in A. C. Fraser, ed., *The Works of George Berkeley* (1901). Oxford: Oxford University Press.

Berkeley, G. (1732). *Alciphron: or, the Minute Philosopher*. London: J. Tonson. Reproduced in A. C. Fraser, ed., *The Works of George Berkeley* (1901). Oxford: Oxford University Press.

Berlucchi, G., and Rizzolatti, G. (1968). Binocularly driven neurons in visual cortex of split-chiasm cats. *Science* 159: 308–310.

Berman, N. E., and Payne, B. R. (1983). Alterations in connections of the corpus callosum following convergent and divergent strabismus. *Brain Res.* 274: 201–212.

Berns, G. S., Cohen, J. D., and Mintun, M. A. (1997). Brain regions responsive to novelty in the absence of awareness. *Science* 276: 1272–1276.

Berry, D. C. (1994). Implicit learning: Twenty-five years on a tutorial. In C. Umiltà and M. Moscovitch, eds., *Attention and Performance XV*, 755–781. Cambridge, MA: MIT Press.

Bertini, G., Karni, A., De Weerd, P., Desimone, R., and Ungerleider, L. (1995). A behavioral and electrophysiological study of monkey visual cortex plasticity. *Soc. Neurosc. Abstr.* 21: 276.

Bertini, G., Karni, A., De Weerd, P., Desimone, R., and Ungerleider, L. (1996). Electro-physiological study of monkey visual cortex plasticity: Comparison of V1 and V2. *Soc. Neurosci. Abstr.* 22: 1614.

Best, F. (1900). Ueber die Grenze der Erkennbarkeit von Lagenunterschieden. *Graefes Arch. Ophthal.* 51: 453–460.

Beymer, D., and Poggio, T. A. (1996). Image representations for visual learning. *Science* 272: 1905–1909.

Bialek, W., Ruderman, D. L., and Zee, A. (1991). Optimal sampling of natural images: A design principle for the visual system? In D. Touretzky, ed., *Advances in Neural Information Processing Systems*, vol. 1. San Francisco: Morgan-Kaufmann.

Biederman, I. (1987). Recognition-by-components: A theory of human image understanding. *Psychol. Rev.* 94: 115–147.

Biederman, I., and Gerhardstein, P. C. (1993). Recognizing depth-rotated objects: Evidence and conditions for three-dimensional viewpoint invariance. *J. Exp. Psychol. Hum. Percep. Perform.* 19: 1162–1182.

Biedermann, I., and Shiffrar, M. M. (1995). Sexing day-old chicks: A case study and expert systems analysis of a difficult perceptual-learning task. *J. Exp. Psychol. Learn. Mem. Cogn.* 13: 640–645.

Bienenstock, E. L., Cooper, L. N., and Munro, P. W. (1982). Theory for the development of neuron selectivity: Orientation specificity and binocular interaction in visual cortex. *J. Neurosci.* 2: 32–48.

Birbaumer, N., Lutzenberger, W., Monotya, P., Larbig, W., Unertl, K., Töpfner, S., Grodd, W., Taub, E., and Flor, H. (1997). Effects of regional anesthesia on phantom limb pain are mirrored in changes in cortical reorganization. *J. Neurosci.* 17(14): 5503–5508.

Bishop, C. (1995). *Neural Networks for Pattern Recognition.* Oxford: Oxford University Press.

Bjordahl, T. S., Dimyan, M. A., and Weinberger, N. M. (1998). Induction of long-term receptive field plasticity in the auditory cortex of the waking guinea pig by stimulation of the nucleus basalis. *Behav. Neurosci.* 112: 467–479.

Blakemore, C., and Campbell, F. W. (1969). On the existence of neurones in the human visual system selectively sensitive to the orientation and size of retinal images. *J. Physiol. (Lond.)* 203: 237–260.

Blakemore, C., and Cooper, G. F. (1970). Development of the brain depends on the visual environment. *Nature* 228: 477–478.

Blakemore, C., Diao, Y., Pu, M., Wang, Y., and Xiao, Y. (1983). Possible functions of interhemispheric connections between visual cortical areas in the cat. *J. Physiol. (Lond.)* 337: 331–348.

Blakemore, C. B., and Nachmias, J. (1971). The orientational specificity of two visual after-effects. *J. Physiol. (Lond.)* 213: 157–174.

Blakemore, C. B., Nachmias, J., and Sutton, P. (1970). The perceived spatial frequency shift: Evidence for frequency-selective neurons in the human brain. *J. Physiol. (Lond.)* 210: 727–750.

Blakemore, C. B., and Sutton, P. (1969). Size adaptation: A new after-effect. *Science* 166: 245–247.

Blakemore, C., and Tobin, E. A. (1972). Lateral inhibition between orientation detectors in the cat's visual cortex. *Exp. Brain Res.* 15: 439–440.

Blamey, P., Arndt, P., Bergeron, S., Bredberg, G., Brimacombe, J., Facer, G., Larky, J., Lindström, B., Nedzelski, J., Peterson, A., Shipp, D., Staller, S., and Whitford, L. (1996). Factors affecting auditory performance of postlinguistically deaf adults using cochlear implants. *Audiol. Neuro-otol.* 1: 293–306.

Blamey, P. J., Pyman, B. C., Gordon, M., Clark, G. M., Brown, A. M., Dowell, R. C., and Hollow, R. D. (1992). Factors predicting postoperative sentence scores in postlinguistically deaf adult cochlear implant patients. *Ann. Otol. Rhinol. Laryngol.* 101: 342–348.

Blasdel, G. G., and Salama, G. (1986). Voltage-sensitive dyes reveal a modular organization in monkey striate cortex. *Nature* 321: 579–585.

Bolz, J., and Gilbert, C. D. (1990). The role of horizontal connections in generating long receptive fields in the cat visual cortex. *Eur. J. Neurosci.* 1: 263–268.

Bonneh, Y., and Sagi, D. (1998). Effects of spatial configuration on contrast detection. *Vision Res.* 38: 3541–3553.

Bonneh, Y., and Sagi, D. (1999). Configuration saliency revealed in short duration binocular rivalry. *Vision Res.* 39: 271–281.

Booth, M. C. A., and Rolls, E. T. (1998). View-invariant representations of familiar objects by neurons in the inferior temporal visual cortex. *Cereb. Cortex* 8: 510–523.

Boring, E. G. (1930). A new ambiguous figure. *Am. J. Psychol.* 42: 444–445.

Bornstein, M. H., and Korda, N. O. (1984). Discrimination and matching within and between hues measured by reaction times: Some implications for categorical perception and levels of information processing. *Psychol. Res.* 46: 207–222.

Bosking, W. H., Zhang, Y., Schofield, B., and Fitzpatrick, D. (1997). Orientation selectivity and the arrangement of horizontal connections in tree shrew striate cortex. *J. Neurosci.* 17: 2112–2127.

Boutet, I., Intriligator, J., and Rivest, J. (1995). The influence of attention on visual learning. *Invest. Ophthalmol. Vis. Sci.* 35: 1769.

Boyd, J., and Matsubara, J. (1991). Intrinsic connections in cat visual cortex: A combined anterograde and retrograde tracing study. *Brain Res.* 560: 207–215.

Braastad, B. O., and Heggelund, P. (1985). Development of spatial receptive-field organization and orientation selectivity in kitten striate cortex. *J. Neurophysiol.* 53: 1158–1178.

Braddick, O., Campbell, F. W., and Atkinson, J. (1978). Channels in vision. In *Handbook of Sensory Physiology.* Vol. 8, *Perception,* ed. R. Held, H. W. Leibowitz, and H. L. Teuber, 1–38 Berlin: Springer.

Bradley, A., Switkes, E., and De Valois, K. (1988). Orientation and spatial frequency selectivity of adaptation to colour and luminance gratings. *Vision Res.* 28: 841–859.

Bradlow, A. R, Pisoni, D. B, Akahane-Yamada, R., and Tohkura, Y. (1997). Training Japanese listeners to identify English /r/ and /l/: IV. Some effects of perceptual learning on speech production. *J. Acoust. Soc. Am.* 101: 2299–2310.

Bradshaw, M., and Rogers, B. (1996). The interaction of binocular disparity and motion parallax in the computation of depth. *Vision Res.* 36(21): 3457–3468.

Brady, M., and Yuille, A. (1983). An extremum principle for shape from contour. AI Memo 711. MIT AI Laboratory.

Brady, M., and Yuille, A. (1984). An extremum principle for shape from contour. *IEEE Trans. Patt. Anal. Mach. Intell.* 6: 288–301.

Braitenberg, V. (1986). Two views of the cerebral cortex. In: G. Palm, and A. Aertsen eds., *Brain Theory,* 81–96. Berlin: Springer.

Brasil-Neto, J. P., Cohen, L. G., Pascual-Leone, A., Jabir, F. K., Wall, R. T., and Hallett, M. (1992). Rapid reversible modulation of human motor outputs after transient deafferentation of the forearm. *Neurology* 42: 1302–1306.

Brasil-Neto, J. P., Valls-Solé, J., Pascual-Leone, A., Cammarota, A., Amassian, V. E., Cracco, R., Maccabee, P., Cracco, J., Hallett, M., and Cohen, L. G. (1993). Rapid modulation of human cortical motor outputs following ischemic nerve block. *Brain* 116: 511–525.

Braun, C., Schweizer, R., Elbert, T., Birbaumer, N., and Taub, E. (1999). Differential reorganization in somatosensory cortex for different discrimination tasks. *J. Neurosci.* 20: 446–450.

Braun, J., and Sagi, D. (1991). Texture-based tasks are little affected by second tasks requiring peripheral or central attentive fixation. *Perception* 20: 483–500.

Bregler, C., and Omohundro, S. M. (1995). Nonlinear image interpolation using manifold learning. In D. S. T. Tesauro and T. K. Leen, eds., *Advances in Neural Information Processing,* vol. 7, pp. 973–980. Cambridge, MA: MIT Press.

Brennan, S. E. (1985). The caricature generator. *Leonardo* 18: 170–178.

Brigham, J. C. (1986). The influence of race on face recognition. In H. D. Ellis, M. A. Jeeves, F. Newcombe, and A. Young, eds., *Aspects of Face Processing*. Dordrecht: Nijhoff.

Broadbent, D. E. (1956). Successive responses to simultaneous stimuli. *Q. J. Exp. Psychol.* 8: 145–152.

Brodlie, J. F., and Burke, J. (1971). Perceptual learning disabilities in blind children. *Percept. Mot. Skills* 32: 313–314.

Brodmann, K. (1909). *Vergleichende Lokalisationslehre der Großhirnrinde in ihren Prinzipien dargestellt auf Grund des Zellenbaues*. Leipzig: Barth.

Brooks, R. (1981). Symbolic reasoning among 3-D and 2-D images. *Artif. Intell.* 17: 205–244.

Brosvic, G. M, Rowe-Boyer, M. M., and Dihoff, R. E. (1991). Acquisition and retention of perceptual learning and the horizontal-vertical illusion. *Percept. Mot. Skills* 72: 587–592.

Brown, T. H., Kairiss, E. W., and Keenan, C. L. (1990). Hebbian synapses: Biophysical mechanisms and algorithms. *Annu. Rev. Neurosci.* 13: 475–511.

Bruce, C., Desimone, R., and Gross, C. G. (1981). Visual properties of neurons in a polysensory area in superior temporal sulcus of the macaque. *J. Neurophysiol.* 46: 369–384.

Bruce, V. (1982). Changing faces: Visual and non-visual coding processes in face recognition. *Br. J. Psychol.* 73: 105–116.

Bruce, V. (1994). Stability from variation: The M. D. Vernon memorial lecture. *Q. J. Exp. Psychol.* 47A: 5–28.

Bruce, V. (1998). Fleeting images of shade: Identifying people caught on video. *Psychologist* 11: 331–337.

Bruce, V., Burton, A. M., Carson, D., Hanna, E., and Mason, O. (1994). Repetition priming of face recognition. In Carlo Umiltà and Morris Moskovitch, eds., *Attention and Performance XV*. Cambridge, MA: MIT Press.

Bruce, V., Campbell, R. N., Doherty-Sneddon, G., Import, A., Langton, S., McAuley, S., and Wright, R. (2000). Testing face processing skills in children. *Br. J. Dev. Psychol.* 18: 319–333.

Bruce, V., Carson, D., Burton, A. M., and Ellis, A. W. (2000). Perceptual priming is not a necessary consequence of semantic classification of pictures. *Q. J. Exp. Psychol. A.* 53: 289–323.

Bruce, V., Carson, D., Burton, A. M., and Kelly, S. (1998). Prime-time advertisements: Repetition priming of faces seen on recruitment posters *Mem. Cognit.* 26: 502–515.

Bruce, V., Doyle, T., Dench, N., and Burton, A. M. (1991). Remembering facial configurations. *Cognition* 38: 109–144.

Bruce, V., Hanna, E., Dench, N., Healey, P., and Burton, M. (1992). The importance of "mass" in line-drawings of faces. *Appl. Cogn. Psychol.* 6: 619–628.

Bruce, V., Healey, P., Burton, A. M., Doyle, T., Coombes, A., and Linney, A. (1991). Recognising facial surfaces. *Perception* 20: 755–769.

Bruce, V., Henderson, Z., Greenwood, K., Hancock, P. J. B., Burton, A. M., and Miller, P. (1999). Verification of face identities from images captured on video. *J. Exp. Psychol. A.*

Bruce, V., Henderson, Z., Newman, C., and Burton, A. M. (2001). Matching identities of familiar and unfamiliar faces caught on CCTV images. *J. Exp. Psychol. A.* 7: 207–218.

Bruce, V., and Humphreys, G. W. (1994). Recognising objects and faces. *Vis. Cognit.* 1: 141–180.

Bruce, V., and Langton, S. (1994). The use of pigmentation and shading information in recognising the sex and identities of faces. *Perception* 23: 803–822.

Bruce, V., Terry, D., and Smith, K. (1998). Visual and non-visual factors affecting repetition priming of faces. Paper presented at the Tenth Congress of the European Society for Cognitive Psychology, Jerusalem, September.

Bruce, V., and Young, A. W. (1986). Understanding face recognition. *Br. J. Psychol.* 77: 305–327.

Bruner, J. S. (1951). Personality dynamics and the process of perceiving. In R. R. Blake and G. V. Ramsey, eds., *Perception: An Approach to Personality*. New York: Ronald Press.

Bruner, J. S. (1957). On perceptual readiness. *Psychol. Rev.* 64: 123–152.

Bruner, J. S., and Goodman, C. C. (1947). Value and need as organizing factors in perception. *J. Abnorm. Soc. Psychol.* 42: 33–44.

Bruner, J. S., and Postman, L. (1947). Emotional selectivity in perception and reaction. *J. Pers.* 16: 69–77.

Büchel, C., Price, C., Frackowiak, R. S. J., and Friston, K. (1998). Different activation patterns in the visual cortex of late and congenitally blind subjects. *Brain* 121: 404–419.

Buchner, H., Reinartz, U., Waberski, T. D., Gobbele, R., Noppeney, U., and Scherg, M. (1999). Sustained attention modulates the immediate effect of de-afferentiation on the cortical representation of the digits: Source localization of somatosensory evoked potentials in humans. *Neurosci. Lett.* 260: 57–60.

Buhmann, J., Lades, M., and von der Malsburg, C. (1990). Size- and distortion-invariant object recognition by hierarchical graph matching. In *International Joint Conference on Neural Networks*, 411–416. New York: IEEE Press.

Bülthoff, H. H., and Edelman, S. (1992). Psychophysical support for a two-dimensional view interpolation theory of object recognition. *Proc. Natl. Acad. Sci. U S A* 89: 60–64.

Bülthoff, H., and Yuille, A. (1996). A Bayesian framework for the integration of visual modules. In J. McClelland and T. Inui, eds., *Attention and Performance XVI: Information Integration in Perception and Communication*, 49–70. Cambridge, MA: MIT Press.

Bülthoff, I., Bülthoff, H. H., and Sinha, P. (1998). Top-down influences on stereoscopic depth-perception. *Nat. Neurosci.* 1: 254–257.

Bülthoff, I., Sinha, P., and Bülthoff, H. H. (1996). Top-down influence of recognition on stereoscopic depth perception. *Invest. Ophthalmol. Vis. Sci.* 37: 5168.

Buonomano, D. V. (1999). Distinct functional types of associative long-term potentiation in neocortical and hippocampal pyramidal neurons. *J. Neurosci.* 19: 6748–6754.

Buonomano, D. V., and Merzenich, M. M. (1996). Associative synaptic plasticity in hippocampal CA1 neurons is not sensitive to unpaired presynaptic activity. *J. Neurophysiol.* 76: 631–636.

Buonomano, D. V., and Merzenich, M. M. (1998a). Cortical plasticity: From synapses to maps. *Annu. Rev. Neurosci.* 21: 149–186.

Buonomano, D. V., and Merzenich, M. M. (1998b). Net interaction between different forms of short-term synaptic plasticity and slow IPSPs in the hippocampus and auditory cortex. *J. Neurophysiol.* 80: 1765–1774.

Burkhalter, A., Bernardo, K. L., and Charles, V. (1993). Development of local circuits in human visual cortex. *J. Neurosci.* 13: 1916–1931.

Burr, D. C. (1980). Sensitivity to spatial phase. *Vision Res.* 20: 391–396.

Burr, D. C., Morrone, M. C., and Spinelli, D. (1989). Evidence for edge and bar detectors in human vision. *Vision Res.* 29: 419–431.

Burr, D. C., and Wijesundra, S. (1991). Orientation discrimination depends on spatial frequency. *Vision Res.* 31: 1449–1452.

Burton, A. M. (1994). Learning new faces in an interactive activation and competition model. *Vis. Cognit.* 1: 313–348.

Burton, A. M. (1998). A model of human face recognition. In J. Grainger and A. M. Jacobs, eds., *Localist Connectionist Approaches to Human Cognition*, 75–100. Mahwah, NJ: Erlbaum.

Burton, A. M., Bruce, V., and Hancock, P. J. B. (1999). From pixels to people: A model of familiar face recognition. *Cogn. Sci.* 23: 1–31.

Burton, A. M., Bruce, V., and Johnston, R. A. (1990). Understanding face recognition with an interactive activation model. *Br. J. Psychol.* 81: 361–380.

Burton, A. M., Wilson, S., Cowan, M., and Bruce, V. (1999). Face recognition in poor-quality video: Evidence from security surveillance *Psychol. Sci.* 10: 243–248.

Busby, P. A., and Clark, G. M. (2000). Electrode discrimination by early deafened subjects using the Cochlear Limited multiple-electrode cochlear implant. *Ear Hear.* 21: 291–304.

Busby, P. A., and Clark, G. M. (2000). Pitch estimation by early-deafened subjects using a multiple-electrode cochlear implant. *J. Acoust. Soc. Am.* 107: 547–558.

Bushnell, I. W. R., Sai, F., and Mullin, J. T. (1989). Neonatal recognition of the mother's face. *Br. J. Dev. Psychol.* 7: 3–15.

Byl, N. N., Merzenich, M. M., Cheung, S., Bedenbaugh, P., Nagarajan, S. S., and Jenkins, W. M. (1997). A primate model for studying focal dystonia and repetitive strain injury: Effects on the primary somatosensory cortex. *Phys. Ther.* 77: 269–284.

Byl, N. N., Merzenich, M. M., and Jenkins, W. M. (1996). A primate genesis model of focal dystonia and repetitive strain injury: 1. Learning-induced dedifferentiation of the representation of the hand in the primary somatosensory cortex in adult monkeys. *Neurology* 47: 508–520.

Cabeza, R., Bruce, V., Kato, T., and Oda, M. (1999). The prototype effect in face recognition: Extension and limits. *Mem. Cognit.* 27: 139–151.

Caelli, T. (1997). Perceptual learning and adaptation in man and machine: Part II. *Spatial Vision* 10: 505–508.

Cahusac, P. M. (1995). Synaptic plasticity induced in single neurones of the primary somatosensory cortex in vivo. *Exp. Brain Res.* 107: 241–253.

Calford, M. B., and Tweedale, R. (1988). Immediate chronic changes in responses of somatosensory cortex in adult flying-fox after digit amputation. *Nature* 332: 446–448.

Calford, M. B., and Tweedale, R. (1990). Interhemispheric transfer of plasticity in the cerebral cortex. *Science* 249: 805–807.

Calford, M. B., and Tweedale, R. (1991). Immediate expansion of receptive fields of neurons in area 3b of macaque monkeys after digit denervation. *Somatosens. Mot. Res.* 8(3): 249–260.

Callaway, E. M., and Katz, L. C. (1990). Emergence and refinement of clustered horizontal connections in cat striate cortex. *J. Neurosci.* 10: 1134–1153.

Campbell, F. W., and Gubisch, R. W. (1966). Optical quality of the human eye. *J. Physiol.* 186: 558–578.

Campbell, F. W., and Kulikowski, J. J. (1966). Orientation selectivity of the human visual system. *J. Physiol.* 187: 437–445.

Campbell, F. W., and Maffei, L. (1971). The tilt aftereffect: A fresh look. *Vision Res.* 11: 833–840.

Campbell, F. W., Nachmias, J., and Hukes, J. (1970). Spatial frequency discrimination in human vision. *J. Opt. Soc. Am.* 60: 555–559.

Candia, V., Elbert, T., Altenmüller, E., Rau, H., Schäfer, T., and Taub, E. (1998). A constraint-induced movement therapy for focal hand dystonia in musicians. *Lancet* 353: 52.

Canny, J. F. (1986). A computational approach to edge-detection. *IEEE Trans. Patt. Anal. Mach. Vis.* 8: 679–698.

Carandini, M., and Ferster, D. (1997). A tonic hyper-polarisation underlying contrast adaptation in cat visual cortex. *Science* 276: 949–952.

Carandini, M., Heeger, D. J., and Movshon, J. A. (1997). Linearity and normalization in simple cells of the macaque primary visual cortex. *J. Neurosci.* 17: 8621–8644.

Carbonell, J. G., Michalski, R. S., and Mitchell, T. M. (1983). An overview of machine learning. In R. S. Michalski, J. G. Carbonell, and T. M. Mitchell, eds., *Machine Learning: An Artificial Intelligence Approach*, 3–23. Palo Alto, CA: Tioga.

Cardoso, J.-F., and Laheld, B. (1996). Equivariant adaptive source separation. *IEEE Trans. Signal Proc.* 45: 434–444.

Carew, T. J., Hawkins, R. D., Abrams, T. W., and Kandel, E. R. (1984). A test of Hebb's postulate at identified synapses which mediate classical conditioning in Aplysia. *J. Neurosci.* 4: 1217–1224.

Carey, S., and Diamond, R. (1994). Are faces perceived as configurations more by adults than by children? *Vis. Cognit.* 1: 253–274.

Carpenter, G. A., and Grossberg, S. (1987). A massively parallel architecture for a self-organizing neural pattern recognition machine. *Comput. Vis. Graph. Image Proc.* 37: 54–115.

Carpenter, G. A., and Grossberg, S. (1990). Adaptive resonance theory: Neural network architectures for self-organizing pattern recognition. In R. Eckmiller, G. Hartmann, and G. Hauske, eds., *Parallel Processing in Neural Systems and Computers*, 383–389. Amsterdam: North-Holland.

Carpenter, G. A., Grossberg, S., Markuzon, N., Reynolds, J. H., and Rosen, D. B. (1992). Fuzzy ARTMAP: A neural network architecture for incremental supervised learning of analog multidimensional maps. *IEEE Trans. Neural Networks*, 3: 698–713.

Cavanagh, P. (1991). In *Representations of Vision: Trends and Tacit Assumptions in Vision Research*, ed. A. Gorea. Cambridge: Cambridge University Press.

Changeux, J.-P., and Danchin, A. (1976). Selective stabilisation of developing synapses as a mechanism for the specification of neuronal networks. *Nature* 264: 705–712.

Chen, R., Corwell, B., Yaseen, Z., Hallett, M., and Cohen, L. G. (1998). Mechanisms of cortical reorganization in lower-limb amputees. *J. Neurosci.* 18(9): 3443–3450.

Cheng, K., Saleem, K. S., and Tanaka, K. (1997). Organization of corticostriatal and corticoamygdalar projections arising from the anterior inferotemporal area TE of the macaque monkey: A *Phaseolus vulgaris* leucoagglutinin study. *J. Neurosci.* 15: 7902–7925.

Chino, Y. M. (1995). Adult plasticity in the visual system. *Can. J. Physiol. Pharmacol.* 73: 1323–1338.

Chino, Y. M. (1997). Receptive-field plasticity in the adult visual cortex: Dynamic signal rerouting or experience-dependent plasticity. *Semin. Neurosci.* 9: 34–46.

Chino, Y. M., Kaas, J. H., Smith III, E. L., Langston, A. L., and Cheng, H. (1992). Rapid reorganization of cortical maps in adult cats following restricted deafferentation in retina. *Vision Res.* 32: 789–796.

Chiroro, P., and Valentine, T. (1995). An investigation of the contact hypothesis of the own-race bias in face recognition. *Q. J. Exp. Psychol.* 48A: 879–894

Choi, D. W., and Rothman, S. M. (1990). The role of glutamate neurotoxicity in hypoxic-ischemic neuronal death. *Annu. Rev. Neurosci.* 13: 171–182.

Cholewiak, R. W. (1976). Satiation in cutaneous saltation. *Sens. Processes* 1: 163–175.

Christie, F., and Bruce, V. (1998). The role of movement in the recognition of unfamiliar faces. *Mem. Cognit.* 26: 780–790.

Chung, M. S., and Thomson, D. M. (1995). Development of face recognition. *Br. J. Psychol.* 86: 55–87.

Churchill, J. P., Muja, N., Myers, W., Besheer, W. A., and Garraghty, P. E. (1998). Somatotopic consolidation: A third phase of cortical reorganization after peripheral nerve injury in adult squirrel monkeys. *Exp. Brain Res.* 118: 189–194.

Churchland, P. S., and Sejnowski, T. J. (1988). Perspectives on cognitive neuroscience. *Science* 242: 741–745.

Churs, L., Spengler, F., Jürgens, M., and Dinse, H. R. (1996). Environmental enrichment counteracts decline of sensorimotor performance and deterioration of cortical organization in aged rats. *Soc. Neurosci. Abstr.* 22: 102.

Cichocki, A., Unbehauen, R., and Rummert, E. (1994). Robust learning algorithm for blind separation of signals. *Electron. Lett.* 30: 1386–1387.

Clark, A. (1993). *Sensory Qualities*. Oxford: Clarendon Press.

Clark, G. M. (1986). The University of Melbourne/ Cochlear Corporation (Nucleus) program. *Otolaryngol. Clin. North Am.* 19: 329–354.

Clark, G. M. (1996). Electrical stimulation of the auditory nerve: The coding of frequency, the perception of pitch, and the development of cochlear implant speech processing strategies for profoundly deaf people. *J. Clin. Physiol. Pharm. Res.* 23: 766–776.

Clark, G. M. (1997). Auditory nervous system plasticity: Application to cochlear implantation. In *Abstract Book for Sixteenth World Congress of Otorhinolaryngology Head and Neck Surgery, Sydney, March 2–7, 1997*, vol. 20, pp. 19–23.

Clark, S. A., Allard, T., Jenkins, W. M., and Merzenich, M. M. (1988). Receptive fields in the body-surface map in adult cortex defined by temporally correlated inputs. *Nature* 332: 444–445.

Clothiaux, E. E., Bear, M. F., and Cooper, L. N. (1991). Synaptic plasticity in visual cortex: Comparison of theory with experiment. *J. Neurophysiol.* 66: 1785–1804.

Clowes, M. B. (1971). On seeing things. *Artif. Intell.* 2(1): 79–116.

Cohen, L. G., Bandinelli, S., Findley, T. W., and Hallet, M. (1991a). Motor Reorganization after upper limb amputation in man: A study with focal magnetic stimulation. *Brain* 114: 615–627.

Cohen, L. G., Bandinelli, S., Sato, S., Kufta, C., and Hallett, M. (1991). Attenuation in detection of somatosensory stimuli by transcranial magnetic stimulation. *Electroenc. Clin. Neurophysiol.* 81: 366–376.

Cohen, L. G., Celnik, P., Pascual-Leone, A., Corwell, B., Falz, L., Dambrosia, J., Honda, M., Sadato, N., Gerloff, C., Catala, M. D., and Hallett, M. (1997). Functional relevance of cross-modal plasticity in blind humans. *Nature* 389: 180–183.

Cohen, L. G., Weeks, R. A., Sadato, N., Celnik, P., Ishii, K., and Hallett, M. (1999). Period of susceptibility for cross-modal plasticity in the blind. *Ann. Neurol.* 45: 451–460.

Comon, P. (1994). Independent component analysis, a new concept? *Signal Proc.* 36: 287–314.

Constantine-Paton, M., Cline, H. T., and Debski, E. (1990). Patterned activity, synaptic convergence, and the NMDA receptor in developing visual pathways. *Annu. Rev. Neurosci.* 13: 129–154.

Coq, J. O., and Xerri, C. (1998). Environmental enrichment alters organizational features of the forepaw representation in the primary somatosensory cortex of adult rats. *Exp. Brain Res.* 121: 191–204.

Cottrell, G. W., Munro, P., and Zipser, D. (1987). Learning internal representations from gray-scale images: An example of extensional programming. In *Proceedings of Ninth Annual Conference of the Cognitive Science Society*, 462–473. Hillsdale, NJ: Erlbaum.

Cover, T. M., and Thomas, J. A. (1991). *Elements of Information Theory*. New York: John Wiley.

Cowan, N., and Wood, N. L. (1997). Constraints on awareness, attention, processing, and memory: some recent investigations with ignored speech. *Conscious. Cognit.* 6: 182–203.

Cowan, R. S. C., Brown, C., Whitford, L. A., et al. (1995). Speech perception in children using the advanced Speak speech-processing system. In G. M. Clark and R. S. C. Cowan, eds., *International Cochlear Implant, Speech and Hearing Symposium, Melbourne, 1994*. St. Louis: Annals. *Ann. Otol. Rhinol. Laryngol.* 104, suppl. 166: 318–321.

Cowey, A. (1992). The role of the face-cell area in the discrimination and recognition of faces by monkeys. *Philos. Trans. R. Soc. London B Biol. Sci.* 335: 31–38.

Creutzfeldt, O. D., Garey, L. J., Kuroda, R., and Wolff, J.-R. (1977). The distribution of degenerating axons after small lesions in the intact and isolated visual cortex of the cat. *Exp. Brain Res.* 27: 419–440.

Crick, F., and Koch, C. (1998). Consciousness and neuroscience. *Cereb. Cortex* 8: 97–107.

Crist, R. E., Kapadia, M. K., Westheimer, G., and Gilbert, C. D. (1997). Perceptual learning of spatial localization: Specificity for orientation, position, and context. *J. Neurophysiol.* 78: 2889–2894.

Crist, R. E., Li, W., and Gilbert, C. D. (2001). Learning to see: Experience and attention in primary visual cortex. *Nat. Neurosci.* 4: 519–525.

Crook, J. M., and Eysel, U. T. (1992). GABA-induced inactivation of functionally characterized sites in cat visual cortex (area 18): Effects on orientation tuning. *J. Neurosci.* 12: 1816–1825.

Crook, J. M., Eysel, U. T., and Machemer, H. F. (1991). Influence of GABA-induced remote inactivation on the orientation tuning of cells in area 18 of feline visual cortex: A comparison with area 17. *Neuroscience* 40: 1–12.

Crook, J. M., Kisvárday, Z. F., and Eysel, U. T. (1996). GABA-induced inactivation of functionally characterized sites in cat visual cortex (area 18): Local determinants of direction selectivity. *J. Neurophysiol.* 75: 2071–2088.

Crook, J. M., Kisvárday, Z. F., and Eysel, U. T. (1997). GABA-induced inactivation of functionally characterized sites in cat striate cortex: Effects on orientation tuning and direction selectivity. *Vis. Neurosci.* 14: 141–158.

Crook, J. M., Kisvárday, Z. F., and Eysel, U. T. (1998). Evidence for a contribution of lateral inhibition to orientation tuning and direction selectivity in cat visual cortex: Reversible inactivation of functionally characterized sites combined with neuroanatomical tracing techniques. *Eur. J. Neurosci.* 10: 2056–2075.

Cross, K. D. (1967). Role of practice in perceptual-motor learning. *Am. J. Phys. Med.* 46: 487–510.

Crovitz, H. F., Harvey, M. T., and McClanahan, S. (1981). Hidden memory: A rapid method for the study of amnesia using perceptual learning. *Cortex* 17: 273–278.

Crowley, J. C., Bosking, W. H., Foster, M., and Fitzpatrick, D. (1996). Development of horizontal connections in layer 2/3 of tree shrew striate cortex: Relation to maps of orientation preference. *Soc. Neurosci. Abstr.* 22: 404.10.

Cruikshank, S. J., and Weinberger, N. M. (1996a). Evidence for the Hebbian hypothesis in experience-dependent physiological plasticity of neocortex: A critical review. *Brain Res. Rev.* 22: 191–228.

Cruikshank, S. J., and Weinberger, N. M. (1996b). Receptive-field plasticity in the adult auditory cortex induced by Hebbian covariance. *J. Neurosci.* 16: 861–875.

Cusick, C. G., Wall, J. T., Jr., Whiting, J. H., and Wiley, R. G. (1990). Temporal progression of cortical reorganization following nerve injury. *Brain Res.* 537: 355–358.

Cutting, J. (1986). *Perception with an Eye for Motion*. Cambridge, MA: MIT Press.

Cynader, M., Lepore, F., and Guillemot, J. P. (1981). Interhemispheric competition during postnatal development. *Nature* 290: 139–140.

D'Amelio, F., Fox, R. A., Wu, L. C., and Daunton, N. G. (1996). Quantitative changes of GABA-immunoreactive cells in the hindlimb representation of the rat somatosensory cortex after 14-day hindlimb unloading by tail suspension. *J. Neurosci. Res.* 44: 532–539.

Daniel, W. F, Crovitz, H. F., and Weiner, R. D. (1984). Perceptual learning with right unilateral versus bilateral electroconvulsive therapy. *Br. J. Psychiatry* 145: 394–400.

Darian-Smith, C., and Gilbert, C. D. (1994). Axonal sprouting accompanies functional reorganization in adult cat striate cortex. *Nature* 368: 737–740.

Darian-Smith, C., and Gilbert, C. D. (1995). Topographic reorganization in the striate cortex of the adult cat and monkey is cortically mediated. *J. Neurosci.* 15: 1631–1647.

Das, A., and Gilbert, C. D. (1995a). Long-range horizontal connections and their role in cortical reorganization revealed by optical recording of cat primary visual cortex. *Nature* 375: 780–784.

Das, A., and Gilbert, C. D. (1995b). Receptive field expansion in adult visual cortex is linked to dynamic changes in strength of cortical connections. *J. Neurophysiol.* 74: 779–792.

Das, A., and Gilbert, C. D. (1999). Topography of contextual modulations mediated by short-range interactions in primary visual cortex. *Nature* 399: 655–661.

Daugman, J. G. (1985). Uncertainty relation for resolution in space, spatial frequency, and orientation optimized by two-dimensional visual cortical filters. *J. Opt. Soc. Am. A* 2(7): 1160–1169.

Daum, I., and Ackermann, H. (1997). [Nondeclarative memory—neuropsychological findings and neuroanatomic principles]. *Fortschr. Neurol. Psychiatr.* 65: 122–132.

Davies, G., Ellis, H., and Shepherd, J. (1978). Face recognition accuracy as a function of mode of representation. *J. Appl. Psychol.* 63: 180–187.

Dawson, P. W., and Clark, G. M. (1997). Changes in synthetic and natural vowel perception after specific training for congenitally deafened patients using a multichannel cochlear implant. *Ear Hear.* 18: 488–501.

Dayan, P., Hinton, G. E., Neal, R. M., and Zemel, R. S. (1995). The Helmholtz machine. *Neural Comput.* 7: 889–904.

de Condillac, E. B. (1754). Treatise on the sensations. In *Philosophical Writings of Etienne Bonnot, abbé de Condillac*. 1982. Hillsdale, NJ: Erlbaum.

De Luca, E., and Fahle, M. (1999). Learning of interpolation in 2 and 3 dimensions. *Vision Res.* 39: 2051–2062.

De Renzi, E. (1997). Prosopagnosia. In T. Feinberg and M. Farah, eds., *Behavioral Neurology and Neuropsychology*, 245–255. New York: McGraw-Hill.

De Valois, R. L., Yund, E. W., and Hepler, N. (1982). The orientation and direction selectivity of cells in macaque visual cortex. *Vision Res.* 22: 531–544.

Dean, P. (1976). Effects of inferotemporal lesions on the behavior of monkeys. *Psychol. Bull.* 83: 41–71.

DeAngelis, G. C., Anzai, A., Ohzawa, I., and Freeman, R. D. (1995). Receptive field structure in the visual cortex: Does selective stimulation induce plasticity? *Proc. Natl. Acad. Sci. U S A* 92: 9682–9686.

Demany, L. (1985). Perceptual learning in frequency discrimination. *J. Acoust. Soc. Am.* 78: 1118–1120.

Desimone, R. (1991). Face-selective cells in the temporal cortex of monkeys. *J. Cogn. Neurosci.* 3: 1–8.

Desimone, R. (1992). The physiology of memory: Recordings of things past. *Science* 258: 245–246.

Desimone, R., Albright, T. D., Gross, C. G., and Bruce, C. (1984). Stimulus-selective properties of inferior temporal neurons in the macaque. *J. Neurosci.* 4: 2051–2062.

Desimone, R., Fleming, J., and Gross, C. D. (1980). Prestriate afferents to inferior temporal cortex: An HRP study. *Brain Res.* 184: 41–55.

Desimone, R., and Ungerleider, L. G. (1989). Neural mechanisms of visual processing in monkey. In *Handbook of Neuropsychology*, ed. F. Boller and J. Grafman, vol. 2, pp. 267–299. Amsterdam: Elsevier.

Deutsch, D. (1987). *The Fabric of Reality*. New York: Viking Penguin.

Deutsch, J. A., and Deutsch, D. (1963). Attention: Some theoretical considerations. *Psychol. Rev.* 70: 80–90.

Diamond, M. E., Armstrong-James, M., and Ebner, F. F. (1993). Experience-dependent plasticity in adult rat barrel cortex. *Proc. Natl. Acad. Sci. U S A* 90: 2082–2086.

Diamond, R., and Carey, S. (1986). Why faces are and are not special: An effect of expertise. *J. Exp. Psychol. Gen.* 115: 107–117.

Dill, M., and Fahle, M. (1997). The role of visual field position in pattern-discrimination learning. *Proc. R. Soc. Lond. B Biol. Sci.* 264: 1031–1036.

Dill, M., and Fahle, M. (1999). Display symmetry affects positional specificity in same-different judgement of pairs of novel visual patterns. *Vision Res.* 39: 3752–3760.

Dill, M., and Heisenberg, M. (1995). Visual pattern memory without shape recognition. *Philos. Trans. R. Soc. Lond. B Biol. Sci.* 349: 143–152.

Dinse, H. R. (1994). A time-based approach towards cortical functions: Neural mechanisms underlying dynamic aspects of information processing before and after postontogenetic plastic processes. *Physica* D75: 129–150.

Dinse, H. R., Godde, B., Hilger, T., Haupt, S. S., Spengler, F., and Zepka, R. (1997). Short-term functional plasticity of cortical and thalamic sensory representations and its implication for information processing. *Adv. Neurol.* 73: 159–178.

Dinse, H. R., Recanzone, G., and Merzenich, M. M. (1990). Direct observation of neural assemblies during neocortical representational reorganization. In R. Eckmiller, G. Hartmann, and G. Hauske eds., *Parallel Processing in Neural Systems and Computers*, 65–70. Amsterdam: Elsevier.

Dinse, H. R., Recanzone, G., and Merzenich, M. M. (1993). Alterations in correlated activity parallel ICMS-induced representational plasticity. *Neuroreport* 5: 173–176.

Dinse, H. R., Zepka, R. F., Jürgens, M., Godde, B., Hilger, H., and Berkefeld, T. (1995). Age-dependent changes of cortical and thalamic representations revealed by optical imaging and electrophysiological mapping techniques: Evidence for degenerative and use-disuse-dependent processes. In *Proceedings of the C.I.N.P. Conference on Neuropsychopharmacology. Homeostasis in Health and Disease* 36(Suppl 1): 49.

Doetsch, G. S. (1998). Perceptual significance of somatosensory cortical reorganization following peripheral denervation. *NeuroReport* 9: R29–R35.

Dolan, R. J., Fink, G. R., Rolls, E., Booth, M., Holmes, A., Frackowiak, R. S., and Friston, K. J. (1997). How the brain learns to see objects and faces in an impoverished context. *Nature* 389: 596–599.

Domann, R., Hagemann, G., Kraemer, M., Freund, H. J., and Witte, O. W. (1993). Electrophysiological changes in the surrounding brain tissue of photochemically induced cortical infarcts in the rat. *Neurosci. Lett.* 155: 69–72.

Doniger, G. M., Foxe, J. J., Schroeder, C. E., Murray, M. M., Higgins, B. A., and Javitt, D. C. (2001). Visual perceptual learning in human object recognition areas: A repetition priming study using high-density electrical mapping. *Neuroimage* 13: 305–313.

Donoghue, J. P. (1995). Plasticity of adult sensorimotor representations. *Curr. Opin. Neurobiol.* 5: 749–754.

Dorais, A., and Sagi, D. (1997). Contrast masking effects change with practice. *Vision Res.* 37: 1725–1733.

Dosher, B. A., and Lu, Z. L. (1998). Perceptual learning reflects external noise filtering and internal noise reduction through channel reweighting. *Proc. Natl. Acad. Sci. U S A* 95: 13988–13993.

Dosher, B. A., and Lu, Z. L. (1999). Mechanisms of perceptual learning. *Vision Res.* 39: 3197–3221.

Dowell, R. C., Brown, A. M., Seligman, P. M., and Clark, G. M. (1985). Patient results for a multiple-channel cochlear prosthesis. In R. A. Schindler and M. M. Merzenich, eds., *Cochlear Implants* (Tenth Anniversary Conference on Cochlear Implants. San Francisco, June 22–24, 1983), 421–431. New York: Raven Press.

Dowell, R. C., Dettman, S. J., and Barker, E. J. (1998). Long-term outcomes for children using cochlear implants. Paper presented at Bi-annual Scientific Meeting of the Audiological Society of Australia, Sydney, April 1998. *Aust. J. Audiol.* Suppl. 20: 67.

Dowell, R. C., Mecklenburg, D. J., and Clark, G. M. (1986). Speech recognition for 40 patients receiving multichannel cochlear implants. *Arch. Otolaryngol.* 112: 1054–1059.

Downing, P. E., and Treisman, A. M. (1997). The line-motion illusion: Attention or impletion? *J. Exp. Psychol. Hum. Percept. Perform.* 23: 768–779.

Drasdo, N. (1991). Neural substrates and threshold gradients of peripheral vision. In J. J. Kulikowski, V. Walsh, and I. J. Murray, eds., *Limits of Vision.* Boca Raton, FL: Macmillan.

Dresp, B. (1999). Dynamic characteristics of spatial mechanisms coding contour structures. *Spat. Vis.* 12: 129–142.

Dresp, B., and Bonnet, C. (1991). Psychophysical evidence for low-level processing of illusory contours and surfaces in the Kanizsa square. *Vision Res.* 31: 1813–1817.

Dretske, F. (1995). *Naturalizing the Mind.* Jean Nicod Lectures. Cambridge, MA: MIT Press.

Duda, R. O., and Hart, P. E. (1973). *Pattern Classification and Scene Analysis.* New York: Wiley.

Duke-Elder, S., and Wybar, K. (1973). *System of Ophthalmology.* Vol. 6, *Ocular Motility and Strabismus.* London: Kimpton.

Duncan, P. (1997). Synthesis of intervention trials to improve motor recovery following stroke. *Top. Stroke Rehab.* 3(4): 1–20.

Durack, J. C., and Katz, L. C. (1996). Development of horizontal projections in layer 2/3 of ferret visual cortex. *Cereb. Cortex* 6: 178–183.

Duvdevani-Bar, S., Edelman, S., Howell, A. J., and Buxton, H. (1998). A similarity-based method for the generalization of face recognition over pose and expression. In S. Akamatsu and K. Mase, eds., *Proceedings of the Third International Symposium on Face and Gesture Recognition,* 118–123. Washington, DC: IEEE Press.

Dykes, R. W., Landry, P., Metherate, R., and Hicks, T. P. (1984). Functional role of GABA in cat primary somatosensory cortex: Shaping receptive fields of cortical neurons. *J. Neurophysiol.* 52: 1066–1093.

Eagleman, D. M., Coenen, O. J. M.-D., Mitsner, V., Bartol, T. M., Bell, A. J., and Sejnowski, T. J. (2001). Cerebellar glomeruli: Does limited extracellular calcium implement a sparse coding strategy? In *Proceedings of the 8th Joint Sumposium on Neural Computation.* http://www.its. caltech.edu/~jsnc/Proceedings/Eagleman-D.pdf.

Ebbinghaus, H. (1885). *Memory: A Contribution to Experimental Psychology,* Trans. H. A. Ruger and C. E. Bussenius. 1913. Reprint, New York: Dover, 1964.

Eddington, D. K. (1980). Speech discrimination in deaf subjects with cochlear implants. *J. Acoust. Soc. Am.* 68: 885–891.

Edeline, J. M. (1996). Does Hebbian synaptic plasticity explain learning-induced sensory plasticity in adult mammals? *J. Physiol. Paris* 90: 271–276.

Edeline, J. M., Hars, B., Maho, C., and Hennevin, E. (1994). Transient and prolonged facilitation of tone-evoked responses induced by basal forebrain stimulations in the rat auditory cortex. *Exp. Brain Res.* 97: 373–386.

Edelman, G. M. (1987). *Neural Darwinism: The Theory of Neuronal Group Selection.* New York: Basic Books.

Edelman, G. M., and Finkel, L. (1984). In G. M. Edelman, W. M. Cowan, and W. Gall, eds., *Dynamic Aspects of Neocortical Function.* 653–695. New York: Wiley.

Edelman, S. (1995). Representation of similarity in three-dimensional object discrimination. *Neural Comput.* 7: 408–423.

Edelman, S. (1998a). Representation is representation of similarity. *Behav. Brain Sci.* 21: 449–498.

Edelman, S. (1998b). Spanning the face space. *J. Biol. Syst.* 6: 265–280.

Edelman, S. (1999). *Representation and Recognition in Vision.* Cambridge, MA: MIT Press.

Edelman, S., and Bülthoff, H. (1992). Orientation dependence in the recognition of familiar and novel views of 3D objects. *Vision Res.* 32: 2385–2400.

Edelman, S., and Duvdevani-Bar, S. (1997). A model of visual recognition and categorization. *Philos. Trans. R. Soc. Lond. B Biol. Sci.* 352(1358): 1191–1202.

Edelman, S., and Intrator, N. (1997). Learning as extraction of low-dimensional representations. In D. Medin, R. Goldstone, and P. Schyns, eds., *Mechanisms of Perceptual Learning,* 353–380. San Diego: Academic Press.

Edelman, S., and Intrator, N. (2000). (Coarse Coding of Shape Fragments) + (Retinotopy) ≈ Representation of Structure. *Spat. Vis.* 13: 255–264.

Edelman, S., and Weinshall, D. (1991). A self-organising multiple-view representation of 3D objects. *Biol. Cybern.* 64: 209–219.

Elberger, A. J., Smith III, E. L., and White, J. M. (1983). Spatial dissociation of visual inputs alters the origin of the corpus callosum. *Neurosci. Lett.* 35: 19–24.

Elbert, T. (1998). *Neuromagnetism.* In W. Andrä and H. Novak eds., *Magnetism in Medicine,* 190–262. New York: Wiley.

Elbert, T., Candia, V., Altenmüller, E., Rau, H., Sterr, A., Rockstroh, B., Pantev, C., and Taub, E. (1998). Alteration of digital representations in somatosensory cortex in focal hand dystonia. *Neuroreport* 9: 3571–3575.

Elbert, T., Flor, H., Birbaumer, N., Knecht, S., Hampson, S., Larbig, W., and Taub, E. (1994). Extensive reorganization of the somatosensory cortex in adult humans after nervous system injury. *Neuroreport* 5: 2593–2597.

Elbert, T., Pantev, C., Wienbruch, C., Hoke, M., Rockstroh, B., and Taub, E. (1995). Increased use of the left hand in string players associated with increased cortical representation of the fingers. *Science* 270: 305–307.

Elbert, T., Sterr, A., Flor, H., Rockstroh, B., Knecht, S., Pantev, C., Wienbruch, C., and Taub, E. (1997). Input-increase and input-decrease types of cortical reorganization after upper extremity amputation. *Exp. Brain Res.* 117: 161–164.

Elbert, T., Sterr, A., Rockstroh, B., Pantev, C., Müller, M. M., and Taub, E. (forthcoming). Expansion of the tonotopic area in auditory cortex of the blind.

Ellis, A. W., Young, A. W., and Flude, B. M. (1990). Repetition priming and face recognition: Priming occurs within the system that responds to the identity of a face. *Q. J. Exp. Psychol.* 42A: 495–512.

Ellis, A. W., Young, A. W., Flude, B. M., and Hay, D. C. (1987). Repetition priming of face recognition. *Q. J. Exp. Psychol.* 39A: 193–210.

Ellis, H. (1965). *The Transfer of Learning.* New York: Macmillan.

Ellis, H. D., Shepherd, J. W., and Davies, G. M. (1979). Identification of familiar and unfamiliar faces from internal and external features: Some implications for theories of face recognition. *Perception* 8: 431–439.

Ellison, A., and Walsh, V. (1998). Perceptual learning in visual search: Some evidence of specificities. *Vision Res.* 38: 333–345.

Epstein, W. (1967). Perceptual learning resulting from exposure to a stimulus-invariant. *Am. J. Psychol.* 80: 205–212.

Epstein, W. (1975). Recalibration by pairing: a process of perceptual learning. *Perception* 4: 59–72.

Epstein, W., Hughes, B., Schneider, S. L., and Bach-y-Rita, P. (1989). Perceptual learning of spatiotemporal events: evidence from an unfamiliar modality. *J. Exp. Psychol. Hum. Percept. Perform.* 15: 28–44.

Ergenzinger, E. R., Glasier, M. M., Hahm, J. O., and Pons, T. P. (1998). Cortically induced thalamic plasticity in the primate somatosensory system. *Nat. Neurosci.* 1: 226–229.

Erickson, R. P. (1974). Parallel population coding in feature extraction. In F. O. Schmitt and F. G. Worden eds., *The Neurosciences: Third Study Program*, 155–169. Cambridge, MA: MIT Press.

Espinet, A., Almaraz, J., and Torres, P. M. (1999). Perceptual learning by preschool children using stimuli with varying proportions of common elements. *Percept. Mot. Skills* 89: 935–942.

Esteky, H., and Tanaka, K. (1998). Effects of changes in aspect ratio of stimulus shape on responses of cells in the monkey inferotemporal cortex. *Soc. Neurosci. Abstr.* 24: 899.

Estes, W. K. (1957). Of models and men. *Am. Psychol.* 12: 609–617.

Etcoff, N. L., and Magee, J. J. (1992). Categorical perception of facial expressions. *Cognition* 44: 227–240.

Eulitz, C., Eulitz, H., and Elbert, T. (1997). Differential outcomes from magneto- and electroencephalography for the analysis of human cognition. *Neurosci. Lett.* 227(3): 185–188.

Eurich, C. W., Dinse, H. R., Dicke, U., Godde, B., and Schwegler, H. (1997). Coarse coding accounts for improvement of spatial discrimination after plastic reorganization in rats and humans. In *Artificial Neural Networks: Proceedings of ICANN'97*, ed. W. Gerstner, A. Germond, M. Hasler, and J. D. Nicaud, 55–60. New York: Springer.

Eurich, C. W., and Schwegler, H. (1997). Coarse coding: Calculation of the resolution achieved by a population of large receptive field neurons. *Biol. Cybern.* 76: 357–363.

Eysel, U. T. (1982). Functional reconnections without new axonal growth in a partially denervated visual relay nucleus. *Nature* 299: 442–444.

Eysel, U. T. (1997). Perilesional cortical dysfunction and reorganization. In H. J. Freund, B. A. Sabel, and H. O. Witte, eds., *Brain Plasticity: Advances in Neurology*, vol. 73, pp. 195–206. Philadelphia: Lippincott-Raven.

Eysel, U. T., Crook, J. M., and Machemer, H. F. (1990). GABA-induced remote inactivation reveals cross-orientation inhibition in the cat striate cortex. *Exp. Brain Res.* 80: 626–630.

Eysel, U. T., Eyding, D., and Schweigart, G. (1998). Repetitive optical stimulation elicits fast receptive field changes in mature visual cortex. *NeuroReport* 9: 949–954.

Eysel, U. T., Gonzalez-Aguilar, F., and Mayer, U. (1980). A functional sign of reorganization in the visual system of adult cats: Lateral geniculate neurons with displaced receptive fields after lesions of the nasal retina. *Brain Res.* 181: 285–300.

Eysel, U. T., Gonzalez-Aguilar, F., and Mayer, U. (1981). Time-dependent decrease of the extent of visual deafferentation in the lateral geniculate nucleus of adult cats with small retinal lesions. *Exp. Brain Res.* 41: 256–263.

Eysel, U. T., Kretschmann, U., and Schmidt-Kastner, R. (1993). Changes of neuronal activity and immunohistochemical reactions associated with photochemically induced thrombosis in cat visual cortex. *Soc. Neurosci. Abstr.* 19: 1668.

Eysel, U. T., Muche, T., and Wörgötter, F. (1988). Lateral interactions at direction selective striate neurones in the cat demonstrated by local cortical inactivation. *J. Physiol.* 399: 657–675.

Eysel, U. T., and Schmidt-Kastner, R. (1991). Neuronal dysfunction at the border of focal lesions in cat visual cortex. *Neurosci. Lett.* 131: 45–48.

Eysel, U. T., and Schweigart, G. (1999). Reorganization of receptive fields at the border of chronic visual cortical lesions. *Cereb. Cortex* 9: 101–109.

Eysel, U. T., Schweigart, G., Mittmann, T., Eyding, D., Qu, Y., Vandesande, F., Orban, G. A., and Arckens, L. (1999). Reorganization in the visual cortex after retinal and cortical damage. *Restor. Neurol. Neurosci.* 15: 153–164.

Eysel, U. T., Wörgötter, F., and Pape, H.-C. (1987). Local cortical lesions abolish lateral inhibition at direction selective cells in cat visual cortex. *Exp. Brain Res.* 68: 606–612.

Faggin, B. M., Nguyen, K. T., and Nicolelis, M. A. (1997). Immediate and simultaneous sensory reorganization at cortical and subcortical levels of the somatosensory system. *Proc. Natl. Acad. Sci. U S A* 94: 9428–9433.

Fahle, M. (1991). A new elementary feature of vision. *Invest. Ophthalmol. Vis. Sci.* 32: 2151–2155.

Fahle, M. (1994). Human pattern recognition: Parallel processing and perceptual learning. *Perception* 23: 411–427.

Fahle, M. (1997). Specificity of learning curvature, orientation, and vernier discriminations. *Vision Res.* 37: 1885–1895.

Fahle, M. (1998). Orientation specificity of perceptual learning. *Invest. Ophthalmol. Vis. Sci.* 39: S912.

Fahle, M., and Daum, I. (1997). Visual learning and memory as functions of age. *Neuropsychologia* 35: 1583–1589.

Fahle, M., and Daum, I. (Forthcoming). Perceptual learning in amnesic patients. *Neuropsychologia* (in press).

Fahle, M., and Edelman, S. (1993). Long-term learning in vernier acuity: Effects of stimulus orientation, range, and feedback. *Vision Res.* 33: 397–412.

Fahle, M., Edelman, S., and Poggio, T. (1995). Fast perceptual learning in hyperacuity. *Vision Res.* 35: 3003–3013.

Fahle, M., and Henke-Fahle, S. (1996). Interobserver variance in perceptual performance and learning. *Invest. Ophthalmol. Vis. Sci.* 37: 869–877.

Fahle, M., and Morgan, M. (1996). No transfer of perceptual learning between similar stimuli in the same retinal position. *Curr. Biol.* 6: 292–297.

Fahle, M., and Skrandies, W. (1994). An electrophysiological correlate of learning in motion perception. *Ger. J. Ophthalmol.* 3: 427–432.

Fantz, R. L. (1964). Visual experience in infants: Decreased attention to familiar patterns relative to novel ones. *Science* 146: 668–670.

Farah, M. (1990). *Visual Agnosia: Disorders of Object Recognition and What They Can Tell Us about Normal Vision.* Cambridge, MA: MIT Press.

Farah, M. J., O'Reilly, R. C., and Vecera, S. P. (1993). Dissociated overt and covert recognition as an emergent property of a lesioned neural network. *Psychol. Rev.* 100: 571–588

Fendick, M., and Westheimer, G. (1983). Effects of practice and the separation of test targets on foveal and peripheral stereoacuity. *Vision Res.* 23: 145–150.

Ferster, D., Chung, S., and Wheat, H. (1996). Orientation selectivity of thalamic input to simple cells of cat visual cortex. *Nature* 380: 249–252.

Field, D. J. (1987). Relations between the statistics of natural images and the response properties of cortical cells. *J. Opt. Soc. Am. A* 4(12): 2370–2393.

Field, D. J. (1994). What is the goal of sensory coding? *Neural Comput.* 6: 559–601.

Field, D. J., and Nachmias, J. (1984). Phase reversal discrimination. *Vision Res.* 24: 333–340.

Field, D. J., Hayes, A., and Hess, R. F. (1993). Contour integration by the human visual system: evidence for a local "association field." *Vision Res.* 33: 173–193.

Fine, I., and Jacobs, R. A. (2000). Perceptual learning for a pattern discrimination task. *Vision Res.* 40: 3209–3230.

Finnerty, G. T., Roberts, L. S., and Connors, B. W. (1999). Sensory experience modifies the short-term dynamics of neocortical synapses. *Nature* 400: 367–371.

Fiorentini, A., and Berardi, N. (1980). Perceptual learning specific for orientation and spatial frequency. *Nature* 287: 43–44.

Fiorentini, A., and Berardi, N. (1981). Learning in grating waveform discrimination: Specificity for orientation and spatial frequency. *Vision Res.* 21: 1149–1158.

Fiorentini, A., and Berardi, N. (1997). Visual perceptual learning: A sign of neural plasticity at early stages of visual processing. *Arch. Ital. Biol.* 135: 157–167.

Fiorentini, A., Berardi, N., Falsini, B., and Porciatti, V. (1992). Interhemispheric transfer of visual perceptual learning in callosal agenesis. *Clin. Vis. Sci.* 7: 133–141.

Fischler, M. A., and Leclerc, Y. G. (1992). Recovering 3-D wire frames from line drawings. *Proceedings of the Image Understanding Workshop.* San Francisco: Kantman.

Fiser, J., Biederman, I., and Cooper, E. (1996). To what extent can matching algorithms based on direct outputs of spatial filters account for human object recognition? *Spat. Vis.* 10(3): 237–271.

Fisken, R. A., Garey, L. J., and Powell, T. P. S. (1975). The intrinsic, association and commissural connections of area 17 of the visual cortex. *Philos. Trans. R. Soc. London B Biol. Sci.* 272: 487–536.

Fitzpatrick, D. (1996). The functional organization of local circuits in visual cortex: insights from the study of tree shrew striate cortex. *Cereb. Cortex* 6: 329–341.

Flannagan, M. J., Fried, L. S., and Holyoak, K. J. (1986). Distributional expectations and the induction of category structure. *J. Exp. Psychol. Learn. Mem. Cognit.* 12: 241–256.

Flor, H., Braun, C., Elbert, T., and Birbaumer, N. (1997). Extensive reorganization of primary somatosensory cortex in chronic back pain patients. *Neurosci. Lett.* 224: 5–8.

Flor, H., and Elbert, T. (1998). Maladaptive consequences of cortical reorganization in humans. *Neurosci. News* 1: 4–11.

Flor, H., Elbert, T., Knecht, S., Wienbruch, C., Pantev, C., Birbaumer, N., Larbig, W., and Taub, E. (1995). Phantom-limb pain as a perceptual correlate of cortical reorganization following arm amputation. *Nature* 375: 482–484.

Flor, H., Elbert, T., Muhlnickel, W., Pantev, C., Wien-bruch, C., and Taub, E. (1998). Cortical reorganization and phantom phenomena in congenital and traumatic upper-extremity amputees. *Exp. Brain Res.* 119: 205–212.

Flor, H., Mühlnickel, W., Karl, A., Denke, C., Grüsser, S., and Taub, E. (2000). A neural substrate for non-painful phantom limb phenomena. *NeuroReport* 11: 1407–1411.

Florence, S. L., and Kaas, J. H. (1995). Large-scale reorganization at multiple levels of the somatosensory pathway follows therapeutic amputation of the hand in monkeys. *J. Neurosci.* 15: 8083–8095.

Florence, S. L., Taub, H. B., and Kaas, J. H. (1998). Large-scale sprouting of cortical connections after peripheral injury in adult macaque monkeys. *Science* 282: 1117–1121.

Fodor, J. A., and Pylyshyn, Z. W. (1981). How direct is visual perception? Some reflections on Gibson's "ecological approach." *Cognition* 9: 139–196.

Földiák, P. (1990). Forming sparse representations by local anti-Hebbian learning. *Biol. Cybern.* 64: 165–170.

Földiák, P. (1991). Learning invariance from transformation sequences. *Neural Comput.* 3: 194–200.

Foley, J. M. (1994). Human luminance pattern-vision mechanisms: Masking experiments require a new model. *J. Opt. Soc. Am. A* 11: 1710–1719.

Foulke, E. (1991). Braille. In M. A. Heller and W. Schiff eds., *The Psychology of Touch*, 219–233. Hillsdale, NJ: Erlbaum.

Fox, K. (1994). The cortical component of experience-dependent synaptic plasticity in the rat barrel cortex. *J. Neurosci.* 14: 7665–7679.

Fox, K., and Daw, N. W. (1993). Do NMDA receptors have a critical function in visual cortical plasticity? *Trends Neurosci.* 16: 116–122.

Fox, R. A., Corcoran, M., Daunton, N. G., and Morey-Holton, E. (1994). Effects of spaceflight and hindlimb suspension on the posture and gait of rats. In *Vestibular and Neural Front*, ed. K. Taguchi, M. Igarashi, and S. Mori, 603–606. Amsterdam: Elsevier.

Franzen, U., Lindinger, G., Lang, W., and Deecke, L. (1991). On the functionality of the visually deprived occipital cortex in early blind persons. *Neurosci. Lett.* 124: 256–259.

Freeman, R. B. Jr. (1966). Function of cues in the perceptual learning of visual slant: An experimental and theoretical analysis. *Psychol. Monogr.* 80: 1–29.

Freeman, R. D., and Pettigrew, J. D. (1973). Alteration of visual cortex from environmental asymmetries. *Nature* 246: 359–360.

Frégnac, Y. (1998). Homeostasis or synaptic plasticity. *Nature* 391: 845–855.

Frégnac, Y., Bringuier, V., Chavane, F., Glaeser, L., and Lorenceau, J. (1996). An intracellular study of space and time representation in primary visual cortical receptive fields. *J. Physiol. Paris* 90: 189–197.

Frégnac, Y., and Imbert, M. (1978). Early development of visual cortical cells in normal and dark-reared kittens: Relationship between orientation selectivity and ocular dominance. *J. Physiol.* 278: 27–44.

Frégnac, Y., Shulz, D., Thorpe, S., and Bienenstock, E. (1988). A cellular analogue of visual cortical plasticity. *Nature* 333: 367–370.

Frégnac, Y., and Shulz, D. E. (1999). Activity-dependent regulation of receptive field properties of cat area 17 by supervised Hebbian learning. *J. Neurobiol.* 41: 69–82.

Frégnac, Y., Shulz, D., Thorpe, S., and Bienenstock, E. (1992). Cellular analogs of visual cortical epigenesis: 1. Plasticity of orientation selectivity. *J. Neurosci.* 12: 1280–1300.

Freund, T. F., Martin, K. A. C., and Whitteridge, D. (1985). Innervation of cat visual areas 17 and 18 by physiologically identified X- and Y-type thalamic afferents: 1. Arborization patterns and quantitative distribution of postsynaptic elements. *J. Comp. Neurol.* 242: 263–274.

Fried, I., MacDonald, K. A., and Wilson, C. L. (1997). Single neuron activity in human hippocampus and amygdala during recognition of faces and objects. *Neuron* 18: 753–765.

Friedman, J. (1994). *Flexible Metric Nearest Neighbor Classification.* Technical report. Stanford University.

Fuhr, P., Cohen, L. G., Dang, N., Findley, T. W., Haghighi, S., Oro, J., and Hallett, M. (1992). Physiological analysis of motor reorganization following lower limb amputation. *Electroenc. Clin. Neurophysiol.* 85: 53–60.

Fujita, I., Tanaka, K., Ito, M., and Cheng, K. (1992). Columns for visual features of objects in monkey inferotemporal cortex. *Nature* 360: 343–346.

Furmanski, C. S., and Engel, S. A. (2000). Perceptual learning in object recognition: Object specificity and size invariance. *Vision Res.* 40: 473–484.

Fuster, J. M., and Jervey, J. P. (1981). Inferotemporal neurons distinguish and retain behaviorally relevant features of visual stimuli. *Science* 212: 952–955.

Fyfe, C., and Baddeley, R. (1995). Finding compact and sparse-distributed representations of visual images. *Network* 6: 333–344.

Gabor, D. (1946). Theory of communication. *J. Inst. Elect. Eng. Lond.* 93: 429–457.

Gabrieli, J. D., Milberg, W., Keane, M. M., and Corkin, S. (1990). Intact priming of patterns despite impaired memory. *Neuropsychologia* 28: 417–427.

Gaffan, D. (1996). Associative and perceptual learning and the concept of memory systems. *Brain Res. Cogn. Brain Res.* 5: 69–80.

Gallant, J. L., Braun, J., and Van Essen, D. C. (1993). Selectivity for polar, hyperbolic, and cartesian gratings in macaque visual cortex. *Science* 259: 100–103.

Gallant, J. L., Connor, C. E., Rakshit, S., Lewis, J. W., and Van Essen, D. C. (1996). Neural responses to polar, hyperbolic, and Cartesian gratings in area V4 of the macaque monkey. *J. Neurophysiol.* 76: 2718–2739.

Gallistel, C. R. (1990). *The Organization of Learning.* Cambridge, MA: MIT Press.

Galper, R. E. (1970). Recognition of faces in photographic negative. *Psychonom. Sci.* 19: 207–208.

Galton, F. (1883). *Inquiries into Human Faculty and Its Development.* London: Macmillan.

Galuske, R. A. W., and Singer, W. (1996). The origin and topography of long-range intrinsic projections in cat visual cortex: A developmental study. *Cereb. Cortex* 6: 417–430.

Gardner, D. (1993). Static determinants of synaptic strength. In Gardner, ed., *The Neurobiology of Neural Networks.* Cambridge, MA: MIT Press.

Gardner, E. P., and Costanzo, R. M. (1980). Temporal integration of multiple-point stimuli in primary somatosensory cortical receptive fields of alert monkeys. *J. Neurophysiol.* 43: 444–468.

Garraghty, P. E., and Kaas, J. H. (1991). Functional reorganization in adult monkey thalamus after peripheral nerve injury. *NeuroReport* 2: 747–750.

Garraghty, P. E., and Kaas, J. H. (1992). Dynamic features of sensory and motor maps. *Curr. Opin. Neurobiol.* 2: 522–527.

Gauthier, I., and Tarr, M. J. (1997). Becoming a "greeble" expert: Exploring mechanisms for face recognition. *Vision Res.* 37: 1673–1682.

Gauthier, I., Tarr, M. J., Anderson, A. W., Skudlarski, P., and Gore, J. C. (1999). Activation of the middle fusiform "face area" increases with expertise in recognizing novel objects. *Nat. Neurosci.* 2: 568–573.

Geisler, W. S., and Albrecht, D. G. (1992). Cortical neurons: Isolation of contrast gain control. *Vision Res.* 32: 1409–1410.

Geisler, W. S., and Albrecht, D. G. (1997). Visual cortex neurons in monkeys and cats: Detection, discrimination and identification. *Vis. Neurosci.* 14: 897–919.

Geldard, F. A., and Sherrick, C. E. (1972). The cutaneous "rabbit": A perceptual illusion. *Science* 178: 178–179.

Gellatly, A. R. (1982). Perceptual learning of illusory contours and colour. *Perception* 11: 655–661.

Georgopoulos, A. P., Schwartz, A. B., and Kettner, R. E. (1986). Neural population coding of movement direction. *Science* 233: 1416–1419.

Gerrits, H. J. M., and Timmermann, G. J. M. E. (1969). The filling-in process in patients with retinal scotomata. *Vision Res.* 9: 439–442.

Gerrits, H. J. M., de Haan, B., Vendrick, A. J. H. (1966). Experiments with retinal stabilized images: Relations between the observations and neural data. *Vision Res.* 6: 427–440.

Gerrits, H. J. M., and Vendrik, A. J. H. (1970). Simultaneous contrast, filling-in process and information processing in man's visual system. *Exp. Brain Res.* 11: 411–430.

Ghazanfar, A. A., Stambaugh, C. R., and Nicolelis, M. A. (2000). Encoding of tactile stimulus location by somatosensory thalamocortical ensembles. *J. Neurosci.* 20: 3761–3775.

Gibson, E. J. (1969). *Principles of Perceptual Learning and Development.* New York: Appleton-Century-Crofts.

Gibson, E. J. (1941). Retroactive inhibition as a function of the degree of generalization between tasks. *J. Exp. Psychol.* 28: 93–115.

Gibson, E. J. (1953). Improvement in perceptual judgements as a function of controlled practice or training. *Psychol. B* 50: 401–431.

Gibson, E. J. (1963). Perceptual learning. *Annu. Rev. Psychol.* 14: 29–56.

Gibson, E. J., and Walk, R. D. (1956). The effect of prolonged exposure to visually presented patterns on learning to discriminate them. *J. Comp. Physiol. Psychol.* 49: 239–242.

Gibson, E., Owsley, C., and Johnston, J. (1978). Perception of invariants by five-month-old infants. *Dev. Psychol.* 14: 407–415.

Gibson, J. J., and Gibson, E. J. (1955). Perceptual learning: Differentiation or enrichment? *Psychol. Rev.* 62: 32–41.

Gick, M., and Holyoak, K. (1980). Analogical problem solving. *Cogn. Psychol.* 12: 306–355

Gilbert, C. D. (1983). Microcircuitry of the visual cortex. *Annu. Rev. Neurosci.* 6: 217–247.

Gilbert, C. D. (1992). Horizontal integration and cortical dynamics. *Neuron* 9: 1–13.

Gilbert, C. D. (1993). Circuitry, architecture and functional dynamics of visual cortex. *Cerebr. Cortex* 3: 373–386.

Gilbert, C. D. (1994). Early perceptual learning. *Proc. Natl. Acad. Sci. U S A* 91: 1195–1197.

Gilbert, C. D. (1994). Neuronal dynamics and perceptual learning. *Curr. Biol.* 4: 627–629.

Gilbert, C. D. (1998). Adult cortical dynamics. *Physiol. Rev.* 78: 467–485.

Gilbert, C. D., and Wiesel, T. N. (1979). Morphology and intracortical projections of functionally characterised neurones in the cat visual cortex. *Nature* 280: 120–125.

Gilbert, C. D., and Wiesel, T. N. (1983). Clustered intrinsic connections in cat visual cortex. *J. Neurosci.* 3: 1116–1133.

Gilbert, C. D., and Wiesel, T. N. (1985). Intrinsic connectivity and receptive field properties in visual cortex. *Vision Res.* 25: 365–374.

Gilbert, C. D., and Wiesel, T. N. (1989). Columnar specificity of intrinsic horizontal and corticocortical connections in cat visual cortex. *J. Neurosci.* 9: 2432–2442.

Gilbert, C. D., and Wiesel, T. N. (1992). Receptive field dynamics in adult primary visual cortex. *Nature* 356: 150–152.

Gilbert, C. D., Das, A., Ito, M., Kapadia, M., and Westheimer, G. (1996). Spatial integration and cortical dynamics. *Proc. Natl. Acad. Sci. U S A* 93: 615–622.

Gilbert, C. D., Ito, M., Kapadia, M., and Westheimer, G. (2000). Interactions between attention, context and learning in primary visual cortex. *Vision Res.* 40: 1217–1226.

Gilbert, C. D., Sigman, M., and Crist, R. E. (2001). The neural basis of perceptual learning. *Neuron* 31: 681–697.

Gilbert, D. K., and Rogers, W. A. (1996). Age-related differences in perceptual learning. *Hum. Factors* 38: 417–424.

Girosi, F., Jones, M., and Poggio, T. (1995). Regularization theory and neural networks architectures. *Neural Comput.* 7: 219–269.

Gliner, J. A., Mihevic, P. M., and Horvath, S. M. (1983). Spectral analysis of electroencephalogram during perceptual-motor learning. *Biol. Psychol.* 16: 1–13.

Gluck, M. A., and Granger, R. (1993). Computational models of the neural bases of learning and memory. *Annu. Rev. Neurosci.* 16: 667–706.

Godde, B., Spengler, F., and Dinse, H. R. (1996). Associative pairing of tactile stimulation induces somatosensory cortical reorganization in rats and humans. *NeuroReport* 8: 281–285.

Godde, B., Stauffenberg, B., Spengler, F., and Dinse, H. R. (2000). Tactile coactivation induced changes in spatial discrimination performance. *J. Neurosci.* 20: 1597–1604.

Godecke, I., and Bonhoeffer, T. (1996). Development of identical orientation maps for two eyes without common visual experience. *Nature* 379: 251–254.

Gold, J., Bennett, P. J., and Sekuler, A. B. (1999). Signal but not noise changes with perceptual learning. *Nature* 402: 176–178.

Goldstein, B. E. (1996). *Sensation and Perception.* Pacific Grove, CA: Brooks/Cole.

Goldstone, R. L. (1998). Perceptual learning. *Annu. Rev. Psychol.* 49: 585–612.

Goldstone, R. L., and Barsalou, L. W. (1998). Reuniting perception and cognition: The perceptual bases of similarity and rules. *Cognition* 65: 231–262.

Gollin, E. S. (1960). Developmental studies of visual recognition of incomplete objects. *Percept. Mot. Skills* 11: 289–298.

Gollin, E. S. (1965). Perceptual learning of incomplete pictures. *Percept. Mot. Skills* 21: 439–445.

Goodale, M. A., and Humphrey, G. K. (1998). The objects of action and perception. *Cognition* 67: 181–207.

Goodale, M., and Milner, A. (1992). Separate visual pathways for perception and action. *Trends Neurosci.* 15: 20–25.

Goodall, M. C. (1960). Performance of stochastic nets. *Nature* 185: 557–558.

Goren, C. C., Sarty, M., and Wu, R. W. K. (1975). Visual following and pattern discrimination of face-like stimuli by new-born infants. *Pediatrics* 56: 544–549.

Gottlieb, G. L., Corcos, D. M., Jaric, S., and Agarwal, G. C. (1988). Practice improves even the simplest movements. *Exp. Brain Res.* 73: 436–440.

Grady, C. L., and Craik, F. I. M. (2000). Changes in memory processing with age. *Curr. Opin. Neurobiol.* 10: 224–231.

Grady, C. L., Horwitz, B., Pietrini, P., Mentis, M. J., Ungerleider, L. G., Rapoport, S. I., and Haxby, J. V. (1996). Effect of task difficulty on cerebral blood flow during perceptual matching of faces. *Hum. Brain Mapp.* 4074: 227–239.

Graham, D. B., and Allison, N. M. (1998). Characterising virtual eigensignatures for general purpose face recognition. In H. Wechsler et al., eds., *Face Recognition: From Theory to Applications*, pp. 446–456. Berlin: Springer.

Graham, S. (1999). Retrospective revaluation and inhibitory associations: does perceptual learning modulate our perception of the contingencies between events? *Q. J. Exp. Psychol. B.* 52: 159–185.

Granger, R., and Lynch, G. (1991). Higher olfactory processes: perceptual learning and memory. *Curr. Opin. Neurobiol.* 1: 209–214.

Granger, R., Whitson, J., Larson, J., and Lynch, G. (1994). Non-Hebbian properties of long-term potentiation enable high-capacity encoding of temporal sequences. *Proc. Natl. Acad. Sci. U S A* 91: 10104–10108.

Gray, C. M., König, P., Engel, A. K., and Singer, W. (1989). Oscillatory responses in cat visual cortex exhibit inter-columnar synchronization which reflects global stimulus parameters. *Nature* 338: 334–337.

Green, J. B., Sora, E., Bialy, Y., Ricamato, A., and Thatcher, R. W. (1998). Cortical sensorimotor reorganization after spinal cord injury. *Neurology* 50: 1115–1121.

Greenspan, S. L., Nusbaum, H. C., and Pisoni, D. B. (1988). Perceptual learning of synthetic speech produced by rule. *J. Exp. Psychol. Learn. Mem. Cogn.* 14: 421–433.

Gregory, R. (1972). *Eye and Brain: The Psychology of Seeing.* 2d ed. London: Weidenfeld and Nicolson.

Gregory, R., and Wallace, J. (1963). *Recovery from Early Blindness: A Case Study.* Experimental Psychology Society Monograph 2. Cambridge: W. Heffer.

Greuel, J. M., Luhmann, H. J., and Singer, W. (1988). Pharmacological induction of use-dependent receptive field modifications in the visual cortex. *Science* 242: 74–77.

Gross, C. G. (1973). Visual functions of inferotemporal cortex. In *Handbook of Sensory Physiology*, vol. 7, part 3B, ed. R. Jung, 451–482. Berlin: Springer.

Gross, C. G. (1992). Representation of visual stimuli in inferior temporal cortex. *Philos. Trans. R. Soc. Lond. B Biol. Sci.* 335: 3–10.

Gross, C. G. (1994). How inferior temporal cortex became a visual area. *Cereb. Cortex* 4: 455–469.

Gross, C. G., Bender, D. B., and Rocha-Miranda, C. E. (1969). Visual receptive fields of neurons in inferotemporal cortex of the monkey. *Science* 166: 1303–1306.

Gross, C. G., Rocha-Miranda, C. E., and Bender, D. B. (1972). Visual properties of neurons in inferotemporal cortex of the macaque. *J. Neurophysiol.* 35: 96–111.

Grossberg, S. (1987). Competitive learning: From interactive activation to adaptive resonance. *Cogn. Sci.* 11: 23–63.

Grossberg, S., and Mingolla, E. (1985). Neural dynamics of perceptual grouping: Textures, boundaries, and emergent segmentations. *Percep. Psychophys.* 38: 141–171.

Grossberg, S., and Williamson, J. R. (2001). A neural model of how horizontal and interlaminar connections of visual cortex develop into adult circuits that carry out perceptual grouping and learning. *Cereb. Cortex* 11: 37–58.

Gruber, H. E. (1995). Insight and affect in the history of science. In *The Nature of Insight*, ed. R. J. Sternberg and J. E. Davidson. Cambridge, MA: MIT Press.

Grunke, M. E., and Pisoni, D. B. (1982). Some experiments on perceptual learning of mirror-image acoustic patterns. *Percept. Psychophys.* 31: 210–218.

Gu, X., and Fortier, P. A. (1996). Early enhancement but no late changes of motor responses induced by intracortical microstimulation in the ketamine-anesthetized rat. *Exp. Brain. Res.* 108: 119–128.

Gunderson, V. M., and Sackett, G. P. (1984). Development of pattern recognition in infant pigtailed macaques (*Macaca nemestrina*). *Dev. Psychol.* 22: 477–480.

Guttman, N. (1963). Laws of behavior and facts of perception. In S. Koch, ed., *Psychology: A study of a Science*, vol. 5, pp. 114–178. New York: McGraw-Hill.

Guzman, A. (1971). Analysis of curved line drawings using context and global information. *Mach. Intell.* 6: 325–375.

Hagemann, G., Redecker, C., Neumann-Haefelin, T., Freund, H.-J., and Witte, O. W. (1998). Increased long-term potentiation in the surround of experimentally induced focal cortical infarction. *Ann. Neurol.* 44: 255–258.

Hall, E. J., Flament, D., Fraser, C., and Lemon, R. N. (1990). Non-invasive brain stimulation reveals reorganized cortical outputs in amputees. *Neurosci. Lett.* 116: 379–386.

Hall, G. (1991). *Perceptual and Associative Learning.* Oxford Psychology Series No.18. Oxford, UK: Clarendon Press.

Halligan, P. W., Marshall, J. C., Wade, D. T., Davey, J., and Morrison, D. (1993). Thumb in cheek? Sensory reorganization and perceptual plasticity after limb amputation. *NeuroReport* 4: 233–236.

Hancock, P. J. B., Baddeley, R. J., and Smith, L. S. (1992). The principal components of natural images. *Network* 3: 61–72.

Hancock, P. J. B., Bruce, V., and Burton, A. M. (1998). A comparison of two computer-based face identification systems with human perceptions of faces. *Vision Res.* 38: 2277–2288.

Hancock, P. J. B., Burton, A. M., and Bruce, V. (1996). Face processing: Human perception and principal components analysis. *Mem. Cognit.* 24: 26–40.

Haralick, R. M. (1980). Edge and region analysis for digital image data. *Comput. Graph. Image Proc.* 12: 60–73.

Harnad, S., ed. (1987). *Categorical Perception: The Groundwork of Cognition.* New York: Cambridge University Press.

Harpur, G. F., and Prager, R. W. (1996). Development of low entropy coding in a recurrent network. *Network* 7: 277–284.

Harpur, J. G., Estabrooks, K. A., Allen, N. J., and Asaph, C. A. (1978). Perceptual versus mediational learning in a total change concept-shift paradigm. *Percept. Mot. Skills* 46: 563–569.

Harris, C. (1963). Adaptation to displaced vision: Visual, motor, or proprioceptive change? *Science* 140: 812–813.

Harris, J. A., and Diamond, M. E. (2000). Ipsilateral and contralateral transfer of tactile learning. *NeuroReport* 11: 263–266.

Hartline, H. K. (1940). The receptive fields of optic nerve fibers. *Am. J. Physiol.* 130: 690–699.

Hasselmo, M. E., Rolls, E. T., and Baylis, G. C. (1989). The role of expression and identity in the face-selective responses of neurons in the temporal visual cortex of the monkey. *Behav. Brain Res.* 32: 203–218.

Hata, Y., Tsumoto, T., Sato, H., and Tamura, H. (1991). Horizontal interactions between visual cortical neurones studied by cross-correlation analysis in the cat. *J. Physiol. (Lond.)* 441: 593–614.

Hatfield, G., and Epstein, W. (1985). The status of the minimum principle in the theoretical analysis of vision. *Psychol. Bull.* 97: 155–186.

Haykin, S., ed. (1994). *Blind Deconvolution.* Englewood Cliffs, NJ: Prentice-Hall.

Hebb, O. D. (1949). *The Organization of Behavior. A Neuropsychological Theory.* New York: Wiley.

Heeger, D. J. (1992). Normalization of cell responses in cat striate cortex. *Vis. Neurosci.* 9: 181–197.

Heinen, S. J., and Skavenski, A. A. (1991). Recovery of visual responses in foveal V1 neurons following bilateral foveal lesions in adult monkey. *Exp. Brain Res.* 83: 670–674.

Held, R. (1999). Visual development in infants. In G. Adelman and B. H. Smith, eds., *Encyclopedia of Neuroscience*, 2nd ed., vol. 2., pp. 2124–2127. New York: Elsevier.

Helmholtz, H. von (1866/1911). *Helmholtz's Physiological Optics.* 3d ed., trans. and ed. J. P. Southwell. Rochester, NY: Optical Society of America.

Hering, E. (1861). *Beiträge zur Physiologie: Zur Lehre vom Ortsinne der Netzhaut.* Leipzig: Engelmann.

Hershberger, W. (1970). Attached-shadow orientation perceived as depth by chickens reared in an environment illuminated from below. *J. Comp. Physiol. Psychol.* 73: 407–411.

Hertz, J., Krogh, A., and Palmer, R. G. (1991). *Introduction to the Theory of Neural Computation.* Redwood City, CA: Addison-Wesley and Santa Fe Institute.

Herzog, M. H., and Fahle, M. (1994). Learning without attention? In N. Elsner and H. Breer, eds., *Proceedings of the Twenty-second Göttingen Neurobiology Conference*, 1994, vol. II, no. 817. Stuttgart: Thieme.

Herzog, M. H., and Fahle, M. (1997). The role of feedback in learning a vernier discrimination task. *Vision Res.* 37: 2133–2141.

Herzog, M. H., and Fahle, M. (1998). Modeling perceptual learning: Difficulties and how they can be overcome. *Biol. Cybern.* 78: 107–117.

Herzog, M. H., and Fahle, M. (1999). Effects of biased feedback on learning and deciding in a vernier discrimination task. *Vision Res.* 39: 4232–4243.

Herzog, M. H., Broos, A. H., and Fahle, M. (1999). Practicing a vernier discrimination task with non-uniformly distributed stimuli influences decision but not learning processes. *Invest. Ophthalmol. Vis. Sci.* 40: 3077.

Hietanen, J. K., Perrett, D. I., Oram, M. W., Benson, P. J., and Dittrich, W. H. (1992). The effects of lighting conditions on responses of cells selective for face views in the macaque temporal cortex. *Exp. Brain Res.* 89: 157–171.

Hikosaka, O., Miyauchi, S., and Shimojo, S. (1993). Visual attention revealed by an illusion of motion. *Neurosci. Res.* 18: 11–18.

Hikosaka, O., Miyauchi, S., and Shimojo, S. (1996). Orienting a spatial attention: Its reflexive, compensatory, and voluntary mechanisms. *Cogn. Brain Res.* 5: 1–9.

Hill, H., and Bruce, V. (1996). Effects of lighting on matching facial surfaces. *J. Exp. Psychol. Hum. Percept. Perform.* 22: 986–1004.

Hinton, G. E. (1989). Connectionist learning procedures. *Artif. Intell.* 40: 185–234.

Hinton, G. E., McClelland, J. L., and Rumelhart, D. E. (1986). Distributed representations. In J. A. Feldman, P. J. Hayes, and D. E. Rumelhart, eds., *Parallel Distributed Processing: Exploration in the Microstructure of Cognition.* Vol. 1, *Foundations.* 77–109. Cambridge, MA: MIT Press.

Hinton, G., Williams, C., and Revow, M. (1992). Adaptive elastic models for hand-printed character recognition. In J. Moody, S. Hanson, and R. Lippman, eds., *Advances in Neural Information-Processing Systems,* vol. 4, pp. 512–519. San Meteo, CA: Morgan Kaufmann.

Hintzman, D. L. (1994). Twenty-five years of learning and memory: Was the cognitive revolution a mistake? In C. Umiltà and M. Moscovitch, eds., *Attention and Performance XV,* 360–391. Cambridge, MA: MIT Press.

Hirsch, J. A., and Gilbert, C. D. (1993). Long-term changes in synaptic strength along specific intrinsic pathways in the cat visual cortex. *J. Physiol.* 461: 247–262.

Hochberg, J. E., and Brooks, V. (1958). Effects of previously associated annoying stimuli (auditory) on visual recognition thresholds. *J. Exp. Psychol.* 55: 490–491.

Hochmair-Desoyer, I. J., and Burian, K. (1985). Reimplantation of a modulated scala tympani electrode: Impact on psychophysical and speech discrimination abilities. *Ann. Otol. Rhinol. Laryngol.* 94: 65–70.

Hochstein, S., Lobovsky, S., Laiwand, R., and Ahissar, M. (2000). Dual-task performance within and across dimensions for spatially overlapping and non-overlapping tasks. *Invest. Ophthalmol. Vis. Sci.* 41(4): 1048.

Hock, H. S., Webb, E., and Cavedo, L. C. (1987). Perceptual learning in visual category acquisition. *Mem. Cognit.* 15: 544–556.

Hoffman, W. (1966). The lie algebra of visual perception. *J. Math. Psychol.* 3: 65–98.

Hollins, M. (1989). *Understanding Blindness.* Hillsdale, NJ: Erlbaum.

Honey, R. C., and Bateson, P. (1996). Stimulus comparison and perceptual learning: Further evidence and evaluation from an imprinting procedure. *Q. J. Exp. Psychol. B.* 49: 259–269.

Honey, R. C., Bateson, P., and Horn, G. (1994). The role of stimulus comparison in perceptual learning: An investigation with the domestic chick. *Q. J. Exp. Psychol. B.* 47: 83–103.

Honig, M. G., and Hume, R. I. (1989). DiI and diO: Versatile fluorescent dyes for neuronal labelling and pathway tracing. *Trends Neurosci.* 12: 333–341.

Horel, J. A., Pytko-Joiner, D. E., Voytko, M. L., and Salsbury, K. (1987). The performance of visual tasks while segments of the inferotemporal cortex are suppressed by cold. *Behav. Brain Res.* 23: 29–42.

Horn, B. K. P. (1975). Obtaining shape from shading information. In *The Psychology of Computer Vision,* ed. P. H. Winston. New York: McGraw-Hill.

Houzel, J.-C., Milleret, C., and Innocenti, G. (1994). Morphology of callosal axons interconnecting areas 17 and 18 of the cat. *Eur. J. Neurosci.* 6: 898–917.

Howard, I. P. (1971). Perceptual learning and adaptation. *Br. Med. Bull.* 27: 248–252.

Hubel, D. H. (1995). *Eye, Brain, and Vision.* New York: Scientific American Library.

Hubel, D. H., and Wiesel, T. N. (1959). Receptive fields of single neurones in the cat's striate cortex. *J. Physiol.* 148: 574–591.

Hubel, D. H., and Wiesel, T. N. (1962). Receptive fields, binocular interaction and functional architecture in the cat's visual cortex. *J. Physiol.* 160: 106–154.

Hubel, D. H., and Wiesel, T. N. (1965). Binocular interaction in striate cortex of kittens reared with artificial squint. *J. Neurophysiol.* 28: 1041–1059.

Hubel, D. H., and Wiesel, T. N. (1967). Cortical and callosal connections concerned with the vertical meridian of visual fields in the cat. *J. Neurophysiol.* 30: 1561–1573.

Hubel, D. H., and Wiesel, T. N. (1968). Receptive fields and functional architecture of monkey striate cortex. *J. Physiol. (Lond.)* 195: 215–243.

Hubel, D. H., and Wiesel, T. N. (1970). The period of susceptibility to the physiological effects of unilateral eye closure in kittens. *J. Physiol.* 206: 419–436.

Hubel, D. H., and Wiesel, T. N. (1974). Uniformity of monkey striate cortex: A parallel relationship between field size, scatter, and magnification factor. *J. Comp. Neurol.* 158: 295–306.

Hubel, D. H., and Wiesel, T. N. (1977). Functional architecture of macaque monkey visual cortex. *Proc. R. Soc. Lond. B.* 198: 1–59.

Hubel, D. H., and Wiesel, T. N. (1998). Early exploration of the visual cortex. *Neuron* 20: 401–412.

Hubel, D. H., Wiesel, T. N., and LeVay, S. (1977). Plasticity of ocular dominance columns in monkey striate cortex. *Philos. Trans. R. Soc. Lond. B Biol. Sci.* 278: 377–409.

Huber, P. J. (1985). Projection pursuit (with discussion). *Ann. Stat.* 13: 435–475.

Hubscher, C. H., and Johnson, R. D. (1999). Changes in neuronal receptive field characteristics in caudal brain stem following chronic spinal cord injury. *J. Neurotrauma* 16: 533–541.

Hughes, B., Epstein, W., Schneider, S., and Dudock, A. (1990). An asymmetry in transmodal perceptual learning. *Percept. Psychophys.* 48: 143–150.

Hume, D. (1738/1956). *A Treatise of Human Nature.* London: Everyman's Library.

Humphrey, N. K., and Keeble, G. R. (1976). How monkeys acquire a new way of seeing. *Perception* 5: 51–56.

Humphreys, G. W., and Riddoch, M. J. (1987). *To See but Not to See: A Case Study of Visual Agnosia.* Hillsdale, NJ: Erlbaum.

Huntley, G. W. (1997). Correlation between patterns of horizontal connectivity and the extent of short-term representational plasticity in rat motor cortex. *Cereb. Cortex* 7: 143–156.

Hupé, J. M., James, A. C., Payne, B. R., Lomber, S. G., Girard, P., and Bullier, J. (1998). Cortical feedback improves discrimination between figure and background by V1, V2, and V3 neurons. *Nature* 394: 784–787.

Hurlbert, A. (2000). Visual perception: Learning to see through noise. *Curr. Biol.* 10: R231–233.

Imbert, M., and Buisseret, P. (1975). Receptive field characteristics and plastic properties of visual cortical cells in kittens reared with or without visual experience. *Exp. Brain Res.* 22: 25–36.

Ingram, D. K. (1988). Motor performance variability during aging in rodents. *Ann. N. Y. Acad. Sci.* 515: 70–95.

Innocenti, G. M. (1986). Postnatal development of corticocortical connections. *Ital. J. Neurol. Sci.* 5: 25–28.

Innocenti, G. M., and Caminiti, R. (1980). Postnatal shaping of callosal connections from sensory areas. *Exp. Brain Res.* 38: 381–394.

Innocenti, G. M., and Frost, D. O. (1979). Effects of visual experience on the maturation of the efferent system to the corpus callosum. *Nature* 280: 231–234.

Innocenti, G. M., Fiore, L., and Caminiti, R. (1977). Exuberant projection into the corpus callosum from the visual cortex of newborn cats. *Neurosci. Lett.* 4: 237–242.

Intrator, N. (1992). Feature extraction using an unsupervised neural network. *Neural Comput.* 4: 98–107.

Intrator, N. (1993). Combining exploratory projection pursuit and projection pursuit regression. *Neural Comput.* 5: 443–455.

Intrator, N., and Edelman, S. (1997). Learning low-dimensional representations of visual objects with extensive use of prior knowledge. *Network* 8: 259–281.

Ippolito, M. F., and Tweney, R. (1995). The inception of insight. In *The Nature of Insight*, ed. R. J. Sternberg and J. E. Davidson. Cambridge, MA: MIT Press.

Irvine, D. R. F., and Rajan, R. (1996). Injury- and use-related plasticity in the primary sensory cortex of adult mammals: possible relationship to perceptual learning. *Clin. Exp. Pharmacol. Physiol.* 23: 939–947.

Irvine, D. R., Martin, R. L., Klimkeit, E., and Smith, R. (2000). Specificity of perceptual learning in a frequency discrimination task. *J. Acoust. Soc. Am.* 108: 2964–2968.

Ishai, A., and Sagi, D. (1995). Common mechanisms of visual imagery and perception. *Science* 268: 1772–1774.

Ito, M., Fujita, I., Tamura, H., and Tanaka, K. (1994). Processing of contrast polarity of visual images in inferotemporal cortex of the macaque monkey. *Cereb. Cortex* 5: 499–508.

Ito, M., Tamura, H., Fujita, I., and Tanaka, K. (1995). Size and position invariance of neuronal responses in monkey inferotemporal cortex. *J. Neurophysiol.* 73: 218–226.

Ito, M., Westheimer, G., and Gilbert, C. D. (1998). Attention and perceptual learning modulate contextual influences on visual perception. *Neuron* 20: 1191–1197.

Jacoby, L. L., and Dallas, M. (1981). On the relationship between autobiographical memory and perceptual learning. *J. Exp. Psychol. Gen.* 110: 306–340.

Jain, N., Catania, K. C., and Kaas, J. H. (1997). Deactivation and reactivation of somatosensory cortex after dorsal spinal cord injury. *Nature* 368: 495–498.

Jain, N., Florence, S. L., Qi, H. X., and Kaas, J. H. (2000). Growth of new brainstem connections in adult monkeys with massive sensory loss. *Proc. Natl. Acad. Sci. U S A* 97: 5546–5550.

James, W. (1890/1950). *Principles of Psychology*. Vol. 1. New York: Dover.

Jancke, J., Erlhagen, W., Dinse, H. R., Akhavan, A. C., Giese, M., Steinhage, A., and Schöner, G. (1999). Parametric population representation of retinal location: Neuronal interaction dynamics in cat primary visual cortex. *J. Neurosci.* 19: 9016–9028.

Jenkins, W. M., and Merzenich, M. M. (1987). Reorganization of neocortical representations after brain injury: A neurophysiological model of the bases of recovery from stroke. *Prog. Brain Res.* 71: 249–266.

Jenkins, W. M., Merzenich, M. M., Ochs, M. T., Allard, T., and Guic-Robles, E. (1990). Functional reorganization of primary somatosensory cortex in adult owl monkeys after behaviorally controlled tactile stimulation. *J. Neurophysiol.* 63: 82–104.

Jensen, A. R. (1966). Social class and perceptual learning. *Ment. Hyg.* 50: 226–239.

Johansson, G. (1973). Visual perception of biological motion and a model of its analysis. *Percept. Psychophys.* 14: 201–211.

Johnson, M. H., Dziurawiec, S., Ellis, H., and Morton, J. (1991). Newborns' preferential tracking of face-like stimuli and its subsequent decline. *Cognition* 40: 1–19.

Johnston, A., Hill, H., and Carman, N. (1992). Recognising faces: Effects of lighting direction, inversion and brightness reversal. *Perception* 21: 365–375.

Johnston, R. A., and Ellis, H. D. (1995). Age effects in the processing of typical and distinctive faces. *Q. J. Exp. Psychol.* 48: 447–465.

Johnston, R. A., Milne, A. B., Williams, C., and Hosie, J. (1997). Do distinctive faces come from outer space? An investigation of the status of a multidimensional face-space. *Vis. Cognit.* 4: 1–112.

Jolicoeur, P. (1990). Orientation congruency effects on the identification of disoriented shapes. *J. Exp. Psychol. Hum. Percept. Perform.* 16: 351–364.

Jones, E. G., and Pons, T. P. (1998). Thalamic and brainstem contributions to large-scale plasticity of primate somatosensory cortex. *Science* 282: 1121–1125.

Jones, M. J., and Poggio, T. A. (1995). Model-based matching by linear combinations of prototypes. In *Proceedings of the Fifth International Conference on Computer Vision*, Los Alamitos, CA: IEEE Press.

Jones, M. J., Sinha, P., Vetter, T., and Poggio, T. (1997). Top-down learning of low-level vision tasks. *Curr. Biol.* 7: 991–994.

Joseph, J. S., Chun, M. M., and Nakayama, K. (1997). Attentional requirements in a 'preattentive' feature search task. *Nature* 387: 805–807.

Joublin, F., Spengler, F., Wacquant, S., and Dinse, H. R. (1996). A columnar model of somatosensory reorganizational plasticity based on Hebbian and non-Hebbian learning rules. *Biol. Cybern.* 74: 275–286.

Juettner, M., Caelli, T., and Rentschler, I. I. (1997). Evidence-based pattern classification: A structural approach to human perceptual learning and generalization. *J. Math. Psychol.* 41: 244–259.

Julesz, B. (1971). *Foundations of Cyclopean Perception*. University of Chicago Press.

Julesz, B. (1981). Textons: The elements of texture perception and their interactions. *Nature* 290: 91–97.

Julesz, B. (1986). Texton gradients: The texton theory revisited. *Biol. Cybern.* 54: 245–251.

Julesz, B. (1990). Early vision is bottom-up except for focal attention. *Cold Spring Harb. Symp. Quant. Biol.* 55: 973–978.

Jürgens, M., and Dinse, H. R. (1995). Spatial and temporal integration properties of cortical somatosensory neurons in aged rats: Lack of age-related cortical changes in behaviorally unimpaired individuals of high age. *Soc. Neurosci. Abstr.* 21: 197.

Jürgens, M., and Dinse, H. R. (1997a). Use-dependent plasticity of SI cortical hindpaw neurons induced by modification of walking in adult rats: A model for age related alterations. *Soc. Neurosci. Abstr.* 23: 1800.

Jürgens, M., and Dinse, H. R. (1997b). Differential effects of the Ca^{2+}-influxblocker nimodipine on receptive field properties and response latencies of somatosensory cortical neurons in aged rats. In *Internal Report 96-10*, 1–23. Institut für Neuroinformatik, Ruhr-University, Bochum.

Jüttner, M., and Rentschler, I. (1996). Reduced perceptual dimensionality in extrafoveal vision. *Vision Res.* 36: 1007–1022.

Jutten, C., and Hérault, J. (1991). Blind separation of sources, part 1. An adaptive algorithm based on neuro-mimetic architecture. *Signal Proc.* 24: 1–10.

Kaas, J. H. (1991). Plasticity of sensory and motor maps in adult mammals. *Annu. Rev. Neurosci.* 14: 137–167.

Kaas, J. H. (1994). The reorganization of sensory and motor maps in adult mammals. In *The Cognitive Neurosciences*, ed. M. A. Gazzaniga. Cambridge, MA: MIT Press.

Kaas, J. H. (1999). Is most of neural plasticity in the thalamus cortical? *Proc. Natl. Acad. Sci. U S A* 96: 7622–7623.

Kaas, J., and Ebner, F. (1998). Intrathalamic connections: A new way to modulate cortical plasticity? *Nat. Neurosci.* 1: 341–342.

Kaas, J. H., and Florence, S. L. (1997). Mechanisms of reorganization in sensory systems of primates after peripheral nerve injury. *Adv. Neurol.* 73: 147–158.

Kaas, J. H., Florence, S. L., and Jain, N. (1999). Subcortical contributions to massive cortical reorganizations. *Neuron* 22: 657–660.

Kaas, J. H., Jain, N., and Florence, S. L. (1998). The re-activation of sensory cortex after deactivation by peripheral nerve or spinal cord injury. *Neurosci. News* 1: 12–17.

Kaas, J. H., Krubitzer, L. A., Chino, Y. M., Langston, A. L., Polley, E. H., and Blair, N. (1990). Reorganization of retinotopic cortical maps in adult mammals after lesions of the retina. *Science* 248: 229–231.

Kalarickal, G. J., and Marshall, J. A. (1999). Models of receptive-field dynamics in visual cortex. *Vis. Neurosci.* 16: 1055–1081.

Kanade, T. (1981). Recovery of the three-dimensional shape of an object from a single view. *Artif. Intell.* 17(1–3): 409–460.

Kandel, E. R., Schwartz, J. H., and Jessel, T. M. (1992). *Principles of Neural Science*, 3rd ed. New York: Elsevier and North-Holland.

Kanizsa, G. (1979). *Organization in Vision*. New York: Praeger.

Kapadia, M. K., Ito, M., Gilbert, C. D., and Westheimer, G. (1995). Improvement in visual sensitivity by changes in local context: Parallel studies in human observes and in V1 of alert monkeys. *Neuron* 15: 843–856.

Kaplan, C. A., and Simon, H. A. (1990). In search of insight. *Cogn. Psychol.* 22: 374–419.

Kapur, N., Abbott, P., Footitt, D., and Millar, J. (1996). Long-term perceptual priming in transient global amnesia. *Brain Cogn.* 31: 63–74.

Karhunen, J., Oja, E., Wang, L., Vigario, R., and Joutsenalo, J. (1997). A class of neural networks for independent component analysis. *IEEE Trans. Neural Networks* 8: 486–504.

Karhunen, J., Wang, L., and Joutsensalo, J. (1995). Neural estimation of basis vectors in independent component analysis. In *Proceedings of the International Conference on Neural Networks*, Paris.

Karni, A., and Bertini, G. (1997). Learning perceptual skills: Behavioral probes into adult cortical plasticity. *Curr. Opin. Neurobiol.* 7: 530–535.

Karni, A., and Sagi, D. (1991). Where practice makes perfect in texture discrimination: Evidence for primary visual cortex plasticity. *Proc. Natl. Acad. Sci. U S A* 88: 4966–4970.

Karni, A., and Sagi, D. (1993). The time-course of learning a visual skill. *Nature* 365: 250–252.

Karni, A., and Sagi, D. (1995). A memory system in the adult visual cortex. In B. Julesz and I. Kovács, eds., *Maturational Windows and Adult Cortical Plasticity*. SFI Studies in the Sciences of Complexity, vol. 24. Reading MA: Addison-Wesley.

Karni, A., Meyer, G., Jazzard, P., Adams, M. M., Turner, R., and Ungerleider, L. G. (1995). Functional MRI evidence for adult motor plasticity during motor skill learning. *Nature* 377: 155–158.

Karni, A., Meyer, G., Rey-Ipolito, C., Jezzard, P., Adams, M. M., Turner, R., and Ungerleider, L. G. (1998). The acquisition of skilled motor performance: Fast and slow experience driven changes in primary motor cortex. *Proc. Natl. Acad. Sci. U S A* 96: 861–868.

Karni, A., Tanne, D., Rubenstein, B. S., Askenasy, J. J., and Sagi, D. (1994). Dependence on REM sleep of overnight improvement of a perceptual skill. *Science* 265: 679–682.

Karni, A., Weisberg, J., Lalonde, F., and Ungerleider, L. G. (1995). An fMRI study of human visual cortex plasticity. *Soc. Neurosci. Abstr.* 21: 276.

Kasten E., and Sabel B. A. (1995). Visual field enlargement after computer training in brain-damaged patients with homonymous deficits: An open pilot trial. *Restor. Neurol. Neurosci.* 8: 113–127.

Kasten, E., Wüst, S., Behrens-Baumann, W., and Sabel, B. A. (1998). Computer-based training for the treatment of partial blindness. *Nat. Med.* 4: 1083–1087.

Katz, L. C., and Callaway, E. M. (1992). Development of local circuits in mammalian visual cortex. *Annu. Rev. Neurosci.* 15: 31–56.

Katz, L. C., and Shatz, C. J. (1996). Synaptic activity and the construction of cortical circuits. *Science* 274: 1133–1138.

Katz, L. C., Burkhalter, A., and Dreyer, W. J. (1984). Fluorescent latex microspheres as a retrograde neuronal marker for in vivo and in vitro studies of visual cortex. *Nature* 310: 498–500.

Kelahan, A. M., and Doetsch, G. S. (1984). Time-dependent changes in the functional organization of so-matosensory cerebral cortex following digit amputation. *Somatosens. Res.* 2: 49–81.

Kemp, R., Pike, G., White, P., and Musselman, A. (1996). Perception and recognition of normal and negative faces: The role of shape from shading and pigmentation cues. *Perception* 25: 37–52.

Kemp, R., Towell, N., and Pike, G. (1997). When seeing should not be believing: Photographs, credit cards and fraud. *Appl. Cogn. Psychol.* 11: 211–222.

Kempermann, G., Kuhn, H. G., and Gage, F. H. (1997). More hippocampal neurons in adult mice living in an enriched environment. *Nature* 386: 493–495.

Kerpelman, L. C. (1967). Stimulus dimensionality and manipulability in visual perceptual learning. *Child Dev.* 38: 563–571.

Kersteen-Tucker, Z. (1991). Long-term repetition priming with symmetrical polygons and words. *Mem. Cognit.* 19: 37–43.

Kew, J. M., Ridding, M. C., Rothwell, J. C., Passingham, R. E., Leigh, P. N., Sooriakumaran, D., Frackowiack, R. S. J., and Brooks, D. J. (1994). Reorganization of cortical blood flow and transcranial magnetic stimulation maps in human subjects after upper limp amputation. *J. Neurophysiol.* 72: 2517–2524.

Kilgard, M. P., and Merzenich, M. M. (1995). Anticipated stimuli across skin. *Nature* 373: 663.

Kilgard, M., and Merzenich, M. M. (1998). Cortical map reorganization enabled by nucleus basalis activity. *Science* 279: 1715–1718.

Killcross, A. S., Kiernan, M. J., Dwyer, D., and Westbrook, R. F. (1998). Effects of retention interval on latent inhibition and perceptual learning. *Q. J. Exp. Psychol. B.* 51: 59–74.

Kimura, A., Melis, F., and Asanuma, H. (1996). Long-lasting changes of neuronal activity in the motor cortex of cats. *NeuroReport* 22: 869–872.

Kimura, F., Nishigori, A., Shirokawa, T., and Tsumoto, T. (1989). Long-term potentiation and n-methyl-d-aspartate receptors in the visual cortex of young rats *J. Physiol.* 414: 125–144.

King, D. L., Shanks, S. C., and Hart, L. L. (1996). Discrimination learning decreases perceived similarity according to an objective measure. *Psychol. Res.* 59: 187–195.

Kirby, M., and Sirovich, L. (1990). Applications of the Karhunen-Loeve procedure for the characterisation of human faces. *IEEE Trans. Patt. Recog. Mach. Intell.* 12: 103–108.

Kirkwood, A., and Bear, M. F. (1994). Hebbian synapses in visual cortex. *J. Neurosci.* 14: 1634–1645.

Kirkwood, A., Rioult, M. G., and Bear, M. F. (1996). Experience-dependent modification of synaptic plasticity in visual cortex. *Nature* 381: 526–528.

Kisvárday, Z. F., and Eysel, U. T. (1992). Cellular organization of reciprocal patchy networks in layer III of cat visual cortex (area 17). *Neuroscience* 46: 275–286.

Kisvárday, Z. F., Cowey, A., Hodgson, A. J., and Somogyi, P. (1986). The relationship between GABA immunoreactivity and labelling by local uptake of [³H]GABA in the striate cortex of monkey. *Exp. Brain Res.* 62: 89–98.

Kisvárday, Z. F., Toth, E., Rausch, M., and Eysel, U. T. (1997). Orientation-specific relationship between populations of excitatory and inhibitory lateral connections in the visual cortex of the cat. *Cereb. Cortex* 7: 605–618.

Kleim, A. J., Swain, R. A., Armstrong, K. A., Napper, R. M. A., Jones, T. A., and Greenough, W. T. (1998). Selective synaptic plasticity within the cortex following complex motor skill learning. *Neurobiol. Learn. Mem.* 69: 274–289.

Knierim, J. J., and Van Essen, D. C. (1992). Neuronal responses to static texture patterns in area V1 of the alert macaque monkey. *J. Neurophysiol.* 67: 961–980.

Knierim, J. J., Kudrimoti, H. S., and McNaughton, B. L. (1995). Place cells, head direction cells, and the learning of landmark stability. *J. Neurosci.* 15: 1648–1659.

Knight, B., and Johnston, A. (1997). The role of movement in face recognition. *Vis. Cognit.* 4: 265–274.

Kobatake, E., and Tanaka, K. (1994). Neuronal selectivities to complex object features in the ventral visual pathway of the macaque cerebral cortex. *J. Neurophysiol* 71: 856–867.

Kobatake, E., and Tanaka, K. (1998). Effects of shape-discrimination training on the selectivity of inferotemporal cells in adult monkeys. *J. Neurophysiol.* 80: 324–330.

Kobatake, E., Wang, G., and Tanaka, K. (1994). Neuronal selectivities to complex object features in the ventral visual pathway of the macaque cerebral cortex. *J. Neurophysiol.* 71: 856–867.

Kobotake, E., Wang, G., and Tanaka, K. (1998). Effects of shape-discrimination training on the selectivity of inferotemporal cells in adult monkeys. *J. Neurophysiol.* 80: 324–330.

Kodman, F. Jr. (1981). Perceptual-motor learning with moderately retarded persons. *Percept. Mot. Skills* 53: 25–26.

Koenderink, J., and Doorn, A. (1991). Affine structure from motion. *J. Opt. Soc. Am. A* 8: 377–385.

Koffka, K. (1935). *Principles of Gestalt Psychology.* New York: Harcourt Brace.

Köhler, W. (1925). *The Mentality of Apes.* London: Routledge and Kegan Paul.

Köhler, W. (1947). *Gestalt Psychology.* New York: Liveright.

Kohonen, T. (1982). Self-organized formation of topologically correct feature maps. *Biol. Cybern.* 43: 59–69.

Kolb, B. (1999). Synaptic plasticity and the organization of behavior after early and late brain injury. *Can. J. Exp. Psychol.* 53: 62–75.

Kolb, B., and Wishaw, I. Q. (1998). Brain plasticity and behavior. *Annu. Rev. Psychol.* 49: 43–64.

König, P., Engel, A. K., Löwel, S., and Singer, W. (1993). Squint affects synchronization of oscillatory responses in cat visual cortex. *Eur. J. Neurosci.* 5: 501–508.

Konorski, J. (1967). *Integrative Activity of the Brain.* Chicago: University of Chicago Press.

Kopp, B., Kunkel, A., Mühlnickel, W., Villringer, K., Taub, E., and Flor, H. (1999). Plasticity in motor system correlated with therapy-induced improvement of movement after stroke. *NeuroReport* 10: 807–810.

Kornblith, H. (1985). *Naturalizing Epistemology.* Cambridge, MA: MIT Press.

Kossel, A., Bonhoeffer, T., and Bolz, J. (1990). Non-Hebbian synapses in rat visual cortex. *NeuroReport* 1: 115–118.

Kovach, J. K. (1985). Constitutional biases in early perceptual learning: III. Similarities and differences between artificially selected and imprinted color preferences in quail chicks (*Coturnix coturnix japonica*). *J. Comp. Psychol.* 99: 35–46.

Kovach, J. K., Fabricius, E., and Fält, L. (1966). Relationships between imprinting and perceptual learning. *J. Comp. Physiol. Psychol.* 61: 449–454.

Krekling, S., Tellevik, J. M., and Nordvik, H. (1989). Tactual learning and cross-modal transfer of an oddity problem in young children. *J. Exp. Child Psychol.* 47: 88–96.

Krüger, J. (1989). Multiple recordings of neuronal properties and spatial distributions in monkey visual cortex. *J. Physiol.* 413.

Krupa, D. J., Ghazanfar, A. A., and Nicolelis, M. A. (1999). Immediate thalamic sensory plasticity depends on corticothalamic feedback. *Proc. Natl. Acad. Sci. U S A* 96: 8200–8205.

Kuffler, S. W. (1953). Discharge patterns and functional organization of the mammalian retina. *J. Neurophysiol.* 16: 37–68.

Kujala, T., Alho, K., Huotilainen, M., Ilmoniemi, R. J., Lehtokoki, A., Leinonen, A., Rinne, T., Salonen, O., Snikkonen, J., Standertskjöld-Nordenstam, C.-G., and Näätänen, R. (1997). Electrophysiological evidence for cross-modal plasticity in humans with early- and late-onset blindness. *Psychophysiology* 34: 213–16.

Kujala, T., Alho, K., Kekoni, J., Hämäläinen, H., Reinikainen, K., Salonen, O., Standertskjöld, C. G., and Näätänen, R. (1995). Auditory and somatosensory event-related potentials in early blind humans. *Exp. Brain Res.* 104: 519–526.

Kulikowski, J. J., Abadi, R., and King-Smith, P. E. (1973). Orientation selectivity of grating and line detectors in human vision. *Vision Res.* 13: 1479–1486.

Kyriazi, H. T., Carvell, G. E., Brumberg, J. C., and Simons, D. J. (1996). Quantitative effects of GABA and bicuculline

methiodide on receptive field properties of neurons in real and simulated whisker barrels. *J. Neurophysiol.* 75: 547–560.

LaBerge, D. (1976). Perceptual learning and attention. In W. K. Estes, ed., *Handbook of Learning and Cognitive Processes*, vol. 4, pp. 237–273. Hillsdale, NJ: Erlbaum.

Lamdan, Y., Schwartz, J., and Wolfson, H. (1988). Object recognition by affine invariant matching. In *Proceedings of the IEEE Conference on Computer Vision and Pattern Recognition*, vol. 1, pp. 335–344.

Land, E. H. (1983). Recent advances in Retinex theory and some implications for cortical computations. *Proc. Natl. Acad. Sci. U S A* 80: 5163–5169.

Land, E. H., and McCann, J. J. (1971). Lightness and Retinex theory. *J. Opt. Soc. Am.* 61: 1–11.

Lander, K. (1999). The role of dynamic information in the recognition of famous faces. Unpublished PhD thesis, University of Stirling.

Lander, K., and Bruce, V. (2000). Recognizing famous faces: Exploring the benefits of facial motion. *Ecol. Psychol.* 12: 259–272.

Lander, K., Christie, F., and Bruce, V. (1999). The role of movement in the recognition of famous faces. *Mem. Cognit.* 27: 974–985.

Landy, M., Maloney, L., Johnston, E., and Young, M. (1995). Measurement and modeling of depth cue combination: In defense of weak fusion. *Vision Res.* 35(3): 389–412.

Laubach, M., Wessberg, J., and Nicolelis, M. A. (2000). Cortical ensemble activity increasingly predicts behaviour outcomes during learning of a motor task. *Nature* 405: 567–571.

Law, C. C., and Cooper, L. N. (1994). Formation of receptive fields in realistic visual environments according to the Bienenstock, Cooper and Munro (BCM) theory. *Proc. Natl. Acad. Sci. U S A* 91: 7797–7801.

Lawrence, D. H. (1952). The transfer of discrimination along a continuum. *J. Comp. Physiol. Psychol.* 45: 511–516.

Layton, A. (1972). Body imagery in perceptual learning. *Am. J. Optom. Arch. Am. Acad. Optom.* 49: 840–846.

Leder, H., and Bruce, V. (1998). Local and relational aspects of facial distinctiveness. *Q. J. Exp. Psychol.* 51: 449–473.

Lee, C. J., and Whitsel, B. L. (1992). Mechanisms underlying somatosensory cortical dynamics: 1. In vivo studies. *Cereb. Cortex* 2: 81–106.

Lee, D. K., Koch, C., and Braun, J. (1997). Spatial vision thresholds in the near absence of attention. *Vision Res.* 37: 2409–2418.

Lee, T.-W., Bell, A. J., and Lambert, R. (1997). Blind separation of delayed and convolved sources. In *Advances in Neural Information Processing Systems*, vol. 9, pp. 758–764. Cambridge, MA: MIT Press.

Lee, T.-W., Girolami, M., and Sejnowski, T. J. (1999). Independent component analysis using an extended infomax algorithm for mixed subgaussian and supergaussian sources. *Neural Comput.* 11: 417–441.

Leek, M. R., and Watson, C. S. (1988). Auditory perceptual learning of tonal patterns. *Percept. Psychophys.* 43: 389–394.

Leen, T. K., and Kambhatla, N. (1994). Fast non-linear dimension reduction. In J. D. Cowan, G. Tesauro, and J. Alspector, eds., *Advances in Neural Information-Processing Systems*, vol. 6, pp. 152–159. San Francisco: Morgan Kaufmann.

Legge, G. E., and Foley, J. M. (1980). Contrast masking in human vision. *J. Opt. Soc. Am.* 70: 1458–1471.

Leonards, U., Rettenbach, R., and Sireteanu, R. (1998). Parallel visual search is not always effortless. *Brain Res. Cogn. Brain Res.* 7: 207–213.

Lepore, F., and Guillemot, J. P. (1982). Visual receptive field properties of cells innervated through the corpus callosum in the cat. *Exp. Brain Res.* 46: 413–424.

Levänen, S., Jousmäki, V., and Hari, R. (1998). Vibration-induced auditory cortex activation in a congenitally deaf adult. *Curr. Biol.* 8: 869–872.

Levi, D. M., and Polat, U. (1996). Neural plasticity in adults with amblyopia. *Proc. Natl. Acad. Sci. U S A* 93: 6830–6834.

Levin, D. T., and Beale, J. M. (2000). Categorical perception occurs in newly learned faces, other-race faces, and inverted faces. *Percept. Psychophys.* 62(2): 386–401.

Levitt, L., and Bennett, T. L. (1975). The effects of crowding under different rearing conditions on emotionality and transfer of perceptual learning. *Behav. Biol.* 15: 65–72.

Levy, W. J., Amassian, V. E., Traad, M., and Cadwell, J. (1990). Focal magnetic coil stimulation reveals motor cortical system reorganized in humans after traumatic hemiplegia. *Brain Res.* 510: 130–134.

Lewicki, M. S., and Olshausen, B. A. (1999). Probabilistic framework for the adaptation and comparison of image codes. *J. Opt. Soc. Am. A* 16: 1587–1601.

Li, L., Miller, E. K., and Desimone, R. (1993). The representation of stimulus familiarity in anterior inferior temporal cortex. *J. Neurophysiol.* 69: 1918–1929.

Liberman, A. M., Harris, K. S., Hoffman, H. S., and Griffith, B. C. (1957). The discrimination of speech sounds within and across phoneme boundaries. *J. Exp. Psychol.* 54: 358–368.

Liepert, J., Miltner, W. H. R., Bauder, H., Sommer, M., Dettmers, C., Taub, E., and Weiller, C. (1998). Motor cortex plasticity during contraint-induced movement therapy in stroke patients. *Neurosci. Lett.* 250: 5–8.

Liepert, J., Tegenthoff, M., and Malin, J. P. (1995). Changes of cortical motor area size during immobilization. *Electroenceph. Clin. Neurophysiol.* 97: 382–386.

Liepert, J., Terborg, C., and Weiller, C. (1999). Motor plasticity induced by synchronized thumb and foot movements. *Exp. Brain Res.* 125: 435–439.

Linsker, R. (1988). Self-organization in a perceptual network. *Computer* 21: 105–117.

Linsker, R. (1992). Local synaptic learning rules suffice to maximize mutual information in a linear network. *Neural Comput.* 4: 691–702.

Lissauer, I. (1890). Ein Fall von Seelenblindheit nebst einem Beitrage zur Theorie derselben. *Archiv für Psychiatrie und Nervenkrankheiten* 21: 222–270.

Liu, Z. (1999). Perceptual learning in motion discrimination that generalizes across motion directions. *Proc. Natl. Acad. Sci. U S A* 96: 14085–14087.

Liu, Z., and Vaina, L. M. (1998). Simultaneous learning of motion discrimination in two directions. *Cogn. Brain Res.* 6: 347–349.

Liu, Z., and Weinshall, D. (2000). Mechanisms of generalization in perceptual learning. *Vision Res.* 40: 97–109.

Livingstone, M. S., and Hubel, D. H. (1984). Specificity of intrinsic connections in primate primary visual cortex. *J. Neurosci.* 4: 2830–2835.

Lobley, K., and Walsh, V. (1998). Perceptual learning in visual conjunction search. *Perception* 27: 1245–1255.

Locke, J. (1690/1939). *An Essay Concerning Human Understanding.* In *The English Philosphers from Bacon to Mill,* ed. E. A. Burtt. New York: Random House.

Locke, J. (1708). *Some Familiar Letters between Mr. Locke and Several of His Friends.* London: A. and J. Churchill.

Locke, J. (1721). *An Essay Concerning Human Understanding,* 8th ed. London: A. Churchill and A. Manship; and Sold by W. Taylor, at the Ship and Black Swan in Paternoster Row.

Lockwood, A. H., Salvi, R. J., Coad, M. L., Towsley, M. L., Wack, D. S., and Murphy, B. W. (1998). The functional neuroanatomy of tinnitus: Evidence for limbic system links and neural plasticity. *Neurology* 50: 114–120.

Logothetis, N. K., and Pauls, J. (1995). Psychophysical and physiological evidence for viewer-centered object representations in the primate. *Cereb. Cortex* 5: 270–288.

Logothetis, N. K., Pauls, J., and Poggio, T. (1995). Shape representation in the inferior temporal cortex of monkeys. *Curr. Biol.* 5: 552–563.

Logothetis, N. K., and Sheinberg, D. L. (1996). Visual object recognition. *Annu. Rev. Neurosci.* 19: 577–621.

Losada, M. A., and Mullen, K. T. (1994). The spatial tuning of chromatic mechanisms identified by simultaneous masking. *Vision Res.* 34: 331–341.

Lotze, M., Grodd, W., Birbaumer, N., Erb, M., Huse, E., and Flor, H. (1999). Does use of a myoelectric prosthesis prevent cortical reorganization and phantom limb pain? *Nat. Neurosci.* 2: 501–502.

Lowe, D. (1984). Perceptual organization and visual recognition. Ph.D. diss., Stanford University.

Löwel, S. (1994). Ocular dominance column development: Strabismus changes the spacing of adjacent columns in cat visual cortex. *J. Neurosci.* 14: 7451–7468.

Löwel, S., and Singer, W. (1992). Selection of intrinsic horizontal connections in the visual cortex by correlated neuronal activity. *Science* 255: 209–212.

Lübke, J., and Albus, K. (1992). Rapid rearrangement of intrinsic tangential connections in the striate cortex of normal and dark-reared kittens: Lack of exuberance beyond the second postnatal week. *J. Comp. Neurol.* 323: 42–58.

Ludvigh, E. (1953). Direction sense of the eye. *Am. J. Ophthalmol.* 36: 139–142.

Lueschow, A., Miller, E. K., and Desimone, R. (1994). Inferior temporal mechanisms for invariant object recognition. *Cereb. Cortex* 5: 523–531.

Luhmann, H. J., and Prince, D. A. (1991). Control of NMDA receptor–mediated activity by GABAergic mechanisms in mature and developing rat neocortex. *Dev. Brain Res.* 54: 287–290.

Luhmann, H. J., Martínez-Millán, L., and Singer, W. (1986). Development of horizontal intrinsic connections in cat striate cortex. *Exp. Brain Res.* 63: 443–448.

Luhmann, H. J., Singer, W., and Martínez-Millán, L. (1990). Horizontal interactions in cat striate cortex: 1. Anatomical substrate and postnatal development. *Eur. J. Neurosci.* 2: 344–357.

Lund, J. S. (1973). Organization of neurons in the visual cortex, area 17, of the monkey (*Macaca mulatta*). *J. Comp. Neurol.* 147: 455–496.

Lund, J. S. (1988). Anatomical organization of macaque monkey striate visual cortex. *Annu. Rev. Neurosci.* 11: 253–288.

Lund, R. D., Mitchell, D. E., and Henry, G. H. (1978). Squint-induced modification of callosal connections in cats. *Brain Res.* 144: 169–172.

Luria, A. R. (1963). *The Working Brain.* Harmondsworth: Penguin.

Lütkenhöner, B. (1996). Current dipole localization with an ideal magnetometer system. *IEEE* 43(11): 1049–1061.

Lütkenhöner, B., Hoke, M., and Pantev, C. (1990). Use of biomagnetic examination procedures in audiology. *Biomed Tech* 35(Suppl. 3): 154–155.

Lutzer, V. D. (1986). Perceptual learning by educable mentally retarded, average, and gifted children of primary school age. *Percept. Mot. Skills* 62: 959–966.

Lutzer, V. D. (1987). Perceptual learning of a non-focal color discrimination between ages three and six. *J. Gen. Psychol.* 114: 273–279.

Mackintosh, N. J., Kaye, H., and Bennett, C. H. (1991). Perceptual learning in flavour aversion conditioning. *Q. J. Exp. Psychol. B.* 43: 297–322.

Maclin, E. L., Rose, D. F., Knight, J. E., Orrison, W. W., and Davis, L. E. (1994). Somatosensory evoked magnetic fields in patients with stroke. *Electroenc. Clin. Neurophysiol.* 91: 468–475.

Maddox, W. T., and Bohil, C. J. (2001). Feedback effects on cost-benefit learning in perceptual categorization. *Mem. Cognit.* 29: 598–615.

Maffei, L., Fiorentini, A., and Bisti, S. (1973). Neural correlate to perceptual adaptation to gratings. *Science* 182: 1036–1103.

Makeig, S. (1993). Auditory event-related dynamics of the EEG spectrum and effects of exposure to tones. *Electroenc. Clin. Neurophysiol.* 86: 283–293.

Malach, R., Amir, Y., Harel, M., and Grinvald, A. (1993). Relationship between intrinsic connections and functional architecture revealed by optical imaging and in vivo targeted biocytin injections in primate striate cortex. *Proc. Natl. Acad. Sci. U S A* 90: 10469–10473.

Malach, R., Tootell, R. B. H., and Malonek, D. (1994). Relationship between orientation domains, cytochrome oxidase stripes, and intrinsic horizontal connections in squirrel monkey area V2. *Cereb. Cortex* 4: 151–165.

Maldonado, P. E., and Gerstein, G. L. (1996a). Reorganization in the auditory cortex of the rat induced by intracortical microstimulation: A multiple single-unit study. *Exp. Brain Res.* 112: 420–430.

Maldonado, P. E., and Gerstein, G. L. (1996b). Neuronal assembly dynamics in the rat auditory cortex during reorganization induced by intracortical microstimulation. *Exp. Brain Res.* 112: 431–441.

Malkova, L., Mishkin, M., and Bachevalier J. (1995). Long-term effects of selective neonatal temporal lobe lesions on learning and memory in monkeys. *Behav. Neurosci.* 109: 212–226.

Marill, T. (1991). Emulating the human interpretation of line-drawings as three-dimensional objects. *Intl. J. Comput. Vis.* 6: 147–161.

Markam, H., Lübke, J., Frotscher, M., and Sakmann, B. (1997). Regulation of synaptic efficacy by coincidence of postsynaptic APs and EPSPs. *Science* 275: 213–15.

Markowitsch, H. J., and Harting, C. (1996). Interdependence of priming performance and brain-damage. *Int. J. Neurosci.* 85: 291–300.

Marks, L. E., Galanter, E., and Baird, J. C. (1995). Binaural summation after learning psychophysical functions for loudness. *Percept. Psychophys.* 57: 1209–1216.

Markson, L., and Bloom, P. (1997). Evidence against a dedicated system for word learning in children. *Nature* 385: 813–815.

Marquet, J., Van Durme, M., Lammens, J., Collier, R., Peeters, S., and Bosiers, W. (1986). Acoustic simulation experiments with preprocessed speech for an 8-channel cochlear implant. *Audiology* 25: 353–362.

Marr, D. (1970). A theory for cerebral neocortex. *Proc. R. Soc. Lond. B Biol. Sci.* 176: 161–234.

Marr, D. (1971). Simple memory: A theory for archicortex. *Philos. Trans. R. Soc. Lond. B Biol. Sci.* 262: 23–81.

Marr, D. (1982). *Vision*. San Francisco: Freeman.

Marr, D., and Hildreth, E. (1980). Theory of edge-detection. *Proc. R. Soc. Lond. B Biol. Sci.* 207: 187–217.

Marr, D., and Nishihara, H. (1978). Representation and recognition of the spatial organization of three-dimensional structure. *Proc. R. Soc. Lond. B Biol. Sci.* 200: 269–294.

Marr, D., and Poggio, T. (1977). From understanding computation to understanding neural circuitry. *Neurosci. Res. Prog. Bull.* 15: 470–488.

Martin, K. A. C., and Whitteridge, D. (1984). Form, function and intracortical projections of spiny neurones in the striate visual cortex of the cat. *J. Physiol.* 253: 463–504.

Martini, P., Girard, P., Morrone, M. C., and Burr, D. (1996). Sensitivity to spatial phase at equiluminance. *Vision Res.* 36: 1153–1162.

Masson, M. E. (1986). Identification of typographically transformed words: Instance-based skill acquisition. *J. Exp. Psychol. Learn. Mem. Cogn.* 12: 479–488.

Mato, G., and Sompolinsky, H. (1996). Neural network models of perceptual learning of angle discrimination. *Neural Comput.* 8: 270–299.

Matthews, N., Liu, Z., Geesaman, B. J., and Qian, N. (1999). Perceptual learning on orientation and direction discrimination. *Vision Res.* 39: 3692–3701.

Mayer, R. E. (1995). The search for insight: Grappling with Gestalt psychology's unanswered questions. In *The Nature of Insight*, ed. R. J. Sternberg and J. E. Davidson. Cambridge, MA: MIT Press.

McClelland, J. L., and Rumelhart, D. E. (1981). An interactive activation model of context effects in letter perception: 1. An account of basic findings. *Psychol. Rev.* 88: 375–407.

McGuire, B. A., Gilbert, C. D., Rivlin, P. K., and Wiesel, T. N. (1991). Targets of horizontal connections in macaque primary visual cortex. *J. Comp. Neurol.* 305: 370–392.

McIntosh, A. R., Rajah, M. N., and Lobaugh, N. J. (1999). Interactions of prefrontal cortex in relation to awareness in sensory learning. *Science* 284: 1531–1533.

McKee, S. P., and Westheimer, G. (1978). Improvement in vernier acuity with practice. *Percept. Psychophys.* 24: 258–262.

McLaren, I. P. (1997). Categorization and perceptual learning: An analogue of the face inversion effect. *Q. J. Exp. Psychol. A.* 50: 257–273.

Medin, D. L. (1989). Concepts and conceptual structure. *Am. Psychol.* 44: 1469–1481.

Meegan, D. V., Aslin, R. N., and Jacobs, R. A. (2000). Motor timing learned without motor training. *Nat. Neurosci.* 3: 860–862.

Meinhardt, G. (2001). Learning a grating discrimination task broadens human spatial frequency tuning. *Biol. Cybern.* 86: 383–400.

Meinhardt, G., and Grabbe, Y. (in press). Attentional control in learning to discriminate bars and gratings. *Exp. Brain Res.*

Melamed, L. E., and Arnett, W. B. (1984). The effect of familial sinistrality on perceptual learning. *Neuropsychologia* 22: 495–502.

Merigan, W. H., Nealy, T. A., and Maunsell, J. H. R. (1993). Visual effects of lesions of cortical area V2 in macaques. *J. Neurosci.* 13: 3180–3191.

Merzenich, M. M., and Jenkins, W. M. (1993). Reorganization of cortical representations of the hand following alterations of skin inputs induced by nerve injury, skin island transfer and experience. *J. Hand Ther.* 6: 89–103.

Merzenich, M. M., and White, M. (1980). Coding considerations in design of cochlear prostheses. *Ann. Otol. Rhinol. Laryngol.* 89: 84–87.

Merzenich, M. M., Jenkins, W. M., Johnston, P., Schreiner, C., Miller, S. L., and Tallal, P. (1996). Temporal processing deficits of language-learning impaired children ameliorated by training. *Nature* 271: 77–80.

Merzenich, M. M., Kaas, J. H., Wall, J., Nelson, R. J., Sur, M., and Felleman, D. (1983a). Topographic reorganization of somatosensory cortical areas 3b and 1 in adult monkeys following restricted deafferentation. *Neuroscience* 8: 33–55.

Merzenich, M. M., Kaas, J. H., Wall, J., Sur, M., Nelson, R. J., and Felleman, D. (1983b). Progression of changes following median nerve section in the cortical representation of the hand in areas 3b and 1 in adult owl and squirrel monkeys. *Neuroscience* 10: 639–665.

Merzenich, M. M., Nelson, R. J., Stryker, M. P., Cynader, M. S., Schoppmann, A., and Zook, J. M. (1984). Somatosensory cortical map changes following digit amputation in adult monkeys. *J. Comp. Neurol.* 224: 591–605.

Merzenich, M. M., Recanzone, G., Jenkins, W. M., Allard, T. T., and Nudo, R. J. (1988). Cortical representational plasticity. In P. Rakic and W. Singer eds., *Neurobiology of Neocortex*, 41–67. New York: Wiley.

Merzenich, M. M., Schreiner, C., Jenkins, W., and Wang, X. (1993). Neural mechanisms underlying temporal integration, segmentation, and input sequence representation: Some implications for the origin of learning disabilities. *Ann. N. Y. Acad. Sci.* 682: 1–22.

Merzenich, M., Wright, B., Jenkins, W., Xerri, C., Byl, N., Miller, S., and Tallal, P. (1996). Cortical plasticity underlying perceptual, motor, and cognitive skill development: implications for neurorehabilitation. *Cold Spring Harb. Symp. Quant. Biol.* 61: 1–8.

Miller, E. K., Li, L., and Desimone, R. (1991). A neural mechanism for working and recognition memory in inferior temporal cortex. *Science* 254: 1377–1379.

Miller, K. D. (1988). Correlation-based models of neural development. In M. Gluck and D. Rumelhart, eds., *Neuroscience and Connectionist Theory*, pp. 267–353. Hillsdale, NJ: Erlbaum.

Miller, K. D., Keller, J. B., and Stryker, M. P. (1989). Ocular dominance column development: Analysis and simulation. *Science* 245: 605–615.

Millodot, M. (1965). Stabilized retinal images and disappearance time. *Br. J. Physiol. Opt.* 22: 148–152.

Miltner, W. H., Braun, C., Arnold, M., Witte, H., and Taub, E. (1999). Coherence of gamma-band EEG activity as a basis for associative learning. *Nature* 397: 434–436.

Minsky, M., and Papert, S. (1969). *Perceptrons.* Cambridge, MA: MIT Press.

Missal, M., Vogels, R., and Orban, G. A. (1997). Responses of macaque inferior temporal neurons to overlapping shapes. *Cereb. Cortex* 7: 758–767.

Mitchison, G., and Crick, F. (1982). Long axons within the striate cortex: Their distribution, orientation, and patterns of connection. *Proc. Natl. Acad. Sci. U S A* 79: 3661–3665.

Mittmann, T., and Eysel, U. T. (2001). Increased synaptic plasticity in the surround of rat visual cortex lesions. *NeuroReport* 12: 3341–3347.

Mittmann, T., Luhmann, H. J., Schmidt-Kastner, R., Eysel, U. T., and Heinemann, U. (1994). Lesion-induced transient suppression of inhibitory function in rat neocortex *in vitro. Neuroscience* 60: 891–906.

Miyashita, Y. (1988). Neural correlate of visual associative long-term memory in the primate temporal cortex. *Nature* 335: 817–820.

Miyashita, Y. (1993). Inferior temporal cortex: Where visual perception meets memory. *Annu. Rev. Neurosci.* 16: 245–263.

Miyashita, Y., Date, A., and Okuno, H. (1993). Configurational encoding of complex visual forms by single neurons of monkey temporal cortex. *Neuropsychologia* 31: 1119–1131.

Miyashita, Y., Okuno, H., Tokuyama, W., Ihara, T., and Nakajima, K. (1996). Feedback signal from medial temporal lobe mediates visual associative mnemonic codes of inferotemporal neurons. *Cogn. Brain Res.* 5: 81–86.

Mogilner, A., Grossman, J. A. I., Ribary, U., Joliot, M., Volkmann, J., Rapaport, D., Beasley, R. W., and Llinás, R. R. (1993). Somatosensory cortical plasticity in adult humans revealed by magnetoencephalography. *Proc. Natl. Acad. Sci. U.S.A.* 90: 3593–3597.

Mollon, J. D., and Danilova, M. V. (1996). Three remarks on perceptual learning. *Spat. Vis.* 10: 51–58.

Montague, P. R., and Sejnowski, T. J. (1994). The predictive brain: Temporal coincidence and temporal order in synaptic learning mechanisms. *Learn. Mem.* 1: 1–33.

Moore, C., and Cavanagh, P. (1998). Recovery of 3D volume from 2-tone images of novel objects. *Cognition* 67: 45–71.

Moore, D. R., and Kowalchuk, N. E. (1988). Auditory brainstem of the ferret: Effects of unilateral cochlear lesions on cochlear nucleus volume, and projections to the inferior colliculus. *J. Comp. Neurol.* 272: 503–515.

Moran, J., and Desimone, R. (1985). Selective attention gates visual processing in extrastriate cortex. *Science* 229: 782–784.

Morgan, M. J., and Baldassi, S. (1997). How the human visual system encodes the orientation of a texture, and why it makes mistakes. *Curr. Biol.* 7: 999–1002.

Morrone, M. C., Burr, D. C., and Maffei, L. (1982). Functional implications of cross-orientation inhibition of cortical visual cells: 1. Neurophysiological evidence. *Proc. R. Soc. Lond. B Biol. Sci.* 216: 335–354.

Morrone, M. C., Burr, D. C., and Spinelli, D. (1989). Discrimination of spatial phase in central and peripheral vision. *Vision Res.* 29: 433–445.

Moses, Y., Schechtman, G., and Ullman, S. (1990). Self-calibrated collinearity detector. *Biol. Cybern.* 63: 463–475.

Motter, B. C. (1993). Focal attention produces spatially selective processing in visual cortical areas V1, V2, and V4 in the presence of competing stimuli. *J. Neurophysiol.* 70: 909–919.

Mountcastle, V. B., Steinmetz, M. A., and Romo, R. (1990). Frequency discrimination in the sense of flutter: Psychophysical measurements correlated with postcentral events in behaving monkeys. *J. Neurosci.* 10: 3032–3044.

Movshon, J. A., and Blakemore, C. B. (1973). Orientation specificity and spatial selectivity in human vision. *Perception* 2: 53–60.

Movshon, J. A., and Lennie, P. (1979). Pattern selective adaptation in visual cortical neurones. *Nature* 278: 850–852.

Mühlnickel, W., Elbert, T., Taub, E., and Flor, H. (1998). Reorganization of auditory cortex in tinnitus. *Proc. Natl. Acad. Sci. U.S.A.* 95: 10340–10343.

Müller, M. M., Bosch, J., Elbert, T., Kreiter, A., Valdes Sosa, M., Valdes Sosa, P., Rockstroh, B. (1996). Visually induced gamma band responses in human EEG. A link to animal studies. *Exp. Brain Res.* 112: 96–112.

Müller, M. M., Junghöfer, M., Elbert, T., and Rockstroh, B. (1997). Visually induced gamma-band responses to coherent and incoherent motion: A replication. *NeuroReport* 8(11): 2575–2579.

Mullen, K. T. (1985). The contrast sensitivity of human colour vision to red-green and blue-yellow gratings. *J. Physiol. (Lond.)* 359: 381–400.

Mumford, D. (1992). On the computational architecture of the neocortex: 2. The role of cortico-cortical loops. *Biol. Cybern.* 66: 241–251.

Mundy, J., and Zisserman, A. (1992). Introduction: Towards a new framework for vision. In J. Mundy and A. Zisserman, eds., *Geometric Invariance in Computer Vision*, pp. 1–39. Cambridge, MA: MIT Press.

Murayama, Y., Fujita, I., and Kato, M. (1997). Contrasting forms of synaptic plasticity in monkey inferotemporal and primary visual cortices. *NeuroReport* 8: 1503–1508.

Murray, E. A., Gaffan, D., and Mishkin, M. (1993). Neural substrates of visual stimulus-stimulus association in rhesus monkeys. *J. Neurosci.* 13: 4549–4561.

Nachmias, J., and Sansbury, R. V. (1974). Grating contrast: Discrimination may be better than detection. *Vision Res.* 14: 1039–1042.

Nachmias, J., and Weber, A. (1975). Discrimination of simple and complex gratings. *Vision Res.* 15: 217–223.

Nadal, J.-P., and Parga, N. (1994). Non-linear neurons in the low noise limit: A factorial code maximizes information transfer. *Network* 5: 565–581.

Nadol, J. B., Young, Y., and Glynn, R. J. (1989). Survival of spiral ganglion cells in profound sensory neural hearing loss: Implications for cochlear implantation. *Ann. Otol. Rhinol. Laryngol.* 98: 411–416.

Nagarajan, S. S., Blake, D. T., Wright, B. A., Byl, N., and Merzenich, M. M. (1998). Practice-related improvements in somatosensory interval discrimination are temporally specific but generalize across skin location, hemisphere, and modality. *J. Neurosci.* 18: 1559–1570.

Nakamura, H., Gattass, R., Desimone, R., and Ungerleider, L. G. (1993). The modular organization of projections from areas V1 and V2 to areas V4 and TEO in macaques. *J. Neurosci.* 13: 3681–3691.

Nakayama, K. (1991). The iconic bottleneck and the tenuous link between early visual processing and perception. In C. Blakemore, ed., *Vision: Coding and Efficiency*, 411–422. Cambridge: Cambridge University Press.

Nazir, T. A., and O'Regan, J. K. (1990). Some results on translation invariance in the human visual system. *Spat. Vis.* 5: 81–100.

Nelson, C. A. (1999). Neural plasticity and human development: The role of early experience in sculpting memory systems. *Psychol. Sci.* 8: 42–45.

Nelson, C. A., and Bloom. F. (1997). Child development and neuroscience. *Child Dev.* 68(5): 970–987.

Nelson, J. I., and Frost, B. J. (1978). Orientation-selective inhibition from beyond the classical receptive field. *Exp. Brain Res.* 139: 359–365.

Nelson, R. B., Friedman, D. P., O'Neill, J. B., Mishkin, M., and Routtenberg, A. (1987). Gratients of protein kinase C substrate phosphorylation in primate visual system peak in visual memory storage areas. *Brain Res.* 416: 387–392.

Nevatia, R., and Binford, T. (1977). Description and recognition of curved objects. *Artif. Intell.* 8: 77–98.

Newell, F., Chiroro, P., and Valentine, T. (1999). Recognising unfamiliar faces: The effects of distinctiveness and view. *Q. J. Exp. Psychol. A* 52: 509–534.

Nicolelis, M. A. L., ed. (1999). *Methods in Neural Ensemble Recordings.* New York: CRC Press.

Nicolelis, M. A., Ghazanfar, A. A., Faggin, B. M., Votaw S., and Oliveira L. M. (1989). Reconstructing the engram: Simultaneous, multisite, many single neuron recordings. *Neuron* 18: 529–537.

Nicolelis, M. A., Ghazanfar, A. A., Stambaugh, C. R., Oliveira, L. M., Laubach, M., Chapin, J. K., Nelson, R. J., and Kaas, J. H. (1998). Simultaneous encoding of tactile information by three primate cortical areas. *Nat. Neurosci.* 1: 621–630.

Nicolelis, M. A., Katz, D., and Krupa, D. J. (1998). Potential circuit mechanisms underlying concurrent thalamic and cortical plasticity. *Rev. Neurosci.* 9: 213–224.

Nicolelis, M. A., Lin, R. C., and Chapin, J. K. (1997). Neonatal whisker removal reduces the discrimination of tactile stimuli by thalamic ensembles in adult rats. *J. Neurophysiol.* 78: 1691–1706.

Nicolelis, M. A., Lin, R. C., Woodward, D. J., and Chapin, J. K. (1993). Induction of immediate spatiotemporal changes in thalamic networks by peripheral block of ascending cutaneous information. *Nature* 361: 533–536.

Niebur, E., and Koch, C. (1994). A model for the neuronal implementation of selective visual attention based on temporal correlation among neurons. *J. Comput. Neurosci.* 1: 141–158.

Nordern, K. W., Killackoy, H. P., and Kitzes, L. M. (1983). Ascending projections to the inferior colliculus following unilateral cochlear ablation in the neonatal gerbil, *Mexiones unguiculatus. J. Comp. Neurol.* 214: 144–153.

Nosofsky, R. M. (1988). Exemplar-based accounts of relations between classification, recognition, and typicality. *J. Exp. Psychol. Learn. Mem. Cognit.* 14: 700–708.

Nothdurft, H. C. (1985). Orientation sensitivity and texture segmentation in patterns with different line orientation. *Vision Res.* 25(4): 551–560.

Nothdurft, H. C. (1992). Feature analysis and the role of similarity in preattentive vision. *Percept. Psychophys.* 52: 355–375.

Nudo, R. J., Jenkins, W. M., and Merzenich, M. M. (1990). Repetitive microstimulation alters the cortical representation of movements in adult rats. *Somatosen. Mot. Res.* 7: 463–483.

Nygaard, L. C., and Pisoni, D. B. (1998). Talker-specific learning in speech perception. *Percept. Psychophys.* 60: 355–376.

Obata, S., Obata, J., Das, A., and Gilbert, C. D. (1999). Molecular correlates of topographic reorganization in primary visual cortex following retinal lesions. *Cereb. Cortex* 9: 238–248.

Odom, R. D., McIntyre, C. W., and Neale, G. S. (1971). The influence of cognitive style on perceptual learning. *Child Dev.* 42: 883–891.

O'Donnell, C., and Bruce, V. (2001). Familiarisation with faces selectively enhances sensitivity to changes made to the eyes. *Perception* 30: 755–764.

Ohl, F., and Scheich, H. (1997). Learning-induced dynamic receptive field changes in primary auditory cortex (A1) of the unanaestetized mongolian gerbil. *J. Comp. Physiol.* A181: 685–696.

Ohzawa, I., Schlar, G., and Freeman, R. D. (1982). Contrast gain control in the cat's visual cortex. *Nature* 298: 5871–5873.

Oja, E. (1989). Neural networks, principal components and linear neural networks. *Neural Networks* 5: 927–935.

O'Keefe, J., and Nadel, L. (1978). *The Hippocampus as a Cognitive Map.* Oxford: Clarendon Press.

Olshausen, B. A., and Field, D. J. (1996). Natural image statistics and efficient coding. *Network Comput. Neural Syst.* 7: 333–339.

Olshausen, B. A., and Field, D. J. (1997). Sparse coding with an overcomplete basis set: a strategy employed by V1? *Vision Res.* 37: 3311–3325.

Omohundro, S. M. (1987). Efficient algorithms with neural network behavior. *Complex Syst.* 1: 273–347.

Oram, M. W., and Perrett, D. I. (1992). Time course of neural responses discriminating different views of the face and head. *J. Neurophysiol.* 68: 70–84.

O Scalaidhe, S. P., Wilson, F. A. W., and Goldman-Rakic, P. S. (1997). Areal segregation of face-processing neurons in prefrontal cortex. *Science* 278: 1135–1138.

Osgood, C. E. (1949). The similarity paradox in human learning: A resolution. *Psychol. Rev.* 56: 132–143.

O'Toole, A. J., and Kersten, D. J. (1992). Learning to see random-dot stereograms. *Perception* 21: 227–243.

Otsu, Y., Kimura, F., and Tsumoto, T. (1995). Hebbian induction of LTP in visual cortex: Perforated patch-clamp study in cultured neurons. *J. Neurophysiol.* 74: 2437–2444.

Owen, D. H., and Machamer, P. K. (1979). Bias-free improvement in wine discrimination. *Perception* 8: 199–209.

Palmer, S., Rosch, E., and Chase, P. (1981). Canonical perspective and the perception of objects. In J. Long and A. Baddeley, eds., *Attention and Performance IX*, 131–151. Hillsdale, NJ: Erlbaum.

Pantev, C., Oostenveld, R., Engelien, A., Ross, B., Roberts, L. E., and Hoke, M. (1998). Increased auditory cortical representation in musicians. *Nature* 392: 811–814.

Papathomas, T. V., Gorea, A., Feher, A., and Conway, T. E. (1999). Attention-based texture segregation. *Percept. Psychophys.* 61: 1399–1410.

Parker, A. J., and Newsome, W. T. (1998). Sense and the single neuron: Probing the physiology of perception. *Annu. Rev. Neurosci.* 21: 227–277.

Pascual-Leone, A., Cammarota, A., Wassermann, E. M., Brasil-Neto, J. P., Cohen, L. G., and Hallett, M. (1993). Modulation of motor cortical outputs to the reading hand of braille readers. *Ann. Neurol.* 34: 33–37.

Pascual-Leone, A., Peris, M., Tormos, J. M., and Catalá, M. D. (1996). Reorganization of human cortical output maps following traumatic forearm amputation. *Neuro-Report* 13(2): 2068–2070.

Pascual-Leone, A., and Torres, F. (1993). Plasticity of the sensorimotor cortex representation of the reading finger in Braille readers. *Brain* 116: 39–52.

Pascual-Leone, A., Wassermann, E. M., Sadato, N., and Hallett, M. (1995). The role of reading activity on the modulation of motor cortical outputs to the reading hand in Braille readers. *Ann. Neurol.* 38: 910–915.

Pashler, H. E. (1998). *The Psychology of Attention.* Cambridge, MA: MIT Press.

Pavlov, I. P. (1927). *Conditioned Reflexes*, pp. 121–122. Oxford: Oxford University Press.

Pei, X., Vidyasagar, T. R., Volgushev, M., and Creutzfeldt, O. D. (1994). Receptive field analysis and orientation selectivity of postsynaptic potentials of simple cells in cat visual cortex. *J. Neurosci.* 14: 7130–7140.

Pellegrino, L. J., Pellegrino, A. S., and Cushman, A. J. (1986). *A Stereotaxic Atlas of the Rat Brain*, 2nd ed. New York: Plenum.

Pelli, D. G. (1985). Uncertainty explains many aspects of visual contrast detection and discrimination. *J. Opt. Soc. Am. A* 2: 1508–1532.

Pentland, A. (1986). Perceptual organization and the representation of natural form. *Artif. Intell.* 28: 293–331.

Peres, R., and Hochstein, S. (1994). Modeling perceptual learning with multiple interacting elements: A neural network model describing early visual perceptual learning. *J. Comput. Neurosci.* 1: 323–338.

Pernberg, J., Jirmann, K. U., and Eysel, U. T. (1998). Structure and dynamics of receptive fields in the visual cortex of the cat (area 18) and the influence of GABAergic inhibition. *Europ. J. Neurosci.* 10: 3596–3606.

Perrett, D., Hietanen, J., Oram, M., and Benson, P. (1992). Organisation and functions of cells responsive to faces in the temporal cortex. *Philos. Trans. R. Soc. Lond. B Biol. Sci.* 335: 23–30.

Perrett, D. I., Mistlin, A. J., and Chitty, A. J. (1987). Visual neurones responsive to faces. *Trends Neurosci.* 10: 358–364.

Perrett, D. I., Rolls, E. T., and Caan, W. (1979). Temporal lobe cells of the monkey with visual responses selective for faces. *Neurosci. Lett. Suppl.* S3: S358.

Perrett, D. I., Rolls, E. T., and Caan, W. (1982). Visual neurones responsive to faces in the monkey temporal cortex. *Exp. Brain Res.* 47: 329–342.

Perrett, D. I., Smith, P. A. J., Potter, D. D., Mistlin, A. J., Head, A. S., Milner, A. D., and Jeeves, M. A. (1984). Neurones responsive to faces in the temporal cortex: Studies of functional organization, sensitivity to identity and relation to perception. *Hum. Neurobiol.* 3: 197–208.

Perrett, D. I., Smith, P. A. J., Potter, D. D., Mistlin, A. J., Head, A. S., Milner, A. D., and Jeeves, M. A. (1985). Visual cells in the temporal cortex sensitive to face view and gaze direction. *Proc. R. Soc. Lond. B Biol. Sci.* 223: 293–317.

Peters, A., and Kaiserman-Abramof, I. R. (1969). The small pyramidal neuron of the rat cerebral cortex: The synapses upon dendritic spines. *Z. Zellforsch. Mikroskop. Anat.* 100: 487–506.

Peters, A., Payne, B. R., and Rudd, J. (1994). A numerical analysis of the geniculocortical input to striate cortex in the monkey. *Cereb. Cortex* 4: 215–229.

Peterson, M. A., and Gibson, B. S. (1993). Shape recognition inputs to figure-ground organization in three-dimensional display. *Cogn. Psychol.* 25: 383–429.

Peterson, M. A., and Gibson, B. S. (1994). Must figure-ground organization precede object recognition? An assumption in peril. *Psychol. Sci.* 5: 253–259.

Petry, S., and Meyer, G., eds. (1987). *The Perception of Illusory Contours.* New York: Springer.

Pettet, M. W., and Gilbert, C. D. (1992). Dynamic changes in receptive-field size in cat primary visual cortex. *Proc. Natl. Acad. Sci. U S A* 89: 8366–8370.

Pettit, M. J., and Schwark, H. D. (1993). Receptive field reorganization in dorsal column nuclei during temporary denervation. *Science* 262: 2054–2056.

Pham, D. T., Garrat, P., and Jutten, C. (1992). Separation of a mixture of independent sources through a maximum likelihood approach. In *Proceedings of European Signal Processing Conference (EUSIPCO)*, pp. 771–774.

Phillips, P. J. (1998). Foundations of face recognition. In H. Wechsler et al., eds., *Face Recognition: From Theory to Applications.* Berlin: Springer.

Phillips, R. J. (1972). Why are faces hard to recognise in photographic negative? *Percept. Psychophys.* 12: 425–426.

Pigarev, I. N., Rizzolatti, G., and Scandolara, C. (1979). Neurons responding to visual stimuli in the frontal lobe of macaque monkeys. *Neurosci. Lett.* 12: 207–212.

Pike, G. E., Kemp, R. I., Towell, N. A., and Phillips, K. C. (1997). Recognising moving faces: The relative contribution of motion and perspective view information. *Vis. Cognit.* 4: 409–438.

Pisoni, D. B. (2000). Cognitive factors and cochlear implants: Some thoughts on perception, learning, and memory in speech perception. *Ear Hear.* 21: 70–78.

Pitts, W. and McCulloch, W. S. (1947/1965). How we know universals: The perception of auditory and visual forms. In *Embodiments of Mind*, 46–66. Reprint, Cambridge, MA: MIT Press, 1965.

Pizlo, Z. (1994). A theory of shape constancy based on perspective invariants. *Vision Res.* 34: 1637–1658.

Plaisted, K., O'Riordan, M., and Baron-Cohen, S. (1998). Enhanced discrimination of novel, highly similar stimuli by adults with autism during a perceptual learning task. *J. Child Psychol. Psychiatry* 39: 765–775.

Pleger, B., Dinse, H. R., Ragert, P., Schwenkreis, P., Malin, J. P., and Tegenthoff, M. (2001). Shifts in cortical representations predict human discrimination improvement. *Proc. Natl. Acad. Sci. U S A* 98: 12255–12260.

Poggio, T. (1990). A theory of how the brain might work. *Cold Spring Harb. Symp. Quant. Biol.* 55: 899–910.

Poggio, T., and Edelman, S. (1990). A network that learns to recognize three-dimensional objects. *Nature* 343: 263–266.

Poggio, T., Edelman, S., and Fahle, M. (1992). Learning of visual modules from examples: A framework for understanding adaptive visual performance. *Comput. Vis. Graph. Image Proc. Image Understand.* 56: 22–30.

Poggio, T., Fahle, M., and Edelman, S. (1992). Fast perceptual learning in visual hyperacuity. *Science* 256: 1018–1021.

Poggio, T., and Girosi, F. (1990). Regularization algorithms for learning that are equivalent to multilayer networks. *Science* 247: 978–982.

Poggio, T. A., and Vetter, T. (1992). Recognition and structure from one 2-D model view: Observations on prototypes, object classes, and symmetries. AI Memo 1347. MIT AI Laboratory.

Polat, U., Mizobe, K., Pettet, M. W., Kasamutsu, T., and Norcia, A. M. (1998). Collinear stimuli regulate visual responses depending on cell's contrast threshold. *Nature* 391: 580–584.

Polat, U., and Sagi, D. (1993). Lateral interactions between spatial channels: Suppression and facilitation revealed by lateral masking experiments. *Vision Res.* 33: 993–999.

Polat, U., and Sagi, D. (1994a). The architecture of perceptual spatial interactions. *Vision Res.* 34: 73–78.

Polat, U., and Sagi, D. (1994b). Spatial interactions in human vision: From near to far via experience-dependent cascades of connections. *Proc. Natl. Acad. Sci. U S A* 91: 1206–1209.

Polat, U., and Sagi, D. (1995). Plasticity of spatial interactions in early vision. In B. Julesz and I. Kovács, eds., *Maturational Windows and Adult Cortical Plasticity*. SFI Studies in the Sciences of Complexity, vol. 24. Reading MA: Addison-Wesley.

Pollen, D. A., and Ronner, S. F. (1981). Phase relationships between adjacent simple cells in the visual cortex. *Science* 212: 1409–1410.

Polley, D. B., Chen-Bee, C. H., and Frostig, R. D. (1999a). Varying the degree of single-whisker stimulation differentially affects phases of intrinsic signals in rat barrel cortex. *J. Neurophysiol.* 81: 692–701.

Polley, D. B., Chen-Bee, C. H., and Frostig, R. D. (1999b). Two directions of plasticity in the sensory-deprived adult cortex. *Neuron* 24: 623–637.

Pollock, W., and Chapais, A. (1952). The apparent length of a line as a function of its inclination. *Q. J. Exp. Psychol.* 4: 170–178.

Pons, T., Garraghty, P. E., Ommaya, A. K., Kaas, J. H., Taub, E., and Mishkin, M. (1991). Massive cortical reorganization after sensory deafferentation in adult macaques. *Science* 252: 1857–1860.

Popper, K. R. (1992). *Conjectures and Refutations: The Growth of Scientific Knowledge*. 5th ed. London: Routledge.

Posner, M. I., and Keele, S. W. (1968). On the genesis of abstract ideas. *J. Exp. Psychol.* 77: 353–363.

Prados, J., Chamizo, V. D., and Mackintosh, N. J. (1999). Latent inhibition and perceptual learning in a swimming-pool navigation task. *J. Exp. Psychol. Anim. Behav. Process.* 25: 37–44.

Prakash, N., Cohen-Cory, S., and Frostig, R. D. (1996). Rapid and opposite effects of BDNF and NGF on the functional organization of the adult cortex *in vivo*. *Nature* 381: 702–706.

Prescott, S. W. (1998). Interactions between depression and facilitation in neural networks: Updating the dual-process theory of plasticity. *Learn. Mem.* 5: 446–466.

Price, D. J. (1986). The postnatal development of clustered intrinsic connections in area 18 of the visual cortex of kittens. *Dev. Brain Res.* 24: 31–38.

Psarrou, A., Gong, S., and Buxton, H. (1995). Modelling spatio-temporal trajectories and face signatures on partially recurrent networks. (1995). In *Proceedings of the International Conference on Neural Networks: ICNN '95*, pp. 2226–2231.

Purves, D., Augustine, G. J., Fitzpatrick, D., Katz, L. C., LaMantia, A.-S., and McNamara, J. O., eds. (1997). *Neuroscience*. Sunderland, MA: Sinauer.

Pustell, T. E. (1957). The experimental induction of perceptual vigilance and defense. *J. Pers.* 25: 425–438.

Pylyshyn, Z. W. (1984). *Computation and Cognition: Toward a Foundation for Cognitive Science*. Cambridge, MA: MIT Press.

Pylyshyn, Z. W. (1999). Is vision continuous with cognition? The case for cognitive impenetrability of visual perception *Behav. Brain Sci.* 22(3): 341–423.

Qian, N., and Matthews, N. (1999). A physiological theory for visual perceptual learning of orientation discrimination. *Soc. Neurosci. Abstr.* 25: 1316.

Quine, W. V. O. (1969). Natural kinds. In *Ontological Relativity and Other Essays*, 114–138. New York: Columbia University Press.

Rainer, G., and Miller, E. K. (2000) Effects of visual experience on the representation of objects in the prefrontal cortex. *Neuron* 27: 179–189.

Rajan, R., Irvine, D. R. F., Wise, L. Z., and Heil, R. (1993). Effect of unilateral partial cochlear lesions in adult cats on the representation of lesioned and unlesioned co-chleas in primary auditory centers. *J. Comp. Neurol.* 338: 17–49.

Ramachandran, V. (1985). The neurobiology of perception. *Perception* 14: 97–103.

Ramachandran, V. (1988). Perception of shape from shading. *Nature* 331: 163–166.

Ramachandran, V. (1994). 2D or not 2D—that is the question. In R. Gregory and J. Harris, eds., *The Artful Eye.* Oxford: Oxford University Press.

Ramachandran, V. S. (1976). Learning-like phenomena in stereopsis. *Nature* 262: 382–384.

Ramachandran, V. S., and Braddick, O. (1973). Orientation-specific learning in stereopsis. *Perception* 2: 371–376.

Ramachandran, V. S., Stewart, M., and Rogers-Ramachandran, D. C. (1992). Perceptual correlates of massive cortical reorganization. *NeuroReport* 3: 583–586.

Rasmusson, D. D., and Dykes, R. W. (1988). Long-term enhancement of evoked potentials in cat somatosensory cortex produced by co-activation of the basal forebrain and cutaneous receptors. *Exp. Brain Res.* 70: 276–286.

Recanzone, G. H., Jenkins, W. M., Hradek, G. T., and Merzenich, M. M. (1992a). Progressive improvements in discriminative abilities in adult owl monkeys performing a tactile frequency discrimination task. *J. Neurophysiol.* 67: 1015–1030.

Recanzone, G. H., Merzenich, M. M., and Dinse, H. R. (1992b). Expansion of the cortical representation of a specific skin field in primary somatosensory cortex by intracortical microstimulation. *Cereb. Cortex* 2: 181–196.

Recanzone, G. H., Merzenich, M. M., and Jenkins, W. M. (1992c). Frequency discrimination training engaging a restricted skin surface results in an emergence of a cutaneous response zone in cortical area 3a. *J. Neurophysiol.* 67: 1057–1070.

Recanzone, G. H., Merzenich, M. M., Jenkins, W. M., Grajski, K., and Dinse, H. R. (1992d). Topographic reorganization of the hand representation in cortical area 3b of owl monkeys trained in a frequency discrimination task. *J. Neurophysiol.* 67: 1031–1056.

Recanzone, G. H., Merzenich, M. M., and Schreiner, C. E. (1992e). Changes in the distributed temporal response properties of SI cortical neurons reflect improvements in performance on a temporally based tactile discrimination task. *J. Neurophysiol.* 67: 1071–1091.

Recanzone, G. H., Schreiner, C. E., and Merzenich, M. M. (1993). Plasticity in the frequency represenation of primary auditory cortex following discrimination training in adult owl monkeys. *J. Neurosci.* 13: 87–103.

Redlich, A. N., Atick, J. J., and Griffin, P. A. (1996). Statistical approach to shape from shading: Deriving 3-D face surfaces from single 2-D images. *Network Comput. Neural Syst.* 7: 1.

Regan, D., and Beverley, K. I. (1985). Postadaptation orientation discrimination. *J. Opt. Soc. Am.* A2: 147–155.

Reicher, G. M. (1969). Perceptual recognition as a function of meaningfulness of stimulus material. *J. Exp. Psychol.* 81: 275–280.

Reinke, H., and Dinse, H. R. (1999). Plasticity in the somatosensory and motor cortex of rats: impact of age and housing conditions. In *Proceedings of the First Göttingen Conference of the German Neuroscience Society 1999: From Molecular Neurobiology to Clinical Neuroscience*, ed. N. Elsner and U. Eysel, vol. 1, pp. 409. Stuttgart: Thieme.

Rentschler, I., Jüttner, M., and Caelli, T. (1994). Probabilistic analysis of human supervised learning and classification. *Vision Res.* 34: 669–687.

Rhodes, G. (1996). *Superportraits: Caricature and Recognition.* Hove, U.K.: Psychology Press.

Rhodes, G., Brake, S., and Atkinson, A. (1993). What's lost in inverted faces? *Cognition* 47: 25–57.

Rhodes, G., Brennan, S., and Carey, S. (1987). Identification and ratings of caricatures: Implications for mental representations of faces. *Cogn. Psychol.* 19: 473–497.

Rhodes, G., Carey, S., Byatt, G., and Proffitt, F. (1998). Coding spatial variations in faces and simple shapes: A test of two models. *Vision Res.* 38: 15–16.

Riches, I. P., Wilson, F. A. W., and Brown, M. W. (1991). The effects of visual stimulation and memory on neurons of the hippocampal formation and the neighboring para-hippocampal gyrus and inferior temporal cortex of the primate. *J. Neurosci.* 11: 1763–1779.

Richmond, B. J., and Optican, L. M. (1987). Temporal encoding of two-dimensional patterns by single units in primate inferior temporal cortex: 2. Quantification of response waveform. *J. Neurophysiol.* 57: 147–161.

Richmond, B. J., Optican, L. M., Podell, M., and Spitzer, H. (1987). Temporal encoding of two-dimensional patterns by single units in primate inferior temporal cortex. 1. Response characteristics. *J. Neurophysiol.* 57: 132–146.

Ridding, M. C., and Rothwell, J. C. (1995). Reorganization in human motor cortex. *Can. J. Physiol. Pharmacol.* 73: 218–222.

Riesenhuber, M., and Poggio, T. (1998). Just one view: Invariances in inferotemporal cell tuning. In M. I. Jordan, M. J. Kearns, and S. A. Solla, eds., *Advances in Neural Information Processing*, vol. 10, pp. 215–221. Cambridge, MA: MIT Press.

Ringach, D., and Shapley, R. (1996). Spatial and temporal properties of illusory contours and amodal boundary completion. *Vision Res.* 36: 3037–3050.

Rivenes, R. S. (1967). Multiple-task transfer effects in perceptual-motor learning. *Res. Q.* 38: 485–493.

Rivest, J., Boutet, I., and Intriligator, J. (1997). Perceptual learning of orientation discrimination by more than one attribute. *Vision Res.* 37: 273–281.

Roberson, E. D., English, J. D., and Sweatt, J. D. (1996). A biochemist's view of long-term potentiation. *Learn. Mem.* 3: 1–24.

Robertson, D., and Irvine, D. R. F. (1989). Plasticity of frequency organization in auditory cortex of guinea pigs with partial unilateral deafness. *J. Comp. Neurol.* 282: 456–471.

Rock, I., and DiVita, J. (1987). A case of viewer-centered object perception. *Cogn. Psychol.* 19: 280–293.

Rockland, K. S. (1985). Anatomical organization of primary visual cortex (area 17) in the ferret. *J. Comp. Neurol.* 241: 225–236.

Rockland, K. S., and Lund, J. S. (1982). Widespread periodic intrinsic connections in the tree shrew visual cortex. *Science* 215: 1532–1534.

Rockland, K. S., and Lund, J. S. (1983). Intrinsic laminar lattice connections in primate visual cortex. *J. Comp. Neurol.* 216: 303–318.

Röder, B., Rösler, F., and Neville, H. J. (1999). Effects of interstimulus interval on auditory event-related potentials in congenitally blind and normally sighted humans. *Neurosci. Lett.* 264: 53–56.

Röder, B., Rösler, F., and Neville, H. J. (2000). Event-related potentials during language processing in congenitally blind and sighted people. *Neuropsychologia* 38: 1482–1502.

Röder, B., Rösler, F., Henninghausen, E., and Nacker, F. (1996). Event-related potentials during auditory and somatosensory discrimination in sighted and blind human subjects. *Cogn. Brain Res.* 4(2): 77–93.

Röder, B., Teder-Sälejärvi, W., Sterr, A., Rösler, F., Hillyard, S. A., and Neville, H. (1999). Improved auditory spatial tuning in blind humans. *Nature* 400: 162–166.

Rösler, F., Röder, B., Heil, M., and Henninghausen, E. (1993). Topographic differences of slow event-related brain potentials in blind and sighted adult human subjects during haptic mental rotation. *Cogn. Brain Res.* 1: 145–159.

Rodman, H. R., and Consuelos, M. J. (1994). Cortical projects to anterior inferior temporal cortex in infant macaque monkeys. *Vis. Neurosci.* 11: 119–133.

Rodman, H. R., O Scalaidhe, S. P., and Gross, C. G. (1993). Response properties of neurons in temporal cortical visual areas of infant monkeys. *J. Neurophysiol.* 70: 1115–1136.

Roelfsema, P. R., Lamme, V. A. F., and Spekreijse, H. (1998). Object-based attention in the primary visual cortex of the macaque monkey. *Nature* 395: 376–381.

Rolls, E. (1992). Neurophysiological mechanisms underlying face processing within and beyond the temporal cortical areas. *Philos. Trans. R. Soc. Lond. B Biol. Sci.* 335: 11–21.

Rolls, E. T. (1984). Neurons in the cortex of the temporal lobe and in the amygdala of the monkey with responses selective for faces. *Hum. Neurobiol.* 3: 209–222.

Rolls, E. T. (1994). Brain mechanisms for invariant visual recognition and learning. *Behav. Processes* 33: 113–138.

Rolls, E. T., and Baylis, G. C. (1986). Size and contrast have only small effects on the responses to faces of neurons in the cortex of the superior temporal sulcus of the monkey. *Exp. Brain Res.* 65: 38–48.

Rolls, E. T., Baylis, G. C., Hasselmo, M. E., and Nalwa, V. (1989). The effect of learning on the face selective responses of neurons in the cortex in the superior temporal sulcus of the monkey. *Exp. Brain Res.* 76: 153–164.

Rolls, E. T., Baylis, G. C., and Leonard, C. M. (1985). Role of low and high spatial frequencies in the face-selective responses of neurons in the cortex in the superior temporal sulcus. *Vision Res.* 25: 1021–1035.

Rolls, E. T., and Tovee, M. J. (1994). Processing speed in the cerebral cortex and the neurophysiology of visual masking. *Proc. R. Soc. Lond. B Biol. Sci.* 257: 9–15.

Rolls, E. T., and Tovee, M. J. (1995). Sparseness of the neuronal representation of stimuli in the primate temporal visual cortex. *J. Neurophysiol.* 73: 713–726.

Rosch, E. (1973). On the internal structure of perceptual and semantic categories. In T. Moore, ed., *Cognitive Development and the Aquisition of Language*, 111–144. New York: Academic Press.

Rosch, E., Mervis, C. B., Gray, W. D., Johnson, D. M., and Boyes-Braem, P. (1976). Basic objects in natural categories. *Cogn. Psychol.* 8: 382–439.

Rosenthal, O., and Hochstein, S. (1994). Effects of stimulus meaning on V1 orientation-tuning properties. *Isr. Soc. Neurosci.* 3: 47.

Rosier, A. M., Arckens, L., Demeulemeester, H., Orban, G. A., Eysel, U. T., Wu, Y.-J., and Vandesande, F. (1995). Effect of sensory deafferentation on immunoreactivity of GABAergic cells and on GABA receptors in the adult cat visual cortex. *J. Comp. Neurol.* 359: 476–489.

Ross, H. (1990). Environmental influences on geometrical illusions. In F. Muller, ed., *Fechner Day '90: Proceedings of the Sixth Annual Meeting of the International Society of Psychophysicists*, 216–221.

Ross, H., and Woodhouse, J. (1979). Genetic and environmental factors in orientation anisotropy: A field study in the British Isles. *Perception* 8: 507–521.

Rossini, P. M., Martino, G., Narici, L., Pasquarelli, A., Peresson, M., Pizzella, V., Tecchio, F., Torrioli, G., and Romani, G. L. (1994). Short-term brain "plasticity" in humans: Transient finger representation changes sensory cortex somatotopy following ischemic anesthesia. *Brain Res.* 642: 169–177.

Rovamo, J., and Virsu, V. (1979). An estimation and application of the human cortical magnification factor. *Exp. Brain Res.* 37: 1–20.

Rubenstein, B. S., and Sagi, D. (1990). Spatial variability as a limiting factor in texture discrimination tasks: Implication for performance asymmetries. *J. Opt. Soc. Am. A* 7: 1632–1643.

Rubin, N., Nakayama, K., and Shapley, R. (1996). Enhanced perception of illusory contours in the lower versus upper visual hemifields. *Science* 271: 651–653.

Rubin, N., Nakayama, K., and Shapley, R. (1997). Abrupt learning and retinal size specifity in illusory-contour perception. *Curr. Biol.* 7: 461–467.

Ruderman, D. L. (1994). The statistics of natural images. *Network* 5: 517–548.

Rumelhart, D. E., and McClelland, J. L., eds. (1986). *Parallel Distributed Processing*. Cambridge, MA: MIT Press.

Rumelhart, D. E., and Todd, P. M. (1993). Learning and connectionist representations. In D. E. Meyer and S. Kornblum, eds., *Attention and Performance XIV*, 3–34. Cambridge, MA: MIT Press.

Rumpel, S., Hoffmann, H., Gottmann, K., Hatt, H., Mittmann, T., and Eysel, U. T. (1999). Lesion-induced changes in transcription levels of NMDA receptor subunit mRNAs in visual cortex of rats. *Soc. Neurosci. Abstr.* 25: 1719.

Russell, G. (1976). Practice effects for auditory localization: A test of a differentiation theory of perceptual learning and development. *Percept. Mot. Skills* 42: 647–653.

Ruthazer, E. S., and Stryker, M. P. (1996). The role of activity in the development of long-range horizontal connections in area 17 of the ferret. *J. Neurosci.* 16: 7253–7269.

Saarinen, J., and Levi, D. M. (1995). Perceptual learning in vernier acuity: What is learned? *Vision Res.* 35: 519–527.

Sachdev, R. N., Lu, S. M., Wiley, R. G., and Ebner, F. F. (1998). Role of the basal forebrain cholinergic projection in somatosensory cortical plasticity. *J. Neurophysiol.* 79: 3216–3228.

Sadato, N., Pascual-Leone, A., Grafman, J., Deiber, M.-P., Ibanez, V., and Hallett, M. (1998). Neural networks for Braille reading in the blind. *Brain* 121: 1213–1229.

Sadato, N., Pascual-Leone, A., Grafman, J., Ibanez, V., Deiber, M. P., Dold, G., and Hallett, M. (1996). Activation of the primary visual cortex by Braille reading in blind subjects. *Nature* 380: 526–528.

Saffran, J. R., Aslin, R. N., and Newport, E. L. (1996). Statistical learning by 8-month-old infants. *Science* 274: 1926–1928.

Sagi, D. (1990). Detection of an orientation singularity in Gabor textures: Effect of signal density and spatial frequency. *Vision Res.* 30: 1377–1388.

Sagi, D. (1996). Early vision: Images, context and memory. In A. Aertsen and V. Braitenberg, eds., *Brain Theory: Biological Basis and Computational Theory of Vision*, 1–15. Amsterdam: Elsevier.

Sagi, D., and Hochstein, S. (1985). Lateral inhibition between spatially adjacent spatial frequency channels? *Percept. Psychophys.* 37: 315–322.

Sagi, D., and Julesz, B. (1987). Short-range limitation on detection of feature differences. *Spat. Vis.* 2: 39–49.

Sagi, D., and Tanne, D. (1994). Perceptual learning: learning to see. *Curr. Opin. Neurobiol.* 4: 195–199.

Saito, S., Kobayashi, S., Ohashi, Y., Igarashi, M., Komiya, Y., and Ando, S. (1994). Decreased synaptic density in aged brains and its prevention by rearing under enriched environment as revealed by synaptophysin contents. *J. Neurosci. Res.* 39: 57–62.

Sakai, K., and Miyashita, Y. (1991). Neural organization for the long-term memory of paired associates. *Nature* 354: 152–155.

Sakai, K., and Miyashita, Y. (1994). Neuronal tuning to learned complex forms in vision. *NeuroReport* 5: 829–832.

Sakai, K., Naya, Y., and Miyashita, Y. (1994). Neuronal tuning and associative mechanisms in form representation. *Learn. Mem.* 1: 83–105.

Saksida, L. M. (1999). Effects of similarity and experience on discrimination learning: A nonassociative connectionist model of perceptual learning. *J. Exp. Psychol. Anim Behav. Process.* 25: 308–323.

Saleem, K. S., and Tanaka, K. (1996). Divergent projections from the anterior inferotemporal area TE to the perirhinal and entorhinal cortices in the macaque monkey. *J. Neurosci.* 16: 4757–4775.

Saleem, K. S., Tanaka, K., and Rockland, K. S. (1993). Specific and columnar projection from area TEO to TE in the macaque inferotemporal cortex. *Cereb. Cortex* 3: 454–464.

Sameshima, K., and Merzenich, M. M. (1993). Cortical plasticity and memory. *Curr. Opin. Neurobiol.* 3: 187–196.

Sanes, J. N., and Donoghue, J. P. (1997). Static and dynamic organization of motor cortex. *Adv. Neurol.* 73: 277–296.

Sanger, T. D. (1989). Optimal unsupervised learning in a single-layer network. *Neural Networks* 2: 459–473.

Sarle, W. S. (1994). Neural networks and statistical models. In *Proceedings of the Nineteenth Annual SAS Users Group International Conference*, 1538–1550, Cary, NC: SAS Institute.

Sary, G., Vogels, R., and Orban, G. A. (1993). Cue-invariant shape selectivity of macaque inferior temporal neurons. *Science* 260: 995–997.

Saslow, M. G. (1967). Latency for saccadic eye movement. *J. Opt. Soc. Am.* 57: 1030–1036.

Sathian, K., and Zangaladze, A. (1997). Tactile learning is task specific but transfers between fingers. *Percept. Psychophys.* 59: 119–128.

Sathian, K., and Zangaladze, A. (1998). Perceptual learning in tactile hyperacuity: Complete intermanual transfer but limited retention. *Exp. Brain Res.* 118: 131–134.

Sato, T. (1988). Effects of attention and stimulus interaction on visual responses of inferior temporal neurons in macaque. *J. Neurophysiol.* 60: 344–364.

Sato, T. (1989). Interactions of visual stimuli in the receptive fields of inferior temporal neurons in awake macaques. *Exp. Brain Res.* 77: 23–30.

Sato, T. (1995). Interactions between two different visual stimuli in the receptive fields of inferior temporal neurons in macaques during matching behaviors. *Exp. Brain Res.* 105: 209–219.

Scannell, J. W., and Young, M. P. (1999). Neuronal population activity and functional imaging. *Proc. R. Soc. Lond. B Biol. Sci.* 266: 875–881.

Schacter, D. L., Cooper, L. A., and Delaney, S. M. (1990). Implicit memory for unfamiliar objects depends on access to structural descriptions. *J. Exp. Psychol. Gen.* 119: 5–24.

Schafer, R., and Murphy, G. (1943). The role of autism in a visual figure-ground relationship. *J. Exp. Psychol.* 32: 335–343.

Scheffler, K., Bilecen, D., Schmid, N., Tschopp, K., and Seelig, J. (1998). Auditory cortical responses in hearing subjects and unilateral deaf patients as detected by functional magnetic resonance imaging. *Cereb. Cortex* 8: 156–163.

Schiene, K., Bruehl, C., Zilles, K., Qü, M., Hagemann, G. Kraemer, M., and Witte, O. W. (1996). Neuronal hyper-excitability and reduction of GABA$_A$-receptor expression in the surround of cerebral photothrombosis. *J. Cereb. Blood Flow Metab.* 16: 906–914.

Schiltz, C., Bodart, J. M., Dubois, S., Dejardin, S., Michel, C., Roucoux, A., Crommelinck, and Orban, G. A. (1999). Neuronal mechanisms of perceptual learning: Changes in human brain activity with training in orientation discrimination. *Neuroimage* 9: 46–62.

Schlaug, G., Jancke, L., Huang, Y., and Steinmetz, H. (1995). In-vivo evidence of structural brain asymmetry in musicians. *Science* 267: 699–701.

Schmid, L. M., Rosa, M. G. P., Calford, M. B., and Ambler, J. S. (1996). Visuotopic reorganization in the primary cortex of adult cats following monocular and binocular retinal lesions. *Cereb. Cortex* 6: 388–405.

Schmidhuber, J., Eldracher, M., and Foltin, B. (1996). Semi-linear predictability minimization produces well-known feature detectors. *Neural Comput.* 8: 773–86.

Schmidt, K. E., Goebel, R., Löwel, S., and Singer, W. (1997). The perceptual grouping criterion of colinearity is reflected by anisotropies of connections in the primary visual cortex. *Eur. J. Neurosci.* 9: 1083–1089.

Schmidt, K. E., Kim, D.-S., Singer, W., Bonhoeffer, T., and Löwel, S. (1997). Functional specificities of long-range and interhemispheric connections in the visual cortex of strabismic cats. *J. Neurosci.* 17: 5480–5492.

Schmidt-Kastner, R., Wietasch, K., Weigel, H., and Eysel, U. T. (1993). Immunohistochemical staining for glial fibrillary acidic protein (GFAP) after deafferentation or ischemic infarction in rat visual system: Features of reactive and damaged astrocytes. *Int. J. Dev. Neurosci.* 11: 157–174.

Schooler, J. W., Fallshore, M., and Fiore, S. M. (1995). Epilogue: Putting insight into perspective. In *The Nature of Insight*, ed. R. J. Sternberg and J. E. Davidson. Cambridge, MA: MIT Press.

Schoups, A. A., and Orban, G. A. (1996). Interocular transfer in perceptual learning of a pop-out discrimination task. *Proc. Natl. Acad. Sci. U S A* 93: 7358–7362.

Schoups, A. A., Vogels, R., and Orban, G. A. (1995). Human perceptual learning in identifying the oblique orientation: Retinotopy, orientation specificity and monocularity. *J. Physiol. (Lond.)* 483: 797–810.

Schoups, A. A., Vogels, R., and Orban, G. A. (1998). Effects of perceptual learning in orientation discrimination on orientation coding in V1. *Invest. Ophthalmol. Vis. Sci.* 39: S684: 3142.

Schoups, A. A., Vogels, R., Qian, N., and Orban, G. A. (2001). Practising orientation identification improves orientation coding in V1 neurons. *Nature* 412: 549–553.

Schroeter, M., Schiene, K., Kraemer, M., Hagemann, G., Weigel, H., Eysel, U. T., Witte, O. W., and Stoll, G. (1995). Astroglial responses in photochemically induced focal ischemia of the rat cortex. *Exp. Brain Res.* 106: 1–6.

Schuurman, T., Klein, H., Beneke, M., and Traber, J. (1987). Nimodipine and motor deficits in the aged rat. *Neurosci. Res. Comm.* 1: 9–15.

Schwartz, E. L., Desimone, R., Albright, T. D., and Gross, C. G. (1983). Shape recognition and inferior temporal neurons. *Proc. Natl. Acad. Sci. U S A* 80: 5776–5778.

Schwartz, O., and Simoncelli, E. P. (1999). Accounting for surround suppression in V1 neurons using a statistically optimized normalization model. *Invest. Ophthalmol. Vis. Sci.* 40: S641.

Schwarz, C., and Bolz, J. (1991). Functional specificity of a long-range horizontal connection in cat visual cortex: A cross-correlation study. *J. Neurosci.* 11: 2995–3007.

Schweigart, G., and Eysel, U. T. (1998). Receptive fields near to excitotoxic lesions in the visual cortex of the cat. *Soc. Neurosci. Abstr.* 24: 647.

Schweigart, G., and Eysel, U. T. (Forthcoming). Activity-dependent receptive field changes in the surround of adult cat visual cortex lesions.

Schweinberger, S. R., and Soukoup, G. R. (1998). Asymmetric relationships between the perception of facial identity, emotion and facial speech. *J. Exp. Psychol. Hum. Percept. Perform.* 24: 1748–1765.

Schyns, P. (1998). Categories and percepts: A bi-directional framework for categorization. *Trends Cogn. Sci.* 1: 183–189.

Schyns, P. G., and Rodet, L. (1997). Categorization creates function features. *J. Exp. Psychol. Learn. Mem. Cogn.* 23: 681–696.

Schyns, P., Goldstone, R., and Thibaut, J.-P. (1998). The development of features in object concepts. *Behav. Brain Sci.* 21: 1–54.

Scott, D. V. (1974). Perceptual learning. *Queens Nurs J.* 17: 2–3.

Searcy, J. H., and Bartlett, J. C. (1996). Inversion and processing of component and spatial-relational information in faces. *J. Exp. Psychol. Hum. Percept. Perform.* 22: 904–915.

Seitz, R. J., Huang, Y., Knorr, U., Tellmann, L., Herzog, H., and Freund, H.-J. (1995). Large-scale plasticity in the human motor cortex. *NeuroReport* 6(5): 742–744.

Selfridge, O. G. (1959). Pandemonium: A paradigm for learning. In *The Mechanisation of Thought Processes*. London: H.M.S.O.

Sengpiel, F., Baddeley, R. J., Freeman, T. C., Harrad, R., and Blakemore, C. (1998). Different mechanisms underlie three inhibitory phenomena in cat area 17. *Vision Res.* 38(14): 2067–2080.

Sengpiel, F., Stawinski, P., and Bonhoeffer, T. (1999). Influence of experience on orientation maps in cat visual cortex. *Nat. Neurosci.* 2: 727–732.

Shannon, C. E. (1948). A mathematical theory of communication. *Bell Sys. Tech. J.* 27: 623–656.

Shapiro, P. N., and Penrod, S. (1986). Meta-analysis of facial identification studies. *Psychol. Bull.* 100: 139–156.

Shapley, R., and Enroth-Cugell, C. (1984). Visual adaptation and retinal gain controls. In *Progress in Retinal Research*, ed. J. G. Osborn and N. N. Chadler, vol. 3, pp. 263–346. Oxford: Pergamon Press.

Shashua, A., and Ullman, S. (1988). Structural saliency. The detection of globally salient structures using a locally connected network. In *Proceedings of the International Conference on Computer Vision*. Los Alamitos, CA: IEEE Press.

Shatz, C. J., Lindström, S., and Wiesel, T. N. (1977). The distribution of afferents representing the right and left eyes in the cat's visual cortex. *Brain Res.* 131: 103–116.

Sheinberg, D. L., and Logothetis, N. K. (1997). The role of temporal cortical areas in perceptual organization. *Proc. Natl. Acad. Sci. U S A* 94: 3408–3413.

Shenoy, K. V., Kaufman, J., McGrann, J. V., and Shaw, G. L. (1993). Learning by selection in the trion model of cortical organization. *Cereb. Cortex* 3: 239–248.

Shepard, R. N. (1967). Recognition memory for words, sentences and pictures. *J. Verb. Learn. Verb. Behav.* 6: 156–163.

Shepard, R. N. (1987). Toward a universal law of generalization for psychological science. *Science* 237: 1317–1323.

Shepard, R., and Cooper, L. (1982). *Mental Images and Their Transforms*. 3d ed. Cambridge, MA: MIT Press.

Shepherd, G. M. (1990). The significance of real neuron architectures for neural network simulations. In E. L. Schwartz, ed., *Computational Neuroscience*. Cambridge, MA: MIT Press.

Shepherd, J., Davies, G., and Ellis, H. (1981). Studies of cue saliency. In G. Davies, H. Ellis, and J. Shepherd, eds., *Perceiving and Remembering Faces*, pp. 105–131. London: Academic Press.

Shiu, L., and Pashler, H. (1992). Improvement in line orientation discrimination is retinally local but dependent on cognitive set. *Percept. Psychophys.* 52: 582–588.

Shouval, H. (1995). Formation and organisation of receptive fields, with an input environment composed of natural scenes. Ph.D. dissertation, Brown University.

Sil'kis, I. G., and Rapoport, S. S. (1995). Plastic reorganizations of the receptive fields of neurons of the auditory cortex and the medial geniculate body induced by microstimulation of the auditory cortex. *Neurosci. Behav. Physiol.* 25: 322–339.

Singer, W. (1990). Search for coherence: A basic principle of cortical self-organization. *Concepts Neurosci.* 1: 1–26.

Singer, W. (1995). Development and plasticity of cortical processing architectures. *Science* 270: 758–764.

Singer, W., Engel, A. K., Kreiter, A. K., Munk, M. H. J., Neuenschwander, S., and Roelfsema, P. R. (1997). Neuronal assemblies: necessity, signature and detectability. *Trends Cogn. Sci.* 1: 252–261.

Singer, W., and Tretter, F. (1976). Unusually large receptive fields in cats with restricted visual experience. *Exp. Brain Res.* 26: 171–184.

Sinha, P. (1994). Object recognition via image invariants. *Invest. Ophthalmol. Vis. Sci.* 35(4): 1735.

Sinha, P. (1995). Perceiving and recognizing three-dimensional forms. Ph.D. diss., Massachusetts Institute of Technology.

Sinha, P., and Adelson, E. H. (1993). Recovering reflectance and illumination in a world of painted polyhedra. In *Proceedings of the IEEE International Conference on Computer Vision*. Los Alamitos, CA: IEEE Press.

Sinha, P., and Poggio, T. A. (1996). Role of learning in three-dimensional form perception. *Nature* 384: 460–463.

Sireteanu, R., and Rettenbach, R. (1995). Perceptual learning in visual search: Fast, enduring, but non-specific. *Vision Res.* 35: 2037–2043.

Sireteanu, R., and Rettenbach, R. (2000). Perceptual learning in visual search generalizes over tasks, locations, and eyes. *Vision Res.* 40: 2925–2949.

Skrandies, W. (1995). Visual information processing: topography of brain electrical activity. *Biol. Psychol.* 40: 1–15.

Skrandies, W., and Fahle, M. (1994). Neurophysiological correlates of perceptual learning in the human brain. *Brain Topog.* 7: 163–168.

Skrandies, W., and Jedynak, A. (1999). Learning to see 3-D: Psychophysics and brain electrical activity. *NeuroReport* 10: 249–253.

Skrandies, W., Jedynak, A., and Fahle, M. (2001). Perceptual learning: Psychophysical thresholds and electrical brain topography. *Int. J. Psychophysiol.* 41: 119–129.

Skrandies, W., Lang, G., and Jedynak, A. (1996). Sensory thresholds and neurophysiological correlates of human perceptual learning. *Spat. Vis.* 9: 475–489.

Smith, D. E. P., and Hochberg, J. E. (1954). The effect of "punishment" (electric shock) on figure-ground perception. *J. Psychol.* 38: 83–87.

Smith, V. C., and Pokorny, J. (1975). Spectral sensitivity of the foveal cone photopigments between 400 and 500 nm. *Vision Res.* 15: 161–171.

Sober, S. J., Stark, J. M., Yamasaki, D. S., and Lytton, W. W. (1997). Receptive field changes after strokelike cortical ablation: A role for activation dynamics. *J. Neurophysiol.* 78: 3438–3443.

Sokoloff, L., Reivich, M., Kennedy, C., DesRosiers, M. H., Patlak, C. S., Pettigrew, K. D., Sakurada, O., and Shinohara, M. (1977). The [^{14}C]deoxyglucose method for the measurement of local cerebral glucose utilization: Theory, procedure, and normal values in the conscious and anesthetized albino rat. *J. Neurochem.* 28: 897–916.

Solso, R., and McCarthy, J. (1981). Prototype formation of faces: A case of pseudo-memory. *Br. J. Psychol.* 72: 499–503.

Somers, D. C., Todorov, E. V., Siapas, A. G., Toth, L. J., Kim, D. S., and Sur, M. (1998). A local circuit approach to understanding integration of long-range inputs in primary visual cortex. *Cerebr. Cortex* 8: 204–217.

Sowden, P. T. (1995). On perceptual learning. PhD thesis, University of Surrey, UK

Sowden, P. T., Davies, I. R., and Roling, P. (2000). Perceptual learning of the detection of features in X-ray images: A functional role for improvements in adults' visual sensitivity? *J. Exp. Psychol. Hum. Percept. Perform.* 26: 379–390.

Sowden, P., Davies, I., Rose, D., and Kaye, M. (1996). Perceptual learning of stereoacuity. *Perception* 25: 1043–1052.

Spelke, E. (1990). Origins of visual knowledge. In D. Osherson and S. M. Kosslyn, eds., *Visual Cognition and Action: An Invitation to Cognitive Science*, vol. 2, pp. 99–127. Cambridge, MA: MIT Press.

Spengler, F., and Dinse, H. R. (1994). Reversible relocation of representational boundaries of adult rats by intracortical microstimulation (ICMS). *NeuroReport* 5: 949–953.

Spengler, F., Godde, B., and Dinse, H. R. (1995). Effects of aging on topographic organization of somatosensory cortex. *NeuroReport* 6: 469–473.

Spengler, F., Roberts, T. P., Poeppel, D., Byl, N., Wang, X., Rowley, H. A., and Merzenich, M. M. (1997). Learning transfer and neuronal plasticity in humans trained in tactile discrimination. *Neurosci. Lett.* 232: 151–154.

Spitzer, H., Desimone, R., and Moran, J. (1988). Increased attention enhances both behavioral and neuronal performance. *Science* 240: 338–340.

Squire, L. R., and Zola, S. M. (1997). Amnesia, memory and brain systems. *Philos. Trans. R. Soc. Lond. B Biol. Sci.* 352: 1663–1673.

Stadler, M. A. (1989). On learning complex procedural knowledge. *J. Exp. Psychol. Learn. Mem. Cogn.* 15: 1061–1069.

Standing, L. (1973). Learning 10,000 pictures. *Q. J. Exp. Psychol.* 25: 207–222.

Stemmler, M., Usher, M., and Niebur, E. (1995). Lateral interactions in primary visual cortex: A model bridging physiology and psychophysics. *Science* 269: 1877–1880.

Stent, G. S. (1973). A physiological mechanism for Hebb's postulate of learning. *Proc. Natl. Acad. Sci. U S A* 70: 997–1001.

Sternberg, R. J., and Davidson, J. E., eds. (1995). *The Nature of Insight*. Cambridge, MA: MIT Press.

Sterr, A., Muller, M. M., Elbert, T., Rockstroh, B., Pantev, C., and Taub, E. (1998a). Perceptual correlates of changes in cortical representation of fingers in blind multifinger Braille readers. *J. Neurosci.* 18: 4417–4423.

Sterr, A., Muller, M. M., Elbert, T., Rockstroh, B., Pantev, C., and Taub, E. (1998b). Changed perceptions in Braille readers. *Nature* 391: 134–135.

Stevenage, S. V. (1998). Which twin are you? A demonstration of induced categorical perception of identical twin faces. *Br. J. Psychol.* 89: 39–58.

Stickgold, R., Whidbee, D., Schirmer, B., Patel, V., and Hobson, J. A. (2000). Visual discrimination task improvement: A multi-step process occurring during sleep. *J. Cogn. Neurosci.* 12: 246–254.

Stoll, S., Dorner, H., Blösch, M., and Platt, R. (1990). Age-dependent differences in the gait of rats. *Arch. Gerontol. Geriatr.* 10: 216–268.

Stone, C. J. (1980). Optimal rates of convergence for nonparametric estimators. *Ann. Stat.* 8: 1348–1360.

Stone, C. J. (1982). Optimal global rates of convergence for nonparametric regression. *Ann. Stat.* 10: 1040–1053.

Stone, C. J. (1985). Additive regression and other nonparametric models. *Ann. Stat.* 13: 689–705.

Stone, C. J. (1986). The dimensionality reduction principle for generalized additive models. *Ann. Stat.* 14: 590–606.

Stone, J. (1998). Object recognition using spatio-temporal signatures. *Vision Res.* 38(7): 947–951.

Stone, J. V. (1996). Learning perceptually salient visual parameters using spatiotemporal smoothness constraints. *Neural Comput.* 8: 1463–1492.

Stone, J. V. (1996). A canonical microfunction for learning perceptual invariances. *Perception* 25: 207–220.

Stone, J. V., and Harper, N. (1999). Temporal constraints on visual learning: A computational model. *Perception* 28: 1089–1104.

Stoney, S. D., Jr., Thompson, W. D., and Asanuma, H. (1968). Excitation of pyramidal tract cells by intracortical microstimulation: Effective extent of stimulating current. *J. Neurophysiol.* 31: 659–669.

Streletz, L. J., Belevich, J. K. S., Jones, S. M., Bhusan, A., Shah, S. H., and Herbison, G. (1995). Transcranial magnetic stimulation: Cortical motor maps in acute spinal cord injury. *Brain Topogr.* 7(3): 245–250.

Stryker, M. (1991). Temporal associations. *Nature* 354: 108–109.

Stryker, M. P., and Sherk, H. (1975). Modification of cortical orientation selectivity in the cat by restricted visual experience: A reexamination. *Science* 190: 904–906.

Stryker, M. P., Sherk, H., Leventhal, A. G., and Hirsch, H. V. (1978). Physiological consequences for the cat's visual cortex of effectively restricting early visual experience with oriented contours. *J. Neurophysiol.* 41: 896–909.

Sugita, Y. (1996). Global plasticity in adult visual cortex following reversal of visual input. *Nature* 380: 523–526.

Sundareswaran, V., and Vaina, L. (1994). Learning direction in global motion: Two classes of psychophysically-motivated models. In G. Tesauro, D. Touretzky, and T. Leen, eds., *Advances in Neural Information Processing Systems*, vol. 7, pp. 917–924, San Francisco: Morgan Kaufmann.

Sutherland, N. S., and Macintosh, N. J. (1971). *Mechanisms of Animal Discrimination Learning*. New York: Academic Press.

Sutherland, N. S., Mackintosh, N. J., and Mackintosh, J. (1963). Simultaneous discrimination training of Octopus and transfer of discrimination along a continuum. *J. Comp. Physiol. Psychol.* 56: 150–156.

Suzuki, W. A., and Amaral, D. G. (1994). Topographic organization of the reciprocal connections between the monkey entorhinal cortex and the perirhinal and para-hippocampal cortices. *J. Neurosci.* 14: 1856–1877.

Suzuki, W. A., and Amaral, D. G. (1995). Perirhinal and parahippocampal cortices of the macaque monkey: Cortical afferents. *J. Comp. Neurol.* 349: 1–36.

Swindale, N. V. (1981). Absence of ocular dominance patches in dark-reared cats. *Nature* 290: 332–333.

Szentágothai, J. (1973). Synaptology of the visual cortex. In R. Jung (ed.), *Handbook of Sensory Physiology*. Vol. 7, *Central Visual Information*, 269–324. Berlin: Springer.

Talairach, J., and Tournoux, P. (1988). *Co-planar Stereotaxic Atlas of the Human Brain*. Stuttgart: Thieme.

Tallal, P., Miller, S. L., Bedi, G., Byma, G., Wang, X., Nagarajan, S. S., Schreiner, C., Jenkins, W. M., and Merzenich, M. M. (1996). Language comprehension in language-learning impaired children improved with acoustically modified speech. *Science* 271: 81–84.

Tallal, P., Miller, S., and Fitch, R. H. (1993). Neurobiological basis of speech: A case for the preeminence of temporal processing. *Ann. N. Y. Acad. Sci.* 682: 27–47.

Tanaka, J. W., and Farah, M. J. (1993). Parts and wholes in face recognition. *Q. J. Exp. Psychol.* 46A: 225–245.

Tanaka, K. (1994). Inferotemporal cortex and object vision. *Annu. Rev. Neurosci.* 19: 101–139.

Tanaka, K., Saito, H., Fukada, Y., and Moriya, M. (1991). Coding visual images of objects in the inferotemporal cortex of the macaque monkey. *J. Neurophysiol.* 66: 170–189.

Tanaka, Y., and Sagi, D. (1998). Long-lasting, long-range detection facilitation. *Vision Res.* 38: 2591–2599.

Tanne, D., and Sagi, D. (1995). Visual learning can be reversed by task. *Invest. Ophthalmol. Vis. Sci.* 36: 376.

Tarr, M., and Bülthoff, H. H. (1995). Is human object recognition better described by geon structural descriptions or by multiple views? *J. Exp. Psychol. Hum. Percept. Perform.* 21: 1494–1505.

Tarr, M., and Pinker, S. (1989). Mental rotation and orientation dependence in shape recognition. *Cogn. Psychol.* 21: 233–282.

Taub, E. (1994). Overcoming learned nonuse: a new behavioral medicine approach to physical medicine. In J. G. Carlson, S. R. Seifert, and N. Birbaumer, eds., *Clinical Applied Psychophysiology*, 185–220. New York: Plenum.

Taub, E., Crago, J. E., and Uswatte, G. (1998). Constraint-induced movement therapy: A new approach to treatment in physical rehabilitation. *Rehab. Psychol.* 43: 152–170.

Taub, E., Miller, N. E., Novack, T. A., Cook, E. W., Fleming, W. C., Nepomuceno, C. S., Connell, J. S., and Crago, J. E. (1993). Technique to improve chronic motor deficit after stroke. *Arch. Phys. Med. Rehab.* 74: 347–354.

Taub, E., Uswatte, G., and Elbert, T. (forthcoming). Stroke rehabilitation and the functional significance of cortical reorganization for behavior and perception. *Am. Psychol.*

Thorek, K., and Sinha, P. (2001). Qualitative representations for recognition. In preparation.

Tighe, T. J., and Tighe, L. S. (1968). Perceptual learning in the discrimination processes of children: An analysis of five variables in perceptual pretraining. *J. Exp. Psychol.* 77: 125–134.

Tinazzi, M., Zanette, G., Polo, A., Volpato, D., Manganotti, P., Bonato, C., Testoni, R., and Fiaschi, A. (1997). Transient deafferentation in humans induces rapid modulation of primary sensory cortex not associated with subcortical changes: A somatosensory evoked potential study. *Neurosci. Lett.* 223: 21–24.

Tolhurst, D. J., and Barfield, L. P. (1978). Interactions between spatial frequency channels. *Vision Res.* 18: 951–958.

Tolhurst, D. J., and Heeger, D. J. (1997). Contrast-normalization and threshold models of the responses of simple cells in cat striate cortex. *Vis. Neurosci.* 14(2): 293–309.

Tolman, E. C. (1948). Cognitive maps in rats and men. *Psych. Rev.* 55: 189–208.

Tomblin, J. B., and Quinn, M. A. (1983). The contribution of perceptual learning to performance on the repetition task. *J. Speech Hear. Res.* 26: 369–372.

Tommerdahl, M., Delemos, K. A., Favorov, O. V., Metz, C. B., Vierck, C. J., Jr., and Whitsel, B. L. (1998). Response of anterior parietal cortex to different modes of same-site skin stimulation. *J. Neurophysiol.* 80: 3272–3283.

Tommerdahl, M., Delemos, K. A., Vierck, C. J., Jr., Favorov, O. V., and Whitsel, B. L. (1996). Anterior parietal cortical response to tactile and skin-heating stimuli applied to the same skin site. *J. Neurophysiol.* 75: 2662–2670.

Tong, Y. C., Black, R. C., Clark, G. M., Forster, I. C., Millar, J. B., O'Loughlin, B. J., and Patrick, J. F. (1979). A preliminary report on a multiple-channel cochlear implant operation. *J. Laryngol. Otol.* 93(7): 679–695.

Tong, Y. C., Millar, J. B., Clark, G. M., Martin, L. F., Busby, P. A., and Patrick, J. F. (1980). Psychophysical and speech perception studies on two multiple-channel cochlear implant patients. *J. Laryngol. Otol.* 94: 1241–1256.

Tootell, R. B. H., Switkes, E., Silverman, M. S. and Hamilton, S. L. (1988). Functional anatomy of macaque striate cortex—II. Retinotopic organization. *J. Neurosci.* 8: 1531–1568.

Topka, H., Cohen, L. G., Cole, R. A., and Hallett, M. (1991). Reorganization of corticospinal pathways following spinal cord injury. *Neurology* 41: 1276–1283.

Torkkola, K. (1996). Blind separation of convolved sources based on information maximization. In *Proceedings of the IEEE Workshop on Neural Networks and Signal Processing*, Kyoto, Japan, September.

Tovee, M. J. (1995). Face recognition: What are faces for? *Curr. Biol.* 5: 480–482.

Tovee, M. J., Rolls, E. T., and Ramachandran, V. S. (1996). Rapid visual learning in neurones of the primate temporal visual cortex. *NeuroReport* 7: 2757–2760.

Tovee, M. J., Rolls, E. T., Trevis, A., and Bellis, R. P. (1993). Information encoding and the responses of single neurons in the primate temporal visual cortex. *J. Neurophysiol.* 70: 640–654.

Traversa, R., Cicinelli, P., Bassi, A., Rossini, P. M., and Bernardi, G. (1997). Mapping motor cortical reorganization after stroke. *Stroke* 28: 110–117.

Treisman A. (1996). The binding problem. *Curr. Opin. Neurobiol.* 6: 171–178.

Treisman, A., and Gelade, G. A. (1980). A feature integration theory of attention. *Cogn. Psychol.* 12: 97–136.

Treisman, A., Vieira, A., and Hayes, A. (1992). Automaticity and preattentive processing. *Am. J. Psychol.* 105: 341–362.

Trobalon, J. B., Chamizo, V. D., and Mackintosh, N. J. (1992). Role of context in perceptual learning in maze discriminations. *Q. J. Exp. Psychol. B.* 44: 57–73.

Trobalon, J. B., Sansa, J., Chamizo, V. D., and Mackintosh, N. J. (1991). Perceptual learning in maze discriminations. *Q. J. Exp. Psychol. B.* 43: 389–402.

Troje, N., and Bülthoff, H. (1996). Face recognition under varying poses: The role of texture and shape. *Vision Res.* 36: 1761–1771.

Troscianko, T., and Harris, J. (1988). Phase discrimination in chromatic compound gratings. *Vision Res.* 28: 1041–1049.

Troyer, T. W., Krukowski, A. E., Priebe, N. J., and Miller, K. D. (1998). Contrast-invariant orientation tuning in cat visual cortex: Thalamocortical input tuning and correlation-based intracortical connectivity. *J. Neurosci.* 18: 5908–5927.

Ts'o, D. Y., and Gilbert, C. D. (1988). The organization of chromatic and spatial interactions in the primate striate cortex. *J. Neurosci.* 8: 1712–1727.

Ts'o, D. Y., Gilbert, C. D., and Wiesel, T. N. (1986). Relationships between horizontal interactions and functional architecture in cat striate cortex as revealed by cross-correlation analysis. *J. Neurosci.* 6: 1160–1170.

Tsotsos, J. K. (1990). Analyzing vision at the complexity level. *Behav. Brain Sci.* 13: 423–469.

Tulving, E., Hayman, C. A., and Macdonald, C. A. (1991). Long-lasting perceptual priming and semantic learning in amnesia: A case experiment. *J. Exp. Psychol. Learn. Mem. Cogn.* 17: 595–617.

Tulving, E., and Schacter, D. L. (1990). Priming and human memory systems. *Science* 247: 301–306.

Turk, M., and Pentland, A. (1991). Eigenfaces for recognition. *J. Cogn. Neurosci.* 3: 71–86

Turnure, C. (1972). Perceptual learning in young children: Varied context and stimulus labels. *Am. J. Psychol.* 85: 339–349.

Turrigiano, G. G., Leslie, K. R., Desai, N. S., Rutherford, L. C., and Nelson, S. B. (1998). Activity-dependent scaling of quantal amplitude in neocortical neurons. *Nature* 391: 892–895.

Tversky, B., and Hemenway, K. (1984). Objects, parts and categories. *J. Exp. Psychol. Gen.* 113: 169–193.

Uhl, F., Kretschmer, T., Lindinger, G., Goldenberg, G., Lang, W., Oder, W., and Deecke, L. (1994). Tactile mental imagery in sighted persons and in patients suffering from blindness early in life. *Electroenc. Clin. Neurophysiol.* 91: 249–255.

Uhl, F., Podreka, I., Steiner, M., and Deecke, L. (1993). Increased regional cerebral blood flow in inferior occipital cortex and cerebellum of early blind humans. *Neurosci. Lett.* 150: 162–164.

Ullman, S. (1979). *The Interpretation of Visual Motion.* Cambridge, MA: MIT Press.

Ullman, S. (1990). 3-dimensional object recognition. *Cold Spring Harb. Symp. Quant. Biol.* 55: 889–898.

Ullman, S. (1995). Sequence seeking and counter streams: A computational model for bidirectional information flow in the visual cortex. *Cereb. Cortex* 5: 1–11.

Ullman, S., and Basri, R. (1991). Recognition by linear combinations of models. *IEEE Trans. Patt. Anal. Mach. Intell.* 13: 992–1005.

Ungerleider, L. G. (1995). Functional brain imaging studies of cortical mechanisms for memory. *Science* 270: 769–775.

Ungerleider, L. G., Gaffan, D., and Pelak, V. S. (1989). Projections from inferior temporal cortex to prefrontal cortex via the uncinate fascicle in rhesus monkeys. *Exp. Brain Res.* 76: 473–484.

Ungerleider, L., and Mishkin, M. (1982). Two cortical visual systems. In D. Ingle, M. Goodale, and R. Mansfield, eds., *Analysis of Visual Behavior*, 549–586. Cambridge, MA: MIT Press.

Uttley, A. M. (1959). The design of conditional probability computers. *Inform. Control* 2: 1–24.

Vaina, L. M., Belliveau J. W., des Roziers, E. B., and Zeffiro, T. (1998). Neural systems underlying learning and representation of global motion. *Proc. Natl. Acad. Sci. U S A* 95: 12657–12662.

Valentine, T. (1988). Upside-down faces: A review of the effect of inversion upon face recognition. *Br. J. Psychol.* 79: 471–491.

Valentine, T. (1991). Representation and process in face recognition. In R. Watt, ed., *Vision and Visual Dysfunction*, vol. 14, pp. 107–124. London: Macmillan.

Valverde, F. (1986). Intrinsic neocortical organization: Some comparative aspects. *Neurosci.* 18: 1–23.

van Ee, R. (2001). Perceptual learning without feedback and the stability of stereoscopic slant estimation. *Perception* 30: 95–114

Van Essen, D. C., Felleman, D. J., DeYoe, E. A., Olavarria, J., and Knierim, J. (1990). Modular and hierarchical organization of extrastriate visual cortex in the macaque monkey. *Cold Spring Harb. Symp. Quant. Biol.* 55: 679–696 van Hateren, J. H. (1992). A theory of maximizing sensory information. *Biol. Cybern.* 68: 23–29.

van Hateren, J. H., Ruderman, D. L. (1998). Independent component analysis of natural image sequences yields spatio-temporal filters similar to simple cells in primary visual cortex. *Proc. R. Soc. Lond.* B 265: 2315–2320.

Van Hoesen, G. W., and Pandya, D. N. (1975). Some connections of the entorhinal (area 28) and perirhinal (area 35) cortices of the rhesus monkey: 1. Temporal lobe afferents. *Brain Res.* 95: 1–24.

van Leeuwen, C. (1990). Perceptual-learning systems as conservative structures: Is economy an attractor? *Psychol. Res.* 52: 145–152.

Van Nes, F. L., and Bouman, M. A. (1967). Spatial modulation transfer in the human eye. *J. Opt. Soc. Am.* 57: 401–406.

Vapnik, V. (1995). *The Nature of Statistical Learning Theory.* Berlin: Springer.

Vasama, J.-P., Mäkelä, J. P., Pyykkö, I., and Hari, R. (1995). Abrupt unilateral deafness modifies function of human auditory pathways. *NeuroReport* 6: 961–964.

Vetter, T., and Poggio, T. (1994). Symmetric 3D objects are an easy case for 2D object recognition. *Spat. Vis.* 8(4): 443–453.

Vetter, T., and Poggio, T. A. (1996). Image synthesis from a single example view. In *Computer Vision—ECCV '96: Notes in Computer Science.* Cambridge, U.K.: Springer.

Vidyasagar, T. R., and Stuart, G. W. (1993). Perceptual learning in seeing form from motion. *Proc. R. Soc. Lond. B Biol. Sci.* 254: 241–244.

Vlek, C. A., and Werner, H. H. (1973). Learning relative frequency distributions: Some perceptual and cognitive factors. *J. Exp. Psychol.* 100: 106–115.

Vogels, R., and Orban, G. A. (1985). The effect of practice on the oblique effect in line orientation judgements. *Vision Res.* 25: 1679–1687.

Vogels, R., and Orban, G. A. (1994). Does practice in orientation discrimination lead to changes in the response properties of macaque inferior temporal neurons? *Eur. J. Neurosci.* 6: 1680–1690.

Volchan, E., and Gilbert, C. D. (1994). Interocular transfer of receptive field expansion in cat visual cortex. *Vision Res.* 35: 1–6.

Volkmann, A. (1858). Über den Einfluss der Übung auf das Erkennen räumlicher Distanzen. *Berichte über die Verhandlungen der Sächsischen Gesellschaft der Wissenschaft zu Leipzig, mathmatische und physische Abtheilung* 10: 38–69.

Volkmann, A. W. (1863). *Physiologische Untersuchungen im Gebiete der Optik.* Leipzig: Breitkopf und Härtel.

Von Bonin, G., and Bailey, P. (1947). *The Neocortex of Macaca mulatta.* Urbana: University of Illinois Press.

Von der Heydt, R., and Peterhans, E. (1989). Mechanisms of contour perception in monkey visual cortex—I. Lines of pattern discontinuity. *J. Neurosci.* 9: 1731–1748.

von der Malsburg, C. (1987). In *The Neural and Molecular Basis of Learning: Dahlem Konferenzen, 1987,* ed. J. P. Changeux and M. Konishi, 411–432. New York: Wiley.

von der Malsburg, C. (1999). The what and why of binding: The modeler's perspective. *Neuron* 24: 95–104.

von Noorden, G. K. (1990). *Binocular Vision and Ocular Motility: Theory and Management of Strabismus.* St. Louis: Mosby.

Vuilleumier, P., and Sagiv, N. (2001). Two eyes make a pair: Facial organization and perceptual learning reduce visual extinction. *Neuropsychologia* 39: 1144–1149.

Wachsmuth, E., Oram, M. W., and Perrett, D. I. (1994). Recognition of objects and their component parts: Responses of single units in the temporal cortex of the macaque. *Cereb. Cortex* 4: 509–522.

Wahba, G. (1979). Convergence rates of "thin plate" smoothing splines when the data are noisy. In T. Gasser and M. Rosenblatt, eds., *Smoothing Techniques for Curve Estimation,* 233–245. Berlin: Springer.

Walk, R. D. (1978). Perceptual learning. In E. C. Carterette and M. P. Friedman, eds., *Handbook of Perception,* vol. 9, pp. 257–298. New York: Academic Press.

Walker, S., Bruce, V., and O'Malley, C. (1995). Facial identity and facial speech processing: Familiar faces and voices in the McGurk effect. *Percept. Psychophys.* 57: 1124–1133.

Wallach, H., and O'Connell, D. N. (1953). The kinetic depth effect. *J. Exp. Psychol.* 45: 205–217.

Wallach, H., O'Connell, D. N., and Neisser, U. (1953). The memory effect of visual perception of three-dimensional form. *J. Exp. Psychol.* 45: 360–368.

Wallis, G., and Baddeley, R. (1997). Optimal unsupervised learning in invariant object recognition. *Neural Comput.* 9(4): 883–894.

Wallis, G., and Bülthoff, H. (1998). Using a "virtual illusion" to put parallax in its place. *Perception* 27 ECVP suppl.: 19.

Wallis, G., and Bülthoff, H. (1999). Learning to recognize objects. *Trends Cogn. Sci.* 3: 22–31.

Wallis, G., and Bülthoff, H. (2001). Effects of temporal association on recognition memory. *Proc. Natl. Acad. Sci. U S A* 98: 4800–4804.

Wallis, G., and Rolls, E. T. (1997). A model of invariant object recognition in the visual system. *Prog. Neurobiol.* 51: 167–194.

Walsh, V., Ashbridge, E., and Cowey, A. (1998). Cortical plasticity in perceptual learning demonstrated by transcranial magnetic stimulation. *Neuropsychologia* 36: 363–367.

Walsh, V., and Booth, M. (1997). Perceptual learning: Insight in sight. *Curr. Biol.* 7: R249–251.

Waltz, D. (1975). Generating semantic descriptions from drawings of scenes with shadows. In P. Winston, ed., *The Psychology of Computer Vision.* New York: McGraw-Hill.

Waltz, D. L. (1972). Generating semantic descriptions from drawings of scenes with shadows. In *The Psychology of Computer Vision*, ed. P. H. Winston New York: McGraw-Hill.

Wang, G., Tanaka, K., and Tanifuji, M. (1996). Optical imaging of functional organization in the monkey inferotemporal cortex. *Science* 272: 1665–1668.

Wang, G., Tanifuji, M., and Tanaka, K. (1998). Functional architecture in monkey inferotemporal cortex revealed by in vivo optical imaging. *Neurosci. Res.* 32: 33–46.

Wang, X., Merzenich, M. M., Sameshima, K., and Jenkins, W. M. (1995). Remodeling of hand representation in adult

cortex determined by timing of tactile stimulation. *Nature* 378: 71–75.

Watanabe, T., Nanez, J. E., and Sasaki, Y. (2001). Perceptual learning without perception. *Nature* 413: 844–848.

Watson, C. S. (1980). Time course of auditory perceptual learning. *Ann. Otol. Rhinol. Laryngol. Suppl.* 89: 96–102.

Watson, C. S. (1991). Auditory perceptual learning and the cochlear implant. *Am. J. Otol.* 12(Suppl.): 73–79.

Waugh, S. J., Levi, D. M., and Carney, T. (1993). Orientation, masking, and vernier acuity for line targets. *Vision Res.* 33: 1619–1638.

Webster, M. A., De Valois, K. K., and Switkes, E. (1990). Orientation and spatial-frequency discrimination for luminance and chromatic gratings. *J. Opt. Soc. Am.* A7: 1034–1049.

Wehrhahn, C., and Rapf, D. (2001). Perceptual learning of apparent motion mediated through ON- and OFF-pathways in human vision. *Vision Res.* 41: 353–358.

Weiller, C., Chollet, F., Friston, K. J., Wise, R. J. S., and Frackowiak, R. S. J. (1992). Functional reorganization of the brain in recovery from striatocapsular infarction in man. *Ann. Neurol.* 31: 463–472.

Weinberger, N. M. (1995). Dynamic regulation of receptive fields and maps in the adult sensory cortex. *Annu. Rev. Neurosci.* 18: 129–158.

Weinberger, N. M., and Bakin, J. S. (1998). Learning-induced physiological memory in adult primary auditory cortex: Receptive field plasticity, model, and mechanisms. *Audiol. Neurootol.* 3: 145–167.

Weiss, I. (1988). Projective invariants of shapes. In *Proceedings of the IEEE Conference on Computer Vision and Pattern Recognition*, pp. 291–297.

Weiss, T., Miltner, W. H., Adler, T., Bruckner, L., and Taub, E. (1999). Decrease in phantom limb pain associated with prosthesis-induced increased use of an amputation stump in humans. *Neurosci. Lett.* 272: 131–134.

Weiss, Y., Edelman, S., and Fahle, M. (1993). Models of perceptual learning in vernier hyperacuity. *Neural Comput.* 5: 695–718.

Wertheimer, M. (1938). *Laws of Organization in Perceptual Forms*. London: Harcourt, Brace, Jovanovich.

Westheimer, G. (1976). Diffraction theory and visual hyperacuity. *Am. J. Optom. Physiol. Opt.* 53: 362–364.

Westheimer, G. (1979). Cooperative neural processes involved in stereoscopic acuity. *Exp. Brain Res.* 36: 585–597.

Westheimer, G. (2001). Is peripheral visual acuity susceptible to perceptual learning in the adult? *Vision Res.* 41: 47–52.

Westheimer, G., Shimamura, K., and McKee, S. P. (1976). Interference with line orientation sensitivity. *J. Opt. Soc. Am.* 66: 332–338.

Whitaker, D., and McGraw, P. V. (2000). Long-term visual experience recalibrates human orientation perception. *Nat. Neurosci.* 3: 13.

Widrow, B., and Stearns, S. D. (1985). *Adaptive Signal Processing*. Englewood Cliffs, NJ: Prentice Hall.

Wiesel, T. N. (1982). Postnatal development of the visual cortex and the influence of environment. *Nature* 299: 583–591.

Wiesel, T. N., and Hubel, D. H. (1963). Single-cell responses in striate cortex of kittens deprived of vision in one eye. *J. Neurophysiol.* 26: 1003–1017.

Wiesel, T. N., and Hubel, D. H. (1965). Comparison of the effects of unilateral and bilateral eye closure on cortical unit responses in kittens. *J. Neurophysiol.* 28: 1029–1040.

Wiesel, T. N., and Hubel, D. H. (1965). Binocular interaction in striate cortex of kittens reared with artificial squint. *J. Neurophysiol.* 28: 1041–1059.

Wiggs, C. L., and Martin, A. (1998). Properties and mechanisms of perceptual priming. *Curr. Opin. Neurobiol.* 8: 227–233.

Williamson, J. R. (1997). A constructive, incremental-learning network for mixture modeling and classification. *Neural Comput.* 9: 1517–1543.

Williamson, J. R. (1999). Learning vernier discrimination with a model of hierarchical map formation. *Invest. Ophthalmol. Vis. Sci.* 3976.

Wills, A. J., and McLaren, I. P. (1998). Perceptual learning and free classification. *Q. J. Exp. Psychol. B.* 51: 235–270.

Willshaw, D. J., Buneman, O. P., and Longuet-Higgins, H. C. (1969). Non-holographic associative memory. *Nature* 222: 960–962.

Wilson, B. S., Finley, C. C., Lawson, D. T., Wolford, R. D., Eddington, D. K., and Rabinowitz, W. M. (1991). Better speech recognition with cochlear implants. *Nature* 352: 236–238.

Wilson, H. R. (1980). A transducer function for threshold and suprathreshold human vision. *Biol. Cybern.* 38: 171–178.

Wilson, H. R., and Humanski, R. (1993). Spatial frequency adaptation and contrast gain control. *Vision Res.* 33: 1133–1149.

Wilson, H. R., and Wilkinson, F. (1997). Evolving concepts of spatial channels in vision: From independence to nonlinear interactions. *Perception* 26: 939–960.

Wilson, M. A., and McNaughton, B. L. (1993). Dynamics of the hippocampal ensemble code for space. *Science* 261: 1055–1058.

Wilson, P., and Snow, P. J. (1987). Reorganization of the receptive fields of spinocervical tract neurons following denervation of a single digit in the cat. *J. Neurophysiol.* 57: 803–818.

Winston, P., ed. (1975). *The Psychology of Computer Vision*. New York: McGraw-Hill.

Wiskott, L. (1998). Learning invariance manifolds. In L. Niklasson, M. Bodén, and T. Ziemke, eds., *Proceedings of the International Conference on Artificial Neural Networks: Perspectives in Neural Computing*, 555–560. Berlin: Springer.

Witkin, A. P. (1981). Recovering surface shape and orientation from texture. *Artif. Intell.* 17(1–3): 17–45.

Wohlwill, J. F. (1966). Perceptual learning. *Annu. Rev. Psychol.* 17: 201–232.

Wolf, S. L., Lecraw, D. E., Barton, L. A., and Jahn, B. B. (1989). Forced use of hemiplegic upper extremities to reverse the effect of learned nonuse among chronic stroke and head injured patients. *Exp. Neurol.* 104: 125–132.

Wolford, G., and Kim, H.-Y. (1992). The role of visible persistence in backward masking. In *From Learning Processes to Cognitive Processes: Essays in Honor of William K. Estes*, ed. A. F. Healy, S. M. Kosslyn, and R. M. Shiffrin, vol. 2, pp. 161–180. Hillsdale, NJ: Erlbaum.

Wolford, G., Marchak, F., and Hughes, H. (1988). Practice effects in backward masking. *J. Exp. Psychol. Hum. Percept. Perform.* 14: 101–112.

Woods, T. M., Cusick, C. G., Pons, T. P., Taub, E., and Jones, E. G. (2000). Progressive transneuronal changes in the brainstem and thalamus after long-term dorsal rhizotomies in adult macaque monkeys. *J. Neurosci.* 20: 3884–3899.

Wright, B. A., Buonomano, D. V., Mahncke, H. W., and Merzenich, M. M. (1997). Learning and generalization of auditory temporal-interval discrimination in humans. *J. Neurosci.* 17: 3956–3963.

Wright, R. L., and Whittlesea, B. W. (1998). Implicit learning of complex structures: Active adaptation and selective processing in acquisition and application. *Mem. Cognit.* 26: 402–420.

Wülfing, E. A. (1892). Ueber den kleinsten Gesichtswinkel. *Zeitschrift für Biologie* 29(11): 199–202.

Wurtz, R., Goldberg, M., and Robinson, D. L. (1982). Brain mechanisms of visual attention. *Sci. Am.* 246(6): 100–107.

Wurtz, R. P., Vorbruggen, J. C., and von der Malsburg, C. (1990). A transputer system for the recognition of human faces by labeled graph matching. In R. Eckmiller, G. Hartmann, and G. Hauske, eds., *Parallel Processing in Neural Systems and Computers*, 37–41. Amsterdam: Elsevier.

Xerri, C., Merzenich, M. M., Jenkins, W., and Santucci, S. (1999). Representational plasticity in cortical area 3b paralleling tactual-motor skill acquisition in adult monkeys. *Cereb. Cortex* 9: 264–276.

Xerri, C., Stern, J. M., and Merzenich, M. M. (1994). Alterations of the cortical representation of the rat ventrum induced by nursing behavior. *J. Neurosci.* 14: 1710–1721.

Xing, J., and Gerstein, G. L. (1996). Networks with lateral connectivity: 3. Plasticity and reorganization of somatosensory cortex. *J. Neurophysiol.* 75: 217–232.

Xu, J., and Wall, J. T. (1997). Rapid changes in brainstem maps of adult primates after peripheral injury. *Brain Res.* 774: 211–215.

Xu, J., and Wall, J. T. (1999). Evidence for brainstem and supra-brainstem contributions to rapid cortical plasticity in adult monkeys. *J. Neurosci.* 19: 7578–7590.

Yaginuma, S., Osawa, Y., Yamaguchi, K., and Iwai, D. (1993). Differential functions of central and peripheral visual field representations in monkey prestriate cortex. In *Brain Mechanisms of Perception and Memory: From Neuron to Behavior*, ed. T. Ono et al., 1–33. New York: Oxford University Press.

Yakovlev, V., Fusi, S., Berman, E., and Zohary, E. (1998). Inter-trial neuronal activity in inferior temporal cortex: A putative vehicle to generate long-term visual associations. *Nat. Neurosci.* 1: 310–317.

Yamashita, H. (1993). Perceptual-motor learning in amnesic patients with medial temporal lobe lesions. *Percept. Mot. Skills* 77: 1311–1314.

Yarbus, A. L. (1957). The perception of an image fixed with respect to the retina. *Biophysics* 2: 683–690.

Yin, R. K. (1969). Looking at upside-down faces. *J. Exp. Psychol. Gen.* 81: 141–145.

Young, A. W., Hay, D. C., and Ellis, A. W. (1985). The faces that launched a thousand slips: Everyday errors and difficulties in recognising people. *Br. J. Psychol.* 76: 495–523.

Young, A. W., Hay, D. C., McWeeny, K. H., Flude, B. M., and Ellis, A. W. (1985). Matching familiar and unfamiliar faces on internal and external features. *Perception* 14: 737–746.

Young, A. W., Hellawell, D., and Hay, D. C. (1987). Configural information in face perception. *Perception* 16: 747–759.

Young, A. W., Rowland, D., Calder, A. J., Etcoff, N., Seth, A., and Perrett, D. I. (1996). Facial expression megamix: Tests of dimensional and categorical accounts of emotion recognition. *Cognition* 63: 271–313.

Young, D., Lawlor, P. A., Leone, P., Dragunow, M., and During, M. J. (1999). Environmental enrichment inhibits spontaneous apoptosis, prevents seizures and is neuroprotective. *Nat. Med.* 5: 448–453.

Young, M. (1992). Objective analysis of the topological organization of the primate cortical visual system. *Nature* 358: 152–155.

Young, M. P., and Yamane, S. (1992). Sparse population coding of faces in the inferotemporal cortex. *Science* 256: 1327–1331.

Yuille, A. (1991). Deformable templates for face recognition. *J. Cogn. Neurosci.* 3(1): 59–71.

Yuille, A. L. (1987). Shape from shading, occlusion and texture. AI Memo 885. MIT AI Laboratory.

Yukie, M., Takeuchi, H., Hasegawa, Y., and Iwai, E. (1990). Differential connectivity of inferotemporal area TE with the amygdala and the hippocampus in the monkey. In *Vision, Memory and the Temporal Lobe*, ed. E. Iwai and M. Mishkin, 129–135. New York: Elsevier.

Zanker, J. M. (1999). Perceptual learning in primary and secondary motion vision. *Vision Res.* 39: 1293–1304.

Zeki, S. (1993). *A Vision of the Brain*. Oxford: Blackwell.

Zelniker, T., and Oppenheimer, L. (1976). Effect of different training methods on perceptual learning in impulsive children. *Child Dev.* 47: 492–497.

Zenger, B., and Sagi, D. (1996). Isolating excitatory and inhibitory nonlinear spatial interactions involved in contrast detection. *Vision Res.* 36: 2497–2513.

Zenger-Landolt, B., and Fahle, M. (2001). Discriminating contrast discontinuities: Asymmetries, dipper functions, and perceptual learning. *Vision Res.* 41: 3009–3021.

Zepka, R. F., Godde, B., and Dinse, H. R. (2000). Synchronous and asynchronous tactile coactivation controls distance between stimulated skin representations in somatosensory cortex of adult rats: An optical imaging study. *Soc. Neurosci. Abstr.* 26: 933.

Zepka, R. F., Jürgens, M., and Dinse, H. R. (1996). Differential time course of use-dependent plastic reorganiz-

ation of cortical and thalamic hindpaw representations by modification of walking in adult rats. *Soc. Neurosci. Abstr.* 22: 1055.

Zernicki, B. (1991). Visual discrimination learning in binocularly deprived cats: 20 years of studies in the Nencki Institute. *Brain Res. Rev.* 16: 1–13.

Zernicki, B. (1999). Visual discrimination learning under switching procedure in visually deprived cats. *Behav. Brain Res.* 100: 237–244.

Ziemann, U., Corwell, B., and Cohen, L. G. (1998). Modulation of plasticity in human motor cortex after forearm ischemic nerve block. *J. Neurosci.* 18(3): 1115–1123.

Zihl, J., and von Cramon, D. (1979). Restitution of visual function in patients with cerebral blindness. *J. Neurol. Neurosurg. Psychiatry* 42: 312–322.

Zihl, J., and von Cramon, D. (1985). Visual field recovery from scotoma in patients with postgeniculate damage. *Brain* 108: 335–365.

Zipser, K., Lamme, V. A. F., and Schiller, P. H. (1996). Contextual modulation in primary visual cortex. *J. Neurosci.* 16: 7376–7389.

Zohary, E., Celebrini, S., Britten, K., and Newsome, W. T. (1994). Neuronal plasticity that underlies improvement in perceptual performance. *Science* 263: 1289–1292.

Zohary, E., and Newsome, W. T. (1994). Perceptual learning in a direction discrimination task is not based upon enhanced neuronal sensitivity in the STS. *Invest. Ophthalmol. Vis. Sci.* 35: 1663.

Contributors

Merav Ahissar
Department of Psychology and Center for Neural
Computation
Hebrew University
Jerusalem, Israel

Anthony J. Bell
Howard Hughes Medical Institute
Computational Neurobiology Laboratory
The Salk Institute
La Jolla, California

Nicoletta Berardi
Department of Psychology
University of Florence
Florence, Italy

Vicki Bruce
Department of Psychology
University of Stirling
Stirling, U.K.

Heinrich Bülthoff
Max-Planck-Institute for Biological Cybernetics
Tübingen, Germany

Mike Burton
Department of Psychology
University of Glasgow
Glasgow, U.K.

Graeme M. Clark
Department of Otolaryngology
University of Melbourne
Melbourne, Australia

Marcus Dill
Visual Science Section
University Eye Clinic Tübingen
Tübingen, Germany

Hubert R. Dinse
Institute for Neurocomputing
Ruhr-University Bochum
Bochum, Germany

Shimon Edelman
Department of Psychology
Cornell University
Ithaca, New York

Thomas Elbert
Department of Psychology
Constance University
Constance, Germany

Ulf T. Eysel
Department of Neurophysiology
Ruhr-University Bochum
Bochum, Germany

Manfred Fahle
Department of Optimetry and Visual Science
City University, London, and
Department of Human Neurobiology
Bremen University
Bremen, Germany

Adriana Fiorentini
Institute of Neurophysiology of the C.N.R.
Pisa, Italy

Michael H. Herzog
Department of Human Neurobiology
Bremen University
Bremen, Germany

Shaul Hochstein
Department of Psychology and Center for Neural
Computation
Hebrew University
Jerusalem, Israel

Nathan Intrator
Department of Computer Science
Tel Aviv University
Tel Aviv, Israel

Nikos K. Logothetis
Max-Planck-Institute for Biological Cybernetics
Tübingen, Germany

Siegrid Löwel
Research Group for Visual Development and
Plasticity
Leibniz Institute for Neurobiology
Magdeburg, Germany

Michael M. Merzenich
Keck Center for Integrative Neurosciences
University of California at San Francisco
San Francisco, California

Ken Nakayama
Department of Psychology
Harvard University
Cambridge, Massachusetts

Tomaso Poggio
Department of Brain and Cognitive Sciences
Massachusetts Institute of Technology
Cambridge, Massachusetts

Brigitte Rockstroh
Department of Psychology
Constance University
Constance, Germany

Nava Rubin
Center for Neural Science
New York University
New York, New York

Dov Sagi
Department of Neurobiology and Brain Research
Weizman Institute of Science
Rehovot, Israel

Aniek Schoups
KUL
Laboratory of Neuro-Psychophysiology
Louvain, Belgium

Terrence J. Sejnowski
Howard Hughes Medical Institute
Computational Neurobiology Laboratory
Salk Institute
La Jolla, California

Robert Shapley
Center for Neural Science
New York University
New York, New York

David L. Sheinberg
Department of Neuroscience
Brown University
Providence, Rhode Island

Wolf Singer
Department of Neurophysiology
Max-Planck-Institute for Brain Research
Frankfurt am Main, Germany

Pawan Sinha
Department of Brain and Cognitive Sciences
Massachusetts Institute of Technology
Cambridge, Massachusetts

Annette Sterr
Department of Cognitive Neuroscience and
Neuropsychology

University of Liverpool
Liverpool, U.K.

Keiji Tanaka
RIKEN Brain Research Institute
Saitama, Japan

Guy Wallis
School of Human Movement Studies
University of Queensland
Brisbane, Australia

Barbara Zenger
Department of Psychology
Stanford University
Stanford, California

Index